T0325385

Disinfection of Root Canal Systems

Disinfection of Root Canal Systems

The Treatment of Apical Periodontitis

Edited by

Nestor Cohenca

Department of Endodontics and Pediatric Dentistry,
University of Washington, Seattle, WA, USA

WILEY Blackwell

This edition first published 2014 © 2014 by John Wiley & Sons, Inc.

Editorial offices: 1606 Golden Aspen Drive, Suites 103 and 104, Ames, Iowa 50010, USA
The Atrium, Southern Gate, Chichester, West Sussex, PO19 8SQ, UK
9600 Garsington Road, Oxford, OX4 2DQ, UK

For details of our global editorial offices, for customer services and for information about how to apply for permission to reuse the copyright material in this book please see our website at www.wiley.com/wiley-blackwell.

Authorization to photocopy items for internal or personal use, or the internal or personal use of specific clients, is granted by Blackwell Publishing, provided that the base fee is paid directly to the Copyright Clearance Center, 222 Rosewood Drive, Danvers, MA 01923. For those organizations that have been granted a photocopy license by CCC, a separate system of payments has been arranged. The fee codes for users of the Transactional Reporting Service are ISBN-13: 978-1-118-36768-1/2014.

Designations used by companies to distinguish their products are often claimed as trademarks. All brand names and product names used in this book are trade names, service marks, trademarks or registered trademarks of their respective owners. The publisher is not associated with any product or vendor mentioned in this book.

Library of Congress Cataloging-in-Publication Data

Disinfection of root canal systems : the treatment of apical periodontitis / edited by Nestor Cohenca.
      p. ; cm.
   Treatment of apical periodontitis
   Includes bibliographical references and index.
   ISBN 978-1-118-36768-1 (cloth)
   I. Cohenca, Nestor, 1968- editor of compilation. II. Title: Treatment of apical periodontitis.
   [DNLM: 1. Periapical Periodontitis–therapy. 2. Root Canal Therapy. 3. Disinfection–methods. 4. Root Canal Irrigants.
   5. Therapeutic Irrigation. WU 230]
   RK351
   617.6′342059–dc23
                                        2014004701

A catalogue record for this book is available from the British Library.

Wiley also publishes its books in a variety of electronic formats. Some content that appears in print may not be available in electronic books.

Cover design by Jen Miller Designs

Typeset in 9.5/11.5 pt PalatinoLTStd by Laserwords Private Limited, Chennai, India
Printed and bound in Malaysia by Vivar Printing Sdn Bhd

1   2014

Contents

Contributors

Alireza Aminlari
Private Practice, Farmington Hills, MI, USA
Department of Cariology, University of Michigan,
Ann Arbor, MI, USA

Bettina Basrani
Discipline of Endodontics, Faculty of Dentistry,
University of Toronto, Toronto, ON, Canada

Rogério de Castilho Jacinto
Department of Semiology and Clinics, Federal
University of Pelotas, Pelotas, RS, Brazil

Nestor Cohenca
Department of Endodontics and Pediatric
Dentistry, University of Washington, Seattle,
WA, USA

Natasha M. Flake
Department of Endodontics, University of
Washington, Seattle, WA, USA

Ashraf F. Fouad
Department of Endodontics, Prosthodontics and
Operative Dentistry, University of Maryland,
Baltimore, MD, USA

Shimon Friedman
Faculty of Dentistry, University of Toronto,
Toronto, ON, Canada

Ana Maria González Amaro
Department of Microbiology, University
Autonomous of San Luis Potosí, San Luis Potosí,
Mexico

Cesar de Gregorio
Department of Endodontics, University of
Washington, Seattle, WA, USA

Markus Haapasalo
Department of Oral Biological and Medical
Sciences, Vancouver, BC, Canada

Carlos Heilborn
Private Practice, Asunción, Paraguay

Eric Herbranson
Private practice, San Leandro, California, USA

James D. Johnson
Department of Endodontics, University of
Washington, Seattle, WA, USA

Anda Kfir
Department of Endodontology, Tel Aviv
University, Tel Aviv, Israel

Anil Kishen
University of Toronto, Toronto, ON, Canada

Ricardo Macedo
The Academic Centre for Dentistry in Amsterdam
(ACTA), University of Amsterdam, Amsterdam,
The Netherlands

Zvi Metzger
Department of Endodontology, Tel Aviv University, Tel Aviv, Israel

Paulo Nelson-Filho
Department of Pediatric Dentistry, School of Dentistry of Ribeirão Preto. University of Sao Paulo, Riberao Preto, Brazil

Frank Paqué
Department of Preventive Dentistry, Periodontology, and Cariology, University of Zurich, Zürich, Switzerland

Avina Paranjpe
Department of Endodontics, University of Washington, Seattle, WA, USA

Ove A. Peters
Department of Endodontics, University of the Pacific, San Francisco, CA, USA

Roberta Pileggi
Department of Endodontics, University of Florida, Gainesville, FL, USA

Richard Rubinstein
Private Practice, Farmington Hills, MI, USA
Department of Cariology, Restorative Sciences, and Endodontics, University of Michigan, Ann Arbor, MI, USA

Christine M. Sedgley
Department of Endodontology, Oregon Health and Science University, Portland, OR, USA

Annie Shrestha
University of Toronto, Toronto, ON, Canada

Lea Assed Bezerra da Silva
Department of Pediatric Dentistry, School of Dentistry of Ribeirão Preto. University of Sao Paulo, Riberao Preto, Brazil

Raquel Assed Bezerra da Silva
Department of Pediatric Dentistry, School of Dentistry of Ribeirão Preto. University of Sao Paulo, Riberao Preto, Brazil

Luc van der Sluis
Department of Conservative Dentistry and Endodontics, University of Toulouse, Toulouse, France

Franklin R. Tay
Department of Endodontics, Georgia Regents University, Augusta, GA, USA

Bram Verhaagen
Research Institute for Biomedical Technology and Technical Medicine, University of Twente, Enschede, The Netherlands

Michel Versluis
Research Institute for Nanotechnology, Research Institute for Biomedical Technology and Technical Medicine, University of Twente, Enschede, The Netherlands

Introduction

During my first endodontic residency, my program director, Professor Ilana Heling, always reminded me that "bacteria" is the reason for all endodontic failures. Back then (24 years ago), I knew all the literature supporting the link between bacteria and apical pathosis but was naive enough to think that biomechanical instrumentation of the root canal will take care of the microbiological status inside the canal, and the immune system (the host) will do the rest at the apical area.

A few years later, the endodontic world underwent a complete reshape of concept and armamentarium. Among them being new techniques, Ni-Ti alloys, rotary systems, using nickel, and the operating microscopes. For all those endodontists trained in the early 1990s or earlier, it meant to learn endodontics almost all over again, and so we did. However, the amazing technological advancement in endodontics had a cost to the consumer, in this case, the endodontists and ultimately the patient.

If we place the financial aspect aside, these advancements were supposed to produce better endodontic therapy, which is measured by a higher outcome and more teeth being saved from extractions. However, despite the "art and science" of current endodontic therapy, current outcome studies have failed to demonstrate an increase in endodontic success. How come? Should we not expect at least a slight improvement? After all, we shape better, we see better, definitely we spend much more, and yet studies demonstrate the same

outcome of apical healing. Something is wrong! In business, we would have used the expression that perhaps we invested our time and money on the wrong market.

After reading most of the outcome studies published between 2005 and 2008, I realized that we will never get any better in healing apical periodontitis until we realize and accept who our real enemy is, what our biological aim is, and what should be our strategy to target the biological reasons of the disease.

Thus, the purpose of this book is to provide the reader with a unique perspective on how to heal apical periodontitis. Successful endodontic therapy depends on the removal of microorganisms and their endotoxins from the root canal system. Toxic metabolites and by-products released from organized biofilms within the canal diffuse into apical tissues and elicit inflammatory responses and bone resorption. Therefore, as endodontists, our main goal should be to focus on the predictable elimination of microorganisms from the root canal system. However, the inherent anatomy and morphology of the root canal system imposes additional inherent challenges making this loyal task of disinfection even tougher. Isthmuses, intercanal and intracanal communications, accessory and lateral canals, curvatures and oval-shaped canals are all part of the anatomical challenges we need to overcome. Yet, the goal remains the same: control of the infection. Bacterial reduction to the extent of a negative culture should be considered the desired "clinical outcome" of endodontic treatment.

In 2004, Bergenholtz and Spangberg claimed that studies must address the fundamental principles of endodontics, rather than the adoption of cutting-edge technology that contributes to the advancement of root canal therapy. To make this statement even stronger, in 2007, Ng et al. published an excellent systematic review on the outcome of primary root canal treatment and reported that the success rates had not improved over the past 40 years. The aforementioned is in complete agreement with the finding by Kakehashi, Stanley, and Fitzgerald. We simply detoured and lost perspective for a few decades, but I believe that it is never too late to make it right.

That is how and why I became interested in the field of root canal disinfection and toward higher healing of apical periodontitis. Another of my mentors, Professor Shimon Friedman – considered one of the best in the field of endodontic outcome – once challenged me on this difficult or impossible task. Although we are not done yet, the results of years of intense research conducted by the authors of this book have produced a significant amount of new data that will provide the reader with a good and current understanding of the etiology of apical periodontitis and the techniques available to obtain a more efficient and predictable disinfection toward better healing and greater outcome. The book discusses the etiology of endodontic disease, especially the endodontic biofilm, and all therapies available to predictably disinfect the root canal system thus increasing endodontic treatment outcome.

I would like to thank the Commissioner of Wiley, Mr. Rick Blanchette, for his vision, trust, and, most of all, his persistence. Last, my gratitude to all authors and co-authors that without much hesitation collaborated with their knowledge, experience, and valuable time. I am extremely proud and blessed for the opportunity I had to work with leaders from around the world who contributed to this book. Not only because of expertise, but because we share the same concerns and passion for endodontics. Together, we joined forces to contribute to our specialty, our peers, and our patients.

Nestor Cohenca
School of Dentistry,
University of Washington,
Seattle, WA, USA

Preface

The passage of time has brought about considerable evolution of the understanding of endodontic disease and its primary cause and the modalities applied to tackle that cause as well as the limitations of those modalities. Driven by an ever-increasing volume of research, this process has seen several shifts in focus that, in turn, have generated technological advances that benefitted almost every aspect of how endodontic therapy is delivered. The rapid pace of those advances challenged the traditional endodontic textbooks to keep up both with the changing focus and the technologies developed to benefit endodontic therapy.

The current focus is the disinfection of the root canal system, widely recognized as a formidable challenge. Confronting this challenge requires specific knowledge, unique technologies developed that apply this knowledge, and updating the clinicians on how to apply those developments in practice. The textbook *Disinfection of Root Canal Systems: The Treatment of Apical Periodontitis* by *Dr. Nestor Cohenca* is designed specifically to provide the knowledge base, the detailed information on current and emerging technological advances, and guidelines on how to clinically apply those technologies. In this regard, it is a most timely addition to the endodontic texts available to clinicians, students, and researchers.

Compared to a decade ago, the understanding of canal disinfection has evolved in ways that impact changes in devices, procedures, protocols, and even concepts. For one, the limitation of endodontic instruments in disinfecting the root canals has been well appreciated, shifting the focus to the anatomical intricacies of the root canal systems as well as the microbial resilience as the ultimate challenges in the clinical practice of endodontic therapy. As a result of this shift, in a relatively short period of time, we have seen development of (the list is not all-inclusive): innovative instrument designs to better address root canal anatomy; new devices for delivery of antimicrobial agents into root canal systems; new antimicrobial agents with dual and triple activity; harnessing of physical effects to distribute and activate antimicrobial agents; optimization of the light energy applied to better address the microbial challenges within the root canal systems; and the use of nanotechnologies to challenge microbial biofilms in ways never tried before in endodontics. Faced with such rapid evolution, compiling a textbook that aims to capture the most recent innovations and concepts is a challenge. On the one hand, the historic context is required to foster a comprehensive understanding of biology and therapeutic concepts. On the other hand, the innovative content needs to remain contemporary for the next few years to come.

To meet those challenges, Dr. Cohenca teamed up with a large panel of experts, allowing the reader to benefit from contributions by 30 educators, researchers, and clinicians from four continents. The result of this collective effort is a unique textbook that highlights like no other the most current concepts of endodontic therapy of the infected teeth. With access to this collective international expertise, the reader gains an in-depth and wide-ranging insight into the current state of disinfection of root canal systems. Under this one cover, the reader will find current research-based information on endodontic infection and resulting disease, microbial challenges facing the host and the clinician, methods and limitations of assessing the efficacy of root canal disinfection, ambivalent relationship between disinfection and healing outcomes of endodontic therapy, anatomic complexities of root canal systems, value of the shaping of root canals, applicable irrigating agents, challenges inherent to flow dynamics in root canals, contrasting approaches to delivery and activation of irrigation agents within root canals, recent and emerging adjuncts to canal disinfection, intracanal medication, kinetics of the healing processes of infection-related endodontic disease, and the complimentary surgical treatment procedure. The specific areas several of its chapters focus on and detailed reviews of research findings that the chapters provide are not commonly found in endodontic textbooks.

This new textbook is organized in a logical sequence. Rather than assigning precedence to treatment techniques, the book first reviews the foundations of biology, anatomy, research methods, and healing assessment, to highlight the challenges facing the clinician and researcher in addressing the disinfection of root canal systems. This is then followed by a comprehensive coverage of the principal disinfection procedures, modalities that have yet to enter the mainstream, and emerging concepts. The lingering challenges of slow healing kinetics and surgical management when disinfection is ineffective are then reviewed to provide an essential perspective.

In compiling this textbook, its editor engaged many talented and knowledgeable individuals within the endodontic community to contribute chapters in their respective areas of undisputed expertise. With collective depth and breadth of experience and knowledge in both endodontic science and art, they possess wide-ranging insight into endodontic research, education, and clinical practice. As a longtime educator, researcher, and clinician, I find it gratifying to see the talent harnessed to collaborate on this textbook.

This textbook has all the potential to become an indispensable resource for dentists and endodontic specialists, endodontic specialty-program students, and for those engaged in endodontic research. They will find its content critical to fostering a sound understanding of the challenges underlining the disinfection of root canal systems, and also as a useful guide to the most current devices, materials, and techniques developed to meet those challenges. It will assist them in achieving sophistication in their selected endeavors.

Shimon Friedman
Faculty of Dentistry, University of Toronto,
Toronto, Ontario, Canada

Acknowledgments

I must confess that I was blessed with one of the best endodontic education any professional can dream of. I was lucky enough to be at the right place and at the right time. Having mentors like Adam Stabholz, Shimon Friedman, Ilana Heling, Anna Fuks, James Simon, James Johnson, Martha Somerman, and Joel Berg impacted my career. Each and every single one of them taught me something different and shaped not only my professional knowledge but also my personality. I want to take this opportunity to thank every one of them and express my gratitude and love. I hope to be able to follow their path and legacy.

Finally, I would like to acknowledge my gratitude and love to my family. First, thanks to my parents who during the first 20 years of my life have motivated me to study hard and excel. Second, I would like to thank my wife Ruti and my children Yair, Natalie, and Daniel who during the past 25 years had to understand and support the hours and days I missed from their lives. I hope that my love and dedication made it up and will serve them as a positive example that in life you need to love what you do and then give your all with passion! From my part, I know that without their love and support I would have never become who I am and this book would have never been written.

Part 1

Background

1 Root Canal Infection and Endodontic Apical Disease

Nestor Cohenca

Department of Endodontics and Pediatric Dentistry, University of Washington, Seattle, WA, USA

Ana Maria González Amaro

Department of Microbiology, University Autonomous of San Luis Potosí, San Luis Potosí, Mexico

Infection control: why now?

The outcome of endodontic treatment depends on the microbiological status of the root canal. In inflamed vital pulps, the infection is commonly limited to the site of exposure causing a localized inflammatory response (1, 2). However, when aseptic technique is used, the effect of endodontic therapy is predictably high as demonstrated by several studies (3–7).

In infected necrotic pulps, microorganisms are present within the root canal system and dentinal tubules, causing a apical inflammatory lesion called *apical periodontitis*. In these cases, endodontic treatment should be essentially directed toward the prevention and control of pulpal and apical infections, as stated by Kakehashi, Stanley, and Fitzgerald nearly 50 years ago (8). Unfortunately, the success of the therapy for these cases is 10–15% lower when compared to non-contaminated teeth (Table 1.1) (3–7, 9–11). What is more concerning is the fact that this lower outcome has not changed or improved despite all the technological advancements the world of endodontics has seen (12). How come that despite the *"art and science"* of current endodontic therapy, outcome studies have failed to demonstrate an increase in endodontic success? Why do we fail to predictably control the infection after so many years of research, experiment, and treatment? The answer might be related to the fact that very few advances have ever targeted the real problem, which continues to be microorganisms, especially in the apical third. The success of the endodontic treatment is possible only with an understanding of the molecular biology of the pathogens, their structures, synergies, and weaknesses. No file will ever disinfect a root canal, nor is it designed for that purpose. Recognizing that our

Disinfection of Root Canal Systems: The Treatment of Apical Periodontitis, First Edition. Edited by Nestor Cohenca.
© 2014 John Wiley & Sons, Inc. Published 2014 by John Wiley & Sons, Inc.

Table 1.1 Outcome of endodontic therapy based on the presence or absence of apical periodontitis.

Author and year	Cases/cohort	Recall	Without apical periodontitis (%)	With apical periodontitis (%)
Strindberg (1956)	258	6 months to 10 years	93	80
Kerekes and Tronstad (1979)	491 Norway, Dental school	3–5 years	92	89
Sjogren et al. (1990)	96 Sweden, Dental school	8–10 years (91%)	96	86
Friedman et al. (2003)	92	4–6 years (20%)	92	74
Farzaneh et al. (2004)	94 Toronto, Grad students	4–6 years (48%)	94	81
Orstravik et al. (2004)	Norway, Dental school	0.5–4 years (83%)	94	79
Ng et al. (2011)	702 London Grad students	4 years (83%)		83
Ricucci et al. (2011)	816 Italy (Ricucci)	5 years (87%)	92.3	82.7

endodontic therapy will end in failure if we do not find a method to completely destroy the microbes within the root canal system, infection control must be our main goal and concern. Therefore, we should focus our research and development on efficient and predictable methods to control the infection and improve the endodontic treatment and healing of apical periodontitis.

Terminology and apical definitions

The term *apical periodontitis* has gained increasing support and is used widely in current literature. The American Association of Endodontists recently published the revised Glossary of Endodontic Terms (13). Some of the terms defined in the glossary are as follows:

Normal apical tissues Teeth with normal apical tissues that are not sensitive to percussion or palpation testing. The lamina dura surrounding the root is intact and the periodontal ligament space is uniform.

Symptomatic apical periodontitis Inflammation, usually of the apical periodontium, producing clinical symptoms including painful response to biting and/or percussion or palpation. It may or may not be associated with an apical radiolucent area.

Asymptomatic apical periodontitis Inflammation and destruction of apical periodontium that is of pulpal origin, appears as an apical radiolucent area and does not produce clinical symptoms.

Acute apical abscess An inflammatory reaction to pulpal infection and necrosis characterized by rapid onset, spontaneous pain, tenderness of the tooth to pressure, pus formation, and swelling of associated tissues.

Chronic apical abscess An inflammatory reaction to pulpal infection and necrosis characterized by gradual onset, little or no discomfort, and the intermittent discharge of pus through an associated sinus tract.

In biological terms, apical periodontitis means "inflammation of the periodontium." This is a broad term to describe an inflammatory reaction in the tissues, including lateral and furcal locations of inflammation; it does not distinguish etymologically pulp-induced periodontitis from marginally derived periodontitis. More specific pathologies such as granulomas and cysts were excluded because they do not represent a "clinical or radiographic" diagnostic reality, but rather a diagnosis based on histological findings. The prevalence of apical periodontitis has increased throughout the years (14, 15), even in the low caries-rate adult Danish population (16).

The evolution of endodontic microbiology

Miller, in 1890 (17), was the first to demonstrate the presence of bacteria in necrotic human pulp tissue. However, the cause and effect relationship is attributed to Kakehashi *et al.* (8) who experimented with gnotobiotic (germ-free) and normal rats. Bacterial contamination in the orally exposed pulp tissue caused necrosis and apical pathoses in normal rats. The study is considered a classic reference as it initiated a new and bright era in endodontic microbiology.

In 1966, Moller (18) established the importance of adequate isolation for microbiological sampling and various culture media for the recovery and identification of anaerobic microorganisms, providing more relevant information regarding the type of bacteria present in root canal systems. Bergenholtz then demonstrated the presence of bacteria in the traumatized teeth. Despite the fact that pulp chambers were not exposed, bacterial growth was observed in 64% of all samples. The flora was dominated by anaerobic microorganisms including *Bacteroides, Corynebacterium, Peptostreptococcus*, and *Fusobacterium* (19). Two years later, Sundqvist (20) demonstrated the prevalence of anaerobic bacteria in root canals, supporting the results obtained by Bergenholtz.

In the 1980s, the studies were more focused on understanding the colonization and interactions within the endodontic microflora. Moller investigated the relationship between uncontaminated necrotic pulp and apical tissues. The study maintained uncontaminated necrotic pulp in the root canal during a period of at least 6 months, and evaluated changes in the microbial flora enclosed in the root canal and its capacity to induce apical periodontitis (21). Using 9 monkeys (Macaca fascicularis), the pulp of 78 teeth was aseptically necrotized. Twenty-six of the pulp chambers were sealed and the pulp chamber remained free. Fifty-two teeth were infected with the indigenous flora. Clinical, radiographic and microbiological data was recorded before and after the completion of the study. The root canals were initially uninfected sterile in the final samples. No inflammatory reactions were found on the 26 control teeth. On the experimental teeth inflammatory reactions were observed clinically (12/52 teeth) and radiographically (47/52 teeth). An average of 8 to 15 bacterial strains were identified as facultative anaerobic bacteria including enterococci, coliforms, and anaerobic bacteria such as *Bacteroides, Eubacterium, Propionibacterium, and Peptococcus, Peptostreptococcus*. Some anaerobic bacteria not present on the

initial microbiological test were isolated on the final samples. Histological examination of the apical tissue confirmed the presence an inflammatory reaction to the bacterial contamination (21).

In 1982, Fabricius *et al.* investigated the pulps of 24 root canals, 8 in each of the 3 monkeys that were experimented on. Teeth were mechanically devitalized and exposed to the oral flora for about 1 week and thereafter sealed. Microbiologic sampling and analysis was performed in 16 teeth (of 2 of the monkeys) after 7 days of closure (initial samples). Afterward, inoculation pulps were sealed for a period of 6 months. Final sampling was taken from the main root canal, the dentin, and the apical region at the same sampling session. All microbiologic analyses were carried out quantitatively. Final root canal samples from the apical region showed a predominance of obligate anaerobic nonsporulating bacteria; in fact 85–98% of the bacterial cells were anaerobic. The most frequently found species were Bacteroides and Gram-positive anaerobic rods. A lower proportion of facultative anaerobic bacteria were found; this was most pronounced for coliform rods in comparison with the strains of *Bacteroides melaninogenicus*.

Today, electron microscopy has become a great technology in many areas of science. Nair (22) studied the structure of the endodontic flora, its relationship to the dentinal wall, microbial interactions, and dynamics of apical inflammatory response. The study was performed on human teeth with granulomas and cysts. The results showed the presence of microorganisms in all the samples. The flora consisted of cocci, bacilli, and spirochetes filamentous organisms. In most cases, the bacteria were restricted to the canal, but in 4 granulomas and 1 cyst, the bacteria were found in the lesion. There was a distinct bacterial plaque adhering to the dentinal wall at the apical foramen. Nair describes this finding as a group or community of one or more types of microorganisms as well as bacterial condensate, suggesting the formation of plaque in the dentinal wall by the flora of the root canal. This finding is considered to be the subject that currently occupies many researchers: the presence of biofilm on root canal walls.

In 1990, Nair (23) analyzed nine therapy-resistant and asymptomatic human apical lesions (4–10 years) removed during surgery using light and electron microscopy. Six out of nine lesions revealed microorganisms in the apical root canal. Four contained bacteria and two contained yeasts. Of the three cases with no microorganisms, one revealed a foreign body giant cell granuloma. In the majority of therapy-resistant apical lesions, microorganisms (bacteria, yeast) and foreign body giant cell granulomas play a significant role in treatment failures.

Although endodontic microbiology has evolved significantly, it still lacks an understanding of the ecology of the root canal and requires an analysis of the bond that develops between microorganisms and their surroundings. This relationship is an essential element that provides a glimpse into the understanding of their behavior and ability to invade an area that is rich in nutrients and whose abiotic and biotic factors determine the distribution and quantity of living organisms that may share the root space. In the early 1990s, Sundqvist (24, 25) published a couple of reviews summarizing the available data. Bacterial flora of the root canal is dominated by obligate anaerobes, comprising up to 90% of the total population. Aerobic bacteria are rarely found initially in the infected root canals but could have been introduced during the treatment. During the course of an infection, interrelationships develop between microbial species, based on their nutritional demands and nutritional interactions, and the pathogenicity of the polymicrobial root flora is dependent on bacterial synergy. Bacteriocins proteins produced by a microorganism enhance their ability to inhibit growth of some species competing for the same ecological niche. Additionally, they promote bacterial coaggregation and interactions establishing the ecology of the apical tissues.

The identification of the endodontic microbiota in the apical third was reported in 1991 by Baumgartner (26) who employed both aerobic and anaerobic cultures in the same study, in order to isolate and identify the microflora of the apical portion of root canals of teeth with carious pulpal exposures and apical lesions. Ten freshly extracted teeth with carious pulpal exposures and apical lesions contiguous with the root apex were placed inside an anaerobic chamber and the apical 5 mm of the root canals cultured. In addition to anaerobic incubation, duplicate cultures were incubated aerobically. Fifty strains of bacteria from the 10 root canals were isolated and identified.

The most prominent bacteria cultured from the 10 root canals were Actinomyces, Lactobacillus, black-pigmented *Bacteroides*, *Peptostreptococcus*, *nonpigmented Bacteroides*, *Veillonella*, *Enterococcus faecalis*, *Fusobacterium nucleatum*, and *Streptococcus mutans*. Of the 50 bacterial isolates, 34 (68%) were strict anaerobes. Baumgartner's study demonstrated the presence of predominantly anaerobic bacteria in the apical 5 mm of infected root canals in teeth with carious pulpal exposures and apical lesions.

Advancements in the identification of endodontic flora by Molander *et al.* in 1998 correlated the clinical outcome, refractory lesions, and the presence of certain strains. Molander and coworkers examined the microbiological status of 100 root-filled teeth with radiographically verified apical periodontitis and 20 teeth without signs of apical pathoses. In teeth with apical periodontitis, 117 strains of bacteria were recovered in 68 teeth. Facultative anaerobic species predominated among these isolates (69% of identified strains). Enterococci were the most frequently isolated genera, showing "heavy" or "very heavy" growth in 25 out of 32 cases (78%). In 11 teeth without signs of apical pathoses, no bacteria were recovered while the remaining 9 yielded 13 microbial strains. Eight of these grew "very sparsely." It was concluded that the microflora of the obturated canal differs from that found normally in the untreated necrotic dental pulp, quantitatively as well as qualitatively.

In 1990, Sha and Collins reclassified the moderately saccharolytic, predominantly oral Bacteroides species, which include *B. melaninogenicus*, *Bacteroides oralis*, and related species. These bacteria form a phenotypically and phylogenetically coherent group of species, which differ so significantly from the emended description of the genus Bacteroides that they should not be classified in the same genus and proposed that these species be reclassified in a new genus, Prevotella (27) (Figure 1.1).

By this time the advent of molecular biology techniques advanced in leaps and bounds in the detection and identification of microorganisms, uncovering the intimacy between genetics, biochemistry, and microbiology. Technique sensitive analyses of nucleic acids extracted from microorganisms directly, or from a sample containing the microorganism in question, have identified

```
┌─────────────────────────────────────────┐
│          New black-pigmented            │
│            classification               │
│                                         │
│  • Porphyromonas (Asaccharolytic)       │
│     – Porphyromonas gingivalis          │
│     – Porphyromonas endodontalis        │
│                                         │
│  • Prevotella (Saccharolytic)           │
│     – Prevotella intermedius            │
│     – Prevotella melaninogenicus        │
│     – Prevotella denticola              │
│     – Prevotella loescheii              │
│     – Prevotella nigrescens             │
│     – Prevotella corporis               │
│                                         │
└─────────────────────────────────────────┘
```

Figure 1.1   Current taxonomy and of black-pigmented bacteria.

endodontic microorganisms of interest; as was the case with Actinomyces. Polymerase chain reaction (PCR) is a biochemical technology in molecular biology used to amplify a single or a few copies of a piece of DNA across several orders of magnitude, generating thousands to millions of copies of a particular DNA sequence. Xia and Baumgartner used PCR with a pair of universal primers for Actinomyces and species-specific primers to evaluate the contents of infected root canals and aspirates from abscesses or cellulitis for the presence of *Actinomyces israelii*, *Actinomyces naeslundii*, and *Actinomyces viscosus*. DNA was extracted from 131 clinical samples (28). DNA reacting with the universal primer for Actinomyces was detected in 72 of 129 (55.8%) clinical samples. Of those, 41 of 51 (80.4%) were from infected root canals, 22 of 48 (45.8%) were from abscesses, and 9 of 30 (30%) were associated with cellulitis.

Since then, Siqueira and Rocas reported hundreds of species obtained from root canals using PCR techniques. In a review article published in 2008, they concluded that bacterial presence in the root canal at the time of filling is a risk factor for posttreatment apical periodontitis (29). About 100 species/phylotypes have already been detected in postinstrumentation and/or postmedication samples, and Gram-positive bacteria are the most dominant. However, it remains to be determined by longitudinal studies if any species/phylotypes persisting after treatment procedures can influence the outcome (29).

Waltimo *et al.* reported the current trend of recurrent yeast in endodontic infections, and their antimicrobial response confirms that yeast may be isolated in about 5–20% of the infected root canals. Their article identifies multiple virulence factors of *Candida* that allow it to infect the dentin–pulp complex and penetrate the dentinal tubules causing an inflammatory reaction and suggesting a pathogenic role of this organism in apical periodontitis (30).

With the discovery and understanding that fungus is present, the complexity of the microbiota became clear. In 2003, Slots *et al.* (31) were the first to report the presence of *cytomegalovirus* and *Epstein–Barr* virus (EBV) in more than 90% of granulomas of symptomatic and large apical lesions (31). Dual infection with cytomegalovirus and EBV is closely associated with symptomatic lesions. *Herpes simplex virus'* (HSV) active infection has no apparent relationship to apical disease.

Another study aimed to identify herpes virus, including *human cytomegalovirus* (HCMV), EBV, HSV-1, and *varicella zoster* virus (VZV) *in-vivo* (32, 33). Patients with acute apical abscesses and cellulitis of endodontic origin were used for the study. The identification was carried out by the primary PCR and nested PCR techniques. The results demonstrated the presence of HCMV, EBV, and HSV-1; however, they indicated that the presence of herpes virus that were identified were very low in their genetic copies, and therefore it was concluded that herpes viruses are present but do not have a direct relation to the development or establishment of pathologies such as acute apical abscess or cellulitis of endodontic origin.

The link between endodontic infection and apical disease

The presence of bacteria within the root canal system is essential for the development of apical inflammation (8). Apical periodontitis is a disease characterized by inflammation and destruction of apical tissues caused by microbial agents of endodontic origin. Initially, the tooth pulp becomes infected and necrotic by an autogenous oral microflora. The microenvironment of root canal systems provides excellent conditions for the establishment of a mixed, predominantly anaerobic, flora. Collectively, this polymicrobial community residing in the root canal has several biological and pathogenic properties, such as antigenicity, mitogenic activity, chemotaxis, enzymatic histolysis, and activation of host cells.

Microorganisms' growth within the root canal is in the form of biofilm. The microbial community develops as a biofilm and colonizes the environment. It occurs first by the deposition of a conditioning film; then there is adhesion and colonization of planktonic microorganisms in a polymeric matrix. The coadhesion of other organisms and the detachment of biofilm microorganisms into their surroundings happen at a later stage (34). Bacterial biofilm has an open architecture with channels traversing from the biofilm surface. The structure of biofilm affects the movement of molecules, and the gradients are key determinants in its development. Bacteria growing on a surface may display a novel phenotype that, consequently, may allow increased resistance to antimicrobial agents. Resistance can result from restricted inhibitor penetration, slower bacterial growth rates, transfer of resistance genes, suboptimal environmental conditions for inhibitor activity, and the expression of a resistant phenotype (35).

This ecological view on the persisting infection in endodontics suggests that the action of individual species in refractory endodontic infections is secondary when compared to the adaptive changes of a polymicrobial biofilm community undergoing physiological and genetic changes in response to changes in the root canal environment (36). The invasion of root dentinal tubules by root canal bacteria is a multifactorial event in which a limited number of oral bacterial species have the required properties to participate. Current literature has demonstrated that biofilms may remain viable in anatomical areas of the root canal system that remain untouched by either mechanical or chemical disinfection (Figure 1.2) (37–39). Scanning electron microscopy (SEM) examination of root tips associated with refractory apical periodontitis has suggested the presence of bacterial biofilm at the apical portion of the root canal (Figure 1.3) (40–42).

SEM analysis revealed bacterial biofilm surrounding the apical foramen and external radicular surface (Figures 1.4a and 1.2c). Careful observation of these structures under higher magnification revealed clumps of coaggregated bacterial cells in a matrix of extracellular polymeric substance (EPS). *E. faecalis* biofilms displayed a complex three-dimensional structure that demonstrated spatial heterogeneity and a typical architecture showing microcolonies with ramifying water channels (Figure 1.4b). Fibrillar structures appeared to be made up of twisted fibers. Larger structures of wrapped sheets were also present and consisted of small numbers of bacteria cells embedded in a matrix of fibers (Figure 1.4d).

Bacterial endotoxins and by-products egress through portals of exit causing the destruction of the apical tissues. In response, the host has an array of defenses consisting of several classes of cells, intercellular messengers, antibodies, and effector molecules. The microbial factors and host defense forces encounter, clash with, and destroy much of the apical tissue, which result in the formation of various categories of apical periodontitis lesions. In spite of the formidable defense, the body is unable to destroy the microbes well-entrenched in the sanctuary of the necrotic root canal, which is beyond the body's immune system. Therefore, the major goal of the root canal debridement is to eliminate the biofilm and bacteria-harboring debris.

Contemporary endodontic microbiology has become even more complex with the discovery of fungi and viruses. Waltimo *et al.* (43) found yeast in 7% of the culture-positive samples from persistent root canal infections. *Candida albicans* was the most frequently isolated yeast (80%). This finding was later confirmed by several studies (44, 45). Attachment to mucosal tissues and to abiotic surfaces and the formation of biofilms are crucial steps for *Candida* survival and proliferation in the oral cavity. *Candida* species possess a wide arsenal of glycoproteins located at the exterior side of the cell wall, many of which play a determining role in these steps. In addition, *C. albicans* secretes signaling molecules that inhibit the yeast-to-hypha transition and biofilm formation. *In-vivo, Candida* species are members of mixed biofilms and subject to various antagonistic and synergistic interactions (Figure 1.5) (46). Recently, Gomes *et al.* (47) confirmed the presence of filamentous fungi, which were isolated *in situ* from 17 of 60 samples (28.3%). The genus *Aspergillus* was isolated from 7/17 samples (41%).

The presence of HCMV, EBV, and HSV was first reported by Sabeti *et al.* (48) in symptomatic apical lesions. In a different study, Slots *et al.* (49) detected

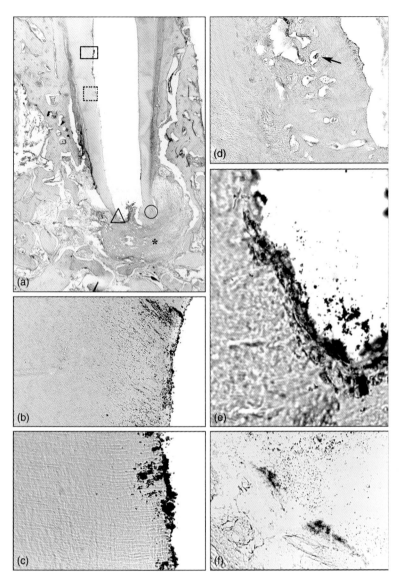

Figure 1.2 Composite figure of photomicrographs representative of microscopic sections of Groups I (EndoVac—ANP), II (Ultrasound—PUI), and III (conventional irrigation—PP) stained by the Brown and Brenn technique, revealing the presence and location of bacteria in the root canal system and apical tissues 180 days after endodontic treatment: (a) Panoramic photomicrograph, showing contamination of the entire extension of the tooth (Zeiss, 1.25×). (b) Detail of panel a (rectangle) in which the cervical root canal third can be visualized with abundant presence of microorganisms inside the dentinal tubules (Zeiss, 20×). (c) Detail of panel a (square) showing the middle root canal third with intense presence of bacteria (Zeiss, 20×). (d) Detail of panel a (circle) revealing the middle root canal third with presence of bacteria in the cemental craters (arrow) (Zeiss, 10×). (e) Detail of panel a (triangle) showing abundant presence of microorganisms in the apical root canal third (Zeiss, 40×). (f) Detail of panel a (asterisk) in which bacteria can be seen in the apical lesion (Zeiss, 20×).

HCMV in 100% of the symptomatic and in 37% of the asymptomatic study lesions (49). EBV was identified only in HCMV-infected apical lesions. The difference of HCMV and EBV between symptomatic and asymptomatic lesions was found to be statistically significant. Current studies confirmed these findings by using primary and nested PCR as well as reverse transcription PCR. (33) EBV DNA and RNA were present in endodontic pathoses in significantly higher percentages (43.9% and 25.6%, respectively) compared with healthy pulp controls.

The DNA of HSV was found in low percentages in endodontic patients (13.4%), and only one patient showed the presence of VZV. In conclusion, the presence of fungi and viruses had been associated with irreversible pulpitis and periodontitis, confirming once again that endodontic micro flora is complex and composed of well-organized biofilms of microorganisms with synergetic interactions.

The host responses to root canal infection have been the subject of much research in recent years. There is great similarity among the pathogenic

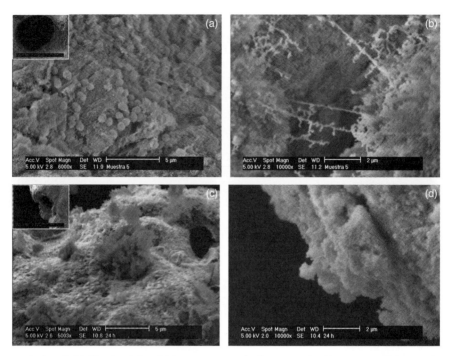

Figure 1.3   *In-vivo E. faecalis* biofilm. (a, c) Cocoidal structures attached to mature biofilm (6000×). (b) Extrapolymeric fibers (10,000×). (d) "Mushroom"-shaped structures (10,000×).

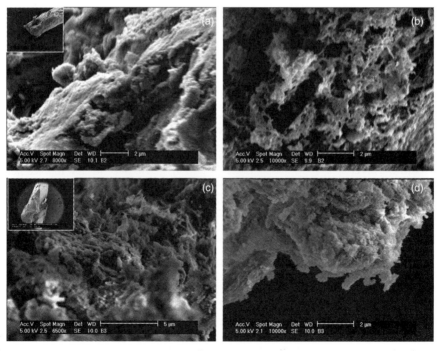

Figure 1.4   *E. faecalis* mature biofilm *in-vivo*. (a, c) Microcolonies wrapped in an extracellular matrix (8000×). (b) Network consisting of fibrillary structures (10,000×). (d) "Mushroom"-shaped structures (10,000×).

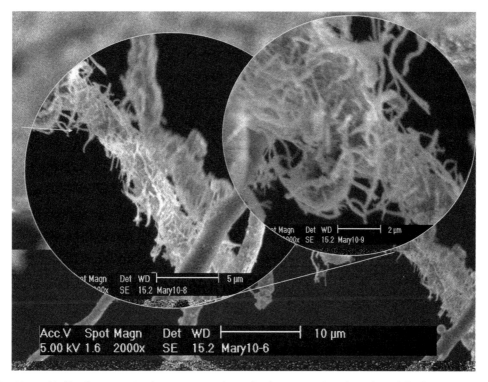

Figure 1.5   Mature biofilm demonstrating the synergistic relationship between *E. faecalis and Candida albicans.*

processes in marginal and apical periodontitis, and many of the findings in periodontal research have direct relevance to apical periodontitis. A clearer concept of the immunological processes involved in the development of apical periodontitis is emerging (50, 51). Microbiological variability and virulence factors in infected root canals have been demonstrated, and specific data indicate that the bacterial flora varies systematically with the clinical condition of the tooth involved (persistent infection, therapy-resistant infection). Different therapeutic strategies of antimicrobial control may have to be applied, depending on the microbiological diagnosis in a given case.

Apical periodontitis is not a self-healing disease (52). Untreated apical periodontitis may lead to a chronic infection of the oral tissues at locations closer to more vital organs than many other oral infections. Although these infections may remain quiescent for decades, they may also develop and spread with serious consequences for the individual (53, 54). In the face of the risks of such chronic infection from the infected teeth, their extraction

and replacement by implants has been put forward and discussed as a viable alternative to endodontic treatment (55, 56). The variable success rates (by strict criteria) of treatment procedures for the cure of apical periodontitis are sometimes used as arguments for the implant "treatment" concept. However, what little evidence there is does not indicate a lower survival rate of endodontically treated teeth, and the superiority of tooth preservation compared to its replacement should be evident as a biological principle of preference. However, the challenge from other treatment concepts, to endodontics as a discipline, should act as a driving force to produce more and scientifically solid evidence for the modalities of cure and prevention applied to our disease of interest, apical periodontitis.

Conclusion

Pulpal and apical inflammation, and the associated pain and the consequences of root canal infection, remain significant aspects of dentistry today. New knowledge and insights provide better treatment opportunities and stimulate further research activities. The prevention and control of apical periodontitis has a solid scientific base but the many variations in the clinical manifestations of the disease still leave technical and biological problems that need to be solved. Despite recent technological advances in treatment, evidence of improved outcome is still lacking. Alternative treatment involving implants is promoted as being better, but the criteria of evaluation of the outcome of the two forms of treatment are dissimilar; there is no true evidence-based comparison. The advancement, and utilization, of our biologic principles will allow a better understanding of the disease process and add to the fundamental truth that the biologic response to disease continues to be a biologic therapy; those therapies will and must continue to advance with our understanding.

References

1. Trowbridge, H.O. (1981) Pathogenesis of pulpitis resulting from dental caries. *Journal of Endodontics*, **7** (**2**), 52–60.
2. Van Hassel, H.J. (1971) Physiology of the human dental pulp. *Oral Surgery, Oral Medicine, and Oral Pathology*, **32** (**1**), 126–134.
3. Friedman, S., Abitbol, S. & Lawrence, H.P. (2003) Treatment outcome in endodontics: the Toronto Study. Phase 1: initial treatment. *Journal of Endodontics*, **29** (**12**), 787–793.
4. Farzaneh, M., Abitbol, S. & Friedman, S. (2004) Treatment outcome in endodontics: the Toronto study. Phases I and II: orthograde retreatment. *Journal of Endodontics*, **30** (**9**), 627–633.
5. Farzaneh, M., Abitbol, S., Lawrence, H.P. & Friedman, S. (2004) Treatment outcome in endodontics – the Toronto Study. Phase II: initial treatment. *Journal of Endodontics*, **30** (**5**), 302–309.
6. Orstavik, D., Qvist, V. & Stoltze, K. (2004) A multivariate analysis of the outcome of endodontic treatment. *European Journal of Oral Sciences*, **112** (**3**), 224–230.
7. Ricucci, D., Russo, J., Rutberg, M., Burleson, J.A. & Spangberg, L.S. (2011) A prospective cohort study of endodontic treatments of 1,369 root canals: results after 5 years. *Oral Surgery, Oral Medicine, Oral Pathology, Oral Radiology, and Endodontics*, **112** (**6**), 825–842.
8. Kakehashi, S., Stanley, H.R. & Fitzgerald, R.J. (1965) The effects of surgical exposures of dental pulps in germ-free and conventional laboratory rats. *Oral Surgery, Oral Medicine, and Oral Pathology*, **20**, 340–349.
9. Strindberg, L. (1956) The dependence of the results of pulp therapy on certain factors. *Acta Odontologica Scandinavica*, **14** (**21**), 1–175.
10. Kerekes, K. & Tronstad, L. (1979) Long-term results of endodontic treatment performed with a standardized technique. *Journal of Endodontics*, **5** (**3**), 83–90.
11. Ng, Y.L., Mann, V. & Gulabivala, K. (2011) A prospective study of the factors affecting outcomes of nonsurgical root canal treatment: part 1: periapical health. *International Endodontic Journal*, **44** (**7**), 583–609.
12. Ng, Y.L., Mann, V., Rahbaran, S., Lewsey, J. & Gulabivala, K. (2007) Outcome of primary root canal treatment: systematic review of the literature – part 1. Effects of study characteristics on probability of success. *International Endodontic Journal*, **40** (**12**), 921–939.
13. Endodontists AAO (2012) *Glossary of Endodontic Terms*, 8 edn. American Association of Endodontists, Chicago.
14. Wayman, B.E., Patten, J.A. & Dazey, S.E. (1994) Relative frequency of teeth needing endodontic treatment in 3350 consecutive endodontic patients. *Journal of Endodontics*, **20** (**8**), 399–401.
15. Boykin, M.J., Gilbert, G.H., Tilashalski, K.R. & Shelton, B.J. (2003) Incidence of endodontic treatment: a 48-month prospective study. *Journal of Endodontics*, **29** (**12**), 806–809.
16. Bjorndal, L. & Reit, C. (2005) The adoption of new endodontic technology amongst Danish general dental practitioners. *International Endodontic Journal*, **38** (**1**), 52–58.
17. Miller, W.D. (1890) *The Microorganisms of the Human Mouth*. The SS White Manufacturing Co, Philadelphia.
18. Moller, A.J. (1966) Microbiological examination of root canals and periapical tissues of human teeth. Methodological studies. *Odontologisk Tidskrift*, **74** (**Suppl. 5**), 1–380.
19. Bergenholtz, G. (1974) Micro-organisms from necrotic pulp of traumatized teeth. *Odontologisk Revy*, **25** (**4**), 347–358.
20. Sundqvist, G. (1976) *Bacteriological studies of necrotic dental pulps*. Umea University, Umea.
21. Moller, A.J., Fabricius, L., Dahlen, G., Ohman, A.E. & Heyden, G. (1981) Influence on periapical tissues of indigenous oral bacteria and necrotic pulp tissue in monkeys. *Scandinavian Journal of Dental Research*, **89** (**6**), 475–484.

22. Nair, P.N. (1987) Light and electron microscope studies of root canal flora and periapical lesions. *Journal of Endodontics*, **13**, 29–39.

23. Nair, P.N., Sjogren, U., Krey, G., Kahnberg, K.E. & Sundqvist, G. (1990) Intraradicular bacteria and fungi in root-filled, asymptomatic human teeth with therapy-resistant periapical lesions: a long-term light and electron microscopic follow-up study. *Journal of Endodontics*, **16 (12)**, 580–588.

24. Sundqvist, G. (1992) Ecology of the root canal flora. *Journal of Endodontics*, **18 (9)**, 427–430.

25. Sundqvist, G. (1994) Taxonomy, ecology, and pathogenicity of the root canal flora. *Oral Surgery, Oral Medicine, and Oral Pathology*, **78 (4)**, 522–530.

26. Baumgartner, J.C. & Falkler, W.A. Jr. (1991) Bacteria in the apical 5 mm of infected root canals. *Journal of Endodontics*, **17 (8)**, 380–383.

27. Shah, H.N. & Collins, D.M. (1990) Prevotella, a new genus to include Bacteroides melaninogenicus and related species formerly classified in the genus Bacteroides. *International Journal of Systematic Bacteriology*, **40 (2)**, 205–208.

28. Xia, T. & Baumgartner, J.C. (2003) Occurrence of Actinomyces in infections of endodontic origin. *Journal of Endodontics*, **29 (9)**, 549–552.

29. Siqueira, J.F. Jr. & Rocas, I.N. (2008) Clinical implications and microbiology of bacterial persistence after treatment procedures. *Journal of Endodontics*, **34 (11)**, 1291–1301, e1293.

30. Waltimo, T.M., Sen, B.H., Meurman, J.H., Orstavik, D. & Haapasalo, M.P. (2003) Yeasts in apical periodontitis. *Critical Reviews in Oral Biology and Medicine*, **14 (2)**, 128–137.

31. Slots, J., Sabeti, M. & Simon, J.H. (2003) Herpesviruses in periapical pathosis: an etiopathogenic relationship? *Oral Surgery, Oral Medicine, Oral Pathology, Oral Radiology, and Endodontics*, **96 (3)**, 327–331.

32. Chen, V., Chen, Y., Li, H., Kent, K., Baumgartner, J.C. & Machida, C.A. (2009) Herpesviruses in abscesses and cellulitis of endodontic origin. *Journal of Endodontics*, **35 (2)**, 182–188.

33. Li, H., Chen, V., Chen, Y., Baumgartner, J.C. & Machida, C.A. (2009) Herpesviruses in endodontic pathoses: association of Epstein–Barr virus with irreversible pulpitis and apical periodontitis. *Journal of Endodontics*, **35 (1)**, 23–29.

34. Svensäter, G. & Bergenholtz, G. (2004) Biofilms in endodontic infections. *Endodontic Topics*, **9**, 27–36.

35. Marsh, P.D. (2003) Plaque as a biofilm: pharmacological principles of drug delivery and action in the sub- and supragingival environment. *Oral Diseases*, **9 (Suppl. 1)**, 16–22.

36. Chavez de Paz, L.E. (2007) Redefining the persistent infection in root canals: possible role of biofilm communities. *Journal of Endodontics*, **33 (6)**, 652–662.

37. Nair, P.N., Henry, S., Cano, V. & Vera, J. (2005) Microbial status of apical root canal system of human mandibular first molars with primary apical periodontitis after "one-visit" endodontic treatment. *Oral Surgery, Oral Medicine, Oral Pathology, Oral Radiology, and Endodontics*, **99 (2)**, 231–252.

38. Ricucci, D. & Siqueira, J.F. Jr. (2010) Biofilms and apical periodontitis: study of prevalence and association with clinical and histopathologic findings. *Journal of Endodontics*, **36 (8)**, 1277–1288.

39. Ricucci, D. & Siqueira, J.F. Jr. (2010) Fate of the tissue in lateral canals and apical ramifications in response to pathologic conditions and treatment procedures. *Journal of Endodontics*, **36 (1)**, 1–15.

40. Lin, L.M., Ricucci, D., Lin, J. & Rosenberg, P.A. (2009) Nonsurgical root canal therapy of large cyst-like inflammatory periapical lesions and inflammatory apical cysts. *Journal of Endodontics*, **35 (5)**, 607–615.

41. Noiri, Y., Ehara, A., Kawahara, T., Takemura, N. & Ebisu, S. (2002) Participation of bacterial biofilms in refractory and chronic periapical periodontitis. *Journal of Endodontics*, **28 (10)**, 679–683.

42. Ricucci, D., Lin, L.M. & Spangberg, L.S. (2009) Wound healing of apical tissues after root canal therapy: a long-term clinical, radiographic, and histopathologic observation study. *Oral Surgery, Oral Medicine, Oral Pathology, Oral Radiology, and Endodontics*, **108 (4)**, 609–621.

43. Waltimo, T.M., Siren, E.K., Torkko, H.L., Olsen, I. & Haapasalo, M.P. (1997) Fungi in therapy-resistant apical periodontitis. *International Endodontic Journal*, **30 (2)**, 96–101.

44. Peciuliene, V., Reynaud, A.H., Balciuniene, I. & Haapasalo, M. (2001) Isolation of yeasts and enteric bacteria in root-filled teeth with chronic apical periodontitis. *International Endodontic Journal*, **34 (6)**, 429–434.

45. Baumgartner, J.C., Watts, C.M. & Xia, T. (2000) Occurrence of Candida albicans in infections of endodontic origin. *Journal of Endodontics*, **26 (12)**, 695–698.

46. ten Cate, J.M., Klis, F.M., Pereira-Cenci, T., Crielaard, W. & de Groot, P.W. (2009) Molecular and cellular mechanisms that lead to Candida biofilm formation. *Journal of Dental Research*, **88 (2)**, 105–115.

47. Gomes, C., Fidel, S., Fidel, R. & de Moura Sarquis, M.I. (2010) Isolation and taxonomy of filamentous fungi in endodontic infections. *Journal of Endodontics*, **36 (4)**, 626–629.

48. Sabeti, M., Simon, J.H., Nowzari, H. & Slots, J. (2003) Cytomegalovirus and Epstein–Barr virus active infection in periapical lesions of teeth with intact crowns. *Journal of Endodontics*, **29 (5)**, 321–323.

49. Slots, J., Nowzari, H. & Sabeti, M. (2004) Cytomegalovirus infection in symptomatic periapical pathosis. *International Endodontic Journal*, **37** (**8**), 519–524.

50. Kawashima, N., Okiji, T., Kosaka, T. & Suda, H. (1996) Kinetics of macrophages and lymphoid cells during the development of experimentally induced periapical lesions in rat molars: a quantitative immunohistochemical study. *Journal of Endodontics*, **22** (**6**), 311–316.

51. Stashenko, P., Wang, C.Y., Tani-Ishii, N. & Yu, S.M. (1994) Pathogenesis of induced rat periapical lesions. *Oral Surgery, Oral Medicine, and Oral Pathology*, **78** (**4**), 494–502.

52. Nair, P.N. (1997) Apical periodontitis: a dynamic encounter between root canal infection and host response. *Periodontology 2000*, **13**, 121–148.

53. Wang, C.H., Chueh, L.H., Chen, S.C., Feng, Y.C., Hsiao, C.K. & Chiang, C.P. (2011) Impact of diabetes mellitus, hypertension, and coronary artery disease on tooth extraction after nonsurgical endodontic treatment. *Journal of Endodontics*, **37** (**1**), 1–5.

54. Seppanen, L., Lemberg, K.K., Lauhio, A., Lindqvist, C. & Rautemaa, R. (2011) Is dental treatment of an infected tooth a risk factor for locally invasive spread of infection? *Journal of Oral and Maxillofacial Surgery: Official Journal of the American Association of Oral and Maxillofacial Surgeons*, **69** (**4**), 986–993.

55. Torabinejad, M. & Goodacre, C.J. (2006) Endodontic or dental implant therapy: the factors affecting treatment planning. *Journal of the American Dental Association*, **137** (**7**), 973–977, quiz 1027–1028.

56. Gatten, D.L., Riedy, C.A., Hong, S.K., Johnson, J.D. & Cohenca, N. (2011) Quality of life of endodontically treated versus implant treated patients: a University-based qualitative research study. *Journal of Endodontics*, **37** (**7**), 903–909.

2

The Anatomy of the Root Canal System as a Challenge to Effective Disinfection

Eric Herbranson

Private practice, San Leandro, California, USA

Introduction

Nair in a 2006 review of the causes of persistent apical periodontitis in endodontically treated teeth identified six biological factors that lead to asymptomatic radiolucencies persisting after root canal treatment. These are (i) intraradicular infection persisting in the complex apical root canal system; (ii) extraradicular infection, generally in the form of apical actinomycosis; (iii) extruded root canal filling or other exogenous materials that cause a foreign body reaction; (iv) accumulation of endogenous cholesterol crystals that irritate apical tissues; (v) true cystic lesions, and (vi) scar tissue (1). He identified intraradicular infection as the main cause of unresolved apical periodontitis. The infectious agents are located in the uninstrumented recess of the internal anatomy of the root canal system and exist primarily as biofilms. The internal anatomy can be notoriously complex, especially in molars, and includes extra canals, recesses, fins, isthmuses, and accessory canals that provide space for the biofilms to reside. In addition, biofilms are difficult to eradicate. It has been reported that biofilms are a thousand times more difficult to eradicate than planktonic organisms floating in an aqueous environment (2–4). It is because of the combination of anatomical hiding places and the difficulty of destroying the biofilm that complete debridement of the canal space is probably impossible with our current treatment protocols.

The complexity of the root canal system

Root canal configuration and classification

There is great complexity and variation to the pulp space as it travels from the coronal to the apex. There are multiple canals that join and separate at unpredictable places in the tooth. All the anatomical studies from Hess forward have demonstrated this. The flatter or more ovoid the root cross-section, the greater the propensity for complexity. In the maxilla, the most variation will be found in the premolars, especially the second and the mesiobuccal (MB) root of the molars. In the mandible, anterior, premolar, and molar teeth

Disinfection of Root Canal Systems: The Treatment of Apical Periodontitis, First Edition. Edited by Nestor Cohenca.
© 2014 John Wiley & Sons, Inc. Published 2014 by John Wiley & Sons, Inc.

Weine (6)

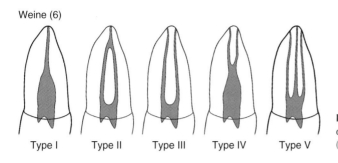

Type I   Type II   Type III   Type IV   Type V

Figure 2.1   Weine's canal classification. Originally described as four types but later expanded to five types. (Reproduced with permission of E. Herbranson.)

Vertucci (7)

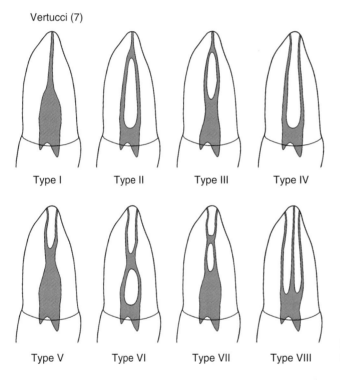

Type I   Type II   Type III   Type IV

Type V   Type VI   Type VII   Type VIII

Figure 2.2   Vertucci's canal classification. (Reproduced with permission of E. Herbranson.)

are the ones that will show the greatest variation. The mandibular premolar is a bit of an enigma as it is usually a round root form with a single canal but it will exhibit multiple canals and great complexity on occasion. There is some ethnic variation in anatomy. For instance, blacks have the highest percentage of complex premolar, with Trope *et al.* (5) reporting a 32.8% incidence of two canals in the first premolar.

Weine (6) attempted to classify these into four types and later five (Figure 2.1). This was expanded by Vertucci (7) with eight different canal morphologies (Figure 2.2). These classifications were further developed by Gulabivala *et al.* (8, 9) to nine types, and Sert and Bayirli (10) reported an additional 14 configurations in a small subset of a Turkish population. This chasing of more and more classification points to the fundamental fact that there is great complexity in the pulp configuration in teeth. It is worth the time for a clinician to look at the Weine or Vertucci classification and then play the mental game of how one would detect, instrument, and obturate these various configurations. It will also help the clinician to appreciate the difficulty of debriding and disinfecting these shapes.

Even with multiple angles these canal variations are difficult to detect with conventional 2D radiographs. The use of small field cone beam computed tomography (CBCT) scans are a valuable adjunct to help the clinician to detect and mentally image the canal system shape.

Root canal morphology

Pulp space shape is conceptualized by many to be a round hole. The reality is they mimic the external shape of the root. If it is round, the pulp shape will be round. If the root is ovoid, the pulp shape will be ovoid (Figure 2.3). There are a family of minor complexities in anatomy that are difficult to categorize. They include fins, niches, loops, and other oddities. They are a reflection of the unlimited variations in pulp space anatomy that exists.

Accessory canals

Accessory and lateral canals extend from the pulp to the periodontium. They are found in all teeth and are formed when Hertwigs's epithelium root sheath traps the periodontal vessels during tooth formation. Vertucci, in 1984 (7), reported their incident was 24–30% in maxillary anterior teeth, 50–60% in maxillary premolars, and 30–50% in maxillary molars with the MB root showing the highest incidence. He reported lateral canals in 18–30% of mandibular anterior teeth and almost half of lower premolars and molars. Lateral canals are found most commonly in the apical third, anywhere from 60% to 90%, with 10–16% occurring in the middle third of the root and the cervical third with a lower percentage. Complex multirooted teeth have more cervical lateral canals and may present patent accessory canals in the furcation region in 29.4% in mandibular molars, and 27.4% in maxillary molars (11).

Isthmuses and intracanal communications

Any root that has more than one canal will always present some degree of communication between those canals spaces. These features are really a variation of the complexity described by the Vertucci classification (Figure 2.4). They occur in a significant number of these types of roots with incidence as high as 71% of the maxillary first molars (12). These communications and isthmuses were respectively in 42% and 54% of the cases in the coronal third, in 59% and 79% of the cases in the middle third, and in 24% and 50% of the cases in the apical third (12). In mandibular first molars, the presence of isthmus communications averaged 54.8% on the mesial and 20.2% on the distal root (13). This anatomical communications should be taken into consideration during endodontic treatment as well as during apical surgery (14).

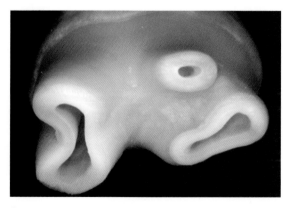

Figure 2.3 A sectioned, partially developed upper first molar showing how the internal pulp space follows the external root form. (Courtesy of Dr. David Clark.)

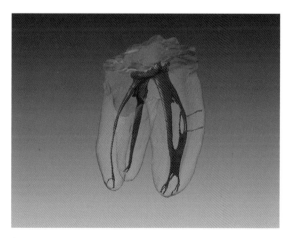

Figure 2.4 A high-resolution micro-CT scan of a three-rooted lower first molar illustrating many of the anatomical challenges facing endodontic therapy. (Reproduced with permission of E. Herbranson.)

Figure 2.4 shows many of the complexity features discussed here illustrated in a single tooth. It has an extra root on the distolingual (DL), Vertucci type IV anatomy on the mesial root with a loop feature, later canals, and isthmus and apical deltas. All are areas for biofilm to hide in. Debridement, disinfection, and obturation of these types of spaces are difficult or impossible. This tooth could be the poster child for the anatomical challenges facing the clinician.

Apical delta

An apical delta is a pattern of small accessory canals at the apex of some teeth that looks like a river delta. The complexity and multiple portals of exit of the pulp system make these areas very hard to debride and disinfect.

C-shaped canals

C-shaped canals are an anatomic variation to keep in mind when treating maxillary and mandibular molars with adjoining or fused roots, which results in a C-shaped configuration of the canal spaces (15).

The etiology of the C-shaped canal is the fusion of the buccal aspect of the mesial and distal roots. Classification systems have been proposed by Melton et al. (16) and more recently by Fan et al. (17, 18). The anatomical variations of the C-shaped canal are numerous as the canal can vary from one distinct ribbon-shaped canal from pulp chamber to apex to three distinct separate canals with interconnections between the canals. The C-shaped canal has been reported in mandibular premolars and molars as well as in maxillary molars and its prevalence seems to be related to the ethnicity, with higher incidence of C-shaped canals in Asian populations. Zheng et al. (19) evaluated a total of 608 patients of Chinese descent with healthy, well-developed mandibular second molars and reported the presence of C-shaped canal system in 39% of the teeth.

The challenge in treating C-shaped canals lies in the thorough debridement and complete obturation because of the irregular areas of the canal house debris and necrotic tissue that is difficult to clean and fill. Mechanical instrumentation is

unpredictable for disinfection, and caution should be taken when preparing the isthmus area as it is frequently very thin leading to a strip perforation. Thus, disinfection is accomplished chemically delivering and activating irrigants with ultrasonic and negative pressure irrigation with the purpose of enhancing debridement and disinfection.

The source of complexity

The anatomy complexity has its source in the development of teeth. Internal pulp anatomy is a reflection of the external anatomy of the root. This is due to the tooth formation process. Primary dentin apposition by the odontoblasts occurs at a relatively constant rate so the wall thickness of the dentin in a partially developed root will be similar around the perimeter. If the external shape is ovoid, the canal will be ovoid. If the external shape resembles a kidney bean, the internal shape will also be the same. Figure 2.3 that shows the cross-section anatomy of a partially developed upper molar illustrates this point. As the tooth reaches its full development, this kidney bean shaped root will end up with two canals with fins, inter and intracanal communications between the canals. This is shown in Figure 2.5, with the

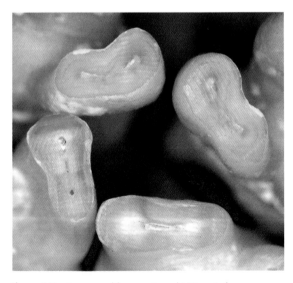

Figure 2.5 A group of four sectioned MB roots from upper first molars. Note how the roots with concavities have two canals. (Reproduced with permission of E. Herbranson.)

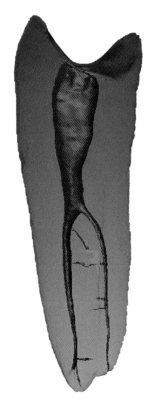

Figure 2.6   A two-rooted lower first premolar with multiple accessory canals including one in the furcation. (Reproduced with permission of E. Herbranson.)

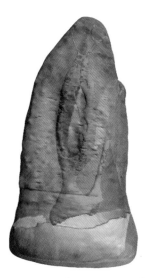

Figure 2.7   Micro-CT scan of a 65,000-year-old Neanderthal upper second molar. Note the anatomical complexity. (Reproduced with permission of E. Herbranson.)

cross-sections of four MB roots of upper first molars. The three that are kidney bean shaped have two canals and isthmus anatomy. As a general rule, any tooth with a concavity in its root form has the potential for multiple canals and aberrant internal anatomy. This goes for almost all the teeth. All maxillary molars and premolars have root concavities. Most mandibular anterior and molar teeth have root concavities. Although lower premolars are typically round in shape, a percentage of them have very complex anatomy (Figure 2.6).

Detecting anatomy

This complex internal anatomy has been around for eons (Figure 2.7) but has been recognized and appreciated by the dental community only slowly. Hess (20) published a landmark book in

1925 demonstrating the complexity of the internal anatomy using cleared teeth with ink dye penetrations of the pulp spaces (Figure 2.8) but this work languished in obscurity until Dr. Herbert Schilder resurrected it to demonstrate the need for 3D obturation of the pulp space (21). This anatomy has been demonstrated in a number of ways since then. The author, during his graduate endodontic training, showed the complexity of posterior tooth anatomy using silicon rubber casts of the pulp space (Figure 2.9). Other methods include careful cutdowns to the obturated canal space (Figure 2.10a,b) and chemically demineralizing the dentin to reveal the internal anatomy (Figure 2.11). All these are revealing and valuable educational tools, but these methods are labor intensive and consequently the sample sizes are small. It was not until the advent of research grade micro-CT technology that it was possible to do this work on a broader sample size.

Micro-CT scanners have resolutions that can produce around 10 μm voxel data. This is high enough resolution to demonstrate much of the complexity of the anatomy. For instance, a typical lateral canal will have a diameter of 20–30 μm (22). Ten micron voxel data can resolve a feature of that size. In addition, because the data

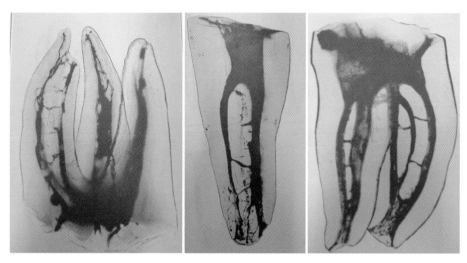

Figure 2.8   Examples of Hess original ink stained pulps in cleared teeth. (Reproduced with permission of E. Herbranson.)

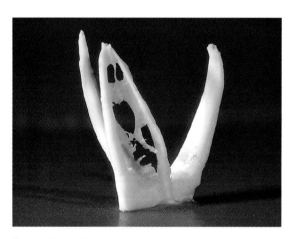

Figure 2.9   A silicon cast of an upper first molar. Note the communication between the MB canals. (Reproduced with permission of E. Herbranson.)

is computer based, it can be manipulated and presented in a variety of visualization formats. Interactivity, transparency, cutting planes, stereopsis are all possible adjuncts to visualization. Dr. Steve Buchanan demonstrated, in a lecture, the first micro-CT data from teeth. The protocols for micro-CT imaging lend themselves to "production line" collection and processing of data. A project started in 1998 by Brown and Herbranson Imaging and funded by NIH was the first attempt to do that on a significant numbers of teeth. This group ultimately micro-CT scanned about 600 teeth. The data is currently available in the 3D Tooth Atlas v7 (23). Artistic rendering of tooth anatomy typically grossly oversimplifies the complexity of the actual anatomy (Figure 2.12a,b). It is this simplification that unfortunately leads to a limited understanding of the complexity. Micro-CT machines currently produce the gold standard images for visualizing the internal anatomy of teeth. As they become more common, other datasets will become available, which will lead to a better understanding.

Although the micro-CT machine produces very useful images, there is a level of anatomy that these machines do not have the ability to resolve. Figure 2.13 shows an upper first premolar image from a typical 10 μm pixel size resolution scan. Note the apparently simple anatomy at the apexes of the buccal roots. Figure 2.14 shows the same apexes at a 1.8 μm pixel resolution using a synchrotron (Advance Light Source, Lawrence Berkeley National Laboratory) as the radiation

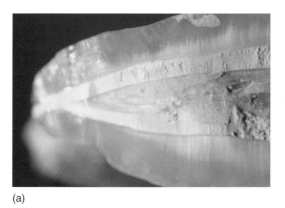
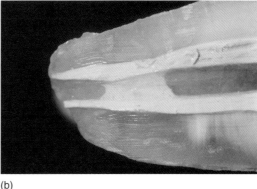

(a)   (b)

Figure 2.10   (a,b) Root canal filling of two different teeth obturated using warm vertical condensation. The root were shaved back to reveal the anatomy and extension of the gutta-percha. Note the significant but incomplete fill of the isthmus between the canals. (Courtesy of Dr. Robert Sharp.)

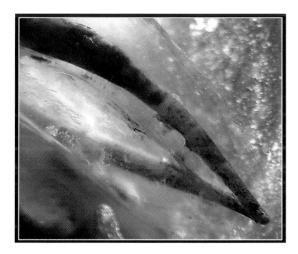

Figure 2.11   A cleared MB root of an upper first molar that was extracted. (Courtesy of Dr. Craig Barrington.)

source (Figure 2.14). This much higher resolution scan shows small apical anatomy and inclusions that are not evident on the lower resolution scan. It is important that we realize that our micro-CT "gold standard," as good as it is, does not reveal all the complexity that exists (Figures 2.15 and 2.16).

The importance of understanding anatomy toward better outcomes

The anatomical variations discussed present significant challenges to irrigation, disinfection, and obturation of the root canal space.

Extra canals require an awareness of the potential for their existence and a strategy to detect and treat them. This requires a high-level understanding of the anatomy, understanding how these variations present themselves, and a commitment to locating it. Without treatment, extra canals will lead to unresolved problems and poorer outcomes. Many cases that present to clinicians for retreatment have problems that can be traced to missed canals. Dealing with these is really a clinical expertise issue. To be successful, these cases demand that the clinician apply all the available armamentarium to the problem, including a studied approach, microscopes, CBCT scans, and a commitment to solving the problem.

Micro anatomy variations such as fins, deltas, accessory canals is anatomy that is beyond the reach of mechanical debridement and puts the burden for resolution on the irrigation protocols we use and to a lesser degree the obturation protocols we use. These spaces is the difficult challenge in

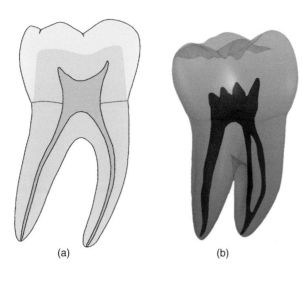

(a)   (b)

Figure 2.12   (a,b) Two examples of the artistic rendering of pulp anatomy. Although dimensionally accurate, they still exhibit a simplicity that does not reflect the complexity of a real tooth. (Reproduced with permission of E. Herbranson.)

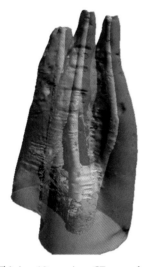

Figure 2.13   This is a 10μm micro-CT scan of a three-rooted upper first premolar. The endodontic procedure was done extraorally. (Reproduced with permission of E. Herbranson.)

endodontics because they are a perfect home for biofilms and a difficult place to access. We must develop and use the most effective protocols for addressing these spaces.

Although many of the current obturation techniques can exhibit what appears to be an effective obturation of lateral anatomy, there are two issues

that need to be highlighted. The first is that even in an impressive-looking obturation, not all the lateral anatomy can be filled (Figure 2.17). You can only see what was obturated, not what was not obturated. The second issue is that the residual debris in the canal can block the effective obturation of a space. Effective obturation depends on the effective debridement of the small anatomy, which is problematic.

There are teeth with such a complexity in anatomy that current orthograde endodontic technology cannot resolve. Figure 2.18 is an example of such a tooth. It is unlikely that a clinician could maneuver a file to the apex of the MB2 canal. A retrograde surgical procedure could adequately treat this MB root if the clinician included the MB2 apex in the apicoectomy prep. A narrow-field CBCT scan would be very useful in ensuring the clinician understood the subtle anatomy challenges presented here.

Clinical cases

Case 1: This endodontic procedure on a mandibular left first molar was done by an experienced endodontist in two appointments with an intermediate $Ca(OH)_2$ dressing and warm vertical obturation. The patient continued to have mild

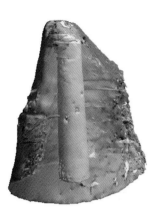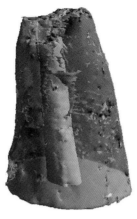

Figure 2.14 These are the apexes of the buccal roots of the tooth shown in Figure 2.13 but scanned at 1.8 μm. Note the fine structures not visible in the lower resolution scans in Figure 2.13. (Reproduced with permission of E. Herbranson.)

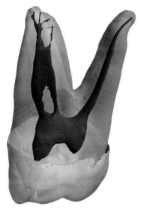

Figure 2.15 A micro-CT scan of an upper first molar showing two canals, isthmus, and delta formation in the MB root. (Reproduced with permission of E. Herbranson.)

discomfort so the tooth was re-treated, again in two appointments, with an intermediate Ca(OH)$_2$ dressing (Figure 2.19a,b). The patient again had mild discomfort. After a discussion of alternative treatment, including apical surgery, the patient decided to have the tooth extracted. Multiple angle 2D radiographs (Figure 2.20) showed nothing extraordinary, but a micro-CT scan revealed the unfilled isthmus and fins in the buccal root (Figure 2.21). This was the result of a failure of our current technology, not a failure of intention or operator skill. This tooth probably could have been salvaged with an apicoectomy

and retrofill on the mesial root but the patient was unwilling to go through the procedure.

Case 2: This is the MB root of an upper first molar that was extracted during periodontal surgery. Note the third canal (in red) that parallels the MB3 canal (Figure 2.22). Locating this canal would be very difficult without a narrow field CBCT scan.

Case 3: This extracted tooth was treated using the hand instrumentation technique see how well the complex D root could be filled with a warm vertical obturation method. Every effort was made to guarantee a solid fill. It is interesting that even though some of the anatomy between the MB and mesiolingual (ML) canals was filled, much of it did not get addressed (Figure 2.23).

In all of these cases, conventional 2D radiographs showed excellent obturations and apparently good technique. It is only the application of micro-CT technology that revealed the unfilled internal anatomy. The clinician must keep in mind the principle that *a radiograph shows what the operator did. It does not show what the operator did not do.* So we must be careful not to make too many assumptions about the quality of the procedure we delivered based on our radiographs.

Conclusions

The ultimate objective of endodontic therapy is the obturation of the prepared root canal space with an

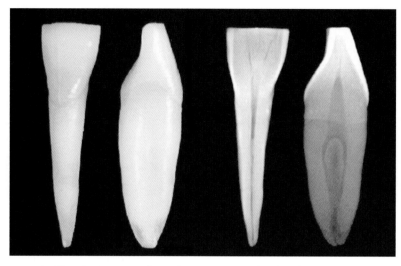

Figure 2.16   A lower central with a classic 1-2-1 pulp configuration. (Reproduced with permission of E. Herbranson.)

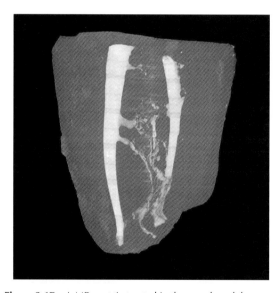

Figure 2.17   A MB root tip treated in the mouth and then amputated during a periodontal procedure. Obturated with a warm vertical gutta-percha technique. Note the impressive obturation of the extra canal anatomy between the two main canals. This is the main sealer, not gutta-percha. (Reproduced with permission of E. Herbranson.)

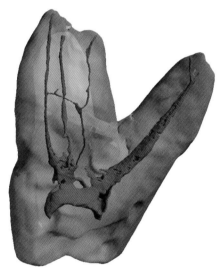

Figure 2.18   An "impossible" tooth on which the MB2 canal would be very difficult to treat and disinfect with nonsurgical orthograde endodontics. (Reproduced with permission of E. Herbranson.)

inert material in order to restore the integrity and health of the treated tooth in the dental arch. Several causes of endodontic failure have been identified, including the failure to disinfect a complex root canal system. Endodontics is a game of eliminating microorganisms from uninstrumented spaces within the internal anatomy of the pulp space. As our knowledge of that space increases, our understanding of the challenge before us increases. Therefore, it is imperative for the endodontist to

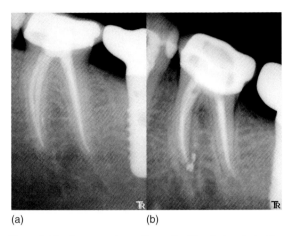

(a)   (b)

Figure 2.19   Postoperative radiograph of the first endodontic treatment of a mandibular left first molar (a). The nonsurgical root canal retreatment (b). The patient was never comfortable with the tooth and eventually had it extracted. (Reproduced with permission of E. Herbranson.)

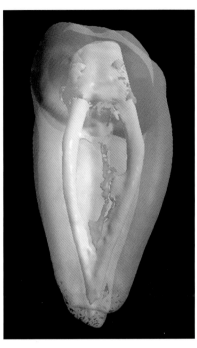

Figure 2.21   Micro-CT scan of the mandibular left first molar. The pink represents unfilled pulp space. (Reproduced with permission of E. Herbranson.)

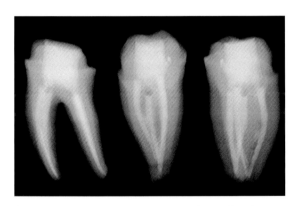

Figure 2.20   After the tooth was extracted, varied angle 2D radiographs taken, including proximal radiograph, demonstrate the complexity of the anatomy such as intracanal isthmus communication. (Reproduced with permission of E. Herbranson.)

be thoroughly familiar with root canal anatomy, including the numbers and locations of canals, in order to clean, shape, and obturate for optimal success. While it is humbling to understand the challenge we face, it is through this understanding that we can design and develop protocols that will help us improve success.

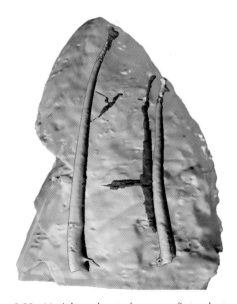

Figure 2.22   Mesiobuccal root of an upper first molar treated in the mouth and amputated during a periodontal surgery. Note the untreated MB2 canal parallel to the MB3. (Reproduced with permission of E. Herbranson.)

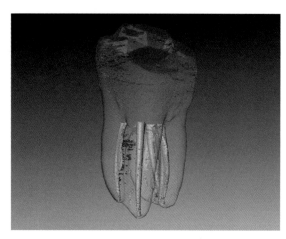

Figure 2.23 An extracted tooth treated extraorally and sealed with warm vertical obturation. The purple is unfilled anatomy between the two main canals in the mesial root. (Reproduced with permission of E. Herbranson.)

References

1. Nair, P.N. (2006) On the causes of persistent apical periodontitis: a review. *International Endodontic Journal*, **39 (4)**, 249–281.
2. Chavez de Paz, L.E. (2007) Redefining the persistent infection in root canals: possible role of biofilm communities. *Journal of Endodontics*, **33 (6)**, 652–662.
3. Estrela, C., Sydney, G.B., Figueiredo, J.A. & Estrela, C.R. (2009) Antibacterial efficacy of intracanal medicaments on bacterial biofilm: a critical review. *Journal of Applied Oral Science*, **17 (1)**, 1–7.
4. Ricucci, D. & Siqueira, J.F. Jr. (2010) Fate of the tissue in lateral canals and apical ramifications in response to pathologic conditions and treatment procedures. *Journal of Endodontics*, **36 (1)**, 1–15.
5. Trope, M., Elfenbein, L. & Tronstad, L. (1986) Mandibular premolars with more than one root canal in different race groups. *Journal of Endodontics*, **12 (8)**, 343–345.
6. Weine, F.S., Healey, H.J., Gerstein, H. & Evanson, L. (1969) Canal configuration in the mesiobuccal root of the maxillary first molar and its endodontic significance. *Oral Surgery, Oral Medicine, and Oral Pathology*, **28 (3)**, 419–425.
7. Vertucci, F.J. (1984) Root canal anatomy of the human permanent teeth. *Oral Surgery, Oral Medicine, and Oral Pathology*, **58 (5)**, 589–599.
8. Gulabivala, K., Opasanon, A., Ng, Y.L. & Alavi, A. (2002) Root and canal morphology of Thai mandibular molars. *International Endodontic Journal*, **35 (1)**, 56–62.
9. Gulabivala, K., Aung, T.H., Alavi, A. & Ng, Y.L. (2001) Root and canal morphology of Burmese mandibular molars. *International Endodontic Journal*, **34 (5)**, 359–370.
10. Sert, S. & Bayirli, G.S. (2004) Evaluation of the root canal configurations of the mandibular and maxillary permanent teeth by gender in the Turkish population. *Journal of Endodontics*, **30 (6)**, 391–398.
11. Gutmann, J.L. (1978) Prevalence, location, and patency of accessory canals in the furcation region of permanent molars. *Journal of Periodontology*, **49 (1)**, 21–26.
12. Somma, F., Leoni, D., Plotino, G., Grande, N.M. & Plasschaert, A. (2009) Root canal morphology of the mesiobuccal root of maxillary first molars: a micro-computed tomographic analysis. *International Endodontic Journal*, **42 (2)**, 165–174.
13. de Pablo, O.V., Estevez, R., Peix Sanchez, M., Heilborn, C. & Cohenca, N. (2010) Root anatomy and canal configuration of the permanent mandibular first molar: a systematic review. *Journal of Endodontics*, **36 (12)**, 1919–1931.
14. de Pablo, O.V., Estevez, R., Heilborn, C. & Cohenca, N. (2012) Root anatomy and canal configuration of the permanent mandibular first molar: clinical implications and recommendations. *Quintessence International*, **43 (1)**, 15–27.
15. Jafarzadeh, H. & Wu, Y.N. (2007) The C-shaped root canal configuration: a review. *Journal of Endodontics*, **33 (5)**, 517–523.
16. Melton, D.C., Krell, K.V. & Fuller, M.W. (1991) Anatomical and histological features of C-shaped canals in mandibular second molars. *Journal of Endodontics*, **17 (8)**, 384–388.
17. Fan, B., Cheung, G.S., Fan, M., Gutmann, J.L. & Fan, W. (2004) C-shaped canal system in mandibular second molars: part II – radiographic features. *Journal of Endodontics*, **30 (12)**, 904–908.
18. Fan, B., Cheung, G.S., Fan, M., Gutmann, J.L. & Bian, Z. (2004) C-shaped canal system in mandibular second molars: part I – anatomical features. *Journal of Endodontics*, **30 (12)**, 899–903.
19. Zheng, Q., Zhang, L., Zhou, X. *et al.* (2011) C-shaped root canal system in mandibular second molars in a Chinese population evaluated by cone-beam computed tomography. *International Endodontic Journal*, **44 (9)**, 857–862.

20. Hess, W. (1925) *The Anatomy of the Root-Canals of the Teeth of the Permanent Dentition*. William Wood, New York.

21. Schilder, H. (1967) Filling root canals in three dimensions. *Dental Clinics of North America*, **11**, 723–744.

22. Vertucci, F.J. (2005) Root canal morphology and its relationship to endodontic procedures. *Endodontic Topics*, **10**, 3–29.

23. Herbranson E. (2013) *3D Tooth Atlas* [cited]. Available from: http://www.ehuman.com/products/3d-tooth-atlas-7.

3 Biofilms in Root Canal Infections

Christine M. Sedgley

Department of Endodontology, Oregon Health and Science University, Portland, OR, USA

Rogério de Castilho Jacinto

Department of Semiology and Clinics, Federal University of Pelotas, Pelotas, RS, Brazil

Introduction

Biofilms are microbial communities composed of microcolonies that contain cells irreversibly attached to a substratum, an interface, or each other, as opposed to being suspended in liquid (planktonic mode). Biofilm formation has been described as an ancient prokaryotic adaptation allowing survival in hostile environments (1–3). The process encompasses attachment of microbial cells to a surface, followed by cell proliferation, adherence to other bacteria, production of a matrix, and microcolony maturation (4). Dispersal of cells allows the formation of new biofilm microcolonies (5). A key characteristic of biofilms is their highly heterogeneous composition that can vary greatly under different environmental conditions. Of particular clinical significance is that microbial cells in biofilms can utilize a variety of mechanisms that enable survival under challenging conditions (6–10). For example, biofilms have been regarded as the primary causative agent for many hospital-acquired infections as well as persistent and chronic infections such as cystic fibrosis pneumonia (4, 8).

Seminal studies published several decades ago established the role of microorganisms as the primary etiologic agents of apical infections (11–14). In these and many subsequent evaluations of the root canal (RC) microflora, strains were typically grown as single-species, planktonic cultures. More recently, it has been recognized that microorganisms exist in the RC system as multispecies biofilm communities (15–20). This chapter describes the general characteristics of biofilms and analyzes biofilms associated with RC infections.

General characteristics of biofilms

Components of biofilms

Microbial cells occupy only a small portion of the biofilm. The majority of the biofilm structure is a highly heterogeneous matrix composed of extracellular polymeric substances (EPS) produced by cells within the biofilm. The EPS matrix can account for greater than 90% of the dry mass of most biofilms and provides multiple functions. These include provision of a scaffold for the biofilm, water retention, protection, an energy sink, ionic exchange, sorption of organic and inorganic compounds,

nutrient source, and exchange of genetic information (21). From a clinical perspective, the EPS can act as a physical barrier to antimicrobial agents such as antibiotics and disinfectants (21, 22). The major component of the EPS matrix is water, with channels throughout the biofilm structure facilitating the inflow of nutrients and the outflow of waste materials (23, 24). Other important components of the highly hydrated EPS include extracellular polysaccharides, proteins, and DNA (eDNA, extracellular deoxyribonucleic acid), as well as other elements (5, 21) (Figure 3.1).

Extracellular polysaccharides provide a scaffold for proteins mediating adhesion of the biofilm to

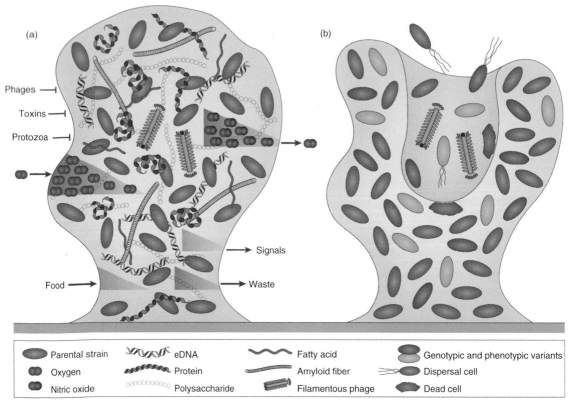

Figure 3.1 Components of biofilms. (a) Microcolonies in the mature biofilm are characterized by an extracellular polymeric substances (EPS) matrix, composed of polysaccharides, proteins, extracellular DNA (eDNA), and other elements. The EPS matrix functions as a shield to protect the bacterial community or population from predators such as protozoa or lytic phages, as well as from chemical toxins (e.g., biocides and antibiotics). The EPS matrix may help to sequester nutrients and, along with the underlying microorganisms, is also responsible for the establishment of gradients (e.g., oxygen and nutrients diffusing inward, and waste products as well as signals such as nitric oxide diffusing outward); (b) at the time of dispersal, microcolonies undergo cell death and lysis along with active dispersal of motile microorganisms to leave behind hollow colonies. (Reprinted by permission from Macmillan Publishers Ltd. from: Nature Reviews in Microbiology (McDougald D, Rice SA, Barraud N, Steinberg PD, Kjelleberg S.)

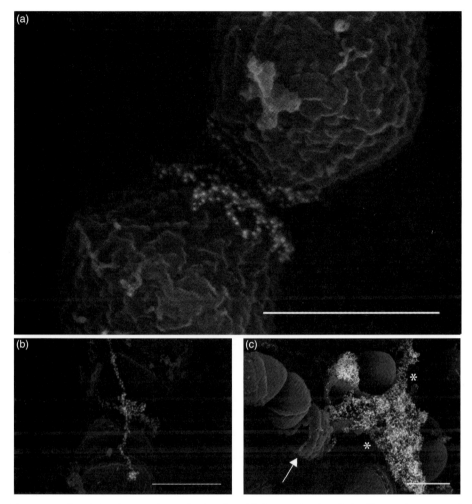

Figure 3.2   Ultrastructural analysis of eDNA during the initial establishment of *E. faecalis* biofilms. (a, b) Immuno-SEM micrographs demonstrating localization of eDNA near the septum in early (4 h) *E. faecalis* biofilms; (c) endogenous lyses of cells in an older (48 h) biofilm display an entirely different morphology from that seen in early biofilms, as DNA (asterisks) is released from a ruptured cell (arrow). Bars, 500 nm. (Barnes et al. (32). Reproduced with permission of Gary Dunny.)

the surface and intercellular attachments (22, 25). They can also contribute to antimicrobial resistance by preventing antibiotics from reaching their site of action (26) and by protecting the biofilm from the host defenses (27). Extracellular proteins supply the essential structural and enzymatic functions. For example, glucan-binding proteins produced by *Streptococcus mutans* provide a link to exopolysaccharides (28). Enzymes within the EPS matrix provide carbon and energy sources by digesting polymers (21) and degrade the EPS matrix to facilitate dispersion of microbial cells that can form new

biofilms (29). eDNA is involved in the adhesion, aggregation, cohesion, and exchange of genetic information (21, 30–32). eDNA also plays a critical role in the initial establishment of biofilms (32) (Figure 3.2).

Cell–cell communication in biofilms

Quorum sensing

The distance between microorganisms and their spatial distribution within biofilms are critical factors for intermicrobial communication processes

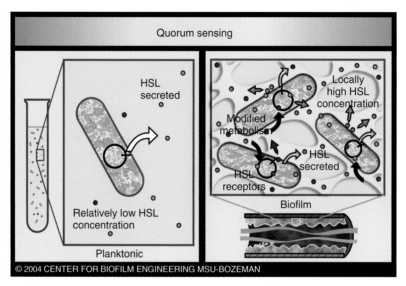

Figure 3.3 Quorum sensing in biofilm and planktonic conditions. Quorum sensing occurs when the concentration of normally low levels of certain signal molecules (e.g., homoserine lactones, or HSLs) becomes high enough to act as autoinducers (AIs) that trigger a synchronized response throughout the biofilm population. As biofilm cells are held together in dense populations, the secreted HSLs attain higher concentrations. HSL molecules then recross the cell membranes and trigger changes in genetic activity. (Reproduced with permission of the Center for Biofilm Engineering, Montana State University.)

in biofilms (1). Certain bacteria communicate and coordinate behavior via the constitutive synthesis of small signaling molecules using an intercellular signaling system called *quorum sensing* (33, 34) (Figure 3.3). Quorum sensing allows the coordinated regulation of the expression of key proteins in biofilms so that when a high density population reaches a certain threshold ("quorum"), the concentration of normally low levels of certain signal molecules becomes high enough to act as autoinducers (AIs) that trigger a synchronized response throughout the biofilm population (35, 36). AI-2 signal is used by both gram-negative and gram-positive bacteria. Gram-negative bacteria also use *N*-acyl homoserine lactone-based signaling while gram-positive bacteria utilize small peptides (33, 37–39).

Horizontal gene transfer (HGT)

Interactions between genetically distinct bacteria are involved in the establishment and maintenance of biofilms (1) and can provide an accommodating environment for the transfer of genetic material (40). Horizontal gene transfer (HGT) occurs by three basic methods: transformation, conjugation, and transduction, and allows the movement of genetic information both within and between species via plasmids, bacteriophages, and transposons (Figure 3.4).

Biofilm growth has been shown to enhance genetic exchange via transformation, as demonstrated in several streptococcal species naturally competent for transformation (42, 43). However, the most efficient HGT process in bacteria is conjugation, with the requirement for cell-to-cell contact distinguishing conjugation from transduction and transformation (Figure 3.4). The ability of plasmids to conjugatively transfer between species has been demonstrated in oral streptococci (44–46), and between *Treponema denticola* and *Streptococcus gordonii* in experimental biofilms (47). In the endodontic microflora, several enterococcal isolates recovered from patients in Sweden exhibited a characteristic response to enterococcal-derived pheromone that supported the possibility of highly efficient pheromone-induced conjugative transfer of genetic elements in RC infections (48). This premise was subsequently supported in an *ex-vivo* model through the demonstration of bidirectional transfer of a conjugative plasmid in RCs occurring between *S. gordonii* and *Enterococcus faecalis* (49)

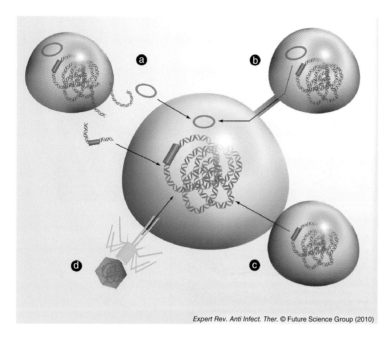

Expert Rev. Anti Infect. Ther. © Future Science Group (2010)

Figure 3.4 Horizontal gene transfer of DNA. The bacterial cells are represented by the green and purple ovals. The DNA is represented by the helix. Transposons and plasmids are either blue bars or circles. The arrows show the direction of transfer of the DNA. (a) Transformation: the donor cell (top left) has lysed and the DNA released into the environment. This can be taken up by competent bacteria and incorporated into the recipient genome; (b) conjugation of plasmids through a pilus; (c) conjugation of transposons via a mating pore; (d) transduction mediated by the injection of DNA by a bacteriophage. (Reprinted with permission from Roberts AP, Mullany P. Oral biofilms: a reservoir of transferable, bacterial, antimicrobial resistance. Expert Review of Anti-Infective Therapy 8(12):1441–1450. Expert Reviews Ltd © 2010.)

(Figure 3.5). Taken together, these findings suggest the feasibility of RC strains containing conjugative plasmids with genes that enhance survival to transfer these properties to other strains in the RC biofilm.

Responses to stress and environmental challenges

In the ever-changing biofilm environment, microbial cells encounter a multitude of stresses and challenges. These include exposure to nutrient limitation, reactive oxygen and nitrogen species, membrane damage, and elevated temperature (10). Exposure to antimicrobial agents also places biofilm communities under stress.

A diverse range of global stress responses by cells exposed to these challenges can facilitate their survival (50). For example, global response systems (GRS) such as the alternative sigma factors RpoS (51) and RpoH (52), gene repressor LexA (53), and small molecule effectors, such as (p)ppGpp that induce the stringent response (54), act by modulating intracellular metabolic processes to enable adaptation and survival. Resultant stress responses include downregulation of error-correcting enzymes, upregulation of error-prone DNA polymerases, and HGT of mobile genetic elements (55, 56). Two-component toxin–antitoxin (TA) systems are also involved in the responses to stress stimuli; the toxins are stable proteins directed against specific intracellular targets, and the antitoxins are degradable proteins or small RNAs that neutralize the toxin or inhibit toxin synthesis (57). TA systems are involved in persister cell formation (58) and quorum sensing (59) and may regulate the switch from planktonic to biofilm lifestyles (60).

As a direct consequence of stresses and the resulting responses, the availability of nutrients and electron acceptors can vary considerably throughout the biofilm, and the growth stage of microbial cells can range from rapidly growing to dormant. This results in variations in metabolic activity, gene expression patterns, and potential phenotypic variations throughout the biofilm community (7). Cells might adapt by turning certain genes on or off or by random gene switching, and fitter mutants might arise as part of a natural selection process (Figure 3.6).

Responses to antimicrobials in biofilms

Microorganisms in biofilm communities have several options available to resist the detrimental

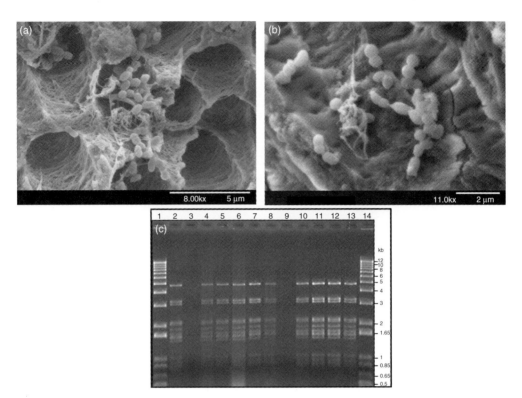

Figure 3.5 Horizontal gene transfer (HGT) in the root canal. Scanning electron micrographs showing accumulations of *E. faecalis* JH2-2/pAM81 and *S. gordonii* Challis-Sm (a) 24 h and (b) 72 h after inoculation into the root canal. Bidirectional HGT of the plasmid pAM81 was confirmed by the purification of the plasmid in transconjugants; (c) confirmation of conjugative transfer of pAM81 from *E. faecalis* to *S. gordonii* (lanes 2–7) and from *S. gordonii* to *E. faecalis* (lanes 8–13): pAM81 plasmid DNA digested with *Hind*III in donor strains (lanes 2 and 8) that were transferred to plasmid-free recipient strains (lanes 3 and 9) that resulted in transconjugant strains with pAM81 (lanes 4–7 and 10–13). Lanes 1 and 14 show molecular size marker. (Reprinted from Journal of Endodontics, 34(5), Sedgley CM, Lee EM, Martin MJ, Flannagan SE. Antibiotic resistance gene transfer between *Streptococcus gordonii* and *Enterococcus faecalis* in root canals of teeth *ex-vivo*, 570–574 © 2008, with permission from Elsevier.)

effects of antimicrobial therapy (4, 61, 62) (Figure 3.7). For example, the thickness of the biofilm, as well as the concentration and ability of the antimicrobial to penetrate the EPS matrix, can determine the extent of exposure of cells in biofilms. Thus, while the superficial cells of the biofilm community are rapidly exposed to high concentrations of antimicrobials, exposure of deeper parts depends on the ability of the antimicrobial to diffuse through the biofilm matrix (61). The EPS matrix can slow down the diffusion of the agent (63) but does not necessarily prevent diffusion (64). Multidrug resistance efflux pumps are also considered to contribute to antibiotic resistance in biofilms (65–67).

Oxygen levels and metabolic rates are reduced at the center of a microcolony compared with near its surface (68, 69). This can result in localized limited or absent metabolic activity of microbial cells deeper in the biofilm as well as induce cells to enter stationary phase and thus lose susceptibility to killing by antibiotics that target dividing cells (70). Persister cells have been associated with recalcitrant biofilm infections (9, 71). Persister cells are phenotypic variants that are genetically identical to the susceptible cells within a clonal population (72, 73). On exposure of the biofilm to antibiotics, persister cells demonstrate very slow or arrested growth ("dormancy") and diminished protein synthesis (9, 74). Following the treatment of biofilms with antibiotics such as β-lactams, the rapidly growing cells are killed, leaving the dormant cells to repopulate the biofilm. The formation of persister cells is thought to be through a combination of continuously occurring random events

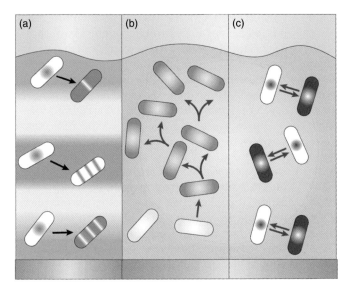

Figure 3.6   Multiplicity of phenotypic states in biofilms. Three hypothesized mechanisms of phenotypic diversification in a biofilm. (a) Physiological adaptation. Cells respond adaptively to local environmental conditions by turning on or off certain genes; the responses depend on the local chemical microenvironment and, therefore, allow for a range of distinct localized adaptations; (b) genotypic variation and natural selection. A mutation or chromosomal rearrangement results in a variant (purple) that multiplies according to its fitness in the biofilm; (c) stochastic gene switching. Cells toggle between discrete physiological states by gene switching, which is random in nature. (Reprinted by permission from Macmillan Publishers Ltd from: Nature Reviews (Stewart PS, Franklin MJ. Physiological heterogeneity in biofilms. Nat Rev Microbiol 6(3):199–210) © 2008.)

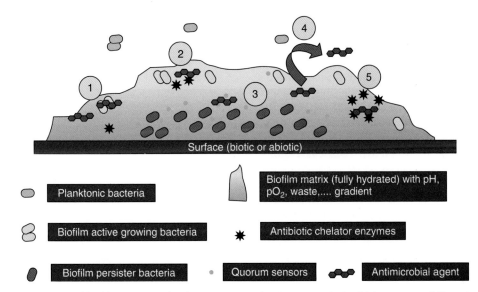

Figure 3.7   Some proposed biofilms associated with resistance mechanisms: (1) antimicrobial agents may fail to penetrate beyond the surface layers of the biofilm. Outer layers of biofilm cells absorb damage. Antimicrobial agents' action may be impaired in areas of waste accumulation or altered environment (pH, pCO_2, pO_2, etc.); (2) antimicrobial agents may be trapped and destroyed by enzymes in the biofilm matrix; (3) altered growth rate inside the biofilm. Antimicrobial agents may not be active against nongrowing microorganisms (persister cells); (4) expression of biofilm-specific resistance genes (e.g., efflux pumps); (5) stress response to hostile environmental conditions (e.g., leading to an overexpression of antimicrobial agent-destroying enzymes). (Reprinted by permission from Macmillan Publishers Ltd: Clinical Pharmacology and Therapeutics (del Pozo JL, Patel R. The challenge of treating biofilm-associated bacterial infections. Clin Pharmacol Ther. 2007 82(2):204–209) © 2007.)

("stochastic"), or in response to an environmental stimulus ("deterministic") (9, 75).

Resistance to antimicrobial treatment is significantly higher in multispecies biofilms compared to single-species biofilms (76–78). Dual-species biofilms of *S. mutans* and *Veillonella parvula* were less susceptible to various antimicrobial agents (chlorhexidine, cetylpyrimidinium chloride, zinc chloride, erythromycin, hydrogen peroxide, and amine chloride) than single-species biofilms of the same microorganisms (76, 79). This may be attributable to the cooperative behavior of the community that enables survival on exposure to the antimicrobial agent (80), and potential advantages to be gained by residing in multispecies biofilms (77).

Root canal biofilms

Evaluation of root canal biofilms

The anatomy of the RC system is intricate and complex. In addition to the main canal(s), there can be lateral canals, accessory canals, apical ramifications, and isthmuses (81). All anatomical areas of the infected RC system have been shown to harbor bacterial cells organized as archetypal biofilm structures (82, 83). In 1987, Nair (15) described infected RCs containing clusters of "self-aggregating" colonies of one distinct type or "coaggregating" communities of several types that would now be described as biofilm structures. Since then, observations of RC biofilms in infected extracted teeth have utilized light microscopy (15, 17, 20, 82, 84), scanning electron microscopy (SEM) (85, 86), environmental SEM (87), transmission electron microscopy (TEM) (18, 88), confocal laser scanning microscopy (CLSM) and fluorescent *in situ* hybridization (FISH) (89), and various combinations of techniques (19, 90) (Figure 3.8). Collectively, these observational studies have shown that RC biofilms are highly variable.

Much effort has gone into the identification of the microbial component of clinical RC infections. Genera cultured from symptomatic and asymptomatic RC infections and aspirates from apical abscesses include *Prevotella*, *Porphyromonas*, *Fusobacterium*, *Peptostreptococcus*, *Streptococcus*, *Lactobacillus*, *Enterococcus*, *Actinomyces*, *Propriobacterium*, and *Candida* (12, 13, 91, 92). Compared to culture methods, molecular analyses of RC samples have shown a substantially more diverse microflora that is composed of a large proportion of unidentifiable and unculturable species (93, 94). Recent analyses using pyrosequencing methods have revealed an even greater microbial diversity (95–98) (Figure 3.9).

The recovery and analyses of the EPS matrix component of RC biofilms during clinical procedures are yet to be described. Considerable challenges exist in obtaining intact RC biofilm samples in a nondestructive manner. From a practical aspect, it is likely that paper points absorb planktonic microorganisms disrupted from the biofilm surface but are less likely to retrieve microorganisms located in the deeper parts of the biofilm or within the dentinal tubules. Similarly, file shavings are also unlikely to provide samples of "intact" RC biofilms. Sampling previously treated RCs poses further obstacles, particularly if the prior restoration and root filling material are difficult to remove.

Primary root canal infections

Many studies have confirmed that infected RCs harbor a multispecies population of facultative and strict anaerobic gram-positive and gram-negative bacteria, spirochetes, yeasts, archaea, and other unidentified species (95–103). In addition, Epstein–Barr virus may be associated with irreversible pulpitis and apical periodontitis (104), and papilloma virus and human herpes virus have been found in exudates from acute apical abscesses (AAAs) (105).

The microflora of carious dentin implicated in endodontic infections subsequent to pulpitis includes significant numbers of lactobacilli (106) and gram-negative bacteria (107). Both innate and adaptive immune responses modulate the relationship between tissue damage and the microflora in advancing caries (108). Many microorganisms cultured from endodontic infections have also been identified as commensals in the oral cavity. The transition from oral "commensal" to RC "pathogen" may reflect an innate ability to switch on genes that encode virulence factors (Figure 3.10) as well as other factors enabling survival and propagation in a different environment.

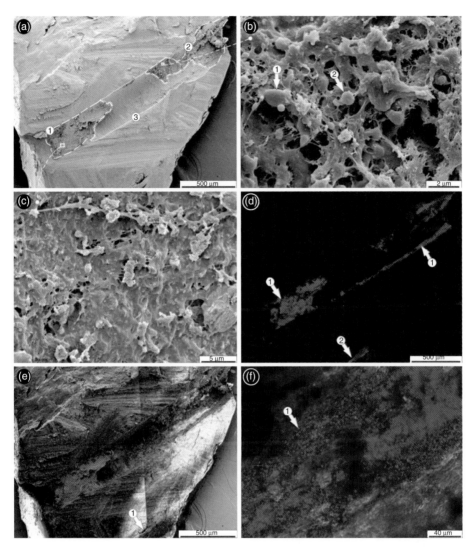

Figure 3.8 Imaging of endodontic biofilms by combined microscopy (FISH/CLSM–SEM). (a) Overview of split root canal. Certain parts of the canal surface were covered with a thick matrix layer (encircled areas 1, 2) whereas other regions showed only sparse and comparatively thin islands of matrix (encircled area 3); (b) the size and shape of some structures of the matrix suggested the presence of bacteria (arrows 1, 2), but without conclusive evidence; (c) other areas of the matrix consisted of so densely composed material that no traces of bacterial presence could be found; (d) After labeling the split tooth with the EUB338 (Cy3) probe, distinct parts of the canal showed a strong red fluorescence signal in the CLSM (arrows 1 and 2); (e) overlay of corresponding SEM and FISH/CLSM (a and d) images of the same regions revealed matching areas of the FISH signal and the amorphous matrix, suggesting the presence of bacterial biofilm. The laterally located FISH signal was within a lateral canal in the root (arrow 1); (f) higher magnifications of FISH-labeled root canal surface with CLSM indicated a biofilm composed of bacteria with short rod or coccus-like morphology (arrow 1). (Reprinted by permission from John Wiley and Sons from Schaudinn C, Carr G, Gorur A, Jaramillo D, Costerton JW, Webster P. Imaging of endodontic biofilms by combined microscopy (FISH/cLSM - SEM). Journal of Microscopy 235(2):124–127 © 2009.)

Bridging, or coaggregation, between two or more bacterial species is an important process in multispecies biofilm formation (1). In dental plaque, *Fusobacterium nucleatum* is considered to be a strategic microorganism as evidenced by its ability to coaggregate with numerous other species and mediate adherence of early and late colonizers (110). Similarly, in infected RCs, the commonly

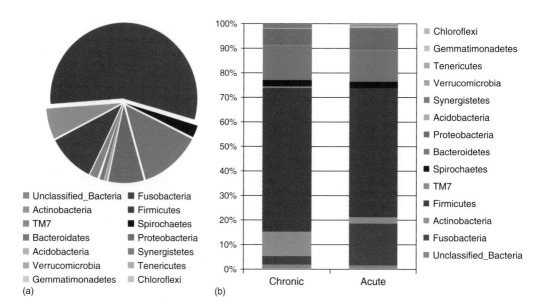

Figure 3.9 Relative abundance of different bacterial phyla in acute and chronic dental root canal infections. (a) Overall data; (b) data according to the clinical condition. Phylogenetic classification was based on Ribosomal Database Project Classifier analyses. (Santos *et al*. (98). Reproduced from PLoS ONE 6(11): e28088. doi:10.1371/journal.pone.0028088.)

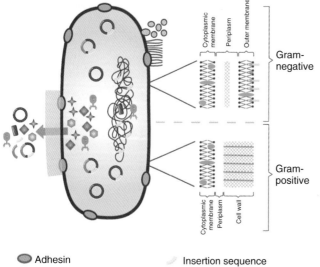

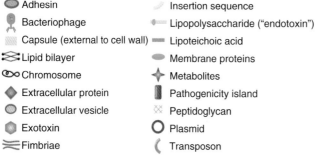

Figure 3.10 Virulence factors and associated genetic elements in bacteria. (From Sedgley CM. Virulence of endodontic bacterial pathogens. Chapter 7;130-51. Endodontic Microbiology. Editor, Fouad AF. Wiley-Blackwell Publishing, Ames, IA. This material is reproduced with permission of John Wiley & Sons, Inc. © 2009.)

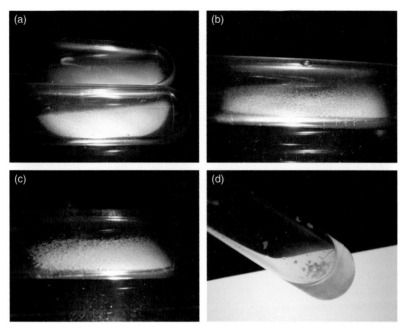

Figure 3.11 Coaggregation assay scoring. (a) Upper tube: "0" no change in turbidity and no evidence of coaggregates in the mixed suspensions; lower tube: "+1" turbid supernatant with finely dispersed coaggregates that did not precipitate immediately; (b) "+2" definite coaggregates easily seen but suspension remained turbid without immediate settling of coaggregates; (c) "+3" slightly turbid supernatant with formation of large precipitating coaggregates; (d) "+4" clear supernatant and large coaggregates that precipitated immediately. (Reprinted from Journal of Endodontics, 32(10), Johnson EM, Flannagan SE, Sedgley CM, Coaggregation interactions between oral and endodontic *Enterococcus faecalis* and bacterial species isolated from persistent apical periodontitis, 946–950, © 2006, with permission from Elsevier.)

recovered *Fusobacterium* species appears to participate in synergistic interactions in RC infections (111). *F. nucleatum* exhibits strong associations with *Peptostreptococcus micros*, *Porphyromonas endodontalis*, and *Campylobacter rectus* (112, 113) and has been shown to enhance the pathogenicity of *Porphyromonas gingivalis* in mouse models (114). In addition, coaggregation assays have shown that fusobacteria form coaggregates with many species including *Prevotella*, *Streptococcus* (115), *E. faecalis*, *Streptococcus anginosus*, *Peptostreptococcus anaerobius*, and *Prevotella oralis* (116) (Figure 3.11). Other positive associations shown to occur in RC strains are between *Prevotella intermedia* and *P. micros*, and between *P. anaerobius* and *Eubacteria* and *P. anaerobius* (113). In addition, in guinea pigs, *Parvimonas micra* enhanced the pathogenicity of *Bacteroides melaninogenicus* (*Prevotella melaninogenica*) and *Bacteroides asaccharolyticus* (*Porphyromonas* spp.) (117).

In contrast to synergistic relationships, interactions between different species and strains of the same species can be antagonistic. For example, some microorganisms produce antimicrobial proteins or peptides collectively termed *bacteriocins* that can be bacteriostatic or bactericidal to other members of the same species (narrow spectrum) or across genera (broad spectrum). Nonvirulent bacteriocin-producing strains have useful applications in the food industry and as probiotics (118). Bacteriocin production is not uncommon in enterococcal strains recovered from endodontic infections (48, 119). However, although the role of bacteriocins in RC biofilms is not known, it is feasible that by changing the composition of the microflora, the production of bacteriocins could modulate the infectious process. This was highlighted by the analysis of the strain *E. faecalis* MC4, originally recovered from an autogenously infected RC of a *Macaca fascicularis* monkey with apical periodontitis (120) and used as part of strain collections in seminal endodontic microbiology studies in monkeys (120–124). In those studies, *E. faecalis* MC4 survived in RCs for at least 2.5 years both as a single species and in combination with other species of an "eight strain collection," and was shown in bacteriologic, radiographic, and histological studies to induce pulpal and apical pathogenesis (inducing the least immune effect when inoculated as a single species). Dahlen and colleagues (119) reported that *E. faecalis* MC4 inhibited other members of the eight strain collections to various degrees. More recent work has shown that the inhibitory activity by *E. faecalis* MC4 is associated with a Class IIa bacteriocin encoded by a pheromone-responsive, multiantibiotic resistance plasmid (125, 126).

In the oral environment, saliva flow impacts the development of biofilms on oral surfaces. However, the RC environment is neither subject to fluid flow nor necessarily fluid-filled. It has been hypothesized that during the initial phase of infection, exudate derived from the inflammatory lesion front may provide the fluid phase during the development of the RC biofilm (16). As such, in those cases where the biofilm is invading vital pulp tissue, nutrients would be available. In contrast, nutrient deprivation would be more likely to occur in RCs containing necrotic pulp tissue and in previously treated RCs. Many microorganisms manage to survive these challenging environments by prompting a starvation response whereby bacteria adjust their metabolic balance away from multiplication and toward the acquisition of energy for survival (127). Therefore, the adoption of a nongrowing state is an important mechanism for survival in the nutrient-deprived milieu of the RC.

As the biofilm progresses apically, it encounters the host's complex and intricately coordinated immune system. Polymorphs attempt to wall off the bacterial biofilm from the remaining canal lumen (128), as can be seen in Figure 3.12 (90). However, *in-vitro* studies have confirmed that biofilms can eventually overwhelm the invading neutrophils (129) and reduce host defense responses as evidenced by a reduced cytokine release from macrophages exposed to *E. faecalis* in biofilm compared to planktonic conditions (130).

Several studies have reported that there are a larger number of species (99) and more diversity (98) in acute compared to chronic infections (Figure 3.9). For example, black-pigmented gram-negative anaerobic bacteria such as *P. endodontalis* and *P. gingivalis* have been associated with symptomatic-infected RCs and endodontic

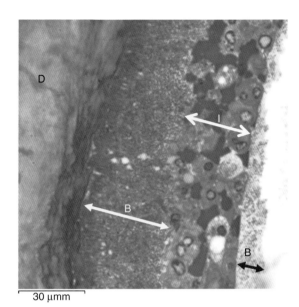

Figure 3.12   Light microscopic view of apical section showing bacterial biofilm (B) adherent to the canal surface dentin (D) and walled in by polymorphonuclear leukocytes and red blood cells (I) beyond which is a further biofilm (1 bar represents 30 μm). (Richardson *et al.* (90). Reproduced with permission of John Wiley and Sons, Inc.)

abscesses (131–134). Molecular fingerprinting of 20 paired samples of RC and AAA exudates showed that, although the mean number of species and the diversity index did not differ, very few species were shared between RC and AAA samples, and microbial communities diverged between subjects (135) (Figure 3.13). Cluster analysis of the same clinical material showed that anaerobic species were distributed in small, complex, and distinctive communities in both RC infections and AAAs, indicating that several microbial profiles can be associated with the development of acute endodontic infections (103).

A classic study on infected RCs in monkeys showed that the microflora was more anaerobic in the apical compared to the coronal part of the canal (122). This is supported by a recent study that used pyrosequencing methods to compare the microbial ecology of the coronal and apical segments of infected RC systems of 23 extracted teeth with apical periodontitis (96) (Figure 3.14). The apical segment harbored more taxa overall and more fastidious obligate anaerobes, leading the authors to conclude that the apical part of the RC

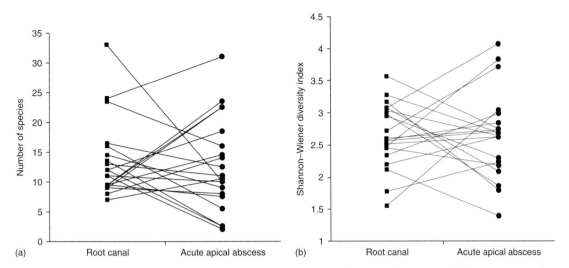

(a)   Root canal   Acute apical abscess   (b)   Root canal   Acute apical abscess

Figure 3.13   Microbial profiles associated with 20 paired samples of root canals (RC) and acute apical abscess (AAA) exudates. (a) Associations between RC and AAA samples in the number of species; (b) diversity index. Pairs of samples are connected by matching lines. (Reprinted from Journal of Endodontics, 36(9), Montagner F, Gomes BP, Kumar PS. Molecular fingerprinting reveals the presence of unique communities associated with paired samples of root canals and acute apical abscesses, 1475–1479 © 2010, with permission from Elsevier.)

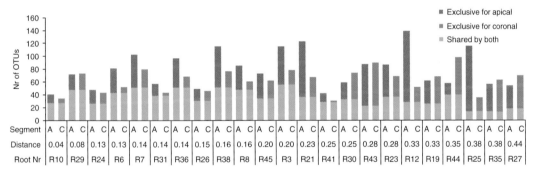

Figure 3.14   Prevalence of exclusive and shared operational taxonomic units (OTUs) (sequences that cluster within 97% similarity level) by the two root segments of 23 root pairs. Only those OTUs that contained at least 10 reads/sample were counted as present in the corresponding sample. The order of the samples (root numbers) from left to right corresponds to the increasing difference in phylogenetic distance (Weighted Unifrac) between the corresponding apical and coronal segments. The distances are shown above the respective root numbers. The two segments from R10 were highly similar (distance = 0.04), while those from R27 differed the most (distance = 0.44) among the corresponding pairs of samples. (Ozok *et al.* (96). Reproduced with permission of John Wiley & Sons, Inc.)

system drives the selection of a more diverse and more anaerobic community than the coronal part.

Persistent and secondary root canal infections

RC treatment aims to eliminate necrotic pulp tissue and bacterial biofilm from the RC system. However, several obstacles to optimal RC disinfection can exist, resulting in persistent infections, or infections arising from the original microflora that have survived RC treatment (84, 136). These obstacles include the anatomical complexities of the RC system (20, 82), the buffering effects of dentin (137), and the physical barrier to antimicrobials provided by the EPS matrix. As a consequence, some species survive endodontic treatment procedures

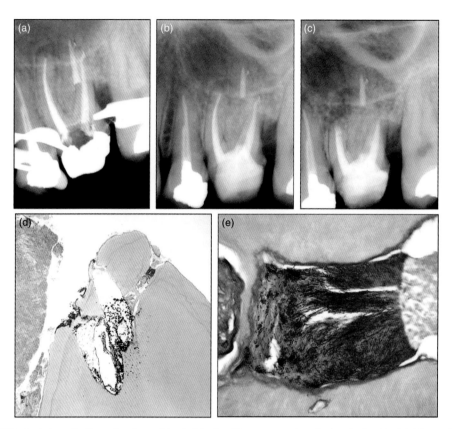

Figure 3.15 Histologic investigation of root-canal-treated teeth with symptomatic apical periodontitis. (a) After endodontic retreatment of tooth 14; (b) follow-up radiograph taken after 1 year. Radiolucency was unchanged. Sinus tract was still present, and the tooth was tender to percussion and palpation; (c) root-end resection was performed of both mesiobuccal and distobuccal roots; (d) overview of the mesiobuccal root tip; (e) magnification of the ramification on the right side in (d). Its lumen is filled with a large biofilm arranged against inflammatory cells (Reprinted from Journal of Endodontics, 35(4), Ricucci D, Siqueira JF, Jr., Bate AL, Pitt Ford TR, Histologic investigation of root canal-treated teeth with apical periodontitis: a retrospective study from twenty-four patients, 493–502, © 2009, with permission from Elsevier.)

(138–143) and persistent infection can ensue (17, 144). As distinct from persistent infections, secondary RC infections are initiated by microorganisms introduced into the RC by disruption in asepsis during treatment, or via coronal leakage and exposure of previously treated RCs to the oral cavity (84, 136).

The primary cause of endodontic treatment failure has been attributed to intraradicular infections, usually in the form of biofilms (145) (Figure 3.15). Ricucci and Siqueira (20) observed biofilms in the apical segment of 31 of 42 previously treated teeth with posttreatment apical periodontitis. They reported that bacteria immediately adjacent to the exit of ramifications were associated with

inflammation of the periodontal ligament. The authors concluded that bacteria present in the apical portion of the RC, apical deltas, and lateral canals have the potential to sustain longstanding infections (20). Those bacteria that survive need to be able to resist periods of starvation and withstand possible disruption of the EPS matrix. If communication with the apical tissues is present, the biofilm is likely to have access to a source of nutrients that facilitates growth and a subsequent host response that sustains or exacerbates apical inflammation and avoids healing (124). Bacterial products from persistent and secondary RC infections diffusing into the apical tissues through RC ramifications and exposed dentinal tubules will induce an inflammatory response with consequent release of cytokines that activate bone resorption mechanisms (146–148).

The composition of the microflora associated with persistent and secondary endodontic infections is significantly different from that associated with primary infections. The most prevalent microorganisms detected include *Enterococcus* (138, 139, 142, 149) and *Streptococcus* species (150), as well as *Lactobacillus* (143), *Actinomyces* (149, 151–153), and *Peptostreptococcus* species (113), *Candida* (154), *Eubacterium alactolyticus* (113), *Propionibacterium propionicum* (155), *Dialister pneumosintes*, and *Filifactor alocis* (94). Studies that use pyrosequencing techniques to evaluate the flora associated with persistent and secondary infections are likely to report a higher diversity than that reported so far.

Bacterial survival after RC treatment might depend in part on how good an adaptor the organism is to the new limiting factors in their niches. For example, *E. faecalis*, a gastrointestinal tract commensal organism commonly recovered from previously treated RCs (138, 156) is an opportunist species that can tolerate adverse environmental conditions, including low nutrient concentrations, high salinity, and high pH (157). *E. faecalis* can survive for extended periods in treated RCs *ex-vivo* (158) (Figure 3.16) and recover from starvation conditions (159). Subramanian and Mickel (160) suggested that *E. faecalis* might contribute to persistent apical infections both by biofilm formation as well as soft-tissue adhesion and invasion. A recent study has shown that both *E. faecalis* biofilm cells and their planktonic counterparts are phagocytosed efficiently by immune cells such as macrophages and dendritic cells; however, once inside the phagocyte, biofilm cells survive better, and proinflammatory cytokines secretion by the host phagocytes is less than that evoked by internalized planktonic cells (161).

The predominance of gram-positive bacteria in persistent endodontic infections has been attributed to their greater resistance to antimicrobials and ability to adapt to harsh environmental conditions. However, it is important to note that the gram-positive *E. faecalis* is by no means the only species recovered from these RC infections (94, 162), nor is there compelling evidence that it is the single causative agent for the failure of endodontic treatment. For example, *E. faecalis* MC4 did not induce a strong apical immune response when left in monkeys' RCs as a single species for 6 months; however, when the strain was inoculated as a mixed species (with *Actinomyces bovis* and *Bacteroides oralis*), more hard tissue resorption and inflammation was seen (121).

Extraradicular biofilms

Several reports have described the presence of extraradicular biofilm in cases of longstanding lesions and persistent RC infections (85, 163–168). Deposition of calculus on the root apex has also been observed in cases with persistent infections with sinus tracts (20, 169, 170); an example is shown in (Figure 3.17).

It is generally accepted that *Actinomyces* species and *P. propionicum* are involved in longstanding apical lesions refractory to endodontic treatment because of their ability to evade the host response, survive in the apical tissues, and prevent apical healing (171–173). In these cases, surgical management that includes apicoectomy and removal of the infected tissue provides a successful outcome (167, 174). Signoretti *et al.* (167) described a case of a lower left first molar that presented with persistent apical infection and sinus tract following retreatment. Bacterial biofilm surrounding the apical foramen and external radicular surface of the resected root was visualized by SEM, and the following species were cultured: *Actinomyces naeslundii*, *Actinomyces meyeri*, *P. propionicum*, *Clostridium botulinum*, *P. micra*, and *Bacteroides ureolyticus* (Figure 3.18).

In contradistinction, extraradicular biofilm infections are not commonly associated with asymptomatic teeth with apical periodontitis (20). In a sample of biopsy specimens from 64 untreated and 42 treated roots of teeth with apical periodontitis, extraradicular biofilms were observed in only 6 out of 100 specimens, all of which were from symptomatic teeth, 3 associated with sinus tracts, and all but one associated with intracanal bacteria (20). The authors concluded that extraradicular biofilm are dependent on intraradicular infections and more likely to be associated with clinically symptomatic teeth.

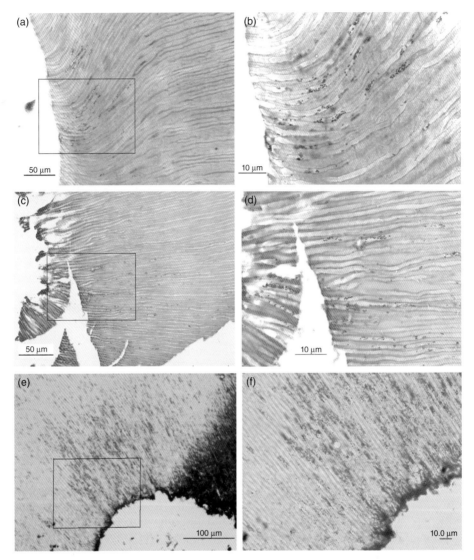

Figure 3.16   Infection of dentinal tubules by *E. faecalis* OG1-S after 48 h incubation (a and inset in b), and after root canal filling followed by 12 months (c and inset in d) and 24 months (e and inset in f) incubation. Brown and Brenn stain. (Sedgley *et al.* (158). Reproduced with permission of John Wiley and Sons, Inc.)

In-vitro models to study root canal biofilms

Several *in-vitro* models have been used to study biofilms of relevance to RC treatment. These studies typically focus on the efficacy of antimicrobial agents against single- or multispecies biofilms. The simplest models have utilized biofilms grown on the surfaces of microtiter plate wells (175, 176) (Figure 3.19) or polystyrene pegs

[minimal biofilm eradication concentration assay (MBEC, Innovotech, Edmonton, Canada)] (177). A major advantage of these simple models is the ability to screen a large number of samples easily and control multiple experimental conditions such as initial inoculum, temperature, and concentration of antimicrobial agents. However, they are "closed" systems, and unless the growth media is regularly replaced, the absence of flow into or out of the wells results in nutrient depletion and other

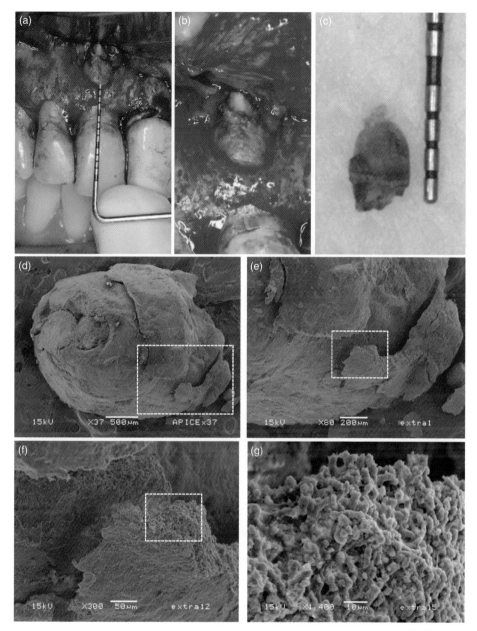

Figure 3.17 Calculus formation on apical root surface of tooth #9 that presented with persistent infection and sinus tract: (a and b) after flap reflection; (c) resected root tip showing calculus; (d) SEM showing root tip (×37); (e) inset of (d) focusing on calculus-like material (×80); (f) inset of (e) (×300); (g) inset of (f) (×1400). (Courtesy Dr. Fernanda GC Signoretti.)

environmental changes such as variations in pH and redox potential.

Flow displacement biofilm devices can in part overcome these limitations by being "open" systems that allow both the flow of nutrients and the removal of waste products. Examples include continuous-flow-stirred tank reactors where a steady state is created by the feed rate being equivalent to the effluent removal rate (e.g., the CDC biofilm reactor), and the plug flow reactor

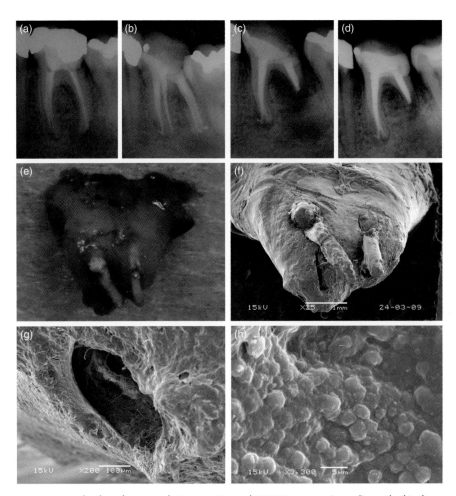

Figure 3.18 Persistent extraradicular infection and sinus tract in tooth 36: (a) preoperative radiograph; (b) after nonsurgical retreatment; (c) postoperative after distal root resection; (d) 24-month recall showing apical healing; (e) resected root; (f) SEM showing extruded gutta-percha (×25); (g) uninstrumented apical foramen (×200); (h) bacterial colonies adhering to external radicular surface (×3300). (Adapted from Journal of Endodontics, 37(12), Signoretti FG, Endo MS, Gomes BP, Montagner F, Tosello FB, Jacinto RC (2011) Persistent extraradicular infection in root-filled asymptomatic human tooth: scanning electron microscopic analysis and microbial investigation after apical microsurgery, 1696–700 © 2011, with permission from Elsevier.)

(PFR) that utilizes unidirectional flow and mixing by diffusion (e.g., the modified Robbins device) (178). There are variations of these open system devices that make them well suited to endodontic biofilm research, an example being flow cells that are a small-scale variation of the PFR (179, 180). Their major advantage is access to real-time, nondestructive microscopic observation, and analyses of biofilms. However, only a low number of biofilms can be observed at any one time. Recently developed microfluidic devices that integrate low-flow-rate channels with multiwell titer plates have the potential to overcome this limitation (181).

In addition to polystyrene, other growth surfaces used in endodontic biofilm investigations include dentin (182), nitrocellulose membranes placed onto agar (183), hydroxyapatite discs (184), and enamel slabs on dental splints (185). The obvious advantage of growing biofilms on dentin is of clinical relevance. However, variations in size, shape, and number of dentinal tubules can occur both between and within teeth, suggesting it might be important

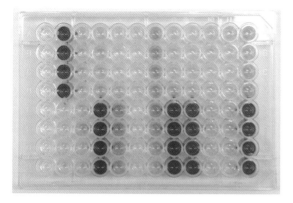

Figure 3.19 Biofilms grown on the surfaces of microtiter plate wells. Representative microtiter plate with 24-h *E faecalis biofilms* after resolubilization of crystal violet used to stain fixed biofilms. More intense coloration represents thicker biofilm formation. The five sets of more intensely stained quadruplicate samples are classified as "moderate" biofilm formers based on OD570 readings. The left column of eight wells are negative controls where no biofilms were detected. (Reprinted from Journal of Endodontics, 33(7), Duggan JM, Sedgley CM, Biofilm formation of oral and endodontic *Enterococcus faecalis*, 815–818 © 2007, with permission from Elsevier.)

less than plaque samples that may differ substantially both between and within subjects (196).

The viability of microbial cells in biofilms has been measured by microbial recovery assays (192, 194, 197) and by evaluating metabolic activity (respiratory activity and mRNA synthesis) and cellular integrity (membrane potential and integrity) (17, 127). Although more technically challenging, methods utilizing CLSM and fluorescent stains have the advantage of providing three-dimensional analyses of viable and nonviable cells in biofilms. Regardless of the *in-vitro* method used, because biofilms are highly heterogeneous and form over multiple stages, standardized and clearly described experimental techniques are essential for meaningful comparisons between studies. Clearly, it is not surprising that the selection of the model system can have a profound influence on the results (198) and therefore should ideally simulate the infected RC environment as closely as possible.

Conclusions

The biofilm structure represents a successful strategy for bacteria to adapt to the RC environment and resist endodontic treatment. From a microbial perspective, biofilm formation is likely to facilitate survival in unfavorable environmental conditions such as the deprived nutritional conditions found in the necrotic or previously treated RC system and under harsh conditions imposed by RC treatment procedures. Although many key mechanisms remain to be elucidated, it is obvious that RC infections are highly heterogeneous and adaptable biofilm communities under the influence of variable local environmental selective pressures, synergistic and antagonistic microbial cell–cell interactions, and a diverse range of host defense responses.

In view of their heterogeneity there are considerable challenges in the development of clinically relevant biofilm models that realistically mimic the RC environment. However, although further work is needed to fully understand antimicrobial resistance in biofilms, the accumulative effects of various processes, rather than their individual involvement, are likely to contribute to increased resistance in biofilm communities.

Finally, although the susceptibility of the host plays a critical role in host–pathogen interactions

to consider these variables when planning *in-vitro* investigations. In addition, biofilm formation on young and old RC dentin may vary (186, 187); "young" teeth (from 18 to 25-year-old patients) had higher numbers of dentinal tubules invaded by bacteria, with deeper invasion, compared with "old" teeth (from patients older than 59 years) (187).

The majority of *in-vitro* investigations has used single-species, or, less commonly, multispecies, biofilms grown on root dentin of extracted human (182, 186, 188–191) or bovine (192–194) teeth. Single-species *E. faecalis* biofilms are commonly utilized for the evaluation of antimicrobial activity of endodontic materials, in part because of its frequent recovery from previously treated RCs (138, 156). A major advantage of *E. faecalis* is its ease of handling relative to obligate anaerobes. However, it is important to recognize that endodontic infections are polymicrobial, and species in addition to *E. faecalis* are routinely recovered from teeth that are re-treated (94). The development of multispecies biofilm models may address this issue (194, 195), although they are likely to present additional challenges in terms of reproducibility, but arguably

(199), recent reports of host resistance and tolerance being complementary defense strategies (200) raise intriguing questions regarding the role of host tolerance in the outcome of RC treatment in the presence of biofilms. It is clear that much remains to be learned about the critical conditions created by the ability of biofilm cells to persist and evade host defense strategies in the RC environment.

References

1. Kolenbrander, P.E., Palmer, R.J. Jr., Periasamy, S. & Jakubovics, N.S. (2010) Oral multispecies biofilm development and the key role of cell–cell distance. *Nature Reviews Microbiology*, **8 (7)**, 471–480.
2. Hall-Stoodley, L., Costerton, J.W. & Stoodley, P. (2004) Bacterial biofilms: from the natural environment to infectious diseases. *Nature Reviews Microbiology*, **2 (2)**, 95–108.
3. Westalla, F., Maarten, J., Dannb, J., van der Gaastc, S., de Ronded, C. & Gernekee, D. (2001) Early Archean fossil bacteria and biofilms in hydrothermally-influenced sediments from the Barberton greenstone belt, South Africa. *Precambrian Research*, **106 (1–2)**, 93–116.
4. Costerton, J.W., Stewart, P.S. & Greenberg, E.P. (1999) Bacterial biofilms: a common cause of persistent infections. *Science*, **284 (5418)**, 1318–1322.
5. McDougald, D., Rice, S.A., Barraud, N., Steinberg, P.D. & Kjelleberg, S. (2012) Should we stay or should we go: mechanisms and ecological consequences for biofilm dispersal. *Nature Reviews Microbiology*, **10 (1)**, 39–50.
6. Fux, C.A., Costerton, J.W., Stewart, P.S. & Stoodley, P. (2005) Survival strategies of infectious biofilms. *Trends in Microbiology*, **13 (1)**, 34–40.
7. Stewart, P.S. & Franklin, M.J. (2008) Physiological heterogeneity in biofilms. *Nature Reviews Microbiology*, **6 (3)**, 199–210.
8. Hoiby, N., Bjarnsholt, T., Givskov, M., Molin, S. & Ciofu, O. (2010) Antibiotic resistance of bacterial biofilms. *International Journal of Antimicrobial Agents*, **35 (4)**, 322–332.
9. Lewis, K. (2010) Persister cells. *Annual Review of Microbiology*, **64**, 357–372.
10. Poole, K. (2012) Bacterial stress responses as determinants of antimicrobial resistance. *The Journal of Antimicrobial Chemotherapy*, **67**, 2069–2089.
11. Kakehashi, S., Stanley, H.R. & Fitzgerald, R.J. (1965) The effects of surgical exposures of dental pulps in germ-free and conventional laboratory rats. *Oral Surgery, Oral Medicine, and Oral Pathology*, **20**, 340–349.
12. Moller, A. (1966) Microbial examination of root canals and periapical tissues of human teeth. *Odontologisk Tidskrift*, **74**, 1–380.
13. Sundqvist, G. (1976) Bacteriological studies of necrotic dental pulps. Dissertation, University of Umea, Umea, Sweden.
14. Moller, A.J., Fabricius, L., Dahlen, G., Ohman, A.E. & Heyden, G. (1981) Influence on periapical tissues of indigenous oral bacteria and necrotic pulp tissue in monkeys. *Scandinavian Journal of Dental Research*, **89 (6)**, 475–484.
15. Nair, P.N.R. (1987) Light and electron microscopic studies of root canal flora and periapical lesions. *Journal of Endodontics*, **13 (1)**, 29–39.
16. Svensater, G. & Bergenholtz, G. (2004) Biofilms in endodontic infections. *Endodontic Topics*, **9**, 27–36.
17. Chavez de Paz, L.C. (2007) Redefining the persistent infection in root canals: possible role of biofilm communities. *Journal of Endodontics*, **33 (6)**, 652–662.
18. Carr, G.B., Schwartz, R.S., Schaudinn, C., Gorur, A. & Costerton, J.W. (2009) Ultrastructural examination of failed molar retreatment with secondary apical periodontitis: an examination of endodontic biofilms in an endodontic retreatment failure. *Journal of Endodontics*, **35 (9)**, 1303–1309.
19. Schaudinn, C., Carr, G., Gorur, A., Jaramillo, D., Costerton, J.W. & Webster, P. (2009) Imaging of endodontic biofilms by combined microscopy (FISH/cLSM–SEM). *Journal of Microscopy*, **235 (2)**, 124–127.
20. Ricucci, D. & Siqueira, J.F. Jr. (2010) Biofilms and apical periodontitis: study of prevalence and association with clinical and histopathologic findings. *Journal of Endodontics*, **36 (8)**, 1277–1288.
21. Flemming, H.C. & Wingender, J. (2010) The biofilm matrix. *Nature Reviews Microbiology*, **8 (9)**, 623–633.
22. Sutherland, I. (2001) Biofilm exopolysaccharides: a strong and sticky framework. *Microbiology*, **147 (Pt 1)**, 3–9.
23. Stewart, P.S. (2012) Mini-review: convection around biofilms. *Biofouling*, **28 (2)**, 187–198.
24. Lawrence, J.R., Korber, D.R., Hoyle, B.D., Costerton, J.W. & Caldwell, D.E. (1991) Optical sectioning of microbial biofilms. *Journal of Bacteriology*, **173 (20)**, 6558–6567.
25. Absalon, C., Van Dellen, K. & Watnick, P.I. (2011) A communal bacterial adhesin anchors biofilm and bystander cells to surfaces. *PLoS Pathogens*, **7 (8)**, e1002210.
26. Mah, T.F., Pitts, B., Pellock, B., Walker, G.C., Stewart, P.S. & O'Toole, G.A. (2003) A genetic basis for Pseudomonas aeruginosa biofilm antibiotic resistance. *Nature*, **426 (6964)**, 306–310.

27. Vuong, C., Voyich, J.M., Fischer, E.R. *et al.* (2004) Polysaccharide intercellular adhesin (PIA) protects Staphylococcus epidermidis against major components of the human innate immune system. *Cellular Microbiology*, **6** (3), 269–275.

28. Lynch, D.J., Fountain, T.L., Mazurkiewicz, J.E. & Banas, J.A. (2007) Glucan-binding proteins are essential for shaping Streptococcus mutans biofilm architecture. *FEMS Microbiology Letters*, **268** (2), 158–165.

29. Sauer, K., Cullen, M.C., Rickard, A.H., Zeef, L.A., Davies, D.G. & Gilbert, P. (2004) Characterization of nutrient-induced dispersion in Pseudomonas aeruginosa PAO1 biofilm. *Journal of Bacteriology*, **186** (21), 7312–7326.

30. Whitchurch, C.B., Tolker-Nielsen, T., Ragas, P.C. & Mattick, J.S. (2002) Extracellular DNA required for bacterial biofilm formation. *Science*, **295** (5559), 1487.

31. Thomas, V.C., Thurlow, L.R., Boyle, D. & Hancock, L.E. (2008) Regulation of autolysis-dependent extracellular DNA release by Enterococcus faecalis extracellular proteases influences biofilm development. *Journal of Bacteriology*, **190** (16), 5690–5698.

32. Barnes, A.M., Ballering, K.S., Leibman, R.S., Wells, C.L. & Dunny, G.M. (2012) Enterococcus faecalis produces abundant extracellular structures containing DNA in the absence of cell lysis during early biofilm formation. *mBio*, **3** (4), 193–212.

33. Parsek, M.R. & Greenberg, E.P. (2005) Sociomicrobiology: the connections between quorum sensing and biofilms. *Trends in Microbiology*, **13** (1), 27–33.

34. Keller, L. & Surette, M.G. (2006) Communication in bacteria: an ecological and evolutionary perspective. *Nature Reviews Microbiology*, **4** (4), 249–258.

35. Duan, K., Dammel, C., Stein, J., Rabin, H. & Surette, M.G. (2003) Modulation of Pseudomonas aeruginosa gene expression by host microflora through interspecies communication. *Molecular Microbiology*, **50** (5), 1477–1491.

36. Dieppois, G., Ducret, V., Caille, O. & Perron, K. (2012) The transcriptional regulator CzcR modulates antibiotic resistance and quorum sensing in Pseudomonas aeruginosa. *PLoS One*, **7** (5), e38148.

37. Fuqua, C. & Greenberg, E.P. (2002) Listening in on bacteria: acyl-homoserine lactone signalling. *Nature Reviews Molecular Cell Biology*, **3** (9), 685–695.

38. Li, Z. & Nair, S.K. (2012) Quorum sensing: how bacteria can coordinate activity and synchronize their response to external signals. *Protein Science*, **21** (10), 1403–1407.

39. Clewell, D.B. & Francia, M.V. (2004) Conjugation in gram-positive bacteria. In: Funnell, B.E. & Phillips, G.J. (eds), *Plasmid Biology*. ASM Press, Washington, D.C., pp. 227–256.

40. Sorensen, S.J., Bailey, M., Hansen, L.H., Kroer, N. & Wuertz, S. (2005) Studying plasmid horizontal transfer in situ: a critical review. *Nature Reviews Microbiology*, **3** (9), 700–710.

41. Roberts, A.P. & Mullany, P. (2010) Oral biofilms: a reservoir of transferable, bacterial, antimicrobial resistance. *Expert Review of Anti-Infective Therapy*, **8** (12), 1441–1450.

42. Li, Y.H., Lau, P.C., Lee, J.H., Ellen, R.P. & Cvitkovitch, D.G. (2001) Natural genetic transformation of Streptococcus mutans growing in biofilms. *Journal of Bacteriology*, **183** (3), 897–908.

43. Li, Y.H., Tang, N., Aspiras, M.B. *et al.* (2002) A quorum-sensing signaling system essential for genetic competence in Streptococcus mutans is involved in biofilm formation. *Journal of Bacteriology*, **184** (10), 2699–2708.

44. Yagi, Y., McLellan, T.S., Frez, W.A. & Clewell, D.B. (1978) Characterization of a small plasmid determining resistance to erythromycin, lincomycin, and vernamycin Balpha in a strain of Streptococcus sanguis isolated from dental plaque. *Antimicrobial Agents and Chemotherapy*, **13** (5), 884–887.

45. Kuramitsu, H.K. & Trapa, V. (1984) Genetic exchange between oral streptococci during mixed growth. *Journal of General Microbiology*, **130** (10), 2497–2500.

46. Fitzgerald, G.F. & Clewell, D.B. (1985) A conjugative transposon (Tn919) in Streptococcus sanguis. *Infection and Immunity*, **47** (2), 415–420.

47. Wang, B.Y., Chi, B. & Kuramitsu, H.K. (2002) Genetic exchange between Treponema denticola and Streptococcus gordonii in biofilms. *Oral Microbiology and Immunology*, **17** (2), 108–112.

48. Sedgley, C.M., Molander, A., Flannagan, S.E. *et al.* (2005) Virulence, phenotype and genotype characteristics of endodontic Enterococcus spp. *Oral Microbiology and Immunology*, **20** (1), 10–19.

49. Sedgley, C.M., Lee, E.H., Martin, M.J. & Flannagan, S.E. (2008) Antibiotic resistance gene transfer between Streptococcus gordonii and Enterococcus faecalis in root canals of teeth ex vivo. *Journal of Endodontics*, **34** (5), 570–574.

50. Boles, B.R., Thoendel, M. & Singh, P.K. (2004) Self-generated diversity produces "insurance effects" in biofilm communities. *Proceedings of the National Academy of Sciences of the United States of America*, **101** (47), 16630–16635.

51. Hengge-Aronis, R. (2002) Signal transduction and regulatory mechanisms involved in control of the sigma(S) (RpoS) subunit of RNA polymerase. *Microbiology and Molecular Biology Reviews*, **66** (3), 373–395.

52. Guisbert, E., Yura, T., Rhodius, V.A. & Gross, C.A. (2008) Convergence of molecular, modeling, and systems approaches for an understanding of the Escherichia coli heat shock response. *Microbiology and Molecular Biology Reviews*, **72** (3), 545–554.

53. Kelley, W.L. (2006) Lex marks the spot: the virulent side of SOS and a closer look at the LexA regulon. *Molecular Microbiology*, **62** (5), 1228–1238.

54. Potrykus, K. & Cashel, M. (2008) (p)ppGpp: still magical? *Annual Review of Microbiology*, **62**, 35–51.

55. Rice, L.B. (1998) Tn916 family conjugative transposons and dissemination of antimicrobial resistance determinants. *Antimicrobial Agents and Chemotherapy*, **42** (8), 1871–1877.

56. Foster, P.L. (2007) Stress-induced mutagenesis in bacteria. *Critical Reviews in Biochemistry and Molecular Biology*, **42** (5), 373–397.

57. Hayes, F. & Van Melderen, L. (2011) Toxins–antitoxins: diversity, evolution and function. *Critical Reviews in Biochemistry and Molecular Biology*, **46** (5), 386–408.

58. Kim, Y., Wang, X., Zhang, X.S. *et al.* (2010) Escherichia coli toxin/antitoxin pair MqsR/MqsA regulate toxin CspD. *Environmental Microbiology*, **12** (5), 1105–1121.

59. Belitsky, M., Avshalom, H., Erental, A. *et al.* (2011) The Escherichia coli extracellular death factor EDF induces the endoribonucleolytic activities of the toxins MazF and ChpBK. *Molecular Cell*, **41** (6), 625–635.

60. Wang, X., Kim, Y., Hong, S.H. *et al.* (2011) Antitoxin MqsA helps mediate the bacterial general stress response. *Nature Chemical Biology*, **7** (6), 359–366.

61. Stewart, P.S. & Costerton, J.W. (2001) Antibiotic resistance of bacteria in biofilms. *Lancet*, **358** (9276), 135–138.

62. del Pozo, J.L. & Patel, R. (2007) The challenge of treating biofilm-associated bacterial infections. *Clinical Pharmacology and Therapeutics*, **82** (2), 204–209.

63. Konig, C., Schwank, S. & Blaser, J. (2001) Factors compromising antibiotic activity against biofilms of Staphylococcus epidermidis. *European Journal of Clinical Microbiology and Infectious Diseases*, **20** (1), 20–26.

64. Spoering, A.L. & Lewis, K. (2001) Biofilms and planktonic cells of Pseudomonas aeruginosa have similar resistance to killing by antimicrobials. *Journal of Bacteriology*, **183** (23), 6746–6751.

65. Li, X.Z. & Nikaido, H. (2009) Efflux-mediated drug resistance in bacteria: an update. *Drugs*, **69** (12), 1555–1623.

66. Kvist, M., Hancock, V. & Klemm, P. (2008) Inactivation of efflux pumps abolishes bacterial biofilm formation. *Applied and Environmental Microbiology*, **74** (23), 7376–7382.

67. Zhang, L. & Mah, T.F. (2008) Involvement of a novel efflux system in biofilm-specific resistance to antibiotics. *Journal of Bacteriology*, **190** (13), 4447–4452.

68. Sternberg, C., Christensen, B.B., Johansen, T. *et al.* (1999) Distribution of bacterial growth activity in flow-chamber biofilms. *Applied and Environmental Microbiology*, **65** (9), 4108–4117.

69. de Beer, D., Stoodley, P., Roe, F. & Lewandowski, Z. (1994) Effects of biofilm structures on oxygen distribution and mass transport. *Biotechnology and Bioengineering*, **43** (11), 1131–1138.

70. Borriello, G., Werner, E., Roe, F., Kim, A.M., Ehrlich, G.D. & Stewart, P.S. (2004) Oxygen limitation contributes to antibiotic tolerance of Pseudomonas aeruginosa in biofilms. *Antimicrobial Agents and Chemotherapy*, **48** (7), 2659–2664.

71. Fauvart, M., De Groote, V.N. & Michiels, J. (2011) Role of persister cells in chronic infections: clinical relevance and perspectives on anti-persister therapies. *Journal of Medical Microbiology*, **60** (Pt 6), 699–709.

72. Keren, I., Kaldalu, N., Spoering, A., Wang, Y. & Lewis, K. (2004) Persister cells and tolerance to antimicrobials. *FEMS Microbiology Letters*, **230** (1), 13–18.

73. Wiuff, C., Zappala, R.M., Regoes, R.R., Garner, K.N., Baquero, F. & Levin, B.R. (2005) Phenotypic tolerance: antibiotic enrichment of noninherited resistance in bacterial populations. *Antimicrobial Agents and Chemotherapy*, **49** (4), 1483–1494.

74. Shah, D., Zhang, Z., Khodursky, A., Kaldalu, N., Kurg, K. & Lewis, K. (2006) Persisters: a distinct physiological state of E. coli. *BMC Microbiology*, **6**, 53.

75. Gefen, O. & Balaban, N.Q. (2009) The importance of being persistent: heterogeneity of bacterial populations under antibiotic stress. *FEMS Microbiology Reviews*, **33** (4), 704–717.

76. Kara, D., Luppens, S.B. & Cate, J.M. (2006) Differences between single- and dual-species biofilms of Streptococcus mutans and Veillonella parvula in growth, acidogenicity and susceptibility to chlorhexidine. *European Journal of Oral Sciences*, **114** (1), 58–63.

77. Burmolle, M., Webb, J.S., Rao, D., Hansen, L.H., Sorensen, S.J. & Kjelleberg, S. (2006) Enhanced biofilm formation and increased resistance to antimicrobial agents and bacterial invasion are caused by synergistic interactions in multispecies biofilms. *Applied and Environmental Microbiology*, **72** (6), 3916–3923.

78. Leriche, V., Briandet, R. & Carpentier, B. (2003) Ecology of mixed biofilms subjected daily to a chlorinated alkaline solution: spatial distribution of bacterial species suggests a protective effect of one

species to another. *Environmental Microbiology*, **5 (1)**, 64–71.

79. Luppens, S.B., Kara, D., Bandounas, L. *et al.* (2008) Effect of Veillonella parvula on the antimicrobial resistance and gene expression of Streptococcus mutans grown in a dual-species biofilm. *Oral Microbiology and Immunology*, **23 (3)**, 183–189.

80. Elias, S. & Banin, E. (2012) Multi-species biofilms: living with friendly neighbors. *FEMS Microbiology Review*, in press. doi: 10.1111/j.1574-6976.2012.00325

81. Peters, O.A., Laib, A., Ruegsegger, P. & Barbakow, F. (2000) Three-dimensional analysis of root canal geometry by high-resolution computed tomography. *Journal of Dental Research*, **79 (6)**, 1405–1409.

82. Nair, P.N., Henry, S., Cano, V. & Vera, J. (2005) Microbial status of apical root canal system of human mandibular first molars with primary apical periodontitis after "one-visit" endodontic treatment. *Oral Surgery, Oral Medicine, Oral Pathology, Oral Radiology, and Endodontics*, **99 (2)**, 231–252.

83. Vieira, A.R., Siqueira, J.F. Jr., Ricucci, D. & Lopes, W.S. (2012) Dentinal tubule infection as the cause of recurrent disease and late endodontic treatment failure: a case report. *Journal of Endodontics*, **38 (2)**, 250–254.

84. Ricucci, D. & Siqueira, J.F. Jr. (2011) Recurrent apical periodontitis and late endodontic treatment failure related to coronal leakage: a case report. *Journal of Endodontics*, **37 (8)**, 1171–1175.

85. Noiri, Y., Ehara, A., Kawahara, T., Takemura, N. & Ebisu, S. (2002) Participation of bacterial biofilms in refractory and chronic periapical periodontitis. *Journal of Endodontics*, **28 (10)**, 679–683.

86. Rocha, C.T., Rossi, M.A., Leonardo, M.R., Rocha, L.B., Nelson-Filho, P. & Silva, L.A. (2008) Biofilm on the apical region of roots in primary teeth with vital and necrotic pulps with or without radiographically evident apical pathosis. *International Endodontic Journal*, **41 (8)**, 664–669.

87. Bergmans, L., Moisiadis, P., Van Meerbeek, B., Quirynen, M. & Lambrechts, P. (2005) Microscopic observation of bacteria: review highlighting the use of environmental SEM. *International Endodontic Journal*, **38 (11)**, 775–788.

88. Nair, P.N., Sjogren, U., Krey, G., Kahnberg, K.E. & Sundqvist, G. (1990) Intraradicular bacteria and fungi in root-filled, asymptomatic human teeth with therapy-resistant periapical lesions: a long-term light and electron microscopic follow-up study. *Journal of Endodontics*, **16 (12)**, 580–588.

89. Sunde, P.T., Olsen, I., Gobel, U.B. *et al.* (2003) Fluorescence in situ hybridization (FISH) for direct visualization of bacteria in periapical lesions of asymptomatic root-filled teeth. *Microbiology*, **149 (Pt 5)**, 1095–1102.

90. Richardson, N., Mordan, N.J., Figueiredo, J.A., Ng, Y.L. & Gulabivala, K. (2009) Microflora in teeth associated with apical periodontitis: a methodological observational study comparing two protocols and three microscopy techniques. *International Endodontic Journal*, **42 (10)**, 908–921.

91. Kantz, W.E. & Henry, C.A. (1974) Isolation and classification of anaerobic bacteria from intact pulp chambers of non-vital teeth in man. *Archives of Oral Biology*, **19 (1)**, 91–96.

92. Baumgartner, J.C. & Falkler, W.A. Jr. (1991) Bacteria in the apical 5 mm of infected root canals. *Journal of Endodontics*, **17 (8)**, 380–383.

93. Rolph, H.J., Lennon, A., Riggio, M.P. *et al.* (2001) Molecular identification of microorganisms from endodontic infections. *Journal of Clinical Microbiology*, **39 (9)**, 3282–3289.

94. Siqueira, J.F. Jr. & Rocas, I.N. (2005) Exploiting molecular methods to explore endodontic infections: part 2—redefining the endodontic microbiota. *Journal of Endodontics*, **31 (7)**, 488–498.

95. Li, L., Hsiao, W.W., Nandakumar, R. *et al.* (2010) Analyzing endodontic infections by deep coverage pyrosequencing. *Journal of Dental Research*, **89 (9)**, 980–984.

96. Ozok, A.R., Persoon, I.F., Huse, S.M. *et al.* (2012) Ecology of the microbiome of the infected root canal system: a comparison between apical and coronal root segments. *International Endodontic Journal*, **45 (6)**, 530–541.

97. Siqueira, J.F. Jr., Alves, F.R. & Rocas, I.N. (2011) Pyrosequencing analysis of the apical root canal microbiota. *Journal of Endodontics*, **37 (11)**, 1499–1503.

98. Santos, A.L., Siqueira, J.F. Jr., Rocas, I.N., Jesus, E.C., Rosado, A.S. & Tiedje, J.M. (2011) Comparing the bacterial diversity of acute and chronic dental root canal infections. *PLoS One*, **6 (11)**, e28088.

99. Jacinto, R.C., Gomes, B.P., Ferraz, C.C., Zaia, A.A. & Filho, F.J. (2003) Microbiological analysis of infected root canals from symptomatic and asymptomatic teeth with periapical periodontitis and the antimicrobial susceptibility of some isolated anaerobic bacteria. *Oral Microbiology and Immunology*, **18 (5)**, 285–292.

100. Waltimo, T.M., Sen, B.H., Meurman, J.H., Orstavik, D. & Haapasalo, M.P. (2003) Yeasts in apical periodontitis. *Critical Reviews in Oral Biology and Medicine*, **14 (2)**, 128–137.

101. Siqueira, J.F. Jr. & Rocas, I.N. (2004) Treponema species associated with abscesses of endodontic origin. *Oral Microbiology and Immunology*, **19 (5)**, 336–339.

102. Vickerman, M.M., Brossard, K.A., Funk, D.B., Jesionowski, A.M. & Gill, S.R. (2007) Phylogenetic analysis of bacterial and archaeal species in symptomatic and asymptomatic endodontic infections. *Journal of Medical Microbiology*, 56 (**Pt 1**), 110–118.

103. Montagner, F., Jacinto, R.C., Signoretti, F.G., Sanches, P.F. & Gomes, B.P. (2012) Clustering behavior in microbial communities from acute endodontic infections. *Journal of Endodontics*, 38 (**2**), 158–162.

104. Li, H., Chen, V., Chen, Y., Baumgartner, J.C. & Machida, C.A. (2009) Herpesviruses in endodontic pathoses: association of Epstein–Barr virus with irreversible pulpitis and apical periodontitis. *Journal of Endodontics*, 35 (**1**), 23–29.

105. Ferreira, D.C., Paiva, S.S., Carmo, F.L. *et al.* (2011) Identification of herpesviruses types 1 to 8 and human papillomavirus in acute apical abscesses. *Journal of Endodontics*, 37 (**1**), 10–16.

106. Chhour, K.L., Nadkarni, M.A., Byun, R., Martin, F.E., Jacques, N.A. & Hunter, N. (2005) Molecular analysis of microbial diversity in advanced caries. *Journal of Clinical Microbiology*, 43 (**2**), 843–849.

107. Martin, F.E., Nadkarni, M.A., Jacques, N.A. & Hunter, N. (2002) Quantitative microbiological study of human carious dentine by culture and real-time PCR: association of anaerobes with histopathological changes in chronic pulpitis. *Journal of Clinical Microbiology*, 40 (**5**), 1698–1704.

108. Hahn, C.L. & Liewehr, F.R. (2007) Relationships between caries bacteria, host responses, and clinical signs and symptoms of pulpitis. *Journal of Endodontics*, 33 (**3**), 213–219.

109. Sedgley, CM (2009) Virulence of endodontic bacterial pathogens. In: Fouad AF, ed. *Endodontic Microbiology*, Ames, IA: Wiley-Blackwell Publishing, pp. 130–151.

110. Kolenbrander, P.E., Andersen, R.N., Blehert, D.S., Egland, P.G., Foster, J.S. & Palmer, R.J. Jr. (2002) Communication among oral bacteria. *Microbiology and Molecular Biology Reviews*, 66 (**3**), 486–505.

111. Jacinto, R.C., Montagner, F., Signoretti, F.G., Almeida, G.C. & Gomes, B.P. (2008) Frequency, microbial interactions, and antimicrobial susceptibility of Fusobacterium nucleatum and Fusobacterium necrophorum isolated from primary endodontic infections. *Journal of Endodontics*, 34 (**12**), 1451–1456.

112. Marsh, P.D. (1986) Host defenses and microbial homeostasis: role of microbial interactions. *Journal of Dental Research*, 68 (**Spec Iss**), 1567–1575.

113. Sundqvist, G. (1992) Associations between microbial species in dental root canal infections. *Oral Microbiology and Immunology*, 7 (**5**), 257–262.

114. Metzger, Z., Lin, Y.Y., Dimeo, F., Ambrose, W.W., Trope, M. & Arnold, R.R. (2009) Synergistic pathogenicity of Porphyromonas gingivalis and Fusobacterium nucleatum in the mouse subcutaneous chamber model. *Journal of Endodontics*, 35 (**1**), 86–94.

115. Khemaleelakul, S., Baumgartner, J.C. & Pruksakom, S. (2006) Autoaggregation and coaggregation of bacteria associated with acute endodontic infections. *Journal of Endodontics*, 32 (**4**), 312–318.

116. Johnson, E.M., Flannagan, S.E. & Sedgley, C.M. (2006) Coaggregation interactions between oral and endodontic Enterococcus faecalis and bacterial species isolated from persistent apical periodontitis. *Journal of Endodontics*, 32 (**10**), 946–950.

117. Sundqvist, G.K., Eckerbom, M.I., Larsson, A.P. & Sjogren, U.T. (1979) Capacity of anaerobic bacteria from necrotic dental pulps to induce purulent infections. *Infection and Immunity*, 25 (**2**), 685–693.

118. Dobson, A., Cotter, P.D., Ross, R.P. & Hill, C. (2012) Bacteriocin production: a probiotic trait? *Applied and Environmental Microbiology*, 78 (**1**), 1–6.

119. Dahlen, G., Fabricius, L., Holm, S.E. & Moller, A. (1987) Interactions within a collection of eight bacterial strains isolated from a monkey dental root canal. *Oral Microbiology and Immunology*, 2 (**4**), 164–170.

120. Fabricius, L., Dahlen, G., Holm, S.E. & Moller, A.J. (1982) Influence of combinations of oral bacteria on periapical tissues of monkeys. *Scandinavian Journal of Dental Research*, 90 (**3**), 200–206.

121. Dahlen, G., Fabricius, L., Heyden, G., Holm, S.E. & Moller, A.J. (1982) Apical periodontitis induced by selected bacterial strains in root canals of immunized and nonimmunized monkeys. *Scandinavian Journal of Dental Research*, 90 (**3**), 207–216.

122. Fabricius, L., Dahlen, G., Ohman, A.E. & Moller, A.J. (1982) Predominant indigenous oral bacteria isolated from infected root canals after varied times of closure. *Scandinavian Journal of Dental Research*, 90 (**2**), 134–144.

123. Moller, A.J., Fabricius, L., Dahlen, G., Sundqvist, G. & Happonen, R.P. (2004) Apical periodontitis development and bacterial response to endodontic treatment. Experimental root canal infections in monkeys with selected bacterial strains. *European Journal of Oral Sciences*, 112 (**3**), 207–215.

124. Fabricius, L., Dahlen, G., Sundqvist, G., Happonen, R.P. & Moller, A.J. (2006) Influence of residual bacteria on periapical tissue healing after chemomechanical treatment and root filling of experimentally infected monkey teeth. *European Journal of Oral Sciences*, 114 (**4**), 278–285.

125. Flannagan, S.E., Clewell, D.B. & Sedgley, C.M. (2008) A "retrocidal" plasmid in Enterococcus faecalis: passage and protection. *Plasmid*, **59** (3), 217–230.

126. Sedgley, C.M., Clewell, D.B. & Flannagan, S.E. (2009) Plasmid pAMS1-encoded, bacteriocin-related "Siblicide" in Enterococcus faecalis. *Journal of Bacteriology*, **191** (9), 3183–3188.

127. Shen, Y., Stojicic, S. & Haapasalo, M. (2010) Bacterial viability in starved and revitalized biofilms: comparison of viability staining and direct culture. *Journal of Endodontics*, **36** (11), 1820–1823.

128. Stashenko, P., Teles, R. & D'Souza, R. (1998) Periapical inflammatory responses and their modulation. *Critical Reviews in Oral Biology and Medicine*, **9** (4), 498–521.

129. Leid, J.G., Shirtliff, M.E., Costerton, J.W. & Stoodley, P. (2002) Human leukocytes adhere to, penetrate, and respond to Staphylococcus aureus biofilms. *Infection and Immunity*, **70** (11), 6339–6345.

130. Mathew, S., Yaw-Chyn, L. & Kishen, A. (2010) Immunogenic potential of Enterococcus faecalis biofilm under simulated growth conditions. *Journal of Endodontics*, **36** (5), 832–836.

131. Gomes, B.P., Jacinto, R.C., Pinheiro, E.T. *et al.* (2005) Porphyromonas gingivalis, Porphyromonas endodontalis, Prevotella intermedia and Prevotella nigrescens in endodontic lesions detected by culture and by PCR. *Oral Microbiology and Immunology*, **20** (4), 211–215.

132. Jacinto, R.C., Gomes, B.P., Shah, H.N., Ferraz, C.C., Zaia, A.A. & Souza-Filho, F.J. (2006) Incidence and antimicrobial susceptibility of Porphyromonas gingivalis isolated from mixed endodontic infections. *International Endodontic Journal*, **39** (1), 62–70.

133. Tomazinho, L.F. & Avila-Campos, M.J. (2007) Detection of Porphyromonas gingivalis, Porphyromonas endodontalis, Prevotella intermedia, and Prevotella nigrescens in chronic endodontic infection. *Oral Surgery, Oral Medicine, Oral Pathology, Oral Radiology, and Endodontics*, **103** (2), 285–288.

134. Siqueira, J.F. Jr. & Rocas, I.N. (2009) The microbiota of acute apical abscesses. *Journal of Dental Research*, **88** (1), 61–65.

135. Montagner, F., Gomes, B.P. & Kumar, P.S. (2010) Molecular fingerprinting reveals the presence of unique communities associated with paired samples of root canals and acute apical abscesses. *Journal of Endodontics*, **36** (9), 1475–1479.

136. Siqueira, J.F. Jr. & Rocas, I.N. (2008) Clinical implications and microbiology of bacterial persistence after treatment procedures. *Journal of Endodontics*, **34** (11), 1291–1301 e3.

137. Haapasalo, H.K., Siren, E.K., Waltimo, T.M., Orstavik, D. & Haapasalo, M.P. (2000) Inactivation of local root canal medicaments by dentine: an in vitro study. *International Endodontic Journal*, **33** (2), 126–131.

138. Molander, A., Reit, C., Dahlen, G. & Kvist, T. (1998) Microbiological status of root-filled teeth with apical periodontitis. *International Endodontic Journal*, **31** (1), 1–7.

139. Sundqvist, G., Figdor, D., Persson, S. & Sjogren, U. (1998) Microbiologic analysis of teeth with failed endodontic treatment and the outcome of conservative re-treatment. *Oral Surgery, Oral Medicine, Oral Pathology, Oral Radiology, and Endodontics*, **85** (1), 86–93.

140. Hancock, H.H. 3rd, Sigurdsson, A., Trope, M. & Moiseiwitsch, J. (2001) Bacteria isolated after unsuccessful endodontic treatment in a North American population. *Oral Surgery, Oral Medicine, Oral Pathology, Oral Radiology, and Endodontics*, **91** (5), 579–586.

141. Chavez De Paz, L.E., Dahlen, G., Molander, A., Moller, A. & Bergenholtz, G. (2003) Bacteria recovered from teeth with apical periodontitis after antimicrobial endodontic treatment. *International Endodontic Journal*, **36** (7), 500–508.

142. Pinheiro, E.T., Gomes, B.P., Ferraz, C.C., Sousa, E.L., Teixeira, F.B. & Souza-Filho, F.J. (2003) Microorganisms from canals of root-filled teeth with periapical lesions. *International Endodontic Journal*, **36** (1), 1–11.

143. Chavez de Paz, L.E., Molander, A. & Dahlen, G. (2004) Gram-positive rods prevailing in teeth with apical periodontitis undergoing root canal treatment. *International Endodontic Journal*, **37** (9), 579–587.

144. Wu, M.K., Dummer, P.M. & Wesselink, P.R. (2006) Consequences of and strategies to deal with residual post-treatment root canal infection. *International Endodontic Journal*, **39** (5), 343–356.

145. Ricucci, D., Siqueira, J.F. Jr., Bate, A.L. & Pitt Ford, T.R. (2009) Histologic investigation of root canal-treated teeth with apical periodontitis: a retrospective study from twenty-four patients. *Journal of Endodontics*, **35** (4), 493–502.

146. Nair, P.N. (2004) Pathogenesis of apical periodontitis and the causes of endodontic failures. *Critical Reviews in Oral Biology and Medicine*, **15** (6), 348–381.

147. Coon, D., Gulati, A., Cowan, C. & He, J. (2007) The role of cyclooxygenase-2 (COX-2) in inflammatory bone resorption. *Journal of Endodontics*, **33** (4), 432–436.

148. Martinho, F.C., Chiesa, W.M., Leite, F.R., Cirelli, J.A. & Gomes, B.P. (2012) Correlation between clinical/radiographic features and inflammatory

cytokine networks produced by macrophages stimulated with endodontic content. *Journal of Endodontics*, **38** (**6**), 740–745.

149. Sjogren, U., Figdor, D., Persson, S. & Sundqvist, G. (1997) Influence of infection at the time of root filling on the outcome of endodontic treatment of teeth with apical periodontitis. *International Endodontic Journal*, **30** (**5**), 297–306.

150. Cheung, G.S. & Ho, M.W. (2001) Microbial flora of root canal-treated teeth associated with asymptomatic periapical radiolucent lesions. *Oral Microbiology and Immunology*, **16** (**6**), 332–337.

151. Kalfas, S., Figdor, D. & Sundqvist, G. (2001) A new bacterial species associated with failed endodontic treatment: identification and description of Actinomyces radicidentis. *Oral Surgery, Oral Medicine, Oral Pathology, Oral Radiology, and Endodontics*, **92** (**2**), 208–214.

152. Figdor, D. (2004) Microbial aetiology of endodontic treatment failure and pathogenic properties of selected species. *Australian Endodontic Journal*, **30** (**1**), 11–14.

153. Chugal, N., Wang, J.K., Wang, R. *et al.* (2011) Molecular characterization of the microbial flora residing at the apical portion of infected root canals of human teeth. *Journal of Endodontics*, **37** (**10**), 1359–1364.

154. Egan, M.W., Spratt, D.A., Ng, Y.L., Lam, J.M., Moles, D.R. & Gulabivala, K. (2002) Prevalence of yeasts in saliva and root canals of teeth associated with apical periodontitis. *International Endodontic Journal*, **35** (**4**), 321–329.

155. Figdor, D. & Davies, J. (1997) Cell surface structures of Actinomyces israelii. *Australian Dental Journal*, **42** (**2**), 125–128.

156. Sedgley, C., Nagel, A., Dahlen, G., Reit, C. & Molander, A. (2006) Real-time quantitative polymerase chain reaction and culture analyses of Enterococcus faecalis in root canals. *Journal of Endodontics*, **32** (**3**), 173–177.

157. Lleo, M.M., Bonato, B., Tafi, M.C., Signoretto, C., Pruzzo, C. & Canepari, P. (2005) Molecular vs culture methods for the detection of bacterial faecal indicators in groundwater for human use. *Letters in Applied Microbiology*, **40** (**4**), 289–294.

158. Sedgley, C.M., Lennan, S.L. & Appelbe, O.K. (2005) Survival of Enterococcus faecalis in root canals ex vivo. *International Endodontic Journal*, **38** (**10**), 735–742.

159. Figdor, D., Davies, J.K. & Sundqvist, G. (2003) Starvation survival, growth and recovery of Enterococcus faecalis in human serum. *Oral Microbiology and Immunology*, **18** (**4**), 234–239.

160. Subramanian, K. & Mickel, A.K. (2009) Molecular analysis of persistent periradicular lesions and root ends reveals a diverse microbial profile. *Journal of Endodontics*, **35** (**7**), 950–957.

161. Daw K, Baghdayan AS, Awasthi S, Shankar N (2012) Biofilm and planktonic Enterococcus faecalis elicit different responses from host phagocytes in vitro. *FEMS immunology and medical microbiology* **65** (**2**), 270–282.

162. Sakamoto, M., Siqueira, J.F. Jr., Rocas, I.N. & Benno, Y. (2008) Molecular analysis of the root canal microbiota associated with endodontic treatment failures. *Oral Microbiology and Immunology*, **23** (**4**), 275–281.

163. Lomcali, G., Sen, B.H. & Cankaya, H. (1996) Scanning electron microscopic observations of apical root surfaces of teeth with apical periodontitis. *Endodontics and Dental Traumatology*, **12** (**2**), 70–76.

164. Leonardo, M.R., Rossi, M.A., Silva, L.A., Ito, I.Y. & Bonifacio, K.C. (2002) EM evaluation of bacterial biofilm and microorganisms on the apical external root surface of human teeth. *Journal of Endodontics*, **28** (**12**), 815–818.

165. Noguchi, N., Noiri, Y., Narimatsu, M. & Ebisu, S. (2005) Identification and localization of extraradicular biofilm-forming bacteria associated with refractory endodontic pathogens. *Applied and Environmental Microbiology*, **71** (**12**), 8738–8743.

166. Su, L., Gao, Y., Yu, C., Wang, H. & Yu, Q. (2010) Surgical endodontic treatment of refractory periapical periodontitis with extraradicular biofilm. *Oral Surgery, Oral Medicine, Oral Pathology, Oral Radiology, and Endodontics*, **110** (**1**), e40–e44.

167. Signoretti, F.G., Endo, M.S., Gomes, B.P., Montagner, F., Tosello, F.B. & Jacinto, R.C. (2011) Persistent extraradicular infection in root-filled asymptomatic human tooth: scanning electron microscopic analysis and microbial investigation after apical microsurgery. *Journal of Endodontics*, **37** (**12**), 1696–1700.

168. Wang, J., Jiang, Y., Chen, W., Zhu, C. & Liang, J. (2012) Bacterial flora and extraradicular biofilm associated with the apical segment of teeth with post-treatment apical periodontitis. *Journal of Endodontics*, **38** (**7**), 954–959.

169. Ricucci, D., Martorano, M., Bate, A.L. & Pascon, E.A. (2005) Calculus-like deposit on the apical external root surface of teeth with post-treatment apical periodontitis: report of two cases. *International Endodontic Journal*, **38** (**4**), 262–271.

170. Yang, C.M., Hsieh, Y.D. & Yang, S.F. (2010) Refractory apical periodontitis associated with a calculus-like deposit at the root apex. *Journal of Dental Sciences*, **5** (**2**), 109–113.

171. Happonen, R.P., Soderling, E., Viander, M., Linko-Kettunen, L. & Pelliniemi, L.J. (1985) Immunocytochemical demonstration of Actinomyces species and Arachnia propionica in periapical infections. *Journal of Oral Pathology*, **14** (5), 405–413.

172. Sjogren, U., Happonen, R.P., Kahnberg, K.E. & Sundqvist, G. (1988) Survival of Arachnia propionica in periapical tissue. *International Endodontic Journal*, **21** (4), 277–282.

173. Sunde, P.T., Olsen, I., Debelian, G.J. & Tronstad, L. (2002) Microbiota of periapical lesions refractory to endodontic therapy. *Journal of Endodontics*, **28** (4), 304–310.

174. Sundqvist, G. & Reuterving, C.O. (1980) Isolation of Actinomyces israelii from periapical lesion. *Journal of Endodontics*, **6** (6), 602–606.

175. Duggan, J.M. & Sedgley, C.M. (2007) Biofilm formation of oral and endodontic *Enterococcus faecalis*. *Journal of Endodontics*, **33**, 815–818.

176. Ozok, A.R., Wu, M.K., Luppens, S.B. & Wesselink, P.R. (2007) Comparison of growth and susceptibility to sodium hypochlorite of mono- and dual-species biofilms of Fusobacterium nucleatum and Peptostreptococcus (micromonas) micros. *Journal of Endodontics*, **33** (7), 819–822.

177. Ferrer-Luque, C.M., Arias-Moliz, M.T., Gonzalez-Rodriguez, M.P. & Baca, P. (2010) Antimicrobial activity of maleic acid and combinations of cetrimide with chelating agents against Enterococcus faecalis biofilm. *Journal of Endodontics*, **36** (10), 1673–1675.

178. Coenye, T. & Nelis, H.J. (2010) In vitro and in vivo model systems to study microbial biofilm formation. *Journal of Microbiological Methods*, **83** (2), 89–105.

179. Dunavant, T.R., Regan, J.D., Glickman, G.N., Solomon, E.S. & Honeyman, A.L. (2006) Comparative evaluation of endodontic irrigants against Enterococcus faecalis biofilms. *Journal of Endodontics*, **32** (6), 527–531.

180. Chavez de Paz, L.E., Bergenholtz, G., Dahlen, G. & Svensater, G. (2007) Response to alkaline stress by root canal bacteria in biofilms. *International Endodontic Journal*, **40** (5), 344–355.

181. Kim, J., Park, H.D. & Chung, S. (2012) Microfluidic approaches to bacterial biofilm formation. *Molecules*, **17** (8), 9818–9834.

182. Norrington, D.W., Ruby, J., Beck, P. & Eleazer, P.D. (2008) Observations of biofilm growth on human dentin and potential destruction after exposure to antibiotics. *Oral Surgery, Oral Medicine, Oral Pathology, Oral Radiology, and Endodontics*, **105** (4), 526–529.

183. Bryce, G., O'Donnell, D., Ready, D., Ng, Y.L., Pratten, J. & Gulabivala, K. (2009) Contemporary root canal irrigants are able to disrupt and eradicate single- and dual-species biofilms. *Journal of Endodontics*, **35** (9), 1243–1248.

184. Shen, Y., Stojicic, S. & Haapasalo, M. (2011) Antimicrobial efficacy of chlorhexidine against bacteria in biofilms at different stages of development. *Journal of Endodontics*, **37** (5), 657–661.

185. Al-Ahmad, A., Maier, J., Follo, M. *et al.* (2010) Food-borne enterococci integrate into oral biofilm: an in vivo study. *Journal of Endodontics*, **36** (11), 1812–1819.

186. Ozdemir, H.O., Buzoglu, H.D., Calt, S., Stabholz, A. & Steinberg, D. (2010) Effect of ethylenediaminetetraacetic acid and sodium hypochlorite irrigation on Enterococcus faecalis biofilm colonization in young and old human root canal dentin: in vitro study. *Journal of Endodontics*, **36** (5), 842–846.

187. Kakoli, P., Nandakumar, R., Romberg, E., Arola, D. & Fouad, A.F. (2009) The effect of age on bacterial penetration of radicular dentin. *Journal of Endodontics*, **35** (1), 78–81.

188. Clegg, M.S., Vertucci, F.J., Walker, C., Belanger, M. & Britto, L.R. (2006) The effect of exposure to irrigant solutions on apical dentin biofilms in vitro. *Journal of Endodontics*, **32** (5), 434–437.

189. Kishen, A., Sum, C.P., Mathew, S. & Lim, C.T. (2008) Influence of irrigation regimens on the adherence of Enterococcus faecalis to root canal dentin. *Journal of Endodontics*, **34** (7), 850–854.

190. Ferrer-Luque, C.M., Conde-Ortiz, A., Arias-Moliz, M.T., Valderrama, M.J. & Baca, P. (2012) Residual activity of chelating agents and their combinations with cetrimide on root canals infected with Enterococcus faecalis. *Journal of Endodontics*, **38** (6), 826–828.

191. Quah, S.Y., Wu, S., Lui, J.N., Sum, C.P. & Tan, K.S. (2012) N-acetylcysteine inhibits growth and eradicates biofilm of Enterococcus faecalis. *Journal of Endodontics*, **38** (1), 81–85.

192. Brandle, N., Zehnder, M., Weiger, R. & Waltimo, T. (2008) Impact of growth conditions on susceptibility of five microbial species to alkaline stress. *Journal of Endodontics*, **34** (5), 579–582.

193. Gubler, M., Brunner, T.J., Zehnder, M., Waltimo, T., Sener, B. & Stark, W.J. (2008) Do bioactive glasses convey a disinfecting mechanism beyond a mere increase in pH? *International Endodontic Journal*, **41** (8), 670–678.

194. Lundstrom, J.R., Williamson, A.E., Villhauer, A.L., Dawson, D.V. & Drake, D.R. (2010) Bactericidal activity of stabilized chlorine dioxide as an endodontic irrigant in a polymicrobial biofilm tooth model system. *Journal of Endodontics*, **36** (11), 1874–1878.

195. Chavez de Paz, L.E. (2012) Development of a multispecies biofilm community by four root canal bacteria. *Journal of Endodontics*, **38** (**3**), 318–323.

196. Aas, J.A., Paster, B.J., Stokes, L.N., Olsen, I. & Dewhirst, F.E. (2005) Defining the normal bacterial flora of the oral cavity. *Journal of Clinical Microbiology*, **43** (**11**), 5721–5732.

197. Persoon, I.F., Hoogenkamp, M.A., Bury, A. *et al.* (2012) Effect of vanadium chloroperoxidase on Enterococcus faecalis biofilms. *Journal of Endodontics*, **38** (**1**), 72–74.

198. Buckingham-Meyer, K., Goeres, D.M. & Hamilton, M.A. (2007) Comparative evaluation of biofilm disinfectant efficacy tests. *Journal of Microbiological Methods*, **70** (**2**), 236–244.

199. Casadevall, A. & Pirofski, L. (2001) Host–pathogen interactions: the attributes of virulence. *The Journal of Infectious Diseases*, **184** (**3**), 337–344.

200. Medzhitov, R., Schneider, D.S. & Soares, M.P. (2012) Disease tolerance as a defense strategy. *Science*, **335** (**6071**), 936–941.

4 Efficacy of Root Canal Disinfection

Ashraf F. Fouad

Department of Endodontics, Prosthodontics and Operative Dentistry, University of Maryland, Baltimore, MD, USA

Goals of endodontic treatment and of root canal disinfection

Root canal disinfection, rather than mere debridement, has become a central goal of endodontic treatment in recent years. This approach developed from the realization that microbial infection is the principal cause for the initiation and persistence of endodontic disease (1, 2). Microbial presence and persistence following treatment is also likely the reason for the differences in clinical outcomes between cases with preoperative apical lesions and cases without lesions (3, 4). It has become evident from the examination of longitudinal outcome studies that this distinction in outcomes between vital cases and cases with preoperative lesions is present despite the fact that many of the cases with vital pulps in these studies are treated by trainees who have less clinical experience (3, 5). Root canal systems in cases with vital pulp are likely to have residual debris in the root canal following the completion of instrumentation, regardless of the instrumentation technique; yet the long-term success remains high. Likewise, retreatment cases without preoperative apical lesions also have a much better outcome compared to those with apical lesions (3, 6), despite numerous studies showing the persistence of debris following the instrumentation of a previously treated case. Thus it is not the debris that is associated with treatment outcome, but rather whether or not there is evidence that the cases involved may have had bacterial biofilms preoperatively. Treatment procedures in these cases may not have completely eliminated the bacterial biofilm in a large number of cases, and despite obturation that may be adequate, the lesions persisted. In fact, a well-performed animal study has documented this relationship between residual bacteria and lesion persistence, by showing that the quality of obturation was an important factor only if bacteria persisted at the time of obturation (2). Another animal study corroborated these findings by showing that instrumented, obturated, and sealed root canals in teeth with apical lesions had similar histological evidence of healing at 6 months to teeth that had instrumentation and coronal seal but without obturation (7).

Clinical outcome studies have documented the association between the presence of intracanal bacteria and the presence and persistence of apical disease. An association may or may not involve a causal relationship. In this case, causation has been demonstrated by several animal studies. These studies have shown the causal relationship between bacteria (8, 9) or bacterial cell wall components (10–12), and the induction and magnitude of apical disease. There have also been other animal studies (2) and clinical studies (13–16) showing improved apical healing in cases in which clinical intervention has resulted in the elimination of cultivable bacteria, although this has not been a universal finding (17).

Given these findings, it could be concluded that one of the main aims of root canal treatments is to provide a bacteria-free space that can be effectively obturated, which will likely improve the outcomes of cases with preexisting apical lesion. However, the root canal space is generally too complex anatomically to allow the clinician to achieve this aim using clinical techniques. In addition, there are areas in the root canal environment, such as surface irregularities, dentinal tubules, and lateral canals, that may become infected, but have a hitherto unknown effect on treatment outcome (18). Finally, the clinician does not have a clinical metric that allows him/her to determine whether root canal disinfection has been adequately accomplished.

Detection of microbial pathogens

In order to adequately discuss the possibility of microbial elimination, one has to have a good understanding of the methods available for microbial detection (Table 4.1). Microbial elimination should be analyzed in the context of how the microorganisms are detected. As different methods of microbial detection have different specificities and sensitivities, it follows that these different methods provide differing thresholds for microbial detection.

Endodontic infections are polymicrobial in nature, and are a result of microbial biofilms that populate the carious lesion causing pulpal inflammation. Following pulpal necrosis, there is microbial transformation and growth in the root canal environment that result in apical disease. These microbial biofilms are primarily bacterial in nature. However, archeal (19–21) and fungal species also have been identified in endodontic infections (22, 23), and viral infections appear to exacerbate apical disease (24–27). Other forms of microbial disease, such as from eukaryotic parasites, have not been described in endodontic infections. As the overwhelming evidence for the causation and persistence of endodontic disease is related to bacterial pathogens, this domain of microorganisms remains the principal target of microbial analyses as well as antimicrobial therapy. Bacterial species in root canal infections appear to be derived from those that populate deep carious lesions, the gingival sulcus, and the rest of the oral cavity (28).

Since 19th century (29), cultivation of bacterial cells has been performed in the majority of studies that have linked bacteria to the initiation of disease or to the healing following treatment. It has been known ever since that what can be cultured in the laboratory is a small fraction of what can be seen in a smear from the root canal under the microscope. Therefore, investigators have always sought to improve bacterial cultivation techniques. In the 1970s, newer cultivation methodologies that involved the use of anaerobic environment have shown that most root canal bacterial species are facultative or strict anaerobes (30–32). Therefore, many studies continue to employ anaerobic cultivation procedures, together with special enriched culture media, in order to maximize the cultivation of bacteria obtained from the root canal environment. However, the advent of molecular studies in the past decade has provided technologies that allow the efficient analyses of much more bacterial species, at a lower amount in the sample (Table 4.1).

These molecular methods rely on the detection of microbial DNA (33), RNA (34), or proteins (35). The detection of microbial DNA depends primarily on the identification of sequences in the 16S rRNA gene (which is uniquely present in bacterial and archeal species (19), other genes in bacteria (36), or the 18S rRNA gene in fungi (37). The analysis of these genes allows the investigators to search public databases that contain tens of thousands of the respective microbial species and thus perform

Table 4.1 Common methods of detection of root canal microorganisms.

Detection method	Description	Limitations
Aerobic and anaerobic culturing	Requires various generic and specific media for specific microorganisms	Many bacteria are not cultivable, or may be rendered viable but uncultivable by temporary stressors in the system
PCR with species-level primers	Enables very specific identification of a particular species	Limited to one species, may detect the DNA of the dead organism
PCR with genus-level primers	Allows identification of a genus, may be followed by direct sequencing of the product to determine the species	Multiple species in the same genus may be present in the specimen, rendering the distinction among them difficult
PCR with broad-range 16S rDNA primers	Identifies the presence or absence of any bacteria, may be followed by cloning and sequencing to identify species	Laborious and expensive; only a limited number of clones could be identified from each sample
DNA–DNA hybridization with molecular probes	Allows identification of selected species or all bacteria	Lacks amplification; only a limited number of species is detectable using this method
Fluorescent *in situ* hybridization	Detects bacteria (or fungi) histologically in their undisturbed sites	Can detect bacteria but not differentiate a lot of individual species
Detection of messenger RNA	Allows detection of live bacteria	Technically difficult and only a limited number of targets available for detection
Proteomics	Allows functional detection of bacterial or fungal proteins, which demonstrate their activities	Complex analysis and differentiation of host and bacterial proteins
Monoclonal antibodies against certain microorganisms	Detects specifically certain microorganisms histologically in tissues	Antibodies may cross-react with other species
Scanning electron micrographs	Shows biofilms and their relationship to substrate	Usable only for hard tissues; industrial SEM needed to avoid distortion of tissues
Transmission electron micrographs	Shows bacteria and fungi *in situ* at very high resolution	Very laborious to perform, particularly for larger specimens
Brown and Brenn histologic bacterial staining	Stains bacteria *in situ*	Cannot stain gram-negative bacteria, and processing of specimens may eliminate many bacteria
BacLight live/dead stains	Stains vital and dead bacteria	Limited to smears or histologic sections
Bacterial luminescence	Uses bacterial species with light emitting characteristics that can be measured in a gradient	Requires use of special dark chamber for minimal light detection
Pyrosequencing	Allows depth of coverage to identify the most amount of taxa of any technique	Does not have resolution to determine individual species with great precision

a more comprehensive analysis of microbial presence. DNA-based molecular procedures generally involve either hybridization methods for identification of DNA signature sequences for specific bacteria (38) or amplification methods that employ the polymerase chain reaction (PCR) technology (33, 39). Amplification, using PCR-based methods, allows the detection of very small amounts of target organisms, thereby remarkably increasing the sensitivity of the test. Depending on the specificity of the primers used in PCR, the test may be used for the detection of specific species, several species in a genus, or for analyzing a large array of microorganisms present in the sample (33, 36, 39). The last method usually employs amplification of a large segment of the 16S rRNA gene that includes conserved regions of the gene thereby amplifying the genes from many different bacterial taxa. This is then followed by cloning the amplified genes into a commercially available vector (such as the ones made in *Escherichia coli*). Allowing the *E. coli* cells to grow then provides colonies of the different bacterial clones amplified. The 16S rRNA gene from each of these colonies can then be sequenced to determine the identity of the bacteria in the original sample from which it was cloned. This process is referred to as *cloning and sequencing with broad-range primers* (40–42).

Contemporary analyses of human microbiome (all bacteria and fungi that populate the human body) revealed that only about 10% of them can be cultivated (43). Current procedures rely on advanced *in silico* sequencing methodologies that avoid the inefficient biological cloning methods, and simultaneously analyze tens of thousands of sequences. This is known as *pyrosequencing* and has revealed a wide diversity of endodontic bacterial taxa, which could not be appreciated from cultivation or even earlier clonal analysis studies (44, 45).

Analyses of functional genes other than the 16S rRNA gene can also be performed, especially to identify certain traits in the specimen, such as virulence factors (46–48) or antibiotic resistance genes (49, 50). However, given the enormity of bacterial genomes and reduced cost of massive sequencing, contemporary studies employ the "shot gun" sequencing approaches to perform the so-called metagenomic analyses of a polymicrobial specimen. This could provide a wealth of information about the virulence of the microorganisms present, the presence of antibiotic resistance genes as well as the host response (51). However, metagenomic analyses have not been extensively performed in endodontic infections. DNA analysis in general, whether for identification or metagenomic analyses, has some limitations despite enabling an extensive examination of microbial presence. These include the fact that DNA may survive after bacterial cells die (52, 53), and that many of the genes present in a specimen may not actually be expressed into RNA and translated into proteins.

Analysis of RNA provides information on genes that have become expressed in the environment and thus can be considered a functional analysis of the specimen. Detection of messenger RNA also provides evidence for the viability of cells, because RNA degrades rapidly after the bacterial or fungal cell from which it is detected dies. Only a limited number of studies have been performed using this method in the endodontic literature (34). Proteomic analysis provides perhaps the most direct evidence for specific microbial activities and virulence, and how the proteins present compare to those of the host. Proteomic analysis is also considered a functional analysis of the specimen and has not been sufficiently utilized in analyzing endodontic infections (35).

With respect to the detection of viable bacterial cells, another method that has been employed frequently is by using the vital stains, most notably the BacLight system (54). This method involves the study of two stains of bacterial cells, of which Syto 9 stains both vital and dead bacteria whereas propidium iodide stains dead cells only. The staining can be performed of smears from the site to be studied, or of histological sections, to observe the cells *in situ*. The imaging is usually performed with a confocal laser scanning microscope, which can visualize the fluorescence of the stains at the appropriate wavelength for each of them. This allows the visualization of viable cells, which will be the ones that stain with Syto 9 but not propidium iodide. In endodontics, this method has been used to demonstrate that calcium hydroxide may render bacterial cells viable but not cultivable (54, 55), and that the biofilm status provides a mechanism for bacterial cells to resist stress from increased alkalinity (56).

Staining of bacteria *in situ* using histobacteriological methods has long been a powerful method to demonstrate the presence and location of bacterial cells. This has traditionally been accomplished using the Brown and Brenn, modified gram staining, method (57–59), or transmission electron microscopy (60, 61).

The observation of bacterial cells *in situ* has also been performed using molecular probes that hybridize with bacterial signatures in the bacterial genome and are attached to fluorescent markers. This method commonly referred to as *fluorescent in situ hybridization (FISH)* has been used to provide elegant staining of bacteria within persistent apical lesions (62). This study demonstrated how this method could identify bacteria within the center of the surgical specimens of apical lesions, without any concerns about the contamination from gingival and oral sources on the periphery of the enucleated lesions.

Histological processing of tissues involves fixation with potent antimicrobials such as formaldehyde or alcohol, followed by decalcification of mineralized tissues in strong acids, or extended soaking in ethylenediaminetetraacetic acid (EDTA), and continued by paraffin embedding, sectioning, and staining, and so on. All these steps may lead to the killing and removal of any bacteria present in the tissues. An ideal *in situ* observation method is one that does not involve the destruction and processing of tissues. An ideal example of the use of bioluminescent bacterial strains in intact teeth to demonstrate the efficacy of root canal preparation and irrigation depth has been presented in Figure 4.1 (63–65).

As noted before, several studies have been performed on the association of cultivated bacteria at the time of root canal obturation and long-term outcomes of treatment. Most of these studies have shown a direct correlation between microbial elimination and healing of apical lesions; however, this conclusion is not unequivocal. Therefore, at the time of writing, it is not known whether the lack of universal predictive nature of cultivation results on treatment outcomes is due to the lack of sensitivity of the technique, its inability to detect many microbial taxa, inability to predict whether the residual microflora will survive and have access to apical tissues, or due to changes that occur with time to root canal microflora following obturation. Very few studies have done these analyses using molecular methods. One animal study referred to earlier has shown that microbial presence at the time of follow-up (which was 2–2.5 years after treatment) showed a much higher association with apical healing than microbial presence at the time of obturation (2).

Sampling as a source of bias

In order to detect microbial presence in root canals, a sample has to be obtained and analyzed, as stated before. The tooth surface involved is typically treated by 30% hydrogen peroxide and disinfected by 5% tincture of iodine (66), with or without 5.25–6% sodium hypochlorite (67). The halides are then inactivated with 5% sodium thiosulfate, so as not to kill root canal bacteria. If the tooth has caries or a defective restoration, this sequence of solutions is repeated after the caries and restoration are removed, but before the canal is entered.

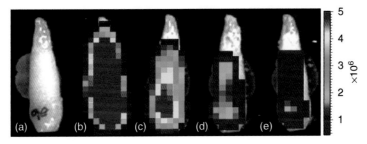

Figure 4.1   Images of representative tooth. (a) Background, no bacteria, (b) 1×10^6 *Pseudomonas fluorescens* 5RL in root canal. Bacterial cell count was determined by culturing the same volume of inoculum. (c–e) After 6 ml irrigation delivered using 28 gauge Max-I-Probe needle positioned 1 mm from WL after root canal instrumented to (c) size 36, (d) size 60, and (e) size 77. Color bar on right gives bioluminescence image units (photons/s/cm^2/sr). (Falk and Sedgley (63). Reproduced with permission of Elsevier.)

A microbiological sample is obtained at this stage to assure the lack of microbial presence. Following access preparation, paper points are used to sample any purulent drainage from the canal. If the necrotic pulp is dry, saline may be delivered without spilling over the margins, in order to enhance sample collection. If the paper points are used at this stage, they will primarily sample planktonic bacteria. Therefore, in order to enhance the sampling of biofilm bacteria, a file may be introduced to the entire length, as determined by an apex locator, and agitated against the walls to disrupt the biofilm. The file itself may be aseptically separated into the sampling vial, together with two to three subsequent paper points. This may be repeated in each canal of a multicanaled tooth (49). If the tooth is previously endodontically treated, the canal contents must be removed by rotary instruments, without the use of any solvents, before the sample is obtained by this method (68). For analyses of the effectiveness of endodontic instrumentation and irrigation methods, hypochlorite or iodine potassium iodide irrigants should first be inactivated by 5% sodium thiosulfate before sampling (49). If chlorhexidine was used for irrigation, it can be inactivated by L-α-lecithin + Tween-80 may be used to inactivate it (69). This inactivator may also be placed in the sampling solution, to prevent interfering with chlorhexidine's substantivity in the root canal, in clinical studies (49).

The microbiological sample obtained by the method described above is typically very meager. For molecular studies, the sample would have much less DNA than that obtained from a periodontal, mucosal, skin, or stool samples, used to study the microbiomes in these sites. In addition, the small file first introduced in an uninstrumented root canal and the paper points have very little contact with the irregular canal walls and do not have access to biofilms in fins, isthmuses, dentinal tubules, and lateral canals. A study that looked at viable bacteria in dentinal tubules showed significant number of bacteria in tubules throughout the thickness of dentin (70). The significance of these bacteria is still not fully understood, although it is well recognized by clinicians that the healing of apical lesions following tooth extraction is usually much more rapid than following endodontic treatment.

These limitations may have significant effects on the adequacy of the endodontic microbial samples, may have implications on the quantification and/or abundance of different microbial taxa, and may lead to false negative responses. They may also lead to significant differences between the endodontic microflora and that of the gingival sulcus of the same tooth, which are not related to true differences, but to sampling bias (71).

In-vitro studies attempt to overcome these limitations by enhancing the sampling of the root canal system. These studies may use more aggressive rotary instruments such as Gates Glidden burs to sample the dentinal wall, split the tooth, and sample the canal surface, or stain and image it directly. Occasionally, artificial models of biofilms are constructed without the need for a tooth altogether. These allow better standardization, and quantification of the results, particularly for the evaluation of standardized biofilms (72).

When it comes to sampling bias, one of the problems in endodontics is that root canal sampling does not differentiate among microflora in different locations in the root canal. It is generally considered that apical flora may not only be different from that in the coronal aspect of the canal, but also may be less accessible to endodontic disinfection procedures, and more likely to affect long-term outcomes (73–75). Evidence for the latter point arises from the fact that many endodontically treated teeth contain bacteria, but show no demonstration of apical lesions (68, 76, 77). Another sampling variation that has been documented in some studies relates to different geographical locations of patients from whom the samples were taken (78, 79).

Therefore, future studies should consider the advantages and disadvantages of *in-vitro* and *in-vivo* sampling and endeavor to improve sampling and reduce sampling bias. Clinical studies are usually the highest level evidence than *in-vitro* studies and better sampling for teeth that will not be extracted as part of the study should be explored in order to determine how this could predict the outcomes of treatment. Potential strategies for enhancing the sampling may be the use of passive ultrasonic activation of a small file in the canal, ultrasonic irrigation of saline or transport medium, and/or the use of the self-adjusting file to sample larger canals, in an attempt to sample as much of the canal anatomy as possible.

Methods for the determination of the efficacy of root canal disinfection

As bacterial presence or persistence in the root canal is causative of apical periodontitis, and several studies have shown the close association between bacterial elimination and long-term outcomes, it follows that determination of the efficacy of root canal disinfection is a reasonable surrogate outcome (Table 4.2). Because of the difficulty of running randomized clinical trials on many of the available technologies, models are sought to screen these technologies, such that only the most promising are tested clinically (80, 81). Scientific research has sought to identify good models of disease, in order to test the effectiveness of various strategies for root canal disinfection. *In-vitro* models allow the efficient testing of several technologies

simultaneously, control a number of variables, and allow direct examination of results by microscopic methods, thus minimizing sampling bias. However, there are many variables in generating these models that call into question their utility in adequately defining the clinical problem and in rendering clinically relevant results.

For example, it has long been recognized that dentin, dentin matrix, and other intracanal proteinaceous material may inhibit the activities of antimicrobials used to disinfect the root canal (82, 83). This shows that it is important to use actual root canals or at least a dentin substrate for conducting these *in-vitro* studies. Moreover, among the important variables recognized recently to play a critical role in the generation of intracanal bacterial biofilms is the length of time the biofilm is allowed to develop (84). So despite the remarkable differences among the different irrigants

Table 4.2 Methods to demonstrate the efficacy of root canal disinfection.

Model system	Description	Limitations
In-vitro biofilms	Standardized biofilms are generated on plastic or other substrates	Loss of buffering effects of dentin and the small volume of root canal environment
Root blocks	Standardized length of roots, with mono- or polymicrobial inoculation	Ideal case scenario, but may not mimic *in-vivo* usage closely
Whole extracted teeth	Usage of the entire canal system is more realistic of clinical situation. May have mono- or polymicrobial inoculation	Teeth have variability in anatomy, canal and tubular dimensions, and curvature. Sterilization techniques of teeth may affect results. Biofilms generated may not mimic natural infections; no validation studies are provided
Whole extracted teeth with natural infections	Naturally occurring bacterial biofilms provide realistic environment for testing antimicrobial strategies	Diversity in microflora from different patients and in tooth-related variables
In-vivo disinfection in animal models of apical lesions	Ideal circumstances of clinical testing, optimal analysis of results including histological analysis of outcomes	Animal teeth may have different anatomy from human teeth (except for primates), cannot measure postoperative symptoms
Clinical disinfection followed by extraction	Ideal circumstances of randomized clinical testing and optimal analysis of results	Does not allow the testing of outcomes of treatment
Clinical disinfection, sampling, and monitoring of long-term outcomes	Ideal circumstances of randomized clinical testing. Allows the demonstration of effects of microbial elimination on treatment outcomes	Subject to sampling limitations and posttreatment infection

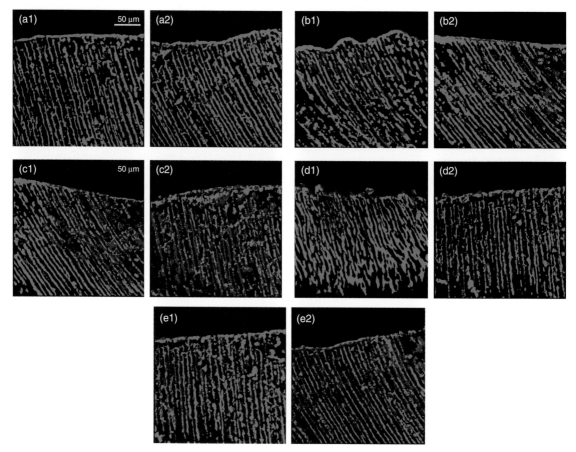

Figure 4.2   Confocal laser scanning micrograph of 3-week-old *E. faecalis*-infected dentinal tubules after exposure to different disinfecting solutions and viability staining. (a1) Sterile water for 1 min; (a2) sterile water for 3 min; (b1) 2% NaOCl for 1 min; (b2) 2% NaOCl for 3 min; (c1) 6% NaOCl for 1 min; (c2) 6% NaOCl for 3 min; (d1) 2% CHX for 1 min; (d2) 2% CHX for 3 min; (e1) QMiX for 1 min; (e2) QMiX for 3 min. All sections stained with BacLight Live/dead bacterial stain. (Wang *et al.* (84). Reproduced with permission of Elsevier.)

demonstrated in that study (Figure 4.2), it was noted that the amount of bacterial killing by the disinfecting agents was 7–21% lower in 3-week-old *Enterococcus faecalis* dentin canal biofilm than in 1-day-old biofilm. Considering that naturally occurring biofilms are polymicrobial, and are likely to have developed over months or years *in-vivo*, it follows that such *in-vitro* testing may not yield the results expected clinically.

Given this difficulty in identifying good *in-vitro* models, the gold standard for antimicrobial testing remains the clinical experimentation (Table 4.2). There are many examples of randomized clinical trials showing the efficacy of various root canal disinfection strategies (85–90). There remains to be a great need for clinical validation of *in-vitro* models to allow testing of newer technologies under a variety of clinically relevant parameters prior to clinical testing (91).

Diversity of conditions requiring disinfection

It is important to realize that the root canal system presents a variety of different clinical conditions and types that require different strategies for optimal disinfection. One of the most notable variables is the size of the root canal, which varies from the large canal with immature apex to the very calcifies that are difficult to negotiate. Large canals in children are also characterized by having larger tubules that permit more bacterial penetration (92). Many roots that have multiple roots are characterized by having isthmuses between the canals, which cannot be effectively negotiated by root canal preparation instruments. Technologies that allow disinfection of these isthmuses may be more effective than other technologies in situations where these are present, and not in other cases (93, 94). In many other situations, root canals present with unusual anatomical variations such as C-shaped canals, dens invaginatus, prominent accessory or lateral canals, and/or pathological changes such as internal resorptions. These variations require the adaptation of specific strategies in order to effectively address the clinical problem.

References

1. Möller, A.J., Fabricius, L., Dahlen, G., Ohman, A.E. & Heyden, G. (1981) Influence on periapical tissues of indigenous oral bacteria and necrotic pulp tissue in monkeys. *Scandinavian Journal of Dental Research*, **89 (6)**, 475–484.

2. Fabricius, L., Dahlen, G., Sundqvist, G., Happonen, R.P. & Moller, A.J. (2006) Influence of residual bacteria on periapical tissue healing after chemomechanical treatment and root filling of experimentally infected monkey teeth. *European Journal of Oral Sciences*, **114 (4)**, 278–285, PubMed PMID: 16911098.

3. Ng, Y.L., Mann, V. & Gulabivala, K. (2011) A prospective study of the factors affecting outcomes of nonsurgical root canal treatment: part 1: periapical health. *International Endodontic Journal*, **44 (7)**, 583–609, PubMed PMID: 21366626.

4. Ricucci, D., Russo, J., Rutberg, M., Burleson, J.A. & Spangberg, L.S. (2011) A prospective cohort study of endodontic treatments of 1,369 root canals: results after 5 years. *Oral Surgery, Oral Medicine, Oral Pathology, Oral Radiology, and Endodontics*, **112 (6)**, 825–842, PubMed PMID: 22099859.

5. de Chevigny, C., Dao, T.T., Basrani, B.R. *et al.* (2008) Treatment outcome in endodontics: the Toronto study–phase 4: initial treatment. *Journal of Endodontics*, **34 (3)**, 258–263, PubMed PMID: 18291271.

6. de Chevigny, C., Dao, T.T., Basrani, B.R. *et al.* (2008) Treatment outcome in endodontics: the Toronto study–phases 3 and 4: orthograde retreatment. *Journal of Endodontics*, **34 (2)**, 131–137, PubMed PMID: 18215667.

7. Sabeti, M.A., Nekofar, M., Motahhary, P., Ghandi, M. & Simon, J.H. (2006) Healing of apical periodontitis after endodontic treatment with and without obturation in dogs. *Journal of Endodontics*, **32 (7)**, 628–633, PubMed PMID: 16793468.

8. Kakehashi, S., Stanley, H.R. & Fitzgerald, R.J. (1965) The effects of surgical exposures of dental pulps in germfree and conventional laboratory rats. *Oral Surgery, Oral Medicine, and Oral Pathology*, **20**, 340–348.

9. Moller, A.J., Fabricius, L., Dahlen, G., Ohman, A.E. & Heyden, G. (1981) Influence on periapical tissues of indigenous oral bacteria and necrotic pulp tissue in monkeys. *Scandinavian Journal of Dental Research*, **89 (6)**, 475–484, PubMed PMID: 6951246.

10. Dahlen, G. & Bergenholtz, G. (1980) Endotoxic activity in teeth with necrotic pulps. *Journal of Dental Research*, **59 (6)**, 1033–1040.

11. Dwyer, T.G. & Torabinejad, M. (1980) Radiographic and histologic evaluation of the effect of endotoxin on the periapical tissues of the cat. *Journal of Endodontics*, **7 (1)**, 31–35.

12. Fouad, A.F. & Acosta, A.W. (2001) Periapical lesion progression and cytokine expression in an LPS hyporesponsive model. *International Endodontic Journal*, **34 (7)**, 506–513, PubMed PMID: 11601767, Epub 2001/10/17. eng.

13. Sjogren, U., Figdor, D., Persson, S. & Sundqvist, G. (1997) Influence of infection at the time of root filling on the outcome of endodontic treatment of teeth with apical periodontitis. *International Endodontic Journal*, **30 (5)**, 297–306, PubMed PMID: 9477818.

14. Sundqvist, G., Figdor, D., Persson, S. & Sjogren, U. (1998) Microbiologic analysis of teeth with failed endodontic treatment and the outcome of conservative re-treatment. *Oral Surgery, Oral Medicine, Oral Pathology, Oral Radiology, and Endodontics*, **85 (1)**, 86–93, PubMed PMID: 9474621.

15. Waltimo, T., Trope, M., Haapasalo, M. & Orstavik, D. (2005) Clinical efficacy of treatment procedures in endodontic infection control and one year follow-up of periapical healing. *Journal of Endodontics*, **31 (12)**, 863–866, PubMed PMID: 16306819.

16. Molander, A., Warfvinge, J., Reit, C. & Kvist, T. (2007) Clinical and radiographic evaluation of one- and two-visit endodontic treatment of asymptomatic necrotic teeth with apical periodontitis: a randomized clinical trial. *Journal of Endodontics*, **33 (10)**, 1145–1148, PubMed PMID: 17889679.

17. Peters, L.B. & Wesselink, P.R. (2002) Periapical healing of endodontically treated teeth in one and two visits obturated in the presence or absence of detectable microorganisms. *International Endodontic Journal*, **35 (8)**, 660–667, PubMed PMID: 12196219.

18. Ricucci, D. & Siqueira, J.F. Jr. (2010) Fate of the tissue in lateral canals and apical ramifications in response to pathologic conditions and treatment procedures. *Journal of Endodontics*, **36 (1)**, 1–15, PubMed PMID: 20003929.

19. Vickerman, M.M., Brossard, K.A., Funk, D.B., Jesionowski, A.M. & Gill, S.R. (2007) Phylogenetic analysis of bacterial and archaeal species in symptomatic and asymptomatic endodontic infections. *Journal of Medical Microbiology*, **56 (Pt 1)**, 110–118, PubMed PMID: 17172525.

20. Vianna, M.E., Conrads, G., Gomes, B.P. & Horz, H.P. (2006) Identification and quantification of archaea involved in primary endodontic infections. *Journal of Clinical Microbiology*, **44 (4)**, 1274–1282, PubMed PMID: 16597851, Pubmed Central PMCID: 1448633.

21. Siqueira, J.F. Jr., Rocas, I.N., Baumgartner, J.C. & Xia, T. (2005) Searching for Archaea in infections of endodontic origin. *Journal of Endodontics*, **31 (10)**, 719–722, PubMed PMID: 16186749.

22. Baumgartner, J.C., Watts, C.M. & Xia, T. (2000) Occurrence of Candida albicans in infections of endodontic origin. *Journal of Endodontics*, **26 (12)**, 695–698, PubMed PMID: 11471635.

23. Waltimo, T.M., Siren, E.K., Torkko, H.L., Olsen, I. & Haapasalo, M.P. (1997) Fungi in therapy-resistant apical periodontitis. *International Endodontic Journal*, **30 (2)**, 96–101, PubMed PMID: 10332243.

24. Sabeti, M., Kermani, V., Sabeti, S. & Simon, J.H. (2012) Significance of human cytomegalovirus and Epstein–Barr virus in inducing cytokine expression in periapical lesions. *Journal of Endodontics*, **38 (1)**, 47–50, PubMed PMID: 22152619.

25. Li, H., Chen, V., Chen, Y., Baumgartner, J.C. & Machida, C.A. (2009) Herpesviruses in endodontic pathoses: association of Epstein-Barr virus with irreversible pulpitis and apical periodontitis. *Journal of Endodontics*, **35 (1)**, 23–29, PubMed PMID: 19084119.

26. Chen, V., Chen, Y., Li, H., Kent, K., Baumgartner, J.C. & Machida, C.A. (2009) Herpesviruses in abscesses and cellulitis of endodontic origin. *Journal of Endodontics*, **35 (2)**, 182–188, PubMed PMID: 19166769, Pubmed Central PMCID: 2661131.

27. Sabeti, M. & Slots, J. (2004) Herpesviral-bacterial coinfection in periapical pathosis. *Journal of Endodontics*, **30 (2)**, 69–72, PubMed PMID: 14977298.

28. Hsiao, W.W., Li, K.L., Liu, Z., Jones, C., Fraser-Liggett, C.M. & Fouad, A.F. (2012) Microbial transformation from normal oral microbiota to acute endodontic infections. *BMC Genomics*, **13**, 345 PubMed PMID: 22839737, Pubmed Central PMCID: 3431219.

29. Miller, W. (1894) An introduction in the study of the bacteriopathology of the dental pulp. *Dental Cosmos*, **36**, 3.

30. Bergenholtz, G. (1974) Micro-organisms from necrotic pulp of traumatized teeth. *Odontologisk Revy*, **25 (4)**, 347–358.

31. Wittgow, W.C. Jr. & Sabiston, C.B. Jr. (1975) Microorganisms from pulpal chambers of intact teeth with necrotic pulps. *Journal of Endodontics*, **1 (5)**, 168–171.

32. Sundqvist, G. (1976) Bacteriological studies of necrotic dental pulps. Odontological dissertation no. 7, University of Umea, Umea, Sweden.

33. Fouad, A.F., Barry, J., Caimano, M. *et al.* (2002) PCR-based identification of bacteria associated with endodontic infections. *Journal of Clinical Microbiology*, **40 (9)**, 3223–3231 PubMed PMID: 12202557, Pubmed Central PMCID: 130810.

34. Williams, J.M., Trope, M., Caplan, D.J. & Shugars, D.C. (2006) Detection and quantitation of E. faecalis by real-time PCR (qPCR), reverse transcription-PCR (RT-PCR), and cultivation during endodontic treatment. *Journal of Endodontics*, **32 (8)**, 715–721, PubMed PMID: 16861068.

35. Nandakumar, R., Madayiputhiya, N. & Fouad, A.F. (2009) Proteomic analysis of endodontic infections by liquid chromatography-tandem mass spectrometry. *Oral Microbiology and Immunology*, **24 (4)**, 347–352, PubMed PMID: 19572900, Pubmed Central PMCID: 2744886.

36. Nandakumar, R., Mirchandani, R. & Fouad, A. (2007) Primer sensitivity: can it influence the results in Enterococcus faecalis prevalence studies? *Oral Surgery, Oral Medicine, Oral Pathology, Oral Radiology, and Endodontics*, **103 (3)**, 429–432, PubMed PMID: 17095258.

37. Siqueira, J.F. Jr. & Rocas, I.N. (2004) Polymerase chain reaction-based analysis of microorganisms associated with failed endodontic treatment. *Oral Surgery, Oral Medicine, Oral Pathology, Oral Radiology, and Endodontics*, **97 (1)**, 85–94, PubMed PMID: 14716262.

38. Siqueira, J.F. Jr., Rocas, I.N., Souto, R., de Uzeda, M. & Colombo, A.P. (2000) Checkerboard DNA-DNA hybridization analysis of endodontic infections. *Oral Surgery, Oral Medicine, Oral Pathology, Oral Radiology, and Endodontics*, **89 (6)**, 744–748, PubMed PMID: 10846131.

39. Fouad, A.F., Kum, K.Y., Clawson, M.L. *et al.* (2003) Molecular characterization of the presence of Eubacterium spp and Streptococcus spp in endodontic infections. *Oral Microbiology and Immunology*, **18 (4)**, 249–255, PubMed PMID: 12823801.

40. Saito, D., Leonardo Rde, T., Rodrigues, J.L., Tsai, S.M., Hofling, J.F. & Goncalves, R.B. (2006) Identification of bacteria in endodontic infections by sequence analysis of 16S rDNA clone libraries. *Journal of Medical Microbiology*, **55 (Pt 1)**, 101–107, PubMed PMID: 16388037.

41. Jacinto, R.C., Gomes, B.P., Desai, M., Rajendram, D. & Shah, H.N. (2007) Bacterial examination of endodontic infections by clonal analysis in concert with denaturing high-performance liquid chromatography. *Oral Microbiology and Immunology*, **22 (6)**, 403–410, PubMed PMID: 17949344.

42. Subramanian, K. & Mickel, A.K. (2009) Molecular analysis of persistent periradicular lesions and root ends reveals a diverse microbial profile. *Journal of Endodontics*, **35 (7)**, 950–957, PubMed PMID: 19567313.

43. Relman, D.A. (2011) Microbial genomics and infectious diseases. *The New England Journal of Medicine*, **365 (4)**, 347–357, PubMed PMID: 21793746, Pubmed Central PMCID: 3412127.

44. Li, L., Hsiao, W.W., Nandakumar, R. *et al.* (2010) Analyzing endodontic infections by deep coverage pyrosequencing. *Journal of Dental Research*, **89 (9)**, 980–984, PubMed PMID: 20519493, Pubmed Central PMCID: 3318071.

45. Siqueira, J., Fouad, A.F. & Rocas, I. (2012) Pyrosequencing as a tool for better understanding of human microbiomes. *J Oral Microbiol*, **4**, 10743, 1–15.

46. Bate, A.L., Ma, J.K. & Pitt Ford, T.R. (2000) Detection of bacterial virulence genes associated with infective endocarditis in infected root canals. *International Endodontic Journal*, **33 (3)**, 194–203.

47. Sedgley, C.M., Molander, A., Flannagan, S.E. *et al.* (2005) Virulence, phenotype and genotype characteristics of endodontic Enterococcus spp. *Oral Microbiology and Immunology*, **20 (1)**, 10–19, PubMed PMID: 15612939.

48. Zoletti, G.O., Pereira, E.M., Schuenck, R.P., Teixeira, L.M., Siqueira, J.F. Jr. & dos Santos, K.R. (2011) Characterization of virulence factors and clonal diversity of Enterococcus faecalis isolates from treated dental root canals. *Research in Microbiology*, **162 (2)**, 151–158, PubMed PMID: 21111042.

49. Jungermann, G.B., Burns, K., Nandakumar, R., Tolba, M., Venezia, R.A. & Fouad, A.F. (2011) Antibiotic resistance in primary and persistent endodontic infections. *Journal of Endodontics*, **37 (10)**, 1337–1344, PubMed PMID: 21924178, Pubmed Central PMCID: 3176416.

50. Rossi-Fedele, G. & Roberts, A.P. (2007) A preliminary study investigating the survival of tetracycline resistant Enterococcus faecalis after root canal irrigation with high concentrations of tetracycline. *International Endodontic Journal*, **40 (10)**, 772–777, PubMed PMID: 17697106.

51. Diaz-Torres, M.L., Villedieu, A., Hunt, N. *et al.* (2006) Determining the antibiotic resistance potential of the indigenous oral microbiota of humans using a metagenomic approach. *FEMS Microbiology Letters*, **258 (2)**, 257–262, PubMed PMID: 16640582.

52. Young, G., Turner, S., Davies, J.K., Sundqvist, G. & Figdor, D. (2007) Bacterial DNA persists for extended periods after cell death. *Journal of Endodontics*, **33 (12)**, 1417–1420, PubMed PMID: 18037049, Epub 2007/11/27. eng.

53. Brundin, M., Figdor, D., Roth, C., Davies, J.K., Sundqvist, G. & Sjogren, U. (2010) Persistence of dead-cell bacterial DNA in ex vivo root canals and influence of nucleases on DNA decay in vitro. *Oral Surgery, Oral Medicine, Oral Pathology, Oral Radiology, and Endodontics*, **110 (6)**, 789–794, PubMed PMID: 21112536.

54. Fouad, A.F. & Barry, J. (2005) The effect of antibiotics and endodontic antimicrobials on the polymerase chain reaction. *Journal of Endodontics*, **31 (7)**, 510–513, PubMed PMID: 15980710.

55. Weiger, R., de Lucena, J., Decker, H.E. & Lost, C. (2002) Vitality status of microorganisms in infected human root dentine. *International Endodontic Journal*, **35 (2)**, 166–171.

56. Chavez de Paz, L.E., Bergenholtz, G., Dahlen, G. & Svensater, G. (2007) Response to alkaline stress by root canal bacteria in biofilms. *International Endodontic Journal*, **40 (5)**, 344–355, PubMed PMID: 17326786.eng.

57. Fouad, A.F., Walton, R.E. & Rittman, B.R. (1992) Induced periapical lesions in ferret canines: histologic and radiographic evaluation. *Endodontics & Dental Traumatology*, **8 (2)**, 56–62, PubMed PMID: 1521506.

58. Ricucci, D. & Siqueira, J.F. Jr. (2011) Recurrent apical periodontitis and late endodontic treatment failure related to coronal leakage: a case report. *Journal of Endodontics*, **37 (8)**, 1171–1175, PubMed PMID: 21763916.

59. Vera, J., Siqueira, J.F. Jr., Ricucci, D. *et al.* (2012) One-versus two-visit endodontic treatment of teeth with apical periodontitis: a histobacteriologic study. *Journal of Endodontics*, **38 (8)**, 1040–1052, PubMed PMID: 22794203.

60. Nair, P. (1987) Light and electron microscopic studies of root canal flora and periapical lesions. *Journal of Endodontics*, **13**, 29–39.

61. Nair, P.N., Henry, S., Cano, V. & Vera, J. (2005) Microbial status of apical root canal system of human mandibular first molars with primary apical periodontitis after "one-visit" endodontic treatment. *Oral Surgery, Oral Medicine, Oral Pathology, Oral Radiology, and Endodontics*, **99 (2)**, 231–252, PubMed PMID: 15660098.

62. Sunde, P.T., Olsen, I., Gobel, U.B. *et al.* (2003) Fluorescence in situ hybridization (FISH) for direct visualization of bacteria in periapical lesions of

asymptomatic root-filled teeth. *Microbiology*, **149 (Pt 5)**, 1095–1102, PubMed PMID: 12724371.

63. Falk, K.W. & Sedgley, C.M. (2005) The influence of preparation size on the mechanical efficacy of root canal irrigation in vitro. *Journal of Endodontics*, **31 (10)**, 742–745, PubMed PMID: 16186754.

64. Nguy, D. & Sedgley, C. (2006) The influence of canal curvature on the mechanical efficacy of root canal irrigation in vitro using real-time imaging of bioluminescent bacteria. *Journal of Endodontics*, **32 (11)**, 1077–1080, PubMed PMID: 17055910.

65. Sedgley, C.M., Nagel, A.C., Hall, D. & Applegate, B. (2005) Influence of irrigant needle depth in removing bioluminescent bacteria inoculated into instrumented root canals using real-time imaging in vitro. *International Endodontic Journal*, **38 (2)**, 97–104, PubMed PMID: 15667631.

66. Möller, A.J.R. (1966) Microbiological examination of root canal and periapical tissues of human teeth. *Odontologisk Tidskrift*, **74 (Suppl. 5)**, 1–380.

67. Ng, Y.L., Spratt, D., Sriskantharajah, S. & Gulabivala, K. (2003) Evaluation of protocols for field decontamination before bacterial sampling of root canals for contemporary microbiology techniques. *Journal of Endodontics*, **29 (5)**, 317–320, PubMed PMID: 12775002.

68. Kaufman, B., Spangberg, L., Barry, J. & Fouad, A.F. (2005) Enterococcus spp. in endodontically treated teeth with and without periradicular lesions. *Journal of Endodontics*, **31 (12)**, 851–856, PubMed PMID: 16306816.

69. Zamany, A. & Spangberg, L.S. (2002) An effective method of inactivating chlorhexidine. *Oral Surgery, Oral Medicine, Oral Pathology, Oral Radiology, and Endodontics*, **93 (5)**, 617–620.

70. Peters, L.B., Wesselink, P.R., Buijs, J.F. & van Winkelhoff, A.J. (2001) Viable bacteria in root dentinal tubules of teeth with apical periodontitis. *Journal of Endodontics*, **27 (2)**, 76–81.

71. Rupf, S., Kannengiesser, S., Merte, K., Pfister, W., Sigusch, B. & Eschrich, K. (2000) Comparison of profiles of key periodontal pathogens in periodontium and endodontium. *Endodontics & Dental Traumatology*, **16 (6)**, 269–275, PubMed PMID: 11202893.

72. Dunavant, T.R., Regan, J.D., Glickman, G.N., Solomon, E.S. & Honeyman, A.L. (2006) Comparative evaluation of endodontic irrigants against Enterococcus faecalis biofilms. *Journal of Endodontics*, **32 (6)**, 527–531, PubMed PMID: 16728243.

73. Baumgartner, J.C. & Falkler, W.A. Jr. (1991) Bacteria in the apical 5 mm of infected root canals. *Journal of Endodontics*, **17 (8)**, 380–383.

74. Siqueira, J.F. Jr., Rocas, I.N., Alves, F.R. & Silva, M.G. (2009) Bacteria in the apical root canal of teeth with primary apical periodontitis. *Oral Surgery, Oral Medicine, Oral Pathology, Oral Radiology, and Endodontics*, **107 (5)**, 721–726, PubMed PMID: 19426923.

75. Rocas, I.N., Alves, F.R., Santos, A.L., Rosado, A.S. & Siqueira, J.F. Jr. (2010) Apical root canal microbiota as determined by reverse-capture checkerboard analysis of cryogenically ground root samples from teeth with apical periodontitis. *Journal of Endodontics*, **36 (10)**, 1617–1621, PubMed PMID: 20850664.

76. Zoletti, G.O., Siqueira, J.F. Jr. & Santos, K.R. (2006) Identification of Enterococcus faecalis in root-filled teeth with or without periradicular lesions by culture-dependent and-independent approaches. *Journal of Endodontics*, **32 (8)**, 722–726, PubMed PMID: 16861069.

77. Zoletti, G.O., Carmo, F.L., Pereira, E.M., Rosado, A.S., Siqueira, J.F. Jr. & Santos, K.R. (2010) Comparison of endodontic bacterial community structures in root-canal-treated teeth with or without apical periodontitis. *Journal of Medical Microbiology*, **59 (Pt 11)**, 1360–1364, PubMed PMID: 20688952.

78. Baumgartner, J.C., Siqueira Junior, J.F., Xia, T. & Rocas, I.N. (2004) Geographical differences in bacteria detected in endodontic infections using polymerase chain reaction. *Journal of Endodontics*, **30 (3)**, 141–144, PubMed PMID: 15055430.

79. Siqueira, J.F. Jr., Rocas, I.N., Debelian, G.J. *et al.* (2008) Profiling of root canal bacterial communities associated with chronic apical periodontitis from Brazilian and Norwegian subjects. *Journal of Endodontics*, **34 (12)**, 1457–1461, PubMed PMID: 19026873.

80. de Gregorio, C., Estevez, R., Cisneros, R., Paranjpe, A. & Cohenca, N. (2010) Efficacy of different irrigation and activation systems on the penetration of sodium hypochlorite into simulated lateral canals and up to working length: an in vitro study. *Journal of Endodontics*, **36 (7)**, 1216–1221, PubMed PMID: 20630302.

81. de Gregorio, C., Paranjpe, A., Garcia, A. *et al.* (2012) Efficacy of irrigation systems on penetration of sodium hypochlorite to working length and to simulated uninstrumented areas in oval shaped root canals. *International Endodontic Journal*, **45 (5)**, 475–481, PubMed PMID: 22283697.

82. Portenier, I., Haapasalo, H., Orstavik, D., Yamauchi, M. & Haapasalo, M. (2002) Inactivation of the antibacterial activity of iodine potassium iodide and chlorhexidine digluconate against Enterococcus faecalis by dentin, dentin matrix, type-I collagen, and heat-killed microbial whole cells. *Journal of Endodontics*, **28 (9)**, 634–637, PubMed PMID: 12236305.

83. Portenier, I., Haapasalo, H., Rye, A., Waltimo, T., Orstavik, D. & Haapasalo, M. (2001) Inactivation of root canal medicaments by dentine, hydroxylapatite and bovine serum albumin. *International*

Endodontic Journal, **34 (3)**, 184–188, PubMed PMID: 12193263.

84. Wang, Z., Shen, Y. & Haapasalo, M. (2012) Effectiveness of Endodontic Disinfecting Solutions against Young and Old Enterococcus faecalis Biofilms in Dentin Canals. *Journal of Endodontics*, **38 (10)**, 1376–1379, PubMed PMID: 22980181.

85. Zamany, A., Safavi, K. & Spangberg, L.S. (2003) The effect of chlorhexidine as an endodontic disinfectant. *Oral Surgery, Oral Medicine, Oral Pathology, Oral Radiology, and Endodontics*, **96 (5)**, 578–581, PubMed PMID: 14600693.

86. Huffaker, S.K., Safavi, K., Spangberg, L.S. & Kaufman, B. (2010) Influence of a passive sonic irrigation system on the elimination of bacteria from root canal systems: a clinical study. *Journal of Endodontics*, **36 (8)**, 1315–1318, PubMed PMID: 20647087.

87. Beus, C., Safavi, K., Stratton, J. & Kaufman, B. (2012) Comparison of the effect of two endodontic irrigation protocols on the elimination of bacteria from root canal system: a prospective, randomized clinical trial. *Journal of Endodontics*, **38 (11)**, 1479–1483, PubMed PMID: 23063221.

88. Pawar, R., Alqaied, A., Safavi, K., Boyko, J. & Kaufman, B. (2012) Influence of an apical negative pressure irrigation system on bacterial elimination during endodontic therapy: a prospective randomized clinical study. *Journal of Endodontics*, **38 (9)**, 1177–1181, PubMed PMID: 22892731.

89. Malkhassian, G., Manzur, A.J., Legner, M. *et al.* (2009) Antibacterial efficacy of MTAD final rinse and two percent chlorhexidine gel medication in teeth with apical periodontitis: a randomized double-blinded clinical trial. *Journal of Endodontics*, **35 (11)**, 1483–1490, PubMed PMID: 19840635.

90. Carver, K., Nusstein, J., Reader, A. & Beck, M. (2007) In vivo antibacterial efficacy of ultrasound after hand and rotary instrumentation in human mandibular molars. *Journal of Endodontics*, **33 (9)**, 1038–1043, PubMed PMID: 17931928.

91. Oliver, C.M. & Abbott, P.V. (2001) Correlation between clinical success and apical dye penetration. *International Endodontic Journal*, **34 (8)**, 637–644, PubMed PMID: 11762501.

92. Kakoli, P., Nandakumar, R., Romberg, E., Arola, D. & Fouad, A.F. (2009) The effect of age on bacterial penetration of radicular dentin. *Journal of Endodontics*, **35 (1)**, 78–81, PubMed PMID: 19084130, Pubmed Central PMCID: 3353976.

93. Ng, R., Singh, F., Papamanou, D.A. *et al.* (2011) Endodontic photodynamic therapy ex vivo. *Journal of Endodontics*, **37 (2)**, 217–222 PubMed PMID: 21238805, Pubmed Central PMCID: 3034089.

94. Burleson, A., Nusstein, J., Reader, A. & Beck, M. (2007) The in vivo evaluation of hand/rotary/ultrasound instrumentation in necrotic, human mandibular molars. *Journal of Endodontics*, **33 (7)**, 782–787, PubMed PMID: 17804312.

5 Impact of Root Canal Disinfection on Treatment Outcome

James D. Johnson and Natasha M. Flake

Department of Endodontics, University of Washington, Seattle, WA, USA

Introduction

Disinfection of the root canal system and its general effect on endodontic outcomes is a complex issue, parts of which have been studied widely, but its specific effect is not well documented in clinical trials with high levels of clinical evidence. Many steps are performed during endodontic therapy and they involve methods that try to disinfect the root canal system. Many of these methods have been investigated, particularly in *in-vitro* testing, but clinical outcome studies are difficult because of the many steps involved. It is difficult to examine which specific steps may improve outcomes. These steps include irrigation, instrumentation, and intracanal medication. Other factors are different irrigating solutions and different concentrations of irrigants; size and length of instrumentation; method of delivery of irrigants; one visit versus two visits; and initial therapy versus retreatment.

Difficulty in assessing clinical outcomes is because of the lack of randomized clinical trials where one specific step is evaluated in terms of outcome and other steps used to disinfect are the same; so there is only one variable. The levels of clinical evidence are listed in Tables 5.1 and 5.2. These high-level studies of clinical outcomes are difficult to perform for a number of reasons, ranging from adequate sample size, different criteria for healing, lack of standardization, differences in study designs, time of recall, adequate number or recalls, and ethical concerns, to name a few. The clinician is left to formulate evidence for treatment techniques that are based on a combination of studies of lower clinical evidence to predict the outcome of treatment for patients. This chapter addresses some of the information that exists for the disinfection of root canal systems, using what evidence is known in the literature to predict outcomes.

It is understood that if a canal system can be filled after a negative culture is obtained, the outcome is better (1). Which steps produce a canal system with a low level of bacteria remaining are of some dispute, and what level is critical to produce a significantly higher outcome is not known.

What is needed is a series of randomized clinical trials, systematic reviews, and meta-analysis of these systematic reviews.

Disinfection of Root Canal Systems: The Treatment of Apical Periodontitis, First Edition. Edited by Nestor Cohenca.
© 2014 John Wiley & Sons, Inc. Published 2014 by John Wiley & Sons, Inc.

Table 5.1   Levels of clinical evidence.

Levels of evidence	Therapy/prevention, etiology/harm
1a	Systematic review of randomized controlled trial (RCT)
1b	RCT (with narrow confidence interval)
1c	All or none
2a	Systematic review of cohort studies
2b	Individual cohort study (including low-quality RCT; i.e., <80%)
2c	"Outcomes" research
3a	Systematic review of case-controlled studies
3b	Individual case-controlled study
4	Case series (and poor-quality cohort and case-control studies)
5	Expert opinion without explicit critical appraisal, or based on physiology, bench research, or "proof of principle study"
	Bench top studies

Journal of Evidence Based Dental Practice. Reproduced with permission of Elsevier.

Nair (2) lists the following causes for persistent apical periodontitis: intraradicular infection (intraradicular bacteria); extraradicular infection found in apical tissues (Actinomyces, Enterococcus, and Propionibacterium, among others); cystic apical periodontitis (radicular cysts that do not heal after nonsurgical endodontic treatment, and may require surgical endodontic treatment, also known as *true cysts*); the presence of cholesterol crystals that may give rise to a foreign body reaction; the presence of foreign bodies in apical tissues that may include gutta-percha, root canal sealers, plant materials, paper points, cotton fibers, amalgam, or other materials; and, finally, the persistent apical lesion may actually heal by scar tissue formation. The presence of intracanal microorganisms is by far the most common cause of persistent apical periodontitis and is most relative to outcomes affected by the disinfection of canals.

Friedman (3) has compared outcome studies and the effects of numerous factors on the outcome of endodontic treatment in terms of healed apical periodontitis, healing of apical periodontitis, and asymptomatic functional teeth.

Friedman reviewed preoperative factors such as the patient's age and gender, the patient's systemic health, tooth location, the presentation of clinical signs and symptoms, the status of the pulp, the presence or absence of apical periodontitis, the size of the radiolucent lesion, and the status of the periodontium, and in the case of endodontic retreatment, the time elapsed from initial treatment to retreatment, the existence of a previous perforation, and the quality of the previous root canal filling.

The intraoperative factors that Friedman (3) examined in outcome studies include the apical extent of treatment, the amount of apical enlargement, negative bacterial cultures before root canal filling, number of treatment sessions (one visit vs. two visits), the occurrence of midtreatment flare-ups, materials and techniques used for treatment, and midtreatment complications.

Friedman also examined postoperative factors, such as the type and presence of an adequate restoration after endodontic treatment.

The findings in most outcome studies examined by Freidman (3) are that the presence of apical periodontitis seems to influence the prognosis to the greatest degree, and that other factors are less defined in terms of outcomes. Apical periodontitis is caused by root canal infection, and the presence of microorganisms within the canal can continue and expand apical periodontitis. In addition, apical periodontitis can be developed if bacteria are reintroduced into the root canal system after initially eliminating them.

Table 5.2   Chart 2: From Oxford Center for Evidenced based Medicine—Levels of Evidence (last edited 16 September 2013). http://www.cebm.net/index.aspx?o=1025.

Level	Therapy/prevention, etiology/harm	Prognosis	Diagnosis	Differential diagnosis/symptom prevalence study	Economic and decision analyses
1a	SR (with homogeneity*) of RCTs	SR (with homogeneity*) of inception cohort studies; CDR[†] validated in different populations	SR (with homogeneity*) of level 1 diagnostic studies; CDR[†] with 1b studies from different clinical centers	SR (with homogeneity*) of prospective cohort studies	SR (with homogeneity*) of level 1 economic studies
1b	Individual RCT (with narrow confidence interval[‡])	Individual inception cohort study with >80% follow-up; CDR[†] validated in a single population	Validating** cohort study with good[†††] reference standards; or CDR[†] tested within one clinical center	Prospective cohort study with good follow-up****	Analysis based on clinically sensible costs or alternatives; systematic review(s) of the evidence; and including multiway sensitivity analyses
1c	All or none[§]	All or none case series	Absolute SpPins and SnNouts[††]	All or none case series	Absolute better-value or worse-value analyses[††††]
2a	SR (with homogeneity*) of cohort studies	SR (with homogeneity*) of either retrospective cohort studies or untreated control groups in RCTs	SR (with homogeneity*) of level >2 diagnostic studies	SR (with homogeneity*) of 2b and better studies	SR (with homogeneity*) of level >2 economic studies
2b	Individual cohort study (including low quality RCT; e.g., <80% follow-up)	Retrospective cohort study or follow-up of untreated control patients in an RCT; Derivation of CDR† or validated on split-sample[§§§] only	Exploratory** cohort study with good[†††] reference standards; CDR[†] after derivation, or validated only on split-sample[§§§] or databases	Retrospective cohort study, or poor follow-up	Analysis based on clinically sensible costs or alternatives; limited review(s) of the evidence, or single studies; and including multiway sensitivity analyses
2c	"Outcomes" research; ecological studies	"Outcomes" research		Ecological studies	Audit or outcomes research
3a	SR (with homogeneity*) of case-control studies		SR (with homogeneity*) of 3b and better studies	SR (with homogeneity*) of 3b and better studies	SR (with homogeneity*) of 3b and better studies
3b	Individual case-control study		Nonconsecutive study; or without consistently applied reference standards	Nonconsecutive cohort study; or very limited population	Analysis based on limited alternatives or costs, poor quality estimates of data, but including sensitivity analyses incorporating clinically sensible variations
4	Case series (and poor quality cohort and case-control studies[§§])	Case series (and poor quality prognostic cohort studies***)	Case-control study, poor or nonindependent reference standard	Case series or superseded reference standards	Analysis with no sensitivity analysis

(continued)

Table 5.2   *(Continued)*

Level	Therapy/prevention, etiology/harm	Prognosis	Diagnosis	Differential diagnosis/symptom prevalence study	Economic and decision analyses
5	Expert opinion without explicit critical appraisal, or based on physiology, bench research, or "first principles"	Expert opinion without explicit critical appraisal, or based on physiology, bench research, or "first principles"	Expert opinion without explicit critical appraisal, or based on physiology, bench research, or "first principles"	Expert opinion without explicit critical appraisal, or based on physiology, bench research, or "first principles"	Expert opinion without explicit critical appraisal, or based on economic theory or "first principles"

Oxford Center for Evidenced-based Medicine—Levels of Evidence (March 2009) http://www.cebm.net/index.aspx?o=1025. Produced by Bob Phillips, Chris Ball, Dave Sackett, Doug Badenoch, Sharon Straus, Brian Haynes, Martin Dawes since November 1998. Updated by Jeremy Howick March 2009.

Notes

Users can add a minus sign "−" to denote the level that fails to provide a conclusive answer because of *either* a single result with a wide confidence interval *or* a systematic review with troublesome heterogeneity.

Such evidence is inconclusive, and therefore can only generate Grade D recommendations.

*By homogeneity we mean a systematic review that is free of worrisome variations (heterogeneity) in the directions and degrees of results between individual studies. Not all systematic reviews with statistically significant heterogeneity need be worrisome, and not all worrisome heterogeneity need be statistically significant. As noted above, studies displaying worrisome heterogeneity should be tagged with a "−" at the end of their designated level.

†Clinical Decision Rule. (These are algorithms or scoring systems that lead to a prognostic estimation or a diagnostic category.)

‡See note above for advice on how to understand, rate, and use trials or other studies with wide confidence intervals.

§Met when all patients died before the Rx became available, but now some survive on it; or when some patients died before the Rx became available, but now none die on it.

§§By poor quality cohort study we mean one that failed to clearly define comparison groups and/or failed to measure exposures and outcomes in the same (preferably blinded), objective way in both exposed and nonexposed individuals and/or failed to identify or appropriately control known confounders and/or failed to carry out a sufficiently long and complete follow-up of patients. By poor quality case-control study we mean one that failed to clearly define comparison groups and/or failed to measure exposures and outcomes in the same (preferably blinded), objective way in both cases and controls and/or failed to identify or appropriately control known confounders.

§§§Split-sample validation is achieved by collecting all the information in a single tranche, then artificially dividing this into "derivation" and "validation" samples.

††An "Absolute SpPin" is a diagnostic finding whose specificity is so high that a positive result rules-in the diagnosis. An "Absolute SnNout" is a diagnostic finding whose sensitivity is so high that a negative result rules out the diagnosis.

‡Good, better, bad, and worse refer to the comparisons between treatments in terms of their clinical risks and benefits.

†††Good reference standards are independent of the test, and applied blindly or objectively to all patients. Poor reference standards are haphazardly applied, but still independent of the test. Use of a nonindependent reference standard (where the "test" is included in the "reference," or where the "testing" affects the "reference") implies a level 4 study.

††††Better-value treatments are clearly as good but cheaper, or better at the same or reduced cost. Worse-value treatments are as good and more expensive, or worse and equal or more expensive.

**Validating studies test the quality of a specific diagnostic test, based on prior evidence. An exploratory study collects information and trawls the data (e.g., using a regression analysis) to find which factors are "significant."

***By poor quality prognostic cohort study, we mean one in which sampling was biased in favor of patients who already had the target outcome, or the measurement of outcomes was accomplished in less than 80% of study patients, or outcomes were determined in an unblinded, nonobjective way, or there was no correction for confounding factors.

****Good follow-up in a differential diagnosis study is greater than 80%, with adequate time for alternative diagnoses to emerge (e.g., 1–6 months acute, 1–5 years chronic).

Grades of recommendation

A   Consistent level 1 studies

B   Consistent level 2 or 3 studies *or* extrapolations from level 1 studies

C   Level 4 studies *or* extrapolations from level 2 or 3 studies

D   Level 5 evidence *or* troublingly inconsistent or inconclusive studies of any level

"Extrapolations" are where data is used in a situation that has potentially clinically important differences than the original study situation.

Kakehashi *et al.* (4) demonstrated the direct correlation between the presence of bacteria and pulpal and apical infection and disease. Sjogren *et al.* (1) showed that the bacteriological status of the root canal at the time of root canal obturation may be a critical factor in determining the outcome of endodontic treatment. Other studies have shown the importance of bacteria on the development of apical periodontitis (5, 6).

Bacteria elimination from root canals, specifically, the effect of irrigation, intracanal interappointment medication, and the effect of apical enlargement during root canal preparation have been investigated. In the subsequent sections, the elimination of bacteria from root canal systems by means of chemicals is discussed, along with the effect of this elimination of bacteria on the outcome of nonsurgical endodontic treatment. Using real-time polymerase chain reaction, it was found that root canals with primary infections contain higher bacterial loads and that chemomechanical root canal preparations can reduce bacterial counts by at least 95% (7).

Irrigation

Irrigation is one of the most important steps in endodontic therapy. It carries out many functions including tissue dissolution, lavage, killing of microorganisms, removal of debris, lubrication of the canal for instrumentation, and smear layer removal (8). Disruption of biofilms is an important factor in reducing endodontic infections (9–11).

The best solution to be used for irrigation has been extensively studied, but, in terms of strong clinical evidence, there is no conclusive evidence. Several solutions have been used ranging from water, saline, sodium hypochlorite (NaOCl), chlorhexidine (CHX), iodine potassium iodide, ethylenediaminetetraacetic acid (EDTA), hydrogen peroxide (H_2O_2), urea peroxide, citric acid, dequalinium acetate, and others (8). The most widely used irrigating solutions are sodium hypochlorite, chlorhexidine, and iodine potassium iodide; and the solution most widely used as a chelating agent for irrigation and for the removal of the inorganic portion of the smear layer is EDTA.

Sodium hypochlorite

NaOCl has a broad antimicrobial spectrum. It dissolves both necrotic and vital pulp tissue. It inactivates endotoxin and dissolves the organic portion of the smear layer (5).

The germicidal ability of NaOCl comes from the formation of hypochlorous acid when it contacts organic debris. Hypochlorous acid oxidizes the sulfhydryl groups of bacterial enzymes, disrupting metabolism(12). Hand *et al.* (13) found that 5.25% NaOCl was significantly more effective as a necrotic tissue solvent than 2.5% NaOCl, 1.0% NaOCl, 0.05% NaOCl, distilled water, normal saline solution, or 3% H_2O_2. Rosenfeld *et al.* (14) discovered that 5.25% NaOCl can dissolve vital pulp tissue, but the ability of NaOCl to dissolve tissues is limited in confined spaces, such as a root canal. Stojicic *et al.* (15) found that optimizing the concentration, temperature, flow, and surface tension can improve the tissue-dissolving effectiveness of NaOCl.

Chlorhexidine

Chlorhexidine (CHX) is a cationic bisbiguanide. Chlorhexidine's antibacterial action is possible following the absorption onto the bacterial surface and disruption of the cytoplasmic membrane (16). CHX solutions have been used as an irrigant, but are unable to dissolve necrotic tissue, and are less effective against gram-negative bacteria than gram-positive bacteria (5). CHX has good substantivity in root canals when used as an irrigant or medicament (17–20). CHX has good antimicrobial action both when used as an irrigant and as a medicament used in conjunction with calcium hydroxide (12, 21–24).

There is some controversy over whether *para*-chloroaniline is formed when CHX is used in combination with NaOCl (25–30).

Iodine potassium iodide

The molecular iodine (I_2) is the active portion of the solution. The iodine has a similar action as chlorine in sodium hypochlorite (31, 32). The iodine does not dissolve necrotic tissue (33); however, it is bactericidal, fungicidal, virucidal, and sporicidal, but to a lesser degree than sodium hypochlorite (34, 35). It is less cytotoxic than sodium hypochlorite (34, 36). Iodine potassium iodide does have a high allergic potential and may also stain dentin.

Clinical evidence to assess the effects of irrigants used in the nonsurgical root canal treatment of teeth

Although there are many studies on irrigants used in endodontics, documentation of the effect of the irrigants on clinical outcomes is lacking.

Fedorowicz et al. (37) performed a systematic review in the Cochrane review and performed a meta-analysis. They found that NaOCl and chlorhexidine are the commonly used irrigating solutions, but there is uncertainty as to which solution is the most effective.

Ng et al. (38) in a prospective study found that the addition of a rinse with 0.2% chlorhexidine with NaOCl irrigation did not improve the odds of success, but actually decreased the odds of success by 53%.

EDTA and other chelators

EDTA is a chelating agent that removes the inorganic portion of the smear layer, softens dentin, and facilitates the removal of calcific obstructions (39–42). The effects of EDTA on dentin may be self-limiting (43), but prolonged contact of EDTA with dentin for 10 min may cause the erosion of dentin (44). Although EDTA may have some antimicrobial activity, the ability of EDTA to remove smear layer and expose bacteria in dentinal tubules to other more potent antimicrobial agents may be its best quality (45–51).

Ng et al. (38), in a prospective study of the factors affecting the outcomes of nonsurgical root canal treatment, found that the use of an EDTA rinse followed with a final rinse of NaOCl had no significant improvement in the outcome of primary endodontic treatment, but it significantly increased the odds of healing by twofold for cases of secondary endodontic treatment.

Effects of various concentrations of solutions

The ultimate concentrations of these various irrigating solutions have also been investigated with regard to their ability to dissolve vital and necrotic tissue, kill microorganisms, remove debris, remove the smear layer, and their biocompatibility with host tissues.

One study compared three strengths of sodium hypochlorite, 1%, 2.5%, and 5% (52). The higher concentration reduced the number of canals with positive cultures. After final irrigation, 10 of 39 (25.8%) samples irrigated with 1% sodium hypochlorite still had positive cultures; 5 of 36 (13.7%) of samples irrigated with 2.5% sodium hypochlorite still had positive cultures; and only 2 out of 36 (6.6%) of samples irrigated with 5% sodium hypochlorite had positive cultures.

The volume of irrigating solution is thought by some to be a very important factor in the successful outcome of endodontically treated teeth, regardless of the solution or concentration. Baker et al. (53) found that the volume of irrigant used was more important than the solution and recommended using the most biologically acceptable irrigating solution. They found that there was no difference in the effectiveness of any solution tested in removing root canal debris. They examined different volumes of the following solutions: saline, 3% H_2O_2, 1% NaOCl, 15% EDTA, glyoxide, and RC-Prep (Premier Dental Products, Morristown, PA). It should be noted that the concentration of 1% NaOCl used was less compared to what many clinicians use in the clinical practice of endodontics. There is, however, general agreement that copious volumes of irrigation during treatment are important for many reasons, especially for the lavage of the area.

Fedorowicz et al. (37) in their systematic review could not find clinical evidence as to which concentration or combination of irrigating solutions would lead to a better clinical outcome.

Effect and efficacy of the delivery of irrigating solutions

Another factor to be considered is how the irrigating solution is delivered to the canal. This would include the depth of the irrigating needle penetration into the canal, size and design of the needle used for irrigation, sonic or ultrasonic agitation of the irrigating solution to produce acoustic streaming, and the use of positive or negative pressure irrigation. Related to the depth of irrigation is the size of canal preparation.

If the irrigating needle can reach the apical few millimeters of the canal, irrigation is more effective in debris removal (54, 55). The ability of the irrigating needle to reach the apical portion of the canal is dependent on the size of the preparation of the canal (55–58). Syringe irrigation has been found to be effective in canals with apical preparations 0.3 mm or greater, and ultrasonic irrigation with NaOCl was more effective than syringe irrigation (59). The 27-gauge notch-tip needle has been found to be effective in canals instrumented to size 30 and 35 (60). A brush-covered irrigating needle produced cleaner coronal thirds than conventional irrigation, as found in one study (61).

Sonic and ultrasonic irrigation, especially passive ultrasonic irrigation, has been found to help eliminate debris and bacteria from instrumented root canals, and is effective in the removal of tissue and debris from isthmus areas (62–67). One clinical study looked at the influence of passive sonic irrigation on the elimination of bacteria from root canal systems and found that there was no significant difference between sonic irrigation and standard syringe irrigation in eliminating bacteria from root canals, but multivisit treatment using calcium hydroxide as an intervisit medication did eliminate cultivable bacteria from canals more than the single visit group (68). One study compared passive ultrasonic irrigation to traditional irrigation, passive sonic irrigation, and apical negative pressure irrigation, and found that passive ultrasonic irrigation moved more irrigant into lateral canals than did the other methods of irrigation, but the apical negative pressure irrigation brought more irrigant into the apical extent of the canal (69).

Perazzi et al. (70) in a systematic review of the literature illustrates a "current lack of published or ongoing randomized controlled trials and the unavailability of high-level evidence, based on clinically relevant outcomes, for the effectiveness of ultrasonic instrumentation used alone or as an adjunct to hand instrumentation for orthograde root canal treatment."

The effectiveness of negative pressure irrigation has been studied and compared to other methods of irrigation. Many investigations have found negative pressure irrigation to be superior in terms of both debris removal and elimination of bacteria, particularly in the apical aspect of the canal (71–75). Cohenca et al. (76), in a randomized controlled clinical trial, found that taper and apical size failed to demonstrate a difference in microbiological reduction of cultivable bacteria, but did find that apical negative pressure irrigation showed a significant difference in the reduction of cultivable bacteria over traditional positive pressure irrigation. Others, who have examined debris removal and the removal of bacteria, have found no differences between negative pressure irrigation and other forms of irrigation (77, 78). One study found that the apical negative pressure irrigation allowed irrigant to reach the apical portions of the canal better than other irrigation regimens (69).

It is recognized that negative pressure irrigation is safer than other forms of irrigation with respect to decreasing or eliminating the possibility of apical extrusion of irrigants (79–81).

As the depth of irrigating needle penetration with traditional irrigation depends on the size of the canal preparation, so does irrigation with negative pressure irrigation (82). Preparation size should be at least to an ISO size 40 with a taper of 0.04 (83). Another study found that with negative pressure irrigation, an apical preparation size of 40 with a 0.06 taper significantly increased the volume and exchange of irrigant at the working length, regardless of canal curvature (84).

Gondim et al. (85) performed a randomized clinical trial to evaluate postoperative pain after irrigation by either endodontic needle irrigation or by negative apical pressure and found that the negative apical pressure device resulted in a significant reduction of postoperative pain as compared to the traditional needle irrigation.

Probably the most desirable quality of irrigating solutions and delivery of irrigating solutions is the elimination of bacteria from the root canal system. This may be easier to link to outcomes, because healing after obtaining a negative culture can be documented. Although obtaining a negative culture is only one of many possible factors determining outcomes, it is one that has been examined (1). Although there is little high-level clinical evidence, there is evidence to point to the fact that there are some clinical procedures that may lead to a significant reduction of bacteria within the root canal system. The use of an adequate volume of irrigant (53), such as sodium hypochlorite, at a sufficient concentration (52) to kill bacteria may lead to negative bacterial cultures. In order to improve the effectiveness of irrigation, it must reach the apical portions of the root canal (54, 55). For this to happen, mechanical preparation must be of sufficient size to allow deeper penetration of irrigating devices (55–58, 60), such as irrigating needles, ultrasonic or sonic devices, or negative pressure irrigation cannulas (76, 83, 84); and these devices need to be small enough to reach the apical 1–3 mm of the canal (54, 60, 69, 83). The combined use of a sodium hypochlorite with EDTA has been shown to be efficient in removing the smear layer and reducing bacterial cultures (38, 45–49, 51). Despite the lack of strong clinical evidence, the elimination of bacteria, through chemical irrigation, will remove the major etiological factor in apical periodontitis.

Although all of these aspects of irrigation have been studied *in-vitro*, on bench tops, and even *in-vivo* during animal and clinical studies, there are many confounding factors that make the comparisons difficult. Robust and specific randomized clinical trials are lacking, but very much needed.

Calcium hydroxide and other interappointment medicaments

Calcium hydroxide is the most widely used intracanal medicament. Other medications that have been used in endodontics include phenolic compounds, essential oils, aldehydes, halogens, quaternary ammonium compounds, antibiotics, and steroids.

Calcium hydroxide has a strong alkaline property with a pH of 12.5. It acts by dissociating in aqueous solution into calcium and hydroxyl ions. Some of the properties of calcium hydroxide including its antimicrobial activity, tissue-dissolving ability, and high pH may aid in inducing hard tissue repair and inhibiting resorption, although not all of these have been proven. The hydroxyl ions create free radicals that may destroy components of the bacterial wall and may also inhibit DNA replication and cell activity in the bacteria (86).

Sjogren *et al.* (87) found that a 7-day application of calcium hydroxide in teeth undergoing endodontic therapy effectively eliminated bacteria from the root canal system. Safavi and Nichols (88) found that calcium hydroxide hydrolyzes the lipid moiety of bacterial lipopolysaccharides in gram-negative bacteria. Calcium hydroxide may also denature proinflammatory cytokines and neuropeptides (89). Calcium hydroxide has also been reported to dissolve tissue, and the tissue-dissolving effect of NaOCl is enhanced with pretreatment with calcium hydroxide (90).

Calcium hydroxide has been shown to be effective in eliminating bacteria from root canals as evaluated by the reduction in bacterial counts, and an increase in negative cultures obtained (87, 91, 92). Another study reported the effects of instrumentation, NaOCl, EDTA, and calcium hydroxide on the reduction of intracanal bacteria and found calcium hydroxide in combination with other factors reduced bacteria within the canal (93).

Other studies have found only a moderate increase in the number of negative cultures, or an actual decrease in the number of negative cultures after interappointment medication with calcium hydroxide (94–96). One systematic review and meta-analysis of the use of calcium hydroxide as an intracanal dressing concluded that calcium hydroxide has limited effectiveness in eliminating bacteria from human root canals when assessed by culture techniques (97).

In a study examining the clinical efficacy of chemomechanical preparation of root canals with sodium hypochlorite and interappointment medication with calcium hydroxide in the control of root canal infection and healing of apical lesions in 1 year, it was found that only minor differences in apical healing were observed between the single visit group for which no calcium hydroxide was used, and the two visit group for which calcium hydroxide was used as a medicament between visits (98). It was found that there is good clinical efficacy of sodium hypochlorite irrigation in the control of root canal infection, and calcium hydroxide dressing between the appointments did not show the expected effect in the disinfection of the root canal system and treatment outcome, indicating the need to develop more efficient interappointment dressings.

Although there is controversy over the effectiveness of calcium hydroxide as an interappointment medicament, it remains the primary medicament to reduce, or at least contain, the number of bacteria between appointments. The usefulness of calcium hydroxide in the future, or some other medicament or combination of medicaments, still requires more studies and more extensive research, including more clinical trials conducted at a high level.

Apical preparation size

The optimal apical preparation size and its effect on treatment outcome is an area of significant interest and debate in endodontics. Two opposing viewpoints exist, with the two camps promoting either large or small apical preparation sizes (99, 100). The rationale for instrumenting to a larger apical size is to remove more bacteria, infected dentin, necrotic tissue, and debris, thus decreasing the risk of post-treatment apical inflammation and/or infection. The rationale for instrumenting to a smaller apical size is to conserve dentin and decrease the risk for subsequent root fracture (101, 102). The majority of research into the effect of apical preparation size on treatment outcome measures surrogate outcomes rather than clinical success. This limitation is likely due to the difficulties in performing high-quality randomized clinical trials with sufficient power on endodontic outcomes, as described earlier in this chapter. The results of these studies generally support the concept that larger apical preparation sizes result in fewer bacteria, bacterial by-products, and debris remaining in the apical portion of the canal. In addition, larger apical sizes result in a greater ability of irrigants to reach the working length of the canal.

Several studies have investigated the amount of debris remaining in the apical portion of the canal after instrumentation to different sizes (103–105). Usman and colleagues (105) instrumented matched pairs of teeth using GT rotary files to an apical size of 20 or 40 and measured the debris remaining after instrumentation using histological techniques at 0.5, 1.5, and 2.5 mm from working length. Teeth instrumented to a size 20 had significantly more debris remaining in the apical third than teeth

instrumented to a size 40 (105). Fornari *et al.* (104) investigated the influence of apical size on the cleaning of the apical third in curved canals. Mesiobuccal canals of maxillary molars were instrumented using 0.02 taper files to size 30, 35, 40, or 45, and the images were analyzed by histological techniques (104). Greater debris remained when teeth were instrumented to size 30 or 35, and there was a significant correlation between the amount of remaining debris and the amount of uninstrumented dentin in the apical third of the root (104). Albrecht *et al.* (103) instrumented teeth to a size 20 or 40 using GT files of varying tapers (0.04, 0.06, 0.08, and 0.10) and measured debris remaining after instrumentation using histological techniques. Significantly greater debris remained in teeth prepared to a size 20 compared to teeth prepared to a size 40 at 1 mm from the apex for all tapers, except 0.10 (103).

Other studies have investigated the amount of bacteria or bacterial by-products remaining in canals after instrumentation to different sizes. Marinho *et al.* (106) investigated the removal of endotoxin after instrumentation of mandibular premolars to progressively larger apical sizes (25/0.06, 30/0.05, 35/0.04, and 40/0.04). Significantly more endotoxin was removed after instrumenting to size 35/0.04 or 40/0.04 compared to size 25/0.06; however, the largest preparation size did not eliminate all endotoxin (106). Mickel and colleagues (107) investigated bacterial reduction in single-rooted extracted teeth after instrumentation to various sizes. The first file to reach working length in a crown down sequence was noted, and then teeth were instrumented to one, two, or three file sizes greater than this file (107). The proportion of teeth with negative bacterial cultures was significantly less after instrumenting to a master apical file size that was three file sizes larger than the first file to reach working length compared to teeth instrumented to one file size larger than the first file to reach working length (107). Rollison *et al.* (108) investigated the removal of radioactive labeled bacteria from canals of extracted teeth after instrumentation to an apical size of 35 or 50, and found that significantly more bacteria were removed when canals were instrumented to a size 50.

Despite multiples lines of evidence from preclinical studies that suggest that larger apical sizes result in more efficient root canal disinfection in the apical aspect of the canal, data do not exist from clinical studies to support the idea that this translates into more successful clinical outcomes. Kerekes and Tronstad (109) investigated the clinical success of over 400 roots treated by dental students in 1971 and found no statistically significant difference between roots treated to a size 20–40 reamer compared to a size 45–100 reamer. Hoskinson *et al.* (110) performed a retrospective evaluation of outcomes of 200 teeth treated by an endodontist and found no significant effect of master apical file size on treatment outcome 4–5 years after treatment. Orstavik and colleagues (111) performed a multivariate analysis on variables that may influence the outcome of endodontic treatment on 498 teeth treated by dental students. The size of reamer used did not have an effect on the outcome; however, teeth with chronic apical periodontitis were instrumented to significantly larger sizes than teeth without apical periodontitis (111). Negishi retrospectively evaluated the success of 114 cases and found no significant effect of master apical file size on treatment success (112). In a prospective study of the factors affecting the outcomes of nonsurgical root canal treatment, Ng and colleagues (113, 38) did not detect a significant effect of apical preparation size (categorized as ≤30 or >30) on either apical health or tooth survival after treatment. As previously stated, a caveat to interpreting the results of these clinical outcomes studies is that they are not designed as prospective, randomized clinical trial with sufficient power to detect differences between groups.

Working length

As with apical preparation size, there is debate in the endodontic community as to the ideal length to which canals should be instrumented and obturated. The rationale for instrumenting and obturating to a longer length is to ensure that the most apical extent of the canal has been cleaned and sealed. The rationale for instrumenting and obturating to a shorter length is to preserve the integrity of the apical tissues and avoid debris extrusion or overfilling the canal. Clinicians' preferences tend to vary between treating to the radiographic apex or the "foramen" reading on an electronic apex locator, up to 0.5 to 1 mm short of one of

these levels. In a review, Wu and colleagues (114) recommended treatment be terminated 2–3 mm short of the radiographic apex in vital cases, and 0–2 mm from the radiographic apex in cases of pulpal necrosis. Several outcomes studies have investigated the influence of the working length on treatment success. However, it should be noted that most of these studies actually measure the level of obturation, not the intended working length (which in most cases should be the same length, unless an error occurred during obturation). Orstavik and colleagues (111) found that the apex-to-filling distance had a significant effect on treatment outcome, with the optimal distance being defined as 0–2 mm. Sjogren *et al.* (115) reported that the level to which a canal could be instrumented had a significant effect on prognosis in necrotic cases; 90% of lesions healed when the canal could be instrumented to the apical constriction, but only 69% of cases healed when the canal could not be instrumented to the apical constriction. The level of obturation also had a significant effect on the outcome in necrotic cases with an apical lesion; 94% of cases that were filled to within 2 mm of the apex healed, but only 76% of cases that were overfilled and 68% of cases that were underfilled healed (115). Peak and colleagues (116) found that root fillings that were less than 2 mm from the radiographic apex had a greater success rate (88%) compared to teeth where the filling was greater than 2 mm from the apex (77%), in a retrospective study of teeth that had been filled for at least 12 months. However, teeth that were overfilled also had a success rate (88%) comparable to those filled less than 2 mm from the apex in this study (116). Ng and colleagues (38) conducted a prospective study of the factors affecting the outcomes of nonsurgical root canal treatment, and they found that the extension of canal cleaning as close as possible to the apical terminus had a significant effect on apical healing. In a systematic review, Ng *et al.* (117) found that root filling extending to within 2 mm of the radiographic apex had a significant positive effect on the outcome of root canal treatment. However, the majority of these studies did not look at obturation level in more detail than the range of 0–2 mm from the radiographic apex, and debate still exists as to what is the ideal working length within that range.

1 versus 2 visits

There is also great debate in the field of endodontics about the number of visits in which root canal treatment should be completed. Consensus exists that a tooth with a vital pulp may have root canal therapy completed in one visit (if time permits) and if the canals are not infected. Consensus also generally exists that teeth should not be obturated when the patient has swelling or the canal cannot be dried because of exudate seepage from the apical tissues. In these cases, the clinician should wait until the swelling has reduced and the canal can be dried completely prior to obturation. However, Southard and Rooney (118) described a one-visit protocol for treating a tooth with an acute apical abscess, which included an incision and drainage prior to root canal therapy as well as prescribing an antibiotic for these patients.

There is disagreement, however, on whether necrotic teeth with asymptomatic apical periodontitis, symptomatic apical periodontitis, or a chronic apical abscess should be treated with single- or multiple-visit root canal therapy. At the core of this debate are the principles of disinfection of the root canal system. The rationale for completing treatment in two visits is that the intracanal medicament placed between visits facilitates disinfection of the root canal system. Sjogren and colleagues (1) investigated the role of infection at the time of obturation in teeth that were treated in one visit; teeth were sampled for bacteria prior to obturation, and all teeth were treated in one visit. Teeth were followed for 5 years, and complete healing occurred in 94% of cases with a negative culture prior to obturation and in 68% of cases with a positive culture prior to obturation. The authors emphasized the importance of completely eliminating bacteria from the root canal system prior to obturation. In a prospective cohort study of a large number of endodontic treatments performed by one operator and followed for 5 years, it was found that when treating teeth with necrotic pulps, teeth treated with a calcium hydroxide intracanal medicament over multiple visits had a significantly better outcome than those treated in a single visit (119).

Despite the sound scientific rationale for completing root canal therapy of necrotic teeth in two visits using an intracanal medicament between visits, the available outcomes studies do not support the idea that two-visit treatment results in a better prognosis. Penesis et al. (120) conducted a randomized clinical trial of treatment of necrotic teeth with apical periodontitis. Sixty-three patients were evaluated after treatment in one visit or two visits with a calcium hydroxide/chlorhexidine intracanal interappointment medicament, and no significant difference was detected in the radiographic healing of these teeth 1 year after treatment (120). In a randomized clinical trial of asymptomatic necrotic teeth with apical periodontitis treated in one or two visits using a calcium hydroxide interappointment medicament, there was no significant difference in clinical and radiographic outcomes 2 years after treatment in 89 teeth (121). Peters and Wesselink (122) evaluated the apical healing of 39 teeth treated in one visit or two visits with a calcium hydroxide intracanal medicament; no significant difference in healing rate was observed. Weiger et al. (123) conducted a prospective study of teeth with a necrotic pulp and apical radiolucency treated in one visit or two visits with a calcium hydroxide intracanal medicament. Of the 67 teeth followed, there was no significant difference in healing rate between groups (123). Trope and colleagues (124) evaluated radiographic healing of teeth with apical periodontitis treated in one visit or two visits with or without a calcium hydroxide intracanal dressing. There was no significant difference in the healing rate between teeth treated in one visit or in two visits with a calcium hydroxide intracanal dressing; however, teeth treated in two visits and left empty between visits had worse results than either of the other two groups (124). In the Toronto Study, no significant difference in the healing rate for 4–6 years was observed after the treatment of teeth treated in one visit compared to two or more visits (125).

Despite the many studies finding no difference in outcomes between one- and two-visit treatment, it should be recognized that these studies are limited in power. In fact, a systematic review and meta-analysis of single- versus multiple-visit treatment of teeth with apical periodontitis found only three randomized clinical trials that could be included, totaling only 146 cases (126). In a Cochrane systematic review, 12 randomized or quasi-randomized clinical trials were included to look at differences in single- versus multiple-visit endodontic treatment, and no significant difference in radiological success of treatment was observed

(127). In another systematic review, Ng and colleagues (117) found no significant effect of the number of treatment visits on radiographic success of root canal therapy. Finally, Su and colleagues (128) performed a systematic review of the healing rate of single- versus multiple-visit treatment of infected root canals and found no significant difference in the healing rate of single- versus multiple-visit treatment.

Preoperative diagnosis

Of the many factors that have been investigated as having potential effects on the prognosis of root canal therapy, the preoperative diagnosis is one that has repeatedly been shown to have a significant effect on outcome. Teeth with preoperative apical radiolucencies have a poorer prognosis than teeth without preoperative apical radiolucencies. This has been demonstrated in several classic studies as well as the contemporary literature and a systematic review. The scientific rationale for this well-documented impact on prognosis stems from the fact that teeth with an apical radiolucency are believed to be infected, whereas teeth without an apical radiolucency may or may not be infected. Thus, teeth with an apical radiolucency would be more difficult to disinfect than teeth with intact apical tissues. In a systematic review and meta-analysis of the literature, Ng and colleagues (117) found 49 studies published between 1922 and 2002 that investigated the effect of apical status on outcome. They concluded that the preoperative absence of an apical radiolucency significantly improved the outcome of root canal treatment (117). Additional studies published since 2002 have corroborated these results. Marending *et al.* (129) found that the initial periapical index (PAI) (23) score had a significant effect on the treatment outcome, with scores of 1 or 2 ("sound" teeth) being predictive of treatment success, also assessed by the PAI. In a prospective study of factors affecting the outcomes of nonsurgical root canal treatment, Ng and colleagues (38) found that factors that significantly increased the probability of apical healing were the absence of an apical lesion, and in the presence of one, the smaller its size. In addition, the results of the Toronto Study demonstrated that teeth without a preoperative apical radiolucency had a higher rate of healing than teeth with a preoperative apical radiolucency (125).

Glossary of Evidence-Based Terms

Case-controlled studies: are studies in which patients who already have a certain condition are compared with people who do not have. Case-controlled studies are less reliable than either randomized controlled trials or cohort studies. Just because there is a statistical relationship between two conditions, it does not mean that one condition actually caused the other.

Case series and case reports: consists either of collection of reports on the treatment of individual patients or of reports on a single patient. Because they use no control group with which to compare outcomes, case series and case reports have no statistical validity.

Cochrane Collaboration: is an international endeavor in which people from different countries systematically find, appraise, and review available evidence from randomized controlled trials (RCT). The Cochrane Collaboration's aims are to develop and maintain systematic, up-to-date reviews of RCTs of all forms of health care and to make this information readily available to clinicians and other decision makers at all levels of health care systems. (http://www.cochrane.org).

Cochrane Database of Systematic Reviews: include the full text of the regularly updated systematic reviews of the effects of health care prepared by the Cochrane Collaboration. The reviews are presented in two types: Complete reviews, and regularly updated Cochrane Reviews, prepared and maintained by Collaborative Review Groups, and Protocols, for reviews currently being prepared (including the expected date of completion). Protocols refer to the background, objectives, and methods of review in preparation.

Cohort Study: a study in which patients who currently have a certain condition, and/or receive a particular treatment are followed up over time and compared with another group who are not affected by the condition under investigation. The disadvantage of cohort studies is that they can take a very long time waiting for the conditions of interest to develop.

Critical appraisal: the process of assessing and interpreting evidence, by systematically considering its validity, results, and relevance to your own work.

Cross-sectional study: an observational study that examines a characteristic (or set of characteristics) and a health outcome in a sample of people at one point in time.

Double-blind study: is one in which neither the patient nor the provider knows whether the patient is receiving the treatment of interest or the control treatment. A double-blind study is the most rigorous clinical research design because, in addition to the randomization of subject that reduces the risk of bias, it can eliminate the placebo effect that is a further challenge to the validity of a study.

Meta-analysis: a statistical process commonly used with systematic reviews. Meta-analysis involves combining the statistical analyses and summarizing the results of several individual studies into one analysis. When data from multiple studies are pooled, the sample size and power usually increase.

Publication bias: results from the fact that studies with "positive" results are more likely to be published than those showing no difference or a negative result.

Randomized controlled trial (RCT): a trial in which subjects are randomly assigned to two groups: one (the experimental group) receiving the intervention that is being tested and the other (the comparison group or controls) receiving an alternative treatment. The two groups are then followed to see if any differences between them result.

Systematic reviews: considered the gold standard for evidence, these reviews provide a summary of individual research studies that have investigated the same phenomenon or question. This scientific technique uses explicit criteria for the retrieval. Assessment and synthesis of evidence from individual randomized controlled trials and other well-controlled methods. Systematic reviews provide a way of managing large quantities of information.

Validity: refers to the soundness or rigor of a study. A Study is valid when the way it is designed and carried out gives results that are unbiased—that is, it gives you a "true" estimate of clinical effectiveness.

References

1. Sjogren, U., Figdor, D., Persson, S. & Sundqvist, G. (1997) Influence of infection at the time of root filling on the outcome of endodontic treatment of teeth with apical periodontitis. *International Endodontic Journal*, **30 (5)**, 297–306.

2. Nair, P.N. (2006) On the causes of persistent apical periodontitis: a review. *International Endodontic Journal*, **39**, 249–281.

3. Friedman S. (2008) Expected outcomes in the prevention and treatment of apical periodontitis IN: *Essential Endodontology*. 2nd ed. Ames, Iowa: Blackwell Publishing Professional. 62 p.

4. Kakehashi, S., Stanley, H.R. & Fitzgerald, R.J. (1965) The effects of surgical exposures of dental pulps in germ-free and conventional laboratory rats. *Oral Surgery*, **20**, 340–348.

5. Siqueira, J.F. Jr., Rocas, I.N., Alves, F.R. & Silva, M.G. (2009) Bacteria in the apical root canal of teeth with primary apical periodontitis. *Oral Surgery, Oral Medicine, Oral Pathology, Oral Radiology, and Endodontics*, **107 (5)**, 721–726.

6. Sundqvist, G. (1992) Ecology of the root canal flora. *Journal of Endodontics*, **18 (9)**, 427–430.

7. Blome, B., Braun, A., Sobarzo, V. & Jepsen, S. (2008) Molecular identification and quantification of bacteria from endodontic infections using real-time polymerase chain reaction. *Oral Microbiology and Immunology*, **23**, 384–390.

8. Zehnder, M. (2006) Root canal irrigants. *Journal of Endodontics*, **32 (5)**, 389–398.

9. Svensater, G. & Bergenholtz, G. (2004) Biofilms in endodontic infection. *Endodontic Topics*, **9**, 27–36.

10. Chavez de Paz, L.E. (2007) Redefining the persistent infection in root canals: possible role of biofilm communities. *Journal of Endodontics*, **33**, 652–662.

11. Ricucci, D. & Siqueira, J.F.J. (2010) Biofilms and apical periodontitis: study of prevalence and association with clinical and histopathologic findings. *Journal of Endodontics*, **36**, 1277–1288.

12. Ohara, P., Torabinejad, M. & Kettering, J.D. (1993) Antibacterial effects of various endodontic irrigants on selected anaerobic bacteria. *Endodontics and Dental Traumatology*, **9 (3)**, 95–100.

13. Hand, R.E., Smith, M.L. & Harrison, J.W. (1978) Analysis of the effect of dilution on the necrotic tissue dissolution property of sodium hypochlorite. *Journal of Endodontics*, **4**, 60–64.

14. Rosenfeld EF, James GA, Burch BS. (1978) Vital pulp tissue response to sodium hypochlorite. *Journal of Endodontics* **4**:140–146.

15. Stojicic, S., Zivkovic, S., Qian, W., Zhang, H. & Haapasalo, M. (2010) Tissue dissolution by sodium hypochlorite: effect of concentration, temperature, agitation, and surfactant. *Journal of Endodontics*, **36**, 1558–1562.

16. Johnson, B.T. (1995) Uses of chlorhexidine in dentistry. *General Dentistry*, **3**, 126–140.

17. Weber, C.D., McClanahan, S.M., Miller, G.A., Diener-West, M. & Johnson, J.D. (2003) The effect of passive ultrasonic activation of 2% chlorhexidine or 5.25% sodium hypochlorite irrigant on residual antimicrobial activity in root canals. *Journal of Endodontics*, **29**, 562–564.

18. Rosenthal S, Spangberg L, Safavi K. Chlorhexidine substantivity in root canal dentin. (2004) *Oral Surgery, Oral Medicine, Oral Pathology, Oral Radiology, and Endodontics* 96:488–492.

19. Souza, M., Cecchin, D., Farina, A.P. *et al.* (2012) Evaluation of chlorhexidine substantivity on human dentin: a chemical analysis. *Journal of Endodontics*, **38**, 1249–1252.

20. White, R.R., Hays, G.L. & Janer, L.R. (1997) Residual antimicrobial activity after canal irrigation with chlorhexidine. *Journal of Endodontics*, **23**, 229–231.

21. Jeansonne MJ, White RR. A comparison of 2.0% chlorhexidine gluconate and 5.25% sodium hypochlorite as antimicrobial endodontic irrigants. (1994) *Journal of Endodontics*. **20**(6):276–278.

22. Zamany A, Safavi K, Spangberg LS. The effect of chlorhexidine as an endodontic disinfectant. *Oral Surgery, Oral Medicine, Oral Pathology, Oral Radiology, and Endodontics* 2003;96:578–581.

23. Siqueira JF Jr, Paiva SS, Rocas IN. Reduction in the cultivable bacterial populations in infected root canals by a chlorhexidine-based antimicrobial protocol. (2007) *Journal of Endodontics*. 33:541–547.

24. Oliveira, D.P., Barbizam, J.V., Trope, M. & Teixeira, F.B. (2007) *In vitro* antibacterial efficacy of endodontic irrigants against *Enterococcus faecalis*. *Oral Surgery, Oral Medicine, Oral Pathology, Oral Radiology, and Endodontics*, **103**, 702–706.

25. Basrani, B.R., Manek, S. & Fillery, E. (2009) Using diazotization to characterize the effect of heat or sodium hypochlorite on 2.0% chlorhexidine. *Journal of Endodontics*, **35**, 1296–1299.

26. Basrani, B.R., Manek, S., Mathers, D., Fillery, E. & Sodhi, R.N. (2010) Determination of 4-chloroaniline and its derivatives formed in the interaction of sodium hypochlorite and chlorhexidine by using gas chromatography. *Journal of Endodontics*, **36**, 312–314.

27. Bui, T.B., Baumgartner, J.C. & Mitchell, J.C. (2008) Evaluation of sodium hypochlorite and chlorhexidine gluconate and its effect on root dentin. *Journal of Endodontics*, **34** (2), 181–185.

28. Thomas, J.E. & Sem, D.S. (2010) An *in vitro* spectroscopic analysis to determine whether para-chloroaniline is produced from mixing sodium hypochlorite and chlorhexidine. *Journal of Endodontics*, **36**, 315–317.

29. Nowicki, J.B. & Sem, D.S. (2011) An *in vitro* spectroscopic analysis to determine the chemical composition of the precipitate formed by mixing sodium hypochlorite and chlorhexidine. *Journal of Endodontics*, **37**, 983–988.

30. Mortenson, D., Sadilek, M., Flake, N.M. *et al.* (2012) The effect of using an alternative irrigant between sodium hypochlorite and chlorhexidine to prevent the formation of para-chloroaniline within the root canal system. *International Endodontic Journal*, **36**, 312–314.

31. Waltimo, T. & Zehnder, M. (2009) Topical antimicrobials in endodontic therapy. In: Fouad, A.F. (ed), *Endodontic Microbiology*. Wiley-Blackwell, Ames, Iowa, pp. 242–260.

32. MacDonnell G, Russell AD. Antiseptics and disinfectants: activity, action, and resistance. (1999) *Clinical Microbiology Reviews*. **12**:147–179.

33. Naenni, N., Thomas, K. & Zehnder, M. (2004) Soft tissue dissolution capacity of currently used and potential endodontic irrigants. *Journal of Endodontics*, **30**, 785–787.

34. Engstrom, B. & Spangberg, L. (1969) Toxic and antimicrobial effects of antiseptics *in vitro*. *Svensk Tandläkare Tidskrift*, **62**, 543–549.

35. Safavi, K., Dowden, W.E., Introcaso, J. & Langland, K. (1985) A comparison of antimicrobial effects of calcium hydroxide and iodine–potassium iodide. *Journal of Endodontics*, **11**, 454–456.

36. Engstrom, B. & Spangberg, L. (1967) Studies on root canal medicaments. II. Cytotoxic effect of root canal antiseptics. *Acta Odontologica Scandinavica*, **25**, 77–84.

37. Fedorowicz, Z., Nasser, M., Sequeira-Byron, P., de Souza, R.F., Carter, B. & Heft, M. (2012) Irrigants for non-surgical root canal treatment in mature permanent teeth (Review). *Cochrane Database of Systematic Reviews*, Cochrane Collaboration, The Cochrane Library, Issue 9. http://www.thecochranelibrary.com.

38. Ng, Y.L., Mann, V. & Gulabivala, K. (2011) A prospective study of the factors affecting outcomes of nonsurgical root canal treatment: part 1: periapical health. *International Endodontic Journal*, **44** (7), 583–609.

39. McComb, D. & Smith, D.C. (1975) A preliminary scanning electron microscope study of root canals after endodontic procedures. *Journal of Endodontics*, **1**, 238–242.

40. Yamada, R.S., Armas, A., Goldman, M. & Lim, P.S. (1983) A scanning electron microscope comparison of high volume flush with several irrigating solutions: part 3. *Journal of Endodontics*, **9**, 137–142.

41. Mader, C.L., Baumgartner, J.C. & Peters, D.D. (1984) Scanning electron microscope investigation of the smeared layer on root canal walls. *Journal of Endodontics*, **10**, 477–483.

42. Baumgartner, J.C. & Mader, C.L. (1987) A scanning electron microscopic evaluation of four root canal irrigation regimens. *Journal of Endodontics*, **13**, 147–157.

43. Seidberg, B.H. & Schilder, H. (1974) An evaluation of EDTA in endodontics. *Oral Surgery*, **37**, 609–620.

44. Calt, S. & Serper, A. (2002) Time-dependent effects of EDTA on dentin structures. *Journal of Endodontics*, **28** (**1**), 17–19.

45. Heling, I., Irani, E., Karni, S. & Steinberg, D. (1999) *In vitro* antimicrobial effect of RC-Prep within dentin tubules. *Journal of Endodontics*, **25**, 782–785.

46. Yoshida, T., Shibata, T., Shinohara, T., Gomyo, S. & Sekine, I. (1995) Clinical evaluation of the efficacy of EDTA solution as an endodontic irrigation. *Journal of Endodontics*, **21**, 592–593.

47. Patterson, S.S. (1963) *In vivo* and *in vitro* studies of the effect of the disodium salt of ethylenediamine tetra-acetic acetate on human dentin and its endodontic implications. *Oral Surgery, Oral Medicine, and Oral Pathology*, **16**, 83–103.

48. Ruff, M.L., McClanahan, S.M. & Babel, B.S. (2006) *In vitro* antifungal efficacy of four irrigants as a final rinse. *Journal of Endodontics*, **32**, 331–333.

49. Chandra, S.S., Miglani, R., Srinivasan, M.R. & Indira, R. (2010) Antifungal efficacy of 5.25% sodium hypochlorite, 2% chlorhexidine gluconate, and 17% EDTA with and without an antifungal agent. *Journal of Endodontics*, **36**, 675–678.

50. Yang, S.E., Cha, J.H., Kim, E.S., Kum, K.Y., Lee, C.Y. & Jung, I.Y. (2006) Effect of smear layer and chlorhexidine treatment on the adhesion of *Enterococcus faecalis* to bovine dentin. *Journal of Endodontics*, **31**, 663–667.

51. Bystrom, A. & Sundqvist, G. (1985) The antibacterial action of sodium hypochlorite and EDTA in 60 cases of endodontic therapy. *International Endodontic Journal*, **18**, 35–40.

52. Soares, J.A. & Pires Junior, D.R. (2006) Influence of sodium hypochlorite-based irrigants on the susceptibility of intracanal microbiota to biomechanical preparations. *Brazilian Dental Journal*, **17** (**4**), 310–316.

53. Baker, N.A., Eleazer, P.D., Averbach, R.E. & Seltzer, S. (1975) Scanning electron microscopic study of the efficacy of various irrigating solutions. *Journal of Endodontics*, **1**, 127–135.

54. Abou-Rass, M. & Piccinino, M.V. (1982) The effectiveness of four clinical irrigation methods on the removal of root canal debris. *Oral Surgery*, **54**, 323–328.

55. Sedgley, C.M., Nagel, A.C., Hall, D. & Applegate, B. (2005) Influence of irrigant needle depth in removing bioluminescent bacteria inoculated into instrumented root canals using real-time imaging *in vitro*. *International Endodontic Journal*, **38** (**2**), 97–104.

56. Falk, K.W. & Sedgley, C.M. (2005) The influence of preparation size on the mechanical efficacy of root canal irrigation in vitro. *Journal of Endodontics*, **31**, 742–745.

57. Khademi, A., Yazdizadeh, M. & Feizianfard, M. (2006) Determination of the minimum instrumentation size for penetration of irrigants to the apical third of root canal systems. *Journal of Endodontics*, **32**, 417–420.

58. Boutsioukis, C., Gogos, C., Verhaagen, B., Versluis, M., Kastrinakis, E. & Van der Sluis, L.W. (2010) The effect of apical preparation size on irrigant flow in root canals evaluated using an unsteady computational fluid dynamics model. *International Endodontic Journal*, **43** (**10**), 874–881.

59. Teplitsky, P.E., Chenail, B.L., Mack, B. & Machnee, C.H. (1987) Endodontic irrigation – a comparison of endosonic and syringe delivery systems. *International Endodontic Journal*, **20**, 233–241.

60. Kahn, F.H., Rosenberg, P.A. & Glicksberg, J. (1995) An *in vitro* evaluation of the irrigating characteristics of ultrasonic and subsonic handpieces and irrigating needles and probes. *Journal of Endodontics*, **21** (**5**), 277–280.

61. Al-Hadlaq SM, Al-Turaiki SA, Al-Sulami U, Saad AY. (2006) Efficacy of a new brush-covered irrigation needle in removing root canal debris: a scanning electron microscopic study. *Journal of Endodontics*. **32**:1181–1184.

62. Archer R, Reader A, Nist R, Beck M, Meyers WJ. An in vitro evaluation of the efficacy of ultrasound after step-back preparation in mandibular molars. *Journal of Endodontics* 1992;**18**:549–552.

63. Gutarts, R., Nusstein, J., Reader, A. & Beck, M. (2005) In vivo debridement efficacy of ultrasonic irrigation following hand-rotary instrumentation in human mandibular molars. *Journal of Endodontics*, **31**, 166–170.

64. Burleson, A., Nusstein, J., Reader, A. & Beck, M. (2007) The in vivo evaluation of hand/rotary/ultrasound instrumentation in necrotic, human mandibular molars. *Journal of Endodontics*, **33** (**7**), 782–787.

65. Jensen, S.A., Walker, T.L., Hutter, J.W. & Nicoll, B.K. (1999) Comparison of the cleaning efficacy of passive sonic activation and passive ultrasonic activation after hand instrumentation in molar root canals. *Journal of Endodontics*, **25**, 735–738.

66. Sabins, R.A., Johnson, J.D. & Hellstein, J.W. (2003) A comparison of the cleaning efficacy of short-term sonic and ultrasonic passive irrigation after hand instrumentation in molar root canals. *Journal of Endodontics*, **29**, 674–678.

67. Spoleti, P., Siragusa, M. & Spoleti, M.J. (2003) Bacteriological evaluation of passive ultrasonic activation. *Journal of Endodontics*, **29**, 12–14.

68. Huffaker, S.K., Safavi, K., Spangberg, L.S. & Kaufman, B. (2010) Influence of a passive sonic irrigation system on the elimination of bacteria from root canal systems: a clinical study. *Journal of Endodontics*, **36 (8)**, 1315–1318.

69. de Gregorio C, Estevez R, Cisneros R, Paranjpe A, Cohenca N. (2010) Efficacy of different irrigation and activation systems on the penetration of sodium hypochlorite into simulated lateral canals and up to working length: an *in vitro* study. *Journal of Endodontics*. **36**:1216–1221.

70. Pedrazzi, V., Oliveira-Neto, J.M., Sequeira, P., Fedorowicz, Z. & Nasser, M. (2008) Hand and ultrasonic instrumentation for orthograde root canal treatment of permanent teeth (Review). *The Cochrane Database of Systematic Reviews, Journal of applied oral science*. **18(3)**:268–272

71. Nielsen, B.A. & Baumgartner, J.C. (2007) Comparison of the endovac system to needle irrigation of root canals. *Journal of Endodontics*, **33**, 611–615.

72. Hockett, J.L., Dommisch, J.K., Johnson, J.D. & Cohenca, N. (2008) Antimicrobial efficacy of two irrigation techniques in tapered and nontapered canal preparations: an in vitro study. *Journal of Endodontics*, **34**, 1374–1377.

73. Siu, C. & Baumgartner, J.C. (2010) Comparison of the debridement efficacy of the endovac irrigation system and conventional needle root canal irrigation in vivo. *Journal of Endodontics*, **36 (11)**, 1782–1785.

74. Fukumoto, Y., Kikuchi, I., Yoshioka, T., Kobayashi, C. & Suda, H. (2006) An *ex vivo* evaluation of a new root canal irrigation technique with intracanal aspiration. *International Endodontic Journal*, **39**, 93–99.

75. Brito PR, Souza LC, Machado de Oliveira JC, Alves FR, De-Deus G, Lopes HP, et al. (2009) Comparison of the effectiveness of three irrigation techniques in reducing intracanal Enterococcus faecalis populations: an in vitro study. *Journal of Endodontics*. **35**:1422–1427.

76. Cohenca, N., Paranjpe, A., Heilborn, C. & Johnson, J.D. (2013) Antimicrobial efficacy of two irrigation techniques in tapered and non-tapered canal preparations. A randomized controlled clinical trial. *Quintessence International*, **44**, 217–228.

77. Miller, T.A. & Baumgartner, J.C. (2010) Comparison of the antimicrobial efficacy of irrigation using the Endovac to endodontic needle delivery. *Journal of Endodontics*, **36**, 509–511.

78. Pawar R, Alqaied A, Safavi K, Boyko J, Kaufman B. (2012) Influence of an apical negative pressure irrigation system on bacterial elimination during endodontic therapy: a prospective randomized clinical study. *Journal of Endodontics*. **38**:1177–1181.

79. Mitchell RP, Yang SE, Baumgartner JC. (2010) Comparison of apical extrusion of NaOCl using the Endovac or needle irrigation of root canals. *Journal of Endodontics*. **36**:338–341.

80. Desai, P. & Himel, V. (2009) Comparative safety of various intracanal irrigation systems. *Journal of Endodontics*, **35**, 545–549.

81. Mitchell, R.P., Baumgartner, J.C. & Sedgley, C.M. (2011) Apical extrusion of sodium hypochlorite using different root canal irrigation systems. *Journal of Endodontics*, **37**, 1677–1681.

82. Shin SJ, Kim HK, Jung IY, Lee CY, Lee SJ, Kim E. (2010) Comparison of the cleaning efficacy of a new apical negative pressure irrigating system with conventional irrigation needles in the root canals. *Oral Surgery, Oral Medicine, Oral Pathology, Oral Radiology, and Endodontics*. **109**:479–484.

83. Brunson M, Heilborn C, Johnson JD, Cohenca N. (2010) Effect of apical preparation size and preparation taper on irrigant volume delivered by using negative pressure irrigation system. *Journal of Endodontics*. **36**:721–724.

84. de Gregorio, C., Arias, A., Navarrete, N., Del Rio, V., Oltra, E. & Cohenca, N. (2013) Effect of apical size and taper on volume of irrigant delivered at working length with apical negative pressure at different root curvatures. *Journal of Endodontics*, **39**, 119–124.

85. Gondim, E. Jr., Setzer, F.C., Dos Carmo, C.B. & Kim, S. (2010) Postoperative pain after the application of two different irrigation devices in a prospective randomized clinical trial. *Journal of Endodontics*, **36 (8)**, 1295–1301.

86. Siqueira JF, Lopes HP. (1999) Mechanisms of antimicrobial activity of calcium hydroxide: a critical review. *International Endodontic Journal*. **32**: 361–369.

87. Sjogren U, Figdor D, Spangberg L, Sundqvist G. (1991) The antimicrobial effect of calcium hydroxide as a short-term intracanal dressing. *International Endodontic Journal*. **24**:119–125.

88. Safavi, K.E. & Nichols, F.C. (1993) Effect of calcium hydroxide on bacterial lipopolysaccharides. *Journal of Endodontics*, **19** (2), 76–78.

89. Khan, A.A., Sun, X. & Hargreaves, K.M. (2008) Effect of calcium hydroxide on proinflammatory cytokines and neuropeptides. *Journal of Endodontics*, **34**, 1360–1363.

90. Hasselgren, G., Olsson, B. & Cvek, M. (1988) Effects of calcium hydroxide and sodium hypochlorite on the dissolution of necrotic porcine muscle tissue. *Journal of Endodontics*, **14**, 125–127.

91. Bystrom, A., Claesson, R. & Sundquist, G. (1985) The antibacterial effect of camphorated paramonochlorophenol, camphorated phenol and calcium hydroxide in the treatment of infected root canals. *Endodontics and Dental Traumatology*, **1**, 170–175.

92. Bystrom, A., Happonen, R.P., Sjogren, U. & Sundqvist, G. (1987) Healing of periapical lesions of pulpless teeth after endodontic treatment with controlled asepsis. *Endodontics and Dental Traumatology*, **3**, 58–63.

93. McGurkin-Smith, R., Trope, M., Caplan, D. & Sigurdsson, A. (2005) Reduction of intracanal bacteria using GT rotary instrumentation, 5.25% NaOCl, EDTA, and Ca(OH)$_2$. *Journal of Endodontics*, **31**, 359–363.

94. Molander A, Reit C, Dahlen G. (1999) The antimicrobial effect of calcium hydroxide in root canals pretreated with 5% iodine potassium iodide. *Endodontics and Dental Traumatology*. **15**:205–209.

95. Orstavik, D., Kerekes, K. & Molven, O. (1991) Effects of extensive apical reaming and calcium hydroxide dressing on bacterial infection during treatment of apical periodontitis: a pilot study. *International Endodontic Journal*, **24**, 1–7.

96. Kvist, T., Molander, A., Dahlen, G. & Reit, C. (2004) Microbiological evaluation of one- and two-visit endodontic treatment of teeth with apical periodontitis: a randomized, clinical trial. *Journal of Endodontics*, **30**, 572–576.

97. Sathorn, C., Parashos, P. & Messer, H. (2007) Antibacterial efficacy of calcium hydroxide intracanal dressing: a systematic review and meta-analysis. *International Endodontic Journal*, **40**, 2–10.

98. Waltimo, T., Trope, M., Haapasalo, M. & Orstavik, D. (2005) Clinical efficacy of treatment procedures in endodontic infection control and one year follow-up of periapical healing. *Journal of Endodontics*, **31**, 683–686.

99. Buchanan, L. & Senia, E. (2010) The 2010 AAE debate continues. *Endodontic Practice*, **3** (4), 18–34.

100. Trope, M. (2010) The Buchanan-Senia debate: who won? *Endodontic Practice*, **3** (4), 1.

101. Mireku, A.S., Romberg, E., Fouad, A.F. & Arola, D. (2010) Vertical fracture of root filled teeth restored with posts: the effects of patient age and dentin thickness. *International Endodontic Journal*, **43** (3), 218–225, Epub 2010/02/18.

102. Wilcox, L.R., Roskelley, C. & Sutton, T. (1997) The relationship of root canal enlargement to finger-spreader induced vertical root fracture. *Journal of Endodontics*, **23** (8), 533–534, Epub 1997/08/01.

103. Albrecht, L.J., Baumgartner, J.C. & Marshall, J.G. (2004) Evaluation of apical debris removal using various sizes and tapers of ProFile GT files. *Journal of Endodontics*, **30** (6), 425–428, Epub 2004/05/29.

104. Fornari, V.J., Silva-Sousa, Y.T., Vanni, J.R., Pecora, J.D., Versiani, M.A. & Sousa-Neto, M.D. (2010) Histological evaluation of the effectiveness of increased apical enlargement for cleaning the apical third of curved canals. *International Endodontic Journal*, **43** (11), 988–994, Epub 2010/08/21.

105. Usman, N., Baumgartner, J.C. & Marshall, J.G. (2004) Influence of instrument size on root canal debridement. *Journal of Endodontics*, **30** (2), 110–112, Epub 2004/02/24.

106. Marinho, A.C., Martinho, F.C., Zaia, A.A., Ferraz, C.C. & Gomes, B.P. (2012) Influence of the apical enlargement size on the endotoxin level reduction of dental root canals. *Journal of Applied Oral Science*, **20** (6), 661–666, Epub 2013/01/19.

107. Mickel, A.K., Chogle, S., Liddle, J., Huffaker, K. & Jones, J.J. (2007) The role of apical size determination and enlargement in the reduction of intracanal bacteria. *Journal of Endodontics*, **33** (1), 21–23, Epub 2006/12/23.

108. Rollison, S., Barnett, F. & Stevens, R.H. (2002) Efficacy of bacterial removal from instrumented root canals in vitro related to instrumentation technique and size. *Oral Surgery, Oral Medicine, Oral Pathology, Oral Radiology, and Endodontics*, **94** (3), 366–371, Epub 2002/09/27.

109. Kerekes, K. & Tronstad, L. (1979) Long-term results of endodontic treatment performed with a standardized technique. *Journal of Endodontics*, **5** (3), 83–90, Epub 1979/03/01.

110. Hoskinson, S.E., Ng, Y.L., Hoskinson, A.E., Moles, D.R. & Gulabivala, K. (2002) A retrospective comparison of outcome of root canal treatment using two different protocols. *Oral Surgery, Oral Medicine, Oral Pathology, Oral Radiology, and Endodontics*, **93** (6), 705–715, Epub 2002/07/27.

111. Orstavik, D., Qvist, V. & Stoltze, K. (2004) A multivariate analysis of the outcome of endodontic treatment. *European Journal of Oral Sciences*, **112** (3), 224–230, Epub 2004/05/25.

112. Negishi, J., Kawanami, M. & Ogami, E. (2005) Risk analysis of failure of root canal treatment for teeth with inaccessible apical constriction. *Journal of Dentistry*, **33** (5), 399–404, Epub 2005/04/19.

113. Ng, Y.L., Mann, V. & Gulabivala, K. (2011) A prospective study of the factors affecting outcomes of non-surgical root canal treatment: part 2: tooth survival. *International Endodontic Journal*, **44** (7), 610–625, Epub 2011/03/04.

114. Wu, M.K., Wesselink, P.R. & Walton, R.E. (2000) Apical terminus location of root canal treatment procedures. *Oral Surgery, Oral Medicine, Oral Pathology, Oral Radiology, and Endodontics*, **89** (1), 99–103, Epub 2000/01/12.

115. Sjogren, U., Hagglund, B., Sundqvist, G. & Wing, K. (1990) Factors affecting the long-term results of endodontic treatment. *Journal of Endodontics*, **16** (10), 498–504, Epub 1990/10/01.

116. Peak, J.D., Hayes, S.J., Bryant, S.T. & Dummer, P.M. (2001) The outcome of root canal treatment. A retrospective study within the armed forces (Royal Air Force). *British Dental Journal*, **190** (3), 140–144, Epub 2001/03/10.

117. Ng, Y.L., Mann, V., Rahbaran, S., Lewsey, J. & Gulabivala, K. (2008) Outcome of primary root canal treatment: systematic review of the literature – part 2. Influence of clinical factors. *International Endodontic Journal*, **41** (1), 6–31, Epub 2007/10/13.

118. Southard, D.W. & Rooney, T.P. (1984) Effective one-visit therapy for the acute periapical abscess. *Journal of Endodontics*, **10** (12), 580–583, Epub 1984/12/01.

119. Ricucci, D., Russo, J., Rutberg, M., Burleson, J.A. & Spangberg, L.S. (2011) A prospective cohort study of endodontic treatments of 1,369 root canals: results after 5 years. *Oral Surgery, Oral Medicine, Oral Pathology, Oral Radiology, and Endodontics*, **112** (6), 825–842, Epub 2011/11/22.

120. Penesis, V.A., Fitzgerald, P.I., Fayad, M.I., Wenckus, C.S., BeGole, E.A. & Johnson, B.R. (2008) Outcome of one-visit and two-visit endodontic treatment of necrotic teeth with apical periodontitis: a randomized controlled trial with one-year evaluation. *Journal of Endodontics*, **34** (3), 251–257, Epub 2008/02/23.

121. Molander, A., Warfvinge, J., Reit, C. & Kvist, T. (2007) Clinical and radiographic evaluation of one- and two-visit endodontic treatment of asymptomatic necrotic teeth with apical periodontitis: a randomized clinical trial. *Journal of Endodontics*, **33** (10), 1145–1148, Epub 2007/09/25.

122. Peters, L.B. & Wesselink, P.R. (2002) Periapical healing of endodontically treated teeth in one and two visits obturated in the presence or absence of detectable microorganisms. *International Endodontic Journal*, **35** (8), 660–667, Epub 2002/08/28.

123. Weiger, R., Rosendahl, R. & Lost, C. (2000) Influence of calcium hydroxide intracanal dressings on the prognosis of teeth with endodontically induced periapical lesions. *International Endodontic Journal*, **33** (3), 219–226, Epub 2001/04/20.

124. Trope M, Delano EO, Orstavik D. (1999) Endodontic treatment of teeth with apical periodontitis: single vs. multivisit treatment *Journal of Endodontics*. **25**(5):345–350, Epub 1999/10/26.

125. de Chevigny, C., Dao, T.T., Basrani, B.R. *et al.* (2008) Treatment outcome in endodontics: the Toronto study – phase 4: initial treatment. *Journal of Endodontics*, **34** (3), 258–263, Epub 2008/02/23.

126. Sathorn, C., Parashos, P. & Messer, H.H. (2005) Effectiveness of single- versus multiple-visit endodontic treatment of teeth with apical periodontitis: a systematic review and meta-analysis. *International Endodontic Journal*, **38** (6), 347–355, Epub 2005/05/25.

127. Figini, L., Lodi, G., Gorni, F. & Gagliani, M. (2008) Single versus multiple visits for endodontic treatment of permanent teeth: a Cochrane systematic review. *Journal of Endodontics*, **34** (9), 1041–1047, Epub 2008/08/23.

128. Su, Y., Wang, C. & Ye, L. (2011) Healing rate and post-obturation pain of single- versus multiple-visit endodontic treatment for infected root canals: a systematic review. *Journal of Endodontics*, **37** (2), 125–132, Epub 2011/01/18.

129. Marending, M., Peters, O.A. & Zehnder, M. (2005) Factors affecting the outcome of orthograde root canal therapy in a general dentistry hospital practice. *Oral Surgery, Oral Medicine, Oral Pathology, Oral Radiology, and Endodontics*, **99** (1), 119–124, Epub 2004/12/16.

Part 2

Nonsurgical Intracanal Disinfection

6 Shaping the Root Canal System to Promote Effective Disinfection

Ove A. Peters

Department of Endodontics, University of the Pacific, San Francisco, CA, USA

Frank Paqué

Department of Preventive Dentistry, Periodontology, and Cariology, University of Zurich, Zürich, Switzerland

Introduction

It has been well established over the past 50 years that the endodontic disease, in other words, the presence of apical periodontitis, has a microbial pathogenesis (1, 2). Consequently, root canal treatment is performed to treat endodontic disease by eradicating bacteria from the root canal space.

Furthermore, it is currently accepted that disinfection and subsequent obturation of the root canal space requires mechanical enlargement of the main canals (3), and the vast majority of techniques and instruments today are based on this objective.

Root canal shaping thus serves two main purposes in canal disinfection: direct mechanistic elimination of intracanal tissue and pathogens and providing optimal space for irrigant and medicament delivery (4–6). Clinical success appears to be enhanced in the presence of better disinfection (7, 8) using antimicrobials delivered into the shaped root canal. Consequently the process of root canal preparation should be considered a main driver of clinical success in endodontics.

Using conventional anaerobic culturing, widely varying clinical preparation techniques have been associated with a reduction of intracanal bacteria to a level of 10–100 CFU/ml (9–14). However, it is highly unlikely that under clinical conditions any root canal will be rendered sterile.

This finding is not incompatible with clinical success. In fact, abundant reports of clinically successful as well as failure cases confirm the presence of bacteria and immune cells inside root canal systems in both healed cases and cases with residual lesions. (15–17). Figure 6.1 illustrates an isthmus area of a mandibular first molar after single-visit endodontic therapy, in which bacteria are present encased in dentin shavings.

The fate of such bacteria remaining in inaccessible canal areas, regardless of clinical technique (18),

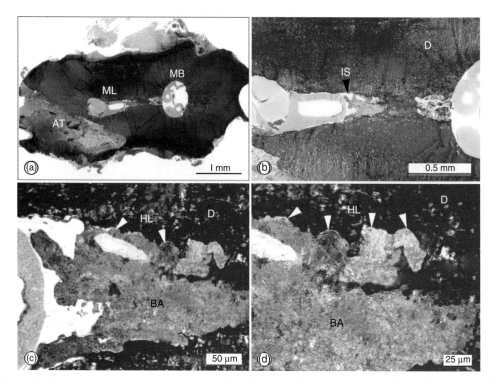

Figure 6.1   Light microscopic view of a transverse section through the apical portion of the mesial root of a right mandibular first molar (a) The surgical artifact (AT) into the root dentin did not reach or damage the instrumented mesiolingual and mesiobuccal canals, which were incompletely obturated with gutta-percha cones. The isthmus (IS) connecting the canals is magnified in (b); the area indicated with the black arrowhead is further magnified in stages in (c) and (d), respectively. Note the un-instrumented isthmus with arcading profiles of Howship's lacunae (HL) clogged with blue-stained bacterial mass (BA). Original magnifications: (a) ×316; (b) ×344; (c) ×3240; (d) ×3400. (Nair *et al.* (17). Reproduced with permission of Mosby, Inc.)

has been a matter of speculation: do they die from starvation (19), are they possibly killed by sealer components (20), or can they persist and cause posttreatment disease (21)?

It was demonstrated that well-filled and hence arguably well-shaped canals may still be associated with failing root canal treatments, mainly because of the fact that microorganisms remain in inaccessible areas of the root canal system (18, 21). Consequently, rather than sterilizing root canal systems, intracanal procedures are tailored to reduce microbial burden so that it becomes compatible with success by creating conditions that prohibit regrowth and persistent infection. It has been held that a threshold exists that may be reached with different canal shaping paradigms depending on numbers, virulence, and location of surviving microorganisms. Therefore, the main objective of root canal shaping is to provide an environment,

in which apical disease is prevented or the body's immune system can achieve the healing of apical disease. At the same time shaping is limited by the overall root anatomy and the deficiencies of currently available instruments.

Effect of canal preparation on intracanal bacteria

Using contemporary instruments, root canals can be prepared to desired shapes without obvious procedural errors as reviewed extensively earlier (4, 5, 22). However, it is obvious that mechanical canal preparation does not create contact with the full radicular surface and therefore all mechanical preparation is incomplete. The areas in red in Figure 6.2 demonstrate the canal surface that was

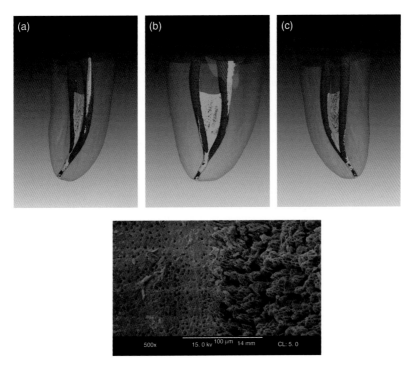

Figure 6.2   (a–c) Microcomputed tomography (MCT) images of the effect of root canal shaping of the mesial root canal system of a mandibular molar, seen from three different angles. Un-instrumented canal areas (static voxels) are depicted in green and instrumented canal areas in red. Note the isthmus area and other sections that were not altered during shaping. Final apical shaping was done with ProTaper Universal F3. Inset shows a scanning electron micrograph (×500 magnification) of areas that were in contact with an endodontic instrument (a) and a section of canal wall that shows the so-called calcospherites of the mineralization front after the removal of the pulp tissue by NaOCl.

not mechanically shaped; more specifically, it did not change by more than 20 µm, which was the resolution of the system. This observation is confirmed by histological and scanning electron microscopic observation that typically reveal mechanically unshaped areas (see inset in Figure 6.2).

Nevertheless, it has been demonstrated that mechanical instrumentation, alone or in combination with an inert flushing solution such as saline, is effective in significantly reducing bacterial load. Several authors have investigated the direct antimicrobial effect of canal instrumentation. First, in 1958, Ingle and Zeldow (23), using aerobic culturing methods, determined that the majority (65/89) of the clinical cases they sampled harbored bacteria prior to instrumentation. Only 13 of those became bacteria-free (=culture negative) after the first appointment. In their study turbidity of the culture medium was used as the sole indicator for

bacterial presence and the authors cautioned that various numbers of microorganisms were needed to cause such turbidity.

Subsequently, Byström and Sundqvist (24) expanded this observation under conditions of anaerobic culturing in a clinical study of 15 single-rooted teeth diagnosed with apical periodontitis. They found that after the first appointment, in which canals were shaped with Hedström files to an apical size 40 to 1 mm short of the radiographic root length, intracanal bacterial numbers were reduced by 10^2–10^3 and even further in subsequent appointments. However, in 8/15 cases, complete elimination of microorganisms was not achieved even after five appointments (24).

Siqueira and colleagues (25) also used saline to irrigate root canal prepared with nickel–titanium (NiTi) hand and rotary instruments *in-vitro*. Utilizing anaerobic culturing, these authors found that mechanical instrumentation was effective in removing more than 90% of bacterial cells from the root canal. This effect appeared to depend on apical sizes since preparation with NiTi K-files to size 40 was significantly more effective in removing bacteria compared to GT hand files or ProFile rotaries used to shape to sizes 20 (0.12 taper) and 28 (0.06 taper), respectively (25).

Falk and Sedgley (26) introduced yet another experimental technique in the laboratory: genetically modified bacteria. They inoculated 30 permanent canines with bioluminescent *Pseudomonas fluorescens* and determined bacterial elimination by the reduction of luminescence, thus waiving the need for culturing. Using saline irrigation, enlarging canals to an apical size 60 was more effective than to size 36 and similarly effective than enlargement to size 77 (all 0.04 taper) (26).

In summary, these data demonstrate that mechanical canal preparation alone is effective in reducing, though not eliminating, bacterial load. Regardless of the study design—benchtop, or *in situ*—the presented evidence does not aid, however, in determining an apical preparation size. There are several reasons for this; first, experimental data that suggest larger preparation size does not take structural weakening or preparation errors into account. Second, the delivery of antimicrobials to remove bacteria more effectively follows different parameters than the purely mechanical removal of canal contents. To conclude, there are other factors to be considered in a clinical setting.

Working length and patency

It has been held that both mechanical removal of microorganisms and irrigation efficacy are dependent on canal shape (27, 28); however, the latter depends also on factors such as sodium hypochlorite turnover, the amount of available chlorine, contact time, and factors such as accessibility (for a more detailed review of endodontic irrigants, see Chapter 7 in this book).

Accessibility of the contaminated root canal areas is key to disinfecting efficacy. Thus, overall canal anatomy and in particular canal dimensions play an integral role in radicular shaping. Two basic concepts govern a numerical approach to root canal shaping procedures: working length (WL)

and apical size, recently also described as working width (WW) (29).

Clinical research has indicated that root canal fillings that are extending beyond the root apex are associated with less success. Therefore, procedures confined to the root canal space (30) seem to be able to address most of the cases of endodontic treatment needs.

Varying concepts have been proposed regarding specific WLs (31), partially depending on preoperative diagnoses. Frequently, vital cases are clinically successful despite apparent short fills. However, with existing apical lesions and contaminated canal systems, WL definitions closer to the apex have been adopted. Classic and more recent studies suggest that a WL between 0 and 2 mm from the radiographic apex results more often in success (healing of apical lesions) than shorter or longer fills (7, 32, 33). However, apical anatomy and the relation between bacterial biofilms and clinical symptoms are complex (34) and can be addressed only partially by mechanical root canal shaping.

Figure 6.3 illustrates that the bacterial colonization in the apical canal portion ends a small distance inside the root canal, probably related to the geometry at that site and specifically the ability for the host defense to interact with microoganisms where blood supply occurs. In consequence WL for teeth with necrotic pulps and apical periodontitis should be set as close as possible the end of the confines of the root canal using radiographs and electronic devices.

Current strategies in this regard include the use of a patency file, e.g. a size #10, K-file, that is gently pushed slightly through an apical foramen without actually enlarging it (35). However, it is not firmly established if patency is beneficial in terms of canal disinfection of even counterproductive.

Indeed, one of the alleged reasons for not using apical patency is possible mechanical injury of apical tissues (36) or extrusion of infected debris through the apical foramen (37), a condition classically related with postoperative pain and with the delay in the healing process of apical pathology (36, 38, 39). On the other hand, *in-vitro* research has indicated that even if a patency file is contaminated, it will be disinfected by the 5.25% NaOCl present in the root canal during the shaping procedures (40).

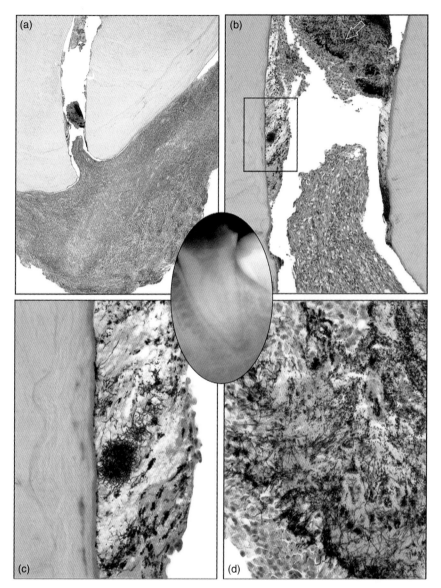

Figure 6.3   Grossly carious single-rooted mandibular second molar extracted with the apical periodontitis lesion attached. The radiographic size of the lesion was less than 5 mm (inset). The tooth was symptomatic. (a) The section passing approximately at the center of the foramen. The overview shows granulomatous tissue ingrowth at the very apical canal (Taylor's modified Brown and Brenn, original magnification ×16). (b) Details of the apical foramen region. A biofilm is present covering the root canal walls, and a dense bacterial aggregate is evidenced more coronally. Empty spaces are shrinkage artifacts (original magnification ×100). (c) Higher magnification of the area demarcated by the rectangle in (b). Bacterial filamentous forms prevail, and the extracellular component is abundant at this level (original magnification ×400). (d) Higher magnification of the bacterial aggregate indicated by the arrow in (b). Different morphotypes are present. Note the concentration of polymorphonuclear neutrophils in contact with the biofilm surface (original magnification ×400). (Ricucci and Siqueira (34). Reproduced with permission of Elsevier, Inc.)

The extrusion of debris appears to be more likely if the apical foramen is patent (41, 42). Certainly, mechanical cleaning of the foramen is unlikely, because the foramen is not enlarged and debris is not mechanically removed with a small file (43).

More recently, it was found that maintaining apical patency did not increase the incidence of postoperative pain (44) and that its benefits exceed the possible injury it might cause. This is because it is intended exclusively to prevent dentinal chips being compacted into the apical region and forming a plug that can interfere with maintaining WL (43). Of note, microcomputed tomography studies have demonstrated that dentin shavings are compacted into canal spaces not directly in contact with instruments (see below).

Other described advantages of this procedure include the sense that it improves apex locator accuracy, helps to maintain WL, reduces preparation errors such as ledges and blockages, and refines the tactile sense of the clinician during apical shaping (45). No apical transportation has been shown in the majority of root canals when using a #8 or a #10 file to maintain apical patency (46); however, using large file diameters for the purpose of apical patency may cause apical transportation (47).

Recently, *in-vivo* studies have suggested that maintaining apical patency may not only help to achieve the mechanical objectives of the shaping procedure of root canal treatments avoiding the accumulation of debris at the apex, but also that the use of a patency file allows better delivery of irrigants to the apical third. However, the mere presence of NaOCl in the apical third does not guarantee the proper cleaning of the root canal.

It should be stressed at this point that the use of a patency file is distinct from "apical clearing," which is defined as a technique to remove loose debris from the apical extent, and involved sequentially rotating files two to four sizes larger than the initial apical file at WL, and then rotating the largest apical file again after a final irrigation and drying (48); this technique may be useful after hand instrumentation (49) but no such effect has been shown after rotary instrumentation.

A major question when defining WL in an attempt to enhance antimicrobial efficacy of canal preparation is where the root canal ends and how close to that point clinicians can estimate their WL. Histological studies indicated the presence of the transition of pulp to apical tissue as well as dentin and cementum in the area of the constriction (50). However, a constriction in the classic sense may be absent (51). In fact, high-resolution tomographic studies suggest more complicated apical canal configurations than previously shown.

The term *working length* is defined in the Glossary of Endodontic Terms as "the distance from a coronal reference point to the point, at which canal preparation and obturation should terminate" (35). The anatomic apex is the tip or the end of the root determined morphologically, whereas the radiographic apex is the tip or end of the root determined radiographically (35).

It is well established that root morphology and radiographic distortion may cause the location of the radiographic apex to vary from the anatomic apex. The apical foramen is the main apical opening of the root canal. It is often eccentrically located away from the anatomic or radiographic apex (50, 51). Kuttler's classic investigation showed that this deviation occurred in 68–80% of teeth (50). An accessory foramen is an orifice on the surface of the root communicating with a lateral or accessory canal (35). They may be found as a single foramen or as multiple foramina. The apical constriction (minor apical diameter) is the apical portion of the root canal with the narrowest diameter.

Probably owing to its importance as a clinical entity, the apical root canal third and the foramen have been the topic of numerous systematic investigations (50, 52) beginning in the middle of the past century. Dummer and coworkers (51) reported four basic variations in the apical canal area that included about 50% of cases where a constriction was present. They also reported 6% of their cases, where the constriction was probably blocked by cementum (51). The cementodentinal junction is the region where the dentin and cementum are united; this is the point at which the cemental surface terminates or refers to the apex of a tooth (35). Of course the cementodentinal junction is a histological landmark that cannot be located clinically or radiographically.

Langeland (53) reported that the cementodentinal junction does not always coincide with the apical constriction. The location of the cementinodential junction also ranges from 0.5 to 3.0 mm short of the anatomic apex (50, 51).

Therefore, it is generally accepted that the apical constriction is most frequently located 0.5–1.0 mm short of the radiographic apex. It has been pointed out by Ricucci (30) that the presence of significant anatomical variation makes the direct clinical use of these average values as end points of canal preparation difficult. Further problems exist in locating apical landmarks and in interpreting their positions on radiographs.

Apical size and taper

The second factor to be considered is the apical width or the preparation size. It is an ongoing matter of debate, which apical enlargement and more specifically shape would lead to an optimal reduction of intracanal microbial load (54).

Principles of a standardized root canal preparation were based on concepts of apical canal geometry developed in the 1950s (50), which suggested apical canal diameters of 0.27–0.33 mm. However, a detailed anatomical assessment indicates that the concept for such a standardized root canal preparation (7) to an apical stop coronal to the constriction may be problematic because the "classical" singular constriction was not present in over 50% of the canals evaluated (51) and because of the possible sequelae of canal overenlargement, in particular vertical root fracture.

To complicate matters, it had been established by Shovelton (55) that intracanal bacteria colonize predentin and penetrate into dentinal tubules, to perhaps half the tubule length or in fact even deeper (56). It was therefore suggested to select a preparation size that removes this infected layer mechanically to maximize chances of success. Unfortunately, it appears that hand instruments and first generation rotaries (e.g., Quantec) were unable to completely remove predentin *in-vitro* (57). Moreover, this goal is likely unattainable even with modern root canal instruments such as the self-adjusting file (SAF, Figure 6.4a,b). For this file, microCT experiments suggested that even in relatively round and straight canals in maxillary anteriors under optimal conditions, about 9% canal area remains un-instrumented (58). More detailed analyses revealed that under these conditions, only about 57% of the canal surface had a dentin layer of 100 μm removed (Figure 6.4c).

This makes the role of irrigation solutions in canal disinfection even more relevant. Generally, irrigants are delivered using a syringe and needle system. Historically, a study using radiopaque liquids indicated that the apical penetration of the irrigants is only 1 mm beyond the needle tip (59). Furthermore, Usman and colleagues (28) demonstrated that the amount of irrigant delivered increased with the number of recapitulations. This information and regularly available needle types (27 and 30 gauge, equivalent to 0.42 and 0.31 mm, respectively) suggest that shaped canal diameter and curvature are relevant in irrigation efficacy.

It is common understanding that bacterial biofilm establishes on root canal surfaces; what is not settled is the best strategy to remove such biofilm. It seems like mechanical forces, such as in canal shaping, irrigant flow, and the selection of suitable irrigation solutions may be required (60).

Whether or not a smaller apical preparation allows sufficient antimicrobial action to take place (12, 61, 62) is a matter of continuous debate. Table 6.1 lists data in support of a variety of apical preparation sizes.

Coldero and colleagues (61), using culturing methods, could not show that larger preparation was any more successful in the reduction of intracanal bacteria from artificially contaminated root canals *in-vitro*. The other end of the spectrum of suggestions is represented by Card and colleagues (12), which was based on *in situ* data recommended sizes as large as #60 or even #80 when shaping molar root canals with LightSpeed instruments.

The majority of findings is somewhere between these extremes with several papers presenting inconclusive results. This is possibly a reflection of very different study designs and research strategies.

Baumgartner's group has frequently attempted to address the question of apical preparation size in well-designed *in-vitro* experiments. They concluded that an apical preparation size #20 would be inferior to size #30 and #40 regarding canal debridement but that a larger taper (e.g., 0.10) may potentially compensate for smaller sizes (27, 28).

This notion is supported by an *in-vitro* study on the efficacy of ultrasonically activated irrigation that demonstrated better debridement with 0.10 taper preparation (85). Similarly, Mickel *et al.*

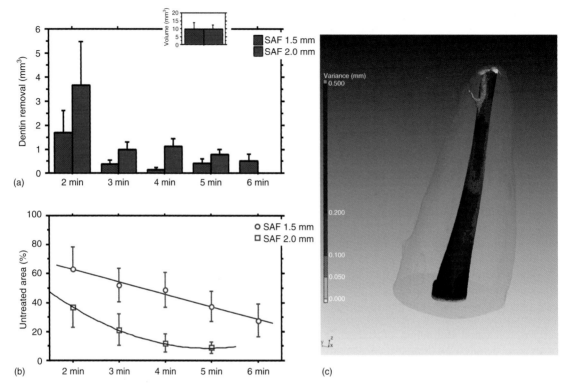

Figure 6.4 Effect of progressive preparation of root canals with the self-adjusting file (SAF) 1.5 and 2.0 mm. Initial canal volumes in both groups (*n* = 10 each) were statistically similar (inset). Preparation was done with 1.5 mm SAF (blue symbols) or 2.0 mm SAF (red symbols). (a) Canal volume increases with preparation over time. (b) Reduction in un-instrumented canal surface with progressive preparation. Data approximated by a linear regression line (blue) and second-order polynomial curve (red; untreated area). (c) Color-coded model for an anterior central incisor that was shaped with the 2 mm SAF for 4 min. Different amounts of surface area changes are indicated. (a and b: Peters *et al.* (58). Reproduced with permission of Elsevier, Inc.)

(84), based on microbiological assays, as well as Khademi *et al.* (66), using scanning electron microscopy, found that apical preparation to size #30 is required to effectively clean root canals. Moreover, recent elegant analyses using a thermal imaging system revealed detailed relationships between master apical file size, needle diameter, and insertion depth (86).

More recently, Cohenca and colleagues (87), using an *in situ* design with randomization, failed to demonstrate any difference in bacterial reduction with different tapers and apical sizes. These parameters varied for cases in the study groups with teeth prepared with LightSpeed or ProTaper but seemed to have less impact than the use of conventional needle irrigation versus negative pressure irrigation (EndoVac) (87).

Earlier, even larger apical preparation sizes were favored, as the results from Trope's group (11, 12, 14) show. Trope and colleagues used anaerobic culturing from teeth that were diagnosed with pulpal necrosis and apical periodontitis to determine sequential reduction in bacterial counts in an *in situ* design. Frequently and despite a significant reduction of bacterial loads, viable bacteria were still detected after several canal shaping appointments. The authors concluded that disinfecting irrigants and intracanal medicaments should be employed to reduce viable bacteria counts (12). Interestingly, larger apical sizes (#40, taper 0.04 compared to #20, taper 0.10) facilitated the application of calcium hydroxide medication *in-vitro* (6).

Taken together, these results suggest that sufficient apical preparation size and the use of

Table 6.1 Summary of evidence published in the past decade to suggest apical preparation geometry. Note that the vast majority of these studies were performed *in-vitro*. Also, there appears to be a very wide variation for favored apical sizes and several studies with inconclusive findings.

Favored size	Article	Conclusion	Design
Small	(63)	Increased apical enlargement of curved canals did not result in a complete apical preparation, whereas it did lead to the unnecessary removal of dentin.	*In-vitro*
Small	(61)	There was no significant difference in intracanal bacterial reduction when Ni–Ti GT rotary preparation with NaOCl and EDTA irrigation was used with or without apical enlargement preparation technique. It may not be necessary therefore to remove dentin in the apical part of the root canal when a suitable coronal taper is achieved to allow satisfactory irrigation of the root canal system with antimicrobial agents.	*In-vitro*
>#20	(64)	Apical canal geometry was affected differently by six preparation techniques; preparations with GT instruments to an apical size #20 left more canal surface untouched, which might affect the ability to disinfect root canals in maxillary molars.	*In-vitro*
#25	(65)	Apical foramen widening (up to a size #25 K-file) and calcium hydroxide-containing sealer were more favorable to the healing of chronic apical lesions.	*Clinical*
#30	(66)	The minimum instrumentation size needed for the penetration of irrigants to the apical third of the root canal is a #30 file.	*In-vitro*
>#25	(67)	Root canal enlargement to sizes larger than #25 appeared to improve the performance of syringe irrigation.	*In-vitro*
Low end of range #30–55	(68)	The larger the foraminal file size, the more difficult the apical foramen instrumentation may be in laterally emerged cemental canals. Note: The diameters compared were from K-files #30 to #55.	*In-vitro*
>#30	(69)	Root canal preparation to apical size #30 and tapers 0.04, 0.06, or 0.08 did not affect canal cleanliness.	*In-vitro*
#40	(70)	Comparing NiTi LightSpeed and NiTi hand instruments both combined with apical preparation size (APS—technique specified in an earlier paper by the same group For distal/palatal canals: APS = DSI + 0.40 mm; for mesiobuccal/mesiolingual/distobuccal canals: APS = DSI + 0.30 mm); both preparation techniques allowed a wide apical preparation with a rather slight risk of procedural errors in molars.	*In-vitro*
#40	(27)	Debris is more effectively removed using 0.04, 0.06, and 0.08 ProFile GT when the apical preparation size is larger (size #40) compared with size #20. When a taper of 0.10 can be produced at the apical extent of the canal, there is no difference in debris removal between the two preparation sizes.	*In-vitro*
#40	(71)	The degree of root canal curvature decreased the volume of irrigant at the working length for a given apical size and taper. An apical preparation of #40.06 significantly increased the volume and exchange of irrigant at the working length regardless of curvature.	*In-vitro*
#40	(72)	An increase in apical preparation size and taper resulted in a statistically significant increase in the volume of irrigant. In addition, an apical enlargement to ISO #40 with a 0.04 taper will allow for tooth structure preservation and maximum volume of irrigation at the apical third when using the apical negative pressure irrigation system.	*In-vitro*

(*continued*)

Table 6.1   (*Continued*)

Favored size	Article	Conclusion	Design
#40	(28)	No differences were found between each level within each apex size group; however, the GT size #20 group left significantly more debris in the apical third compared with the GT size 40 group.	*In-vitro*
#40	(73)	Endotoxin levels of dental root canals could be predicted by increasing the apical enlargement size. Note: The diameters compared were Mtwo sizes #25/0.06, 30/0.05, 35/0.04, 40/0.04.	*In-vitro*
#40–50	(74)	The APS in 2-canal upper premolars and mandibular premolars should be at least 6 sizes larger than the first apically binding file, whereas in upper premolars with a central canal, the APS should be enlarged to 8 sizes larger. Normally, this implies shaping premolars with 1 canal to #60–70 and with 2 canals to #40–50.	*In-vitro*
#50	(62)	The results suggested that instrumentation to an apical size of #50, as performed with the Pow-R instruments, was more effective in debriding infected root canals than instrumentation to an apical size of #35, as performed with the GT and Profile instruments.	*In-vitro*
#60–80	(12)	Typically, molars were instrumented to size #60 and cuspid/bicuspid canals to size #80. It is concluded that simple root canal systems (without multiple canal communications) may be rendered bacteria-free when preparation of this type is utilized.	*In situ*
Large	(75)	The enlargement of the canal to 3 sizes larger than the FABF is adequate, and further enlargement does not provide any additional benefit during endodontic treatment.	*Clinical*
Large	(76)	Root canals should be shaped to larger sizes than normally recommended. Note: Compared diameters of special instruments (SI) ranging 0.08–0.45 mm.	*In-vitro*
Large	(54)	Better microbial removal and more effective irrigation occurred when canals were instrumented to larger apical sizes. Although bacteria may remain viable in dentinal tubules, proper instrumentation and adequate irrigation significantly reduces bacteria from the canal and the dentinal tubules.	*Review*
Large	(77)	An increase in the root canal taper was found to improve irrigant replacement and wall shear stress while reducing the risk for irrigant extrusion. Irrigant flow in a minimally tapered root canal with a large apical preparation size appeared more advantageous than in the tapered root canals with a smaller apical preparation size (size #30, 0.02 taper, 30, 0.04, 30, 0.06, ProTaper F3 or size #60, 0.02 taper root canals were evaluated).	*In-vitro*
Large	(78)	An increase in file size was shown to be important in allowing the NaOCl to be an effective antibacterial irrigant.	*In situ*
Large	(79)	It was concluded that greater apical enlargement using LS rotary instruments is beneficial as an attempt to further debride the apical third region in mesiobuccal canals of mandibular molars.	*In-vitro*
Inconclusive or statistically insignificant	(80)	No apical enlargement size allowed the root canal walls to be prepared completely. The diameters compared were Hero642 instruments sizes #30/0.02, 35/0.04, 40/0.02, 45/0.02.	*In-vitro*

Table 6.1   *(Continued)*

Favored size	Article	Conclusion	Design
Inconclusive or statistically insignificant	(81)	Neither the first K-file nor the first LightSpeed instrument that bound at the working length reflected accurately the diameter of the apical canal in curved mandibular premolars. It is uncertain whether dentine can be removed from the entire circumference of the canal wall by filing the root canal to three sizes larger than the file that binds first.	*In-vitro*
Inconclusive or statistically insignificant	(82)	When comparing ProTaper size #30; taper 0.09–0.055 and Hero Shaper size #30, taper 0.04, both to the full WL, the difference between changes in bacterial numbers achieved with two instrumentation techniques was statistically not significant.	*In-vitro*
Inconclusive or statistically insignificant	(83)	Root canals with mild curvature prepared with the #45.02 instrument to the full WL showed the highest values for extruded material to the apical region (0.87 ± 0.22). It seems more reasonable to establish final instrument diameters based on the anatomic diameter after cervical preparation.	*In-vitro*
Inconclusive or statistically insignificant	(84)	An appropriate apical sizing method can help the operator avoid unnecessary enlargement of the apex while predictably reducing intracanal debris. Method: During crown-down preparation, the first crown-down file to reach the apex during instrumentation was noted (CDF). Teeth were then divided into three master apical file size groups of CDF + 1, CDF + 2, and CDF + 3.	*In-vitro*

a small-caliber irrigation needle are desirable to promote irrigation and hence antimicrobial efficacy. It is a common theme that canal preparation needs to adapt to specific irrigation devices (detailed in Chapters 8–13 in this book). Placement of irrigation needles, ultrasonic activation inserts, and negative pressure devices all have specific requirements for canal space, and canal shaping has to provide this space.

Besides WL and apical size, a third, as yet incompletely understood aspect of canal shape is taper. Some have expressed concerns that the importance of root canal taper should be seen only in conjunction with root canal filling techniques, most notably vertical compaction (88). However, as stated before, there is some experimental evidence that taper may be connected to the ability to clean the root canal system by improving the irrigant action (27, 28, 71, 77, 85).

Limited microbiological data deliver conflicting information regarding the potential of smaller apical preparations with larger taper to disinfect the root canal system (14, 61). Using the amount of instrumented canal area as surrogate outcome for disinfecting capacity, no significant differences were found overall comparing shapes with GT 20

0.10 taper to apical size #40 with smaller tapers (89). However, there were significant differences when the apical canal segment was evaluated for instrumented canal surface area (64).

Potential negative effects of shaping on disinfection

Obviously, a clinician has to carefully decide with which instrument and how wide to shape a given canal in order to achieve antimicrobial efficiency without overly weakening the tooth structure. Most NiTi instruments used according to current guidelines allow wider shapes without major preparation errors and without excessively reducing radicular walls (22, 45). Remaining dentin thickness was in the range of 0.6 mm with various rotary instruments (90, 91). It is currently unknown if and possibly how remaining dentin thickness is correlated to root fractures. However, simulation studies using finite element models (92) suggest that larger tapers may have the potential to increase *von Mises* stresses during masticatory load. Research is ongoing to identify possible canal preparation strategies that may retain more bulk dentin and hence structural strength.

Another possible negative effect of canal preparation is the production of the so-called smear layer that is typically generated in contact between dentin and mechanical instrumentation (see Figure 6.2). This smear layer depends on the type of instrument and irrigation solutions used. Most clinicians remove it in order to promote access of irrigants to dentinal tubules and small accessory canals.

Finally, interest has recently been focused on hard tissue debris that is compacted into canal spaces not directly shaped by root canal instruments, such as isthmuses, apical ramifications, and larger accessory canals. As demonstrated in Figure 6.1 dentin shavings have the potential to encase microorganisms, which may, on contact with the host defense in the periodontal ligament, impede tissue healing and bone fill.

Paqué and colleagues (93) have developed a microCT-based model to assess the amount and distribution of such hard tissue debris. They demonstrated that up to 30% of the volume of regions with accessory anatomy was initially filled with dentin shavings. Figure 6.5 demonstrates that subsequent irrigation fails to completely remove compacted root dentin from these anatomical spaces. Removal of such hard tissue debris is facilitated by various irrigation parameters (94, 95).

Considering the need for sufficient canal shapes that promote disinfection and the limitations of current shaping instruments and procedures, it seems prudent to suggest a compromise between the needed size and avoiding negative consequences of overenlargement. Clinically a variety of different procedures will allow clinicians to achieve their specific shaping objectives.

Clinical data to support specific shaping paradigms

Unfortunately, clinical outcome data is lacking that would support specific canal shaping strategies. Those clinical outcome studies that include the factor "apical preparation size" often present insufficient statistical power and conflicting results (96–98).

A review of the technical aspects of root canal treatments (99) found that apical periodontitis was more frequent with inadequate root canal fillings; however, the author did not find evidence that canal instrumentation methods, and in particular apical sizes, had any measurable effect on outcomes.

Conversely, one result of the *Toronto study* on endodontic outcomes seemed to favor smaller preparations in conjunction with tapered shapes and vertically compacted gutta-percha over step-back preparation to larger apical shapes

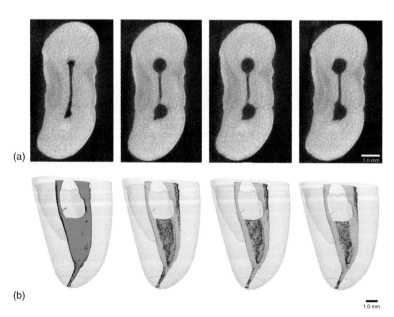

(a)

(b)

Figure 6.5 Debris accumulation in accessory anatomy following instrumentation, illustrated using the same specimen shown in Figure 6.2. Individual MCT slices from the apical third of a typical specimen before and after root canal preparation and irrigation with NaOCl, subsequent irrigation with EDTA, and final passive ultrasonic irrigation using NaOCl (a, from left to right). The corresponding three-dimensional reconstructions of the whole canal system are depicted in (b). (Paqué *et al.* (94). Reproduced with permission of John Wiley & Sons, Inc.)

(90% and 80% success, respectively) (100). Again, in contrast, using PAI scores determined from radiographs, Ørstavik and colleagues (101) did not find any significant impact of the preparation size on outcomes. Similarly Ng and colleagues (32) could not find any effect on clinical outcomes by final canal size (<#30 and >#30) as well as by taper. However, achieving patency was associated with significantly higher clinical success (32).

More recently, a randomized prospective clinical study specifically addressing canal preparation dimension (75) concluded that apical enlargement at least 3 sizes larger than the first file to bind at the apex was adequate for the clinical outcome investigated (change in apical radiolucent areas reflected in decreased PAI scores). They further noted that additional enlargement did not provide additional benefit for clinical outcomes. The authors used the criterion "first file to bind" based on tactile feedback when placing stainless steel hand files to the estimated WL in preflared canal (75).

It is not possible to determine canal diameters from radiographs (29); however, microCT scans may be able to give more detailed information regarding root canal anatomy (102). The resolution of current clinically available small field-of-view cone bean systems is in the range of 80 μm, corresponding to a size #08 F-file, and hence not sufficient to determine canal diameters with precision. Therefore, currently, canals width will still be determined by passing a series of K-files to WL to gauge canal shapes.

This process may depend on file type and the amount of preflaring (102, 79, 81). Clearly, the first instrument that gives the clinician a sense of binding does not correspond to any canal diameter. Wu and colleagues (81) demonstrated that the diameter of the "binding" instrument was smaller than the canals' diameter in 90% of the cases with a difference of up to 0.19 mm. Unexpectedly, Lightspeed instruments that possess a fine noncutting shaft did not perform better than K-files with .02 taper. Therefore, they concluded that it is uncertain whether circumferential removal of dentin occurs based on the criterion that one should prepare 3 sizes larger than the first binding file (81). This fact does not appear to preclude clinical success considering the available clinical outcome data (32, 97–99, 101).

Conclusions

The description of clinical techniques to shape root canals is beyond the scope of this chapter and the reader is referred to current endodontic textbooks for that purpose. Nevertheless, it appears reasonable to briefly state what can be summarized as relevant steps in canal shaping in an attempt to reconcile optimized antimicrobial effects and retained structural strength.

It should be acknowledged that technology and clinical skills must go hand in hand to reach these goals. Experience suggests that success in canal shaping can be promoted by using a systematic approach in shaping stages, regardless of the instruments or technique selected.

Stage 1
1.1. Initial canal exploration with small hand files to gauge canal size, shape, and configuration. Irrigation with antimicrobials, preferably sodium hypochlorite.
1.2. Coronal preflaring to facilitate placing subsequent files to WL (either hand or rotary). Maintaining antimicrobial efficiency by frequent and copious irrigation.

Stage 2 (if there is only one major curve)
2.1. Negotiation to the apical foramen, establishing patency and WL.
2.2. Achieving a predictable glide path to WL.
2.3. Shaping to full canal length with rotary instruments while under frequent irrigation turnover. Hand instrumentation if needed should be done passively involving the balance force technique.
2.4. Determining apical constriction size and correction of final canal size accordingly.

Stage 3 (only needed when there is a major secondary curve, in which case Stage 2 would only instruments to advance allow into the secondary curve).
3.1–3.4. accordingly.

Taking all mentioned studies and clinical experience together, it is not possible to suggest definite dimension or techniques in canal shaping that would fit all anatomical variations. It seems likely though that a clinical technique, including shaping tools, irrigation devices, and obturation materials that overall enhances antimicrobial activity is desirable as long as structural integrity of the treated radicular structure is retained.

Acknowledgment

We are grateful for the helpful comments by Drs Ana Arias and Paul Singh.

References

1. Kakehashi, S., Stanley, H.R. & Fitzgerald, R.J. (1965) The effects of surgical exposures of dental pulps in germ-free and conventional laboratory rats. *Oral Surgery, Oral Medicine, and Oral Pathology*, **20** (3), 340–349.
2. Möller, A.J., Fabricius, L., Dahlén, G., Ohman, A.E. & Heyden, G. (1981) Influence on periapical tissues of indigenous oral bacteria and necrotic pulp tissue in monkeys. *Scandinavian Journal of Dental Research*, **89** (6), 475–484.
3. Schilder, H. (1974) Cleaning and shaping the root canal. *Dental Clinics of North America*, **18** (2), 269–296.
4. Peters, O.A. (2004) Current challenges and concepts in the preparation of root canal systems: a review. *Journal of Endodontics*, **30** (8), 559–567.
5. Hülsmann, M., Peters, O.A. & Dummer, P.M.H. (2005) Mechanical preparation of root canals: shaping goals, techniques and means. *Endodontic Topics*, **10** (1), 30–76.
6. Peters, C.I., Koka, R.S., Highsmith, S. & Peters, O.A. (2005) Calcium hydroxide dressings using different preparation and application modes: density and dissolution by simulated tissue pressure. *International Endodontic Journal*, **38** (12), 889–895.
7. Sjögren, U., Figdor, D., Persson, S. & Sundqvist, G. (1997) Influence of infection at the time of root filling on the outcome of endodontic treatment of teeth with apical periodontitis. *International Endodontic Journal*, **30** (5), 297–306.
8. Fabricius, L., Dahlén, G., Sundqvist, G., Happonen, R.P. & Möller, A.J. (2006) Influence of residual bacteria on periapical tissue healing after chemomechanical treatment and root filling of experimentally infected monkey teeth. *European Journal of Oral Sciences*, **114** (4), 278–285.
9. Sjögren, U. & Sundqvist, G. (1987) Bacteriologic evaluation of ultrasonic root canal instrumentation. *Oral Surgery, Oral Medicine, and Oral Pathology*, **63** (3), 366–370.
10. Yared, G.M. & Dagher, F.E. (1994) Influence of apical enlargement on bacterial infection during treatment of apical periodontitis. *Journal of Endodontics*, **20** (11), 535–537.
11. Dalton, B.C., Ørstavik, D., Phillips, C., Pettiette, M. & Trope, M. (1998) Bacterial reduction with nickel-titanium rotary instrumentation. *Journal of Endodontics*, **24** (11), 763–767.
12. Card, S.J., Sigurdsson, A., Ørstavik, D. & Trope, M. (2002) The effectiveness of increased apical enlargement in reducing intracanal bacteria. *Journal of Endodontics*, **28** (11), 779–783.
13. Peters, L.B., van Winkelhoff, A.J., Buijs, J.F. & Wesselink, P.R. (2002) Effects of instrumentation, irrigation and dressing with calcium hydroxide on infection in pulpless teeth with periapical bone lesions. *International Endodontic Journal*, **35** (1), 13–21.
14. McGurkin-Smith, R., Trope, M., Caplan, D. & Sigurdsson, A. (2005) Reduction of intracanal bacteria using GT rotary instrumentation, 5.25% NaOCl, EDTA, and Ca(OH)$_2$. *Journal of Endodontics*, **31** (5), 359–363.
15. Brynolf, I. (1967) A histological and roentgenological study of the periapical region of human incisors. *Odontologisk Revy*, **18** (**Suppl. 11**), 1–176.
16. Green, T.L., Walton, R.E., Taylor, J.K. & Merrell, P. (1997) Radiographic and histologic periapical findings of root canal treated teeth in cadaver. *Oral Surgery, Oral Medicine, Oral Pathology, Oral Radiology, and Endodontics*, **83** (6), 707–711.
17. Nair, P.N., Henry, S., Cano, V. & Vera, J. (2005) Microbial status of apical root canal system of human mandibular first molars with primary apical periodontitis after "one-visit" endodontic treatment. *Oral Surgery, Oral Medicine, Oral Pathology, Oral Radiology, and Endodontics*, **99** (2), 231–252.
18. Nair, P.N. (2006) On the causes of persistent apical periodontitis: a review. *International Endodontic Journal*, **39** (4), 249–281.
19. Peters, L.B., Wesselink, P.R. & Moorer, W.R. (1995) The fate and the role of bacteria left in root dentinal tubules. *International Endodontic Journal*, **28** (2), 95–99.
20. Saleh, I.M., Ruyter, I.E., Haapasalo, M. & Ørstavik, D. (2004) Survival of *Enterococcus faecalis* in infected dentinal tubules after root canal filling with different root canal sealers in vitro. *International Endodontic Journal*, **37** (3), 193–198.
21. Siqueira, J.F. (2001) The aetiology of root canal treatment failure: why well-treated teeth can fail. *International Endodontic Journal*, **34** (1), 1–10.
22. Peters, O.A. & Paqué, F. (2010) Current developments in rotary root canal instrument technology and clinical use: a review. *Quintessence International*, **41** (6), 479–488.

23. Ingle, J.I. & Zeldow, B.J. (1958) An evaluation of mechanical instrumentation and the negative culture in endodontic therapy. *Journal of the American Dental Association*, **57** (**4**), 471–476.

24. Byström, A. & Sundqvist, G. (1981) Bacteriologic evaluation of the efficacy of mechanical root canal instrumentation in endodontic therapy. *Scandinavian Journal of Dental Research*, **89** (**4**), 321–328.

25. Siqueira, J.F., Lima, K.C., Magalhães, F.A., Lopes, H.P. & de Uzeda, M. (1999) Mechanical reduction of the bacterial population in the root canal by three instrumentation techniques. *Journal of Endodontics*, **25** (**5**), 332–335.

26. Falk, K.W. & Sedgley, C.M. (2005) The influence of preparation size on the mechanical efficacy of root canal irrigation in vitro. *Journal of Endodontics*, **31** (**10**), 742–745.

27. Albrecht, L.J., Baumgartner, J.C. & Marshall, J.G. (2004) Evaluation of apical debris removal using various sizes and tapers of ProFile GT files. *Journal of Endodontics*, **30** (**6**), 425–428.

28. Usman, N., Baumgartner, J.C. & Marshall, J.G. (2004) Influence of instrument size on root canal debridement. *Journal of Endodontics*, **30** (**2**), 110–112.

29. Jou, Y.T., Karabucak, B., Levin, J. & Liu, D. (2004) Endodontic working width: current concepts and techniques. *Dental Clinics of North America*, **48** (**1**), 323–335.

30. Ricucci, D. & Langeland, K. (1998) Apical limit of root canal instrumentation and obturation, part 2. A histological study. *International Endodontic Journal*, **31** (**6**), 394–409.

31. Wu, M.K., Wesselink, P.R. & Walton, R.E. (2000) Apical terminus location of root canal treatment procedures. *Oral Surgery, Oral Medicine, Oral Pathology, Oral Radiology, and Endodontics*, **89** (**1**), 99–103.

32. Ng, Y.L., Mann, V. & Gulabivala, K. (2011) A prospective study of the factors affecting outcomes of nonsurgical root canal treatment: part 1: periapical health. *International Endodontic Journal*, **44** (**7**), 583–609.

33. Ricucci, D., Russo, J., Rutberg, M., Burleson, J.A. & Spångberg, L.S.W. (2011) A prospective cohort study of endodontic treatments of 1,369 root canals: results after 5 years. *Oral Surgery, Oral Medicine, Oral Pathology, Oral Radiology, and Endodontics*, **112** (**6**), 825–842.

34. Ricucci, D. & Siqueira, J.F. (2010) Biofilms and apical periodontitis: study of prevalence and association with clinical and histopathologic findings. *Journal of Endodontics*, **36** (**8**), 1277–1288.

35. American Association of Endodontists (2012) *Glossary of Endodontic Terms*. 8th ed. Chicago, Il.

36. Holland, R., Sant'Anna Junior, A., Souza, V. *et al.* (2005) Influence of apical patency and filling material on healing process of dogs' teeth with vital pulp after root canal therapy. *Brazilian Dental Journal*, **16** (**1**), 9–16.

37. Lambrianidis, T., Tosounidou, E. & Tzoanopoulou, M. (2001) The effect of maintaining apical patency on periapical extrusion. *Journal of Endodontics*, **27** (**11**), 696–698.

38. Yusuf, H. (1982) The significance of the presence of foreign material periapically as a cause of failure of root treatment. *Oral Surgery, Oral Medicine, and Oral Pathology*, **54** (**5**), 566–574.

39. Walton, R.E. & Ardjmand, K. (1992) Histological evaluation of the presence of bacteria in induced periapical lesions in monkeys. *Journal of Endodontics*, **18** (**5**), 216–227.

40. Izu, K.H., Thomas, S.J., Zhang, P., Izu, A.E. & Michalek, S. (2004) Effectiveness of sodium hypochlorite in preventing inoculation of periapical tissues with contaminated patency files. *Journal of Endodontics*, **30** (**2**), 92–94.

41. Beeson, T.J., Hartwell, G.R., Thornton, J.D. & Gunsolley, J.C. (1998) Comparison of debris extruded apically in straight canals: conventional filing versus ProFile .04 taper series 29. *Journal of Endodontics*, **24** (**1**), 18–22.

42. Tinaz, A.C., Alacam, T., Uzun, O., Maden, M. & Kayaoglu, G. (2005) The effect of disruption of the apical constriction on periapical extrusion. *Journal of Endodontics*, **31** (**7**), 533–535.

43. Souza, R.A. (2006) The importance of apical patency and cleaning the apical foramen on root canal preparation. *Brazilian Dental Journal*, **17** (**1**), 6–9.

44. Arias, A., Azabal, M., Hidalgo, J.J. & de la Macorra, J.C. (2009) Relationship between postendodontic pain, tooth diagnostic factors, and apical patency. *Journal of Endodontics*, **35** (**2**), 189–192.

45. Peters OA, Peters CI. Cleaning and shaping of the root canal system. In: Hargreaves KM, Cohen S, editors. *Pathways of the Pulp*. 10th ed. St. Louis, MS: Mosby; 2011. p. 283–348.

46. Sanchez, J.A., Duran-Sindreu, F., Matos, M.A. *et al.* (2010) Apical transportation created using three different patency instruments. *International Endodontic Journal*, **43** (**7**), 560–564.

47. Tsesis, I., Amdor, B., Tamse, A. & Kfir, A. (2008) The effect of maintaining apical patency on canal transportation. *International Endodontic Journal*, **41** (**5**), 431–435.

48. Parris, J., Wilcox, L. & Walton, R. (1994) Effectiveness of apical clearing: histological and radiographical evaluation. *Journal of Endodontics*, **20** (**5**), 219–224.

49. Heard, F. & Walton, R.E. (1997) Scanning electron microscope study comparing four root canal preparation techniques in small curved canals. *International Endodontic Journal*, **30** (**5**), 323–331.

50. Kuttler, Y. (1955) Microscopic investigation of root apexes. *The Journal of the American Dental Association*, **50** (**5**), 544–552.

51. Dummer, P.M.H., McGinn, J.H. & Rees, D.G. (1984) The position and topography of the apical canal constriction and apical foramen. *International Endodontic Journal*, **17** (**4**), 192–198.

52. Green, D. (1956) A stereomicroscopic investigation of the root apices of 400 maxillary and mandibular anterior teeth. *Oral Surgery, Oral Medicine, Oral Pathology, Oral Radiology, and Endodontics*, **9** (**11**), 1224–1232.

53. Langeland, K. (1967) The histopathologic basis in endodontic treatment. *Dental Clinics of North America*, 491–520.

54. Baugh, D. & Wallace, J. (2005) The role of apical instrumentation in root canal treatment: a review of the literature. *Journal of Endodontics*, **31** (**5**), 330–340.

55. Shovelton, D.S. (1964) The presence and distribution of microorganisms within non-vital teeth. *British Dental Journal*, **117** (**3**), 101–107.

56. Love, R.M. (2002) Invasion of dentinal tubules by oral bacteria. *Critical Reviews in Oral Biology and Medicine*, **13** (**2**), 171–183.

57. Evans, G.E., Speight, P.M. & Gulabivala, K. (2001) The influence of preparation technique and sodium hypochlorite on removal of pulp and predentine from root canals of posterior teeth. *International Endodontic Journal*, **34** (**4**), 322–330.

58. Peters, O.A., Boessler, C. & Paqué, F. (2010) Root canal preparation with a novel nickel-titanium instrument evaluated with micro-computed tomography: canal surface preparation over time. *Journal of Endodontics*, **36** (**6**), 1068–1072.

59. Ram, Z. (1977) Effectiveness of root canal irrigation. *Oral Surgery, Oral Medicine, and Oral Pathology*, **44** (**2**), 306–312.

60. Shen, Y., Stojicic, S., Qian, W., Olsen, I. & Haapasalo, M. (2010) The synergistic antimicrobial effect by mechanical agitation and two chlorhexidine preparations on biofilm bacteria. *Journal of Endodontics*, **36** (**1**), 100–104.

61. Coldero, L.G., McHugh, S., MacKenzie, D. & Saunders, W.P. (2002) Reduction in intracanal bacteria during root canal preparation with and without apical enlargement. *International Endodontic Journal*, **35** (**5**), 437–446.

62. Rollison, S., Barnett, F. & Stevens, R.H. (2002) Efficacy of bacterial removal from instrumented root canals in vitro related to instrumentation technique and size. *Oral Surgery, Oral Medicine, Oral Pathology, Oral Radiology, and Endodontology.*, **94** (**3**), 366–371.

63. ElAyouti, A., Dima, E., Judenhofer, M.S., Löst, C. & Pichler, B.J. (2011) Increased apical enlargement contributes to excessive dentin removal in curved root canals: a stepwise microcomputed tomography study. *Journal of Endodontics*, **37** (**11**), 1580–1584.

64. Paqué, F., Ganahl, D. & Peters, O.A. (2009) Effects of root canal preparation on apical geometry assessed by micro-computed tomography. *Journal of Endodontics*, **35** (**7**), 1056–1059.

65. Borlina, S.C., de Souza, V., Holland, R. *et al.* (2010) Influence of apical foramen widening and sealer on the healing of chronic periapical lesions induced in dogs' teeth. *Oral Surgery, Oral Medicine, Oral Pathology, Oral Radiology, and Endodontics*, **109** (**6**), 932–940.

66. Khademi, A., Yazdizadeh, M. & Feizianfard, M. (2006) Determination of the minimum instrumentation size for penetration of irrigants to the apical third of root canal systems. *Journal of Endodontics*, **32** (**5**), 417–420.

67. Boutsioukis, C., Gogos, C., Verhaagen, B., Verslius, M., Kastrinakis, E. & van der Sluis, L.W. (2010) The effect of apical preparation size on irrigant flow in root canals evaluated using an unsteady computational fluid dynamics model. *International Endodontic Journal*, **43** (**10**), 874–881.

68. Souza, R.A., Souza, Y.T.C.S., Figueiredo, J.A.P., Dantas, J.C.P., Colombo, S. & Pecora, J.D. (2012) Influence of apical foramen lateral opening and file size on cemental canal instrumentation. *Brazilian Dental Journal*, **23** (**2**), 122–126.

69. Arvaniti, I.S. & Khabbaz, M.G. (2011) Influence of root canal taper on its cleanliness: a scanning electron microscopic study. *Journal of Endodontics*, **37** (**6**), 871–874.

70. Bartha, T., Kalwitzki, M., Löst, C. & Weiger, R. (2006) Extended apical enlargement with hand files versus rotary NiTi files. Part II. *Oral Surgery, Oral Medicine, Oral Pathology, Oral Radiology, and Endodontics*, **102** (**5**), 692–697.

71. de Gregorio, C., Arias, A., Navarrete, N., Del Rio, V., Oltra, E. & Cohenca, N. (2013) Effect of apical size and taper on volume of irrigant delivered at working length with apical negative pressure at different root curvatures. *Journal of Endodontics*, **39** (**1**), 119–124.

72. Brunson, M., Heilborn, C., Johnson, D.J. & Cohenca, N. (2010) Effect of apical preparation size and preparation taper on irrigant volume delivered by using negative pressure irrigation system. *Journal of Endodontics*, **36** (**4**), 721–724.

73. Marinho, A.C.S., Martinho, F.C., Zaia, A.A., Ferraz, C.C.R. & Gomes, B.P.F.A. (2012) Influence of the apical enlargement size on the endotoxin level

reduction of dental root canals. *Journal of Applied Oral Science : Revista FOB*, **20** (**6**), 661–666.

74. Hecker, H., Bartha, T., Löst, C. & Weiger, R. (2010) Determining the apical preparation size in premolars: part III. *Oral Surgery, Oral Medicine, Oral Pathology, Oral Radiology, and Endodontics*, **110** (**1**), 118–124.

75. Saini, H.R., Tewari, S., Sangwan, P., Duhan, J. & Gupta, A. (2012) Effect of different apical preparation sizes on outcome of primary endodontic treatment: a randomized controlled trial. *Journal of Endodontics*, **38** (**10**), 1309–1315.

76. Weiger, R., Bartha, T., Kalwitzki, M. & Löst, C. (2006) A clinical method to determine the optimal apical preparation size. Part I. *Oral Surgery, Oral Medicine, Oral Pathology, Oral Radiology, and Endodontics*, **102** (**5**), 686–691.

77. Boutsioukis, C., Gogos, C., Verhaagen, B., Versluis, M., Kastrinakis, E. & van der Sluis, L.W. (2010) The effect of root canal taper on the irrigant flow: evaluation using an unsteady computational fluid dynamics model. *International Endodontic Journal*, **43** (**10**), 909–916.

78. Shuping, G.B., Ørstavik, D., Sigurdsson, A. & Trope, M. (2000) Reduction of intracanal bacteria using nickel-titanium rotary instrumentation and various medications. *Journal of Endodontics*, **26** (**12**), 751–755.

79. Tan, B.T. & Messer, H.H. (2002) The quality of apical canal preparation using hand and rotary instruments with specific criteria for enlargement based on initial apical file size. *Journal of Endodontics*, **28** (**9**), 658–664.

80. Fornari, V.J., Silva-Sousa, Y.T., Vanni, J.R., Pecora, J.D., Versiani, M.A. & Sousa-Neto, M.D. (2010) Histological evaluation of the effectiveness of increased apical enlargement for cleaning the apical third of curved canals. *International Endodontic Journal*, **43** (**11**), 988–994.

81. Wu, M.K., Barkis, D., Roris, A. & Wesselink, P.R. (2002) Does the first file to bind correspond to the diameter of the canal in the apical region? *International Endodontic Journal*, **35** (**3**), 264–267.

82. Aydin, C., Tunca, Y.M., Senses, Z., Baysallar, M., Kayaoglu, G. & Orstavik, D. (2007) Bacterial reduction by extensive versus conservative root canal instrumentation in vitro. *Acta Odontologica Scandinavica*, **65** (**3**), 167–170.

83. Borges, M.F., Miranda, C.E., Silva, S.R. & Marchesan, M. (2011) Influence of apical enlargement in cleaning and extrusion in canals with mild and moderate curvatures. *Brazilian Dental Journal*, **22** (**3**), 212–217.

84. Mickel, A.K., Chogle, S., Liddle, J., Huffaker, K. & Jones, J.J. (2007) The role of apical size determination and enlargement in the reduction of intracanal bacteria. *Journal of Endodontics*, **33** (**1**), 21–23.

85. van der Sluis, L.W., Wu, M.K. & Wesselink, P.R. (2005) The efficacy of ultrasonic irrigation to remove artificially placed dentine debris from human root canals prepared using instruments of varying taper. *International Endodontic Journal*, **38** (**10**), 764–768.

86. Hsieh, Y.D., Gau, C.H., Kung Wu, S.F., Shen, E.C., Hsu, P.W. & Fu, E. (2007) Dynamic recording of irrigating fluid distribution in root canals using thermal image analysis. *International Endodontic Journal*, **40** (**1**), 11–17.

87. Cohenca, N., Paranjpe, A., Heilborn, C. & Johnson, J.D. (2013) Antimicrobial efficacy of two irrigation techniques in tapered and non-tapered canal preparations. A randomized controlled clinical trial. *Quintessence International*, **44** (**3**), 217–228.

88. Spångberg, L. (2001) The wonderful world of rotary root canal preparation. *Oral Surgery, Oral Medicine, Oral Pathology, Oral Radiology, and Endodontics*, **92** (**5**), 479.

89. Peters, O.A., Schönenberger, K. & Laib, A. (2001) Effects of four Ni–Ti preparation techniques on root canal geometry assessed by micro computed tomography. *International Endodontic Journal*, **34** (**3**), 221–230.

90. Gluskin, A.H., Brown, D.C. & Buchanan, L.S. (2001) A reconstructed computerized tomographic comparison of Ni–Ti rotary GT files versus traditional instruments in canals shaped by novice operators. *International Endodontic Journal*, **34** (**6**), 476–484.

91. Garala, M., Kuttler, S., Hardigan, P., Steiner-Carmi, R. & Dorn, S. (2003) A comparison of the minimum canal wall thickness remaining following preparation using two nickel–titanium rotary systems. *International Endodontic Journal*, **36** (**9**), 636–642.

92. Rundquist, B.D. & Versluis, A. (2006) How does canal taper affect root stresses? *International Endodontic Journal*, **39** (**3**), 226–237.

93. Paqué, F., Laib, A. & Gautschi, H. (2009) Hard-tissue debris accumulation analysis by high-resolution computed tomography scans. *Journal of Endodontics*, **35** (**7**), 1044–1047.

94. Paqué, F., Boessler, C. & Zehnder, M. (2011) Accumulated hard tissue debris levels in mesial roots of mandibular molars after sequential irrigation steps. *International Endodontic Journal*, **44** (**2**), 148–153.

95. Paqué, F., Rechenberg, D.K. & Zehnder, M. (2012) Reduction of hard-tissue debris accumulation during rotary root canal instrumentation by etidronic

acid in a sodium hypochlorite irrigant. *Journal of Endodontics*, **38** (5), 692–695.

96. Pekruhn, R.B. (1986) The incidence of failure following single-visit endodontic therapy. *Journal of Endodontics*, **12** (2), 68–72.

97. Hoskinson, S.E., Ng, Y.L., Hoskinson, A.E., Moles, D.R. & Gulabivala, K. (2002) A retrospective comparison of outcome of root canal treatment using two different protocols. *Oral Surgery Oral Medicine, Oral Patholology, Oral Radiology, and Endodontics*, **93** (6), 705–715.

98. Peters, O.A., Barbakow, F. & Peters, C.I. (2004) An analysis of endodontic treatment with three nickel–titanium rotary root canal preparation techniques. *International Endodontic Journal*, **37** (12), 849–859.

99. Kirkevang, L.L. & Hørsted-Bindslev, P. (2002) Technical aspects of treatment in relation to treatment outcome. *Endodontic Topics*, **2**, 89–102.

100. Farzaneh, M., Abitbol, S., Lawrence, H.P. & Friedman, S. (2004) Treatment outcome in endodontics – the Toronto study. Phase II: initial treatment. *Journal of Endodontics*, **30** (5), 302–309.

101. Ørstavik, D., Qvist, V. & Stoltze, K. (2004) A multivariate analysis of the outcome of endodontic treatment. *European Journal of Oral Sciences*, **112** (3), 224–230.

102. Paqué, F., Zehnder, M. & Marending, M. (2010) Apical fit of initial K-files in maxillary molars assessed by micro-computed tomography. *International Endodontic Journal*, **43** (4), 328–335.

7 Topical Disinfectants for Root Canal Irrigation

Bettina Basrani
Discipline of Endodontics, University of Toronto, Toronto, ON, Canada

Markus Haapasalo
Department of Oral Biological and Medical Sciences, Unreality of British Columbia, Vancouver, BC, Canada

Introduction

Bacteria have long been recognized as the primary etiologic factors in the development of pulp and apical lesions (1). Successful root canal therapy depends on the thorough chemomechanical debridement of pulpal tissue, dentin debris, and infective microorganisms (2). For a treatment to reach favorable outcomes in endodontic infection management, the recognition of the problem and the removal of the etiological factors is important.

Irrigation is defined as "to wash out a body cavity or wound with water or a medicated fluid" and aspiration as "the process of removing fluids or gases from the body with a suction device." Disinfectant, on the other hand, is defined as an agent that destroys or inhibits the activity of microorganisms that cause a disease (3).

The objectives of irrigation in endodontics are mechanical, chemical, and biological. The mechanical and chemical objectives are as follows: (i) flush out debris, (ii) lubricate the canal, (iii) dissolve organic and inorganic tissue, and (iv) prevent the formation of a smear layer during instrumentation or dissolve it once it has formed. The biological function of the irrigants is related to their antimicrobial effect, more specifically: (i) they have a high efficacy against anaerobic and facultative microorganisms in their planktonic state and in biofilms, (ii) they have the ability to inactivate endotoxin, and (iii) they are nontoxic when they come in contact with vital tissues, are not caustic to periodontal tissues, and have little potential to cause an anaphylactic reaction (4). The characteristics of an ideal irrigant and the classification of current irrigants are shown in Tables 7.1 and 7.2 respectively.

Disinfection of Root Canal Systems: The Treatment of Apical Periodontitis, First Edition. Edited by Nestor Cohenca.
© 2014 John Wiley & Sons, Inc. Published 2014 by John Wiley & Sons, Inc.

Table 7.1 Characteristics of an ideal endodontic irrigant (5–7).

(1) Be an effective germicide and fungicide.
(2) Be nonirritating to the apical tissues.
(3) Remain stable in solution.
(4) Have a prolonged antimicrobial effect and have a sustained antibacterial effect after use.
(5) Be active in the presence of blood, serum, and protein derivate of tissue.
(6) Be able to completely remove the smear layer.
(7) Have low surface tension.
(8) Be able to disinfect the dentin and its tubules.
(9) Do not interfere with repair of apical tissues.
(10) Do not stain tooth structure.
(11) Be capable of inactivation in a culture medium.
(12) Do not induce a cell mediated immune response. Be nonantigenic, nontoxic, and noncarcinogenic to tissue cells surrounding the tooth.
(13) Have no adverse effects on the physical properties of exposed dentin.
(14) Have no adverse effect on the sealing ability of filling materials.
(15) Have convenient application.
(16) Be relatively inexpensive.

Grossman and Meiman (1941) (5). Reproduced with permission of Elsevier.

Table 7.2 Classification of current irrigants.

(A) *Antibacterial agents*: Sodium hypochlorite (NaOCl), chlorhexidine (CHX).
(B) *Decalcifying agents*:
   (a) Weak: Hydroxyethylidene bisphosphonate or etidrona acid (HEBP).
   (b) Strong: Ethylenediaminetetraacetic acid (EDTA).
(C) *Combinations* (antibacterial agents and/or chelating agents + detergent):
   (a) MTAD (Dentsply Tulsa Dental Specialties, Tulsa, OK) and Tetraclean (Ogna Laboratori Farmaceutici, Muggiò, Italy): tetracycline + acid + detergent.
   (b) QMiX (Dentsply Tulsa Dental, Tulsa, OK): CHX, EDTA + detergent.
   (c) Smear Clear (SybronEndo, Orange, CA): EDTA + detergent.
   (d) Chlor-Xtra (Vista Dental, Racine, WI): NaOCl + detergent.
   (e) CH plus (Vista Dental, Racine, WI): CHX + detergent.
(D) *Natural agents*: Green tea, Triphala.

Irrigation solution in endodontics

Sodium hypochlorite (NaOCl)

Sodium hypochlorite is a chemical compound with the formula NaOCl. Sodium hypochlorite solution, commonly known as *bleach*, is frequently used as a disinfectant or a bleaching agent. It is the medicament of choice during root canal treatments following its efficacy against pathogenic organisms and pulp digestion. The main characteristics of sodium hypochlorite are summarized in Table 7.3.

History

Hypochlorite was first produced in 1789 in Javelle, France, by passing chlorine gas through a solution of sodium carbonate. The resulting liquid, known as *Eau de Javelle* or *Javelle water*, was a weak solution of sodium hypochlorite. However, this process was not very efficient and alternative production methods were sought. One such method involved the extraction of chlorinated lime (known as *bleaching powder*) with sodium carbonate to yield low levels of available chlorine. This method was commonly used to produce hypochlorite solutions for use as a hospital antiseptic, which was sold under the trade names "Eusol" and "Dakin's solution." Sodium hypochlorite as a buffered 0.5% solution was recommended for the irrigation of wounds during World War I by Dakin.

Table 7.3 Summary of the characteristics of NaOCl.

Current irrigant of choice
Effective antimicrobial agent
Excellent organic tissue solvent
Lubricant
Fairly quick effective agent

Limitations:

Toxic
Not substantive
Discolors, corrodes, and exudes unpleasant odor
Is ineffective in smear layer removal

Mode of action

When hypochlorite contacts tissue proteins, within a short time, nitrogen, formaldehyde, and acetaldehyde are formed. The peptide links are broken up to dissolve the proteins. During this process, hydrogen in the imino groups (–NH–) is replaced by chlorine (–N·Cl–), forming chloramines, which plays an important role in antimicrobial effectiveness. Thus, the necrotic tissue and pus are dissolved and the antimicrobial agent can better reach and clean the infected areas. In addition to its application as a root canal irrigant, NaOCl is commonly used to deproteinize hard tissues for biomedical applications.

Estrela (8) reported that sodium hypochlorite exhibits a dynamic balance. Sodium hypochlorite acts as an organic and fat solvent that degrades fatty acids and transforms them into fatty acid salts (soap) and glycerol (alcohol), thus reducing the surface tension of the remaining solution (saponification reaction) (Figure 7.1).

Sodium hypochlorite neutralizes amino acids, forming water and salt (neutralization reaction). With the exit of hydroxyl ions, there is a reduction of pH. When chlorine dissolves in water and gets in contact with organic matter, it forms hypochlorous acid. It is a weak acid with the chemical formula HClO. HClO is an oxidizer. This acid acts as a solvent, releasing chlorine that combined with the protein amino group forms chloramines (chloramination reaction). Hypochlorous acid ($HOCl^-$) and hypochlorite ions (OCl^-) lead to amino acid degradation and hydrolysis.

The chloramination reaction between chlorine and the amino group (NH) forms chloramines that interfere in cell metabolism. Chlorine, a strong oxidant, presents antimicrobial action by inhibiting bacterial enzymes, leading to the irreversible oxidation of SH groups (sulfhydryl group) of essential bacterial enzymes (8).

Sodium hypochlorite is a strong base (pH > 11). The antimicrobial effectiveness of sodium hypochlorite, based in its high pH (hydroxyl ions action), is similar to the mechanism of action of calcium hydroxide. The high pH of sodium hypochlorite interferes in the cytoplasmic membrane integrity with an irreversible enzymatic inhibition, biosynthetic alterations in cellular metabolism, and phospholipid degradation observed in lipidic peroxidation (8).

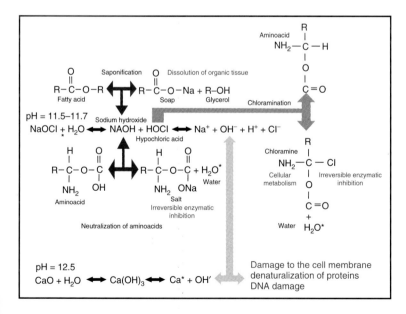

Figure 7.1 Mechanism of the action of NaOCl. (Courtesy of Dr. Manzur.)

Concentrations

As an endodontic irrigant, NaOCl is used in concentrations between 0.5% and 6%. There has been controversy over the use of different concentrations of sodium hypochlorite during root canal treatment. Some *in-vitro* studies have shown that NaOCl in higher concentrations is more effective against *Enterococcus faecalis* and *Candida albicans* (9–11). In contrast, clinical studies have indicated both low and high concentrations to be equally effective in reducing bacteria from the root canal system (2, 12). NaOCl in higher concentrations has a better tissue-dissolving ability (13); however, even in lower concentrations when used in high volumes it can equally be effective (14, 15). Higher concentrations of NaOCl are more toxic than lower concentrations (16); however, because of the confined anatomy of the root canal system, higher concentrations have successfully been used during root canal treatment, with a low incidence of mishaps. Altogether, if lower concentrations are to be used for intracanal irrigation, it is recommended that the solution be used in higher volume and in more frequent intervals to compensate for the limitations of low concentrations (15).

Instrumentation coupled with an antimicrobial irrigant, such as NaOCl, has been shown to yield more negative cultures than instrumentation alone (17–19). However, even with the use of NaOCl, removal of bacteria from the root canal systems following instrumentation remains an elusive goal.

Grossman (20), observing pulp tissue dissolution capacity, reported that 5% sodium hypochlorite dissolves this tissue in between 20 min and 2 h. The dissolution of bovine pulp tissue by sodium hypochlorite (0.5%, 1.0%, 2.5%, and 5.0%) was studied *in-vitro* under different conditions (8). It was concluded that (i) the velocity of dissolution of the bovine pulp fragments was directly proportional to the concentration of the sodium hypochlorite solution and was greater without the surfactant; (ii) the variation of surface tension, from the beginning to the end of pulp dissolution, was directly proportional to the concentration of the sodium hypochlorite solution and was greater in the solutions without surfactant. Solutions without surfactant presented a decrease in surface tension and those with surfactant an increase; (iii) with the

elevation of temperature of the sodium hypochlorite solutions, dissolution of the bovine pulp tissue was more rapid; (iv) the percent variation of the sodium hypochlorite solutions, after dissolution, was inversely proportional to the initial concentration of the solution, or, in other words, the greater the initial concentration of the sodium hypochlorite solutions, the smaller the reduction of its pH (8).

Time of exposure for optimal effect

There is considerable variation in the literature regarding the antibacterial effect of NaOCl (21). In some articles, hypochlorite is reported to kill the target microorganism in seconds, even at low concentrations, although other articles published report considerably longer times for the killing of the same species (21). Such differences are a result of the confounding factors in some of the studies. In the experiments, it was found that the presence of organic matter has a great effect on the antibacterial activity of NaOCl. Haapasalo and colleagues (21) showed that the presence of dentin caused marked delays in the killing of *E. faecalis* by 1% NaOCl. Many of the earlier studies were performed in the presence of an unknown amount of organic matter. When the confounding factors are eliminated, it has been shown that NaOCl kills the target microorganisms rapidly even at low concentrations of less than 0.1% (22, 23). However, *in vivo*, the presence of organic matter (inflammatory exudate, tissue remnants, and microbial biomass) consumes NaOCl and weakens its effect. Therefore, continuous irrigation and time are important factors for the effectiveness of NaOCl (21).

In summary, even fast-acting biocides such as NaOCl require an adequate working time to reach their potential. Chlorine, which is responsible for the dissolving and antibacterial capacity of NaOCl, is unstable and is consumed rapidly during the first phase of tissue dissolution, probably within 2 min (14); therefore, continuous replenishment is essential. This should especially be considered in view of the fact that rotary root canal preparation techniques have expedited the shaping process. The optimal time that a hypochlorite irrigant at a given concentration needs to remain in the canal system is an issue yet to be resolved (24).

Storage and handling

The following points should be considered when handling sodium hypochlorite:

(1) The stability of NaOCl solutions is reduced by lower pH, presence of metallic ions, exposure to light, open containers, and higher temperatures.

(2) To ensure good shelf life, all solutions should be stored in light-proof (opaque glass or polythene), airtight containers, in a cool place.

(3) If diluted, it should be done as soon as possible after purchase, because dilute solutions deteriorate less rapidly than concentrated solutions.

(4) Domestic bleach solutions produced and stored in this manner will deteriorate more rapidly than Milton, because they do not have the added salt, which provides stability.

(5) If undiluted bleach is used, the bottle should always be tightly sealed, and the bleach should be discarded by the "use by" date. The same goes for Milton as well; as long as the container and lid are intact, the product will be effective until the expiry date.

(6) Frequent opening of a container or failure to close it securely would have an effect similar to leaving a container open, and the shelf life would be reduced accordingly.

(7) Metallic containers should never be used for sodium hypochlorite, as the hypochlorite will react with the metal in the containers.

(8) The corrosive nature of sodium hypochlorite must be considered before disposal. As drainage pipes from sinks and dental units may use stainless steel, copper, galvanized steel, poly(vinyl chloride) (PVC), polythene, and perhaps other materials, copious quantities of water should be flushed down all drains at the time of disposal to avoid risk of perforation of drainage traps that have undiluted sodium hypochlorite in them for any period (25).

Safety

Sodium hypochlorite is a nonspecific oxidizing agent. Products of the oxidation reactions are corrosive. Solutions burn skin and cause eye damage, particularly when used in concentrated forms. However, as recognized by the National Fire Protection Association (NFPA), only solutions containing more than 40% sodium hypochlorite by weight are considered hazardous oxidizers. Solutions less than 40% are classified as a moderate oxidizing hazard (NFPA 430, 2000). The toxic effects of NaOCl on vital tissues include hemolysis, epithelial ulceration, and necrosis (4).

Several mishaps during root canal irrigation have been described in the dental literature. These range from damage to the patient's clothing, splashing the irrigant into the patient's or operator's eye, injection through the apical foramen, and allergic reactions to the irrigant, to inadvertent use of an irrigant as an anesthetic solution (4). Preventive measures that should be taken to minimize potential complications with sodium hypochlorite are presented in Table 7.4 (26) (Figure 7.2).

A literature review of inadvertent extrusion of NaOCl beyond the apical foramen found similar symptoms, regardless of the concentration, with tissue responses proportional to the volume of NaOCl extruded (27) (Figure 7.3). Extrusion of NaOCl into the apical tissues can result from several pathways. A wide apical foramen, lack of

Table 7.4 Protective measures during NaOCl irrigation.

- Plastic bib to protect patient's clothing
- Provision of protective eye-wear for both patient and operator
- The use of a sealed rubber dam for isolation of the tooth under treatment
- The use of side exit Luer-Lok needles for root canal irrigation
- Irrigation needle a minimum of 2 mm short of the working length (Figure 7.2)
- Avoidance of binding the needle into the root canal
- Avoidance of excessive pressure during irrigation

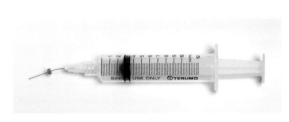

Figure 7.2 Placement of rubber stopper on irrigation needle to prevent NaOCl accident.

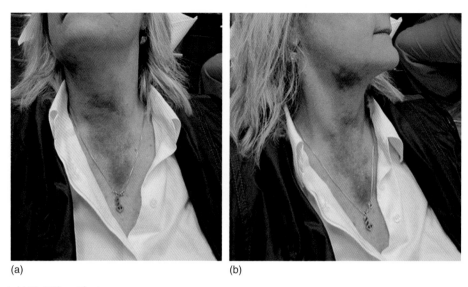

(a)   (b)

Figure 7.3   (a,b) NaOCl accident.

apical constriction, or extreme pressure might all lead to the extrusion of NaOCl. Most complications occur because of the incorrect working length, widening of the apical foramen, lateral perforation, or binding of the irrigating needle (28).

The main symptoms when injected into the apical tissues are immediate severe pain, immediate edema of the neighboring soft tissues, possible extension of edema over the injured side of the face, upper lip and infraorbital region, profuse bleeding from the root canal, profuse interstitial bleeding with hemorrhage of the skin and mucosa (ecchymosis), chlorine taste and irritation of the throat after injection into the maxillary sinus, secondary infection, reversible anesthesia, or paresthesia.

Current treatment protocols for NaOCl accidents have been determined mainly from the numerous case reports published, rather than more evidence-based research efforts. Mehdipour *et al.* (29) suggest early recognition of extrusion, immediate canal irrigation with normal saline, encouragement of bleeding, pain control with local anesthetics and analgesics, and warm compresses and frequent warm mouth rinses for the stimulation of the local systemic circulation, reassurance of the patient, and monitoring the improvement. Cancellous bone is significantly affected by NaOCl, whereas cortical bone is minimally affected. Cancellous bone after a NaOCl accident is less dense, with broken and dissolved architecture. The deeper

penetration of the test needle is interpreted as the result of a disrupture in the structural integrity of the cancellous bone. The principal harm is to the cells, because they are dependent on the specific fluid environment in which they are found; NaOCl changes that environment, causing cellular necrosis and apoptosis. The damaged matrix can then become a nidus for infection. Trabecular bone is damaged by the toxic effects of NaOCl. The less cellular cortical bone is clearly less affected. The results show that the loss of organic content of the bone and demineralization are significant, and no sign of living cellular content remains (30).

Effect of NaOCl on dentin

Dentin is composed of approximately 22% organic material by weight. Most of this consists of type I collagen, which contributes considerably to the mechanical properties of dentin (31). Sodium hypochlorite is known to fragment long peptide chains and to chlorinate protein terminal groups; the resulting *N*-chloramines are broken down into other species (32). Consequently, hypochlorite solutions may affect mechanical dentin properties via the degradation of organic dentin components (33).

A study on bovine dentin suggested that within the time frame of a root canal treatment, concentrated hypochlorite solutions cause untoward effects on dentin biomechanics (34).

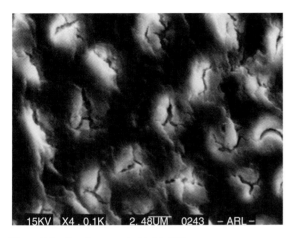

Figure 7.4 Dentin treated with NaOCl.

A 2 h exposure of dentin to NaOCl solutions of more than 3% (w/v) significantly decreases the elastic modulus and flexural strength of human dentin compared to physiological saline (35). However, contrasting results have also been published (36). A recent study showed a clear concentration-dependent effect of NaOCl solutions on the mechanical dentin properties resulting from the disintegration of the organic dentin matrix (37) (Figure 7.4).

There have been several reports of the adverse effects of sodium hypochlorite on physical properties such as flexural strength, elastic modulus, and microhardness of dentin. These changes in the physical properties of dentin come not only from changes in the inorganic phase but also from the organic phase of dentin. Moreover, in their eagerness to ensure "complete" disinfection, dentists vary not only the concentration but also the volume, duration, flow rate, and temperature in their attempts to eliminate all bacteria (37). It is quite clear from the literature that the higher the concentration of sodium hypochlorite, the greater the deleterious effects on dentin. These effects include the reduction of the elastic modulus and the flexural strength.

Sodium hypochlorite penetration of dentinal tubules

Not many studies have analyzed the penetration of NaOCl inside the dentinal tubules. Zou *et al.*

(38) are the first to report hypochlorite penetration into dentin measured with such accuracy (micrometers). Within their experimental setup, the depth of hypochlorite penetration varied between 77 and 300 μm. The three parameters potentially affecting hypochlorite penetration that were evaluated in the present study were concentration, time, and temperature. All of these did have an impact on the penetration, but the effect was generally less than anticipated. Perhaps the most surprising observation was that increasing the concentration from 1% to 6% did not result in more than 30–50% increase in penetration. Longer exposure time in the present study resulted in deeper penetration of hypochlorite, although the speed of penetration declined sharply over time. For example, at 20 °C, penetration depth of 1% NaOCl in 2 min was about 77 μm; after another 18 min at the same temperature, the depth reached about 185 μm. Because the solubilizing abilities of NaOCl solutions are reduced by contact with organic material, it can be speculated that most of its activity is lost after 2 min, and continuous replenishment of fresh solution will be needed. The antibacterial effectiveness of NaOCl is dependent on its concentration, temperature, and volume and contact time in the root canal. The results showed that the three variables all had an effect on NaOCl penetration, but the effect was not very pronounced for any of the factors alone. The penetration depths of 1%, 2%, 4%, and 6% solutions after 2 min at room temperature were 77, 96, 105, and 123 μm, respectively. The highest values, 291 and 300 μm, were found in the groups treated by 6% NaOCl at 37 and 45 °C for 20 min. Within the limitations of this study, temperature, time, and concentration all play a role in determining the depth of hypochlorite penetration into dentinal tubules. Deepest penetration was obtained when these factors were present simultaneously, suggesting an additive effect (Figure 7.5) (38).

Allergic reactions to NaOCl

Although few reports on allergy-like reactions to sodium hypochlorite have been published (39, 40), real allergies to sodium hypochlorite are unlikely to occur as both sodium and chlorine are essential elements in the physiology of the human body. Nevertheless, hypersensitivity and contact dermatitis may occur in rare cases. In cases

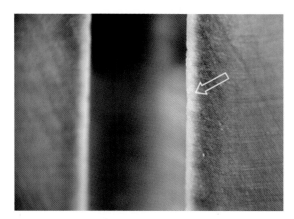

Figure 7.5   Sodium hypochlorite penetration of dentinal tubules.

of hypersensitivity against sodium hypochlorite, chlorhexidine (CHX) should not be used because of the chlorine content. In such cases, the use of an alternative irrigant with high antimicrobial efficacy such as iodine–potassium iodide (IPI) should be considered. Before use, any allergy against iodine must be ruled out. Further irrigants such as alcohol or tap water are less effective against microorganisms and do not dissolve vital or necrotic tissue. Calcium hydroxide could be used as a temporary medicament as it dissolves both vital and necrotic tissues (41, 42).

Effect on biofilm

Biofilm growth over root surfaces has been demonstrated on teeth with chronic apical periodontitis and teeth refractory to root canal treatment. Bacteria organized as biofilms have been found in inaccessible areas of necrotic pulp space and on root surfaces and cemental lacunae. Growing within a competitive environment, the organisms within biofilm generally have a low metabolic rate and tend to be very resistant to antimicrobial substances. The negatively charged polymers within the matrix may neutralize strong oxidizing agents, making it difficult for them to penetrate and kill microorganisms. Because of the close proximity of bacterial cells within the biofilm, DNA exchange readily takes place and can rapidly transfer antibiotic resistance. Therefore, antimicrobial substances that easily kill free-floating organisms have not shown the same effectiveness on the same

organisms originating from a biofilm. In addition, the structure of biofilm offers protection to resident bacteria from immune defenses. These properties of biofilm help to explain the chronic nature and resistance of some endodontic infections (43).

Clegg *et al.* (44), in their classic paper on the effect of NaOCl on biofilms, reported that 6% NaOCl was the only agent capable of both physically removing artificial biofilm and killing bacteria. There was a dose-dependent effect of NaOCl against bacteria, as higher concentrations were more antibacterial. This confirms the results of previous studies that also demonstrated the concentration-dependant antibacterial nature of NaOCl. One percent and 3% NaOCl showed some disruption and physical removal of bacteria when viewed with the scanning electron microscopy (SEM); however, both gave positive cultures when their dentinal shavings were cultured, indicating that bacteria had escaped the effects of the irrigant probably by invading the dentinal tubules. The lower the concentration of NaOCl, the better the chances for more bacteria survival. However, the lower NaOCl concentrations may have been more effective against bacteria if they were replenished or given additional time to exert their antimicrobial properties. The antibiofilm effects of NaOCl may be a result of the removal of organic tissue, eliminating the bacterial attachment to dentin and other organisms (44).

A recent study evaluated the antibacterial effect of a several irrigating solution on 3-week-old *E. faecalis* biofilms. The agents analyzed were QMiX (see the details below in this chapter), 2% CHX, MTAD, 1%, and 2% NaOCl. QMiX and 2% NaOCl killed up to 12 times more biofilm bacteria than 1% NaOCl ($P < 0.01$), 2% CHX ($P < 0.05$; $P < 0.001$), and MTAD ($P < 0.05$; $P < 0.001$) (Figure 7.6) (45).

Increasing the efficacy of NaOCl

Possible ways to improve the efficacy of hypochlorite preparations in tissue dissolution are to increase the pH and the temperature of the solutions, use ultrasonic activation (7), and extend the working time.

Increasing the temperature of sodium hypochlorite

Cunningham (46) and Joseph reported that the collagen-dissolving ability of 2.6% sodium

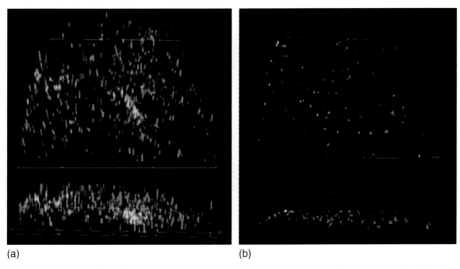

(a)   (b)

Figure 7.6   The three-dimensional confocal laser scanning microscopy reconstruction of the *in-vitro* 7 days' biofilm of *Enterococcus faecalis* subjected to antimicrobial irrigants (inlet shows the sagittal section). These biofilms were stained using Live/Dead BacLight stain (green: viable cell and red: dead cell) (a) the biofilm receiving no treatment, (b) the biofilm exposed to sodium hypochlorite. The biofilm structure in the sodium hypochlorite treated specimen is disrupted. (Courtesy of Dr. Anil Kishen.)

hypochlorite was comparable to that of 5.25% at both 21 and 37 °C. The investigators also compared the solutions' ability to kill bacteria at different temperatures. They tested the ability of 2.6% and 5.25% sodium hypochlorite in reducing a planktonic culture of *Escherichia coli* to below culturable level at 20 and 37 °C. They found that it took less time to kill *E. coli* in both concentrations at 37 °C. Interestingly, it was also reported that increasing the temperature of sodium hypochlorite to 50 °C did not help in making the root canal cleaner. However, at the higher temperature (50 °C), Berutti *et al.* (47) observed a thin, less organized, and less adherent smear layer on the root canal wall. This thinner layer was not evident on root canals irrigated with sodium hypochlorite at 21 °C.

From the above studies, it is apparent that raising the temperature may have some benefit in killing bacteria more quickly. However, raising the temperature to 37 °C did not help dissolve tissues more effectively. Though we may think of raising the temperature of irrigants to kill bacteria more effectively, we should not raise the temperature more than a few degrees above body temperature as this may have harmful effects on the cells of the periodontal ligament (48).

Different devices for warming the NaOCl syringes (Figure 7.7) have been released into the market, but these devices are not capable of maintaining any raise of temperature. The best way of heating up the NaOCl is to do it *in situ* with an ultrasonic device.

A recent study evaluated and compared the effects of concentration, temperature, and agitation on the tissue-dissolving ability of sodium hypochlorite (48). The results showed that weight loss (dissolution) of the tissue increased almost linearly with the concentration of sodium hypochlorite. Higher temperatures and agitation considerably enhanced the efficacy of sodium hypochlorite. The effect of agitation on tissue dissolution was greater than that of temperature; continuous agitation resulted in the fastest tissue dissolution.

Agitation

Moorer and Wesselink (14) found that the impact of mechanical agitation of hypochlorite solutions on tissue dissolution was very important and they emphasized the great impact of violent fluid flow and shearing forces caused by ultrasound on the ability of hypochlorite to dissolve tissue. Stojicic

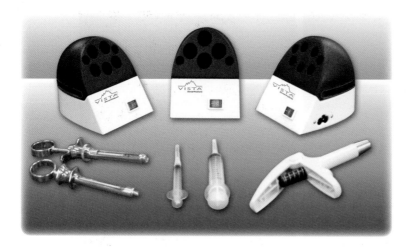

Figure 7.7   Heating devices for NaOCl. (Courtesy of Vista Dental Products.)

et al. (45) found that refreshing the hypochlorite solution at the site of dissolution by agitation, preferably continuous, also resulted in a marked increase of hypochlorite effect. Fabiani (49) also demonstrated that the use of ultrasonic agitation increased the effectiveness of 5% NaOCl in the apical third of the canal wall. Finally, passive ultrasonic irrigation with a nickel–titanium tip produced superior tissue-dissolving effects as compared to sonic irrigant activation (50).

Influence of NaOCl on bond strength

NaOCl irrigation leads to decreased bond strength between dentin and resin cements and may require a reversal agent because of its ability to affect the polymerization of the resin sealer (51).

Chlorhexidine (CHX)

History

CHX (Figure 7.8) was developed more than 50 years ago at Imperial Chemical Industries in England, and was first marketed in the United Kingdom in 1953 as an antiseptic cream (52). Since 1957, it has been used for general disinfection purposes and for the treatment of skin, eye, and throat infections in both humans and animals (52, 53).

Molecular structure

CHX belongs to the polybiguanide antibacterial family, consisting of two symmetric 4-chlorophenyl rings and two biguanide groups connected by a central hexamethylene chain. CHX is a strong basic molecule and is stable as a salt. CHX digluconate salt is easily soluble in water (Figure 7.9) (54).

Mode of action

CHX is a wide-spectrum antimicrobial agent, active against gram-positive and gram-negative bacteria, and yeasts (55). Owing to its cationic nature, CHX is capable of electrostatically binding to the negatively charged surfaces of bacteria (56), damaging the outer layers of the cell wall and rendering it permeable (57–59).

Depending on its concentration, CHX can have both bacteriostatic and bactericidal effects. At high concentration, CHX acts as a detergent, and by damaging the cell membrane it causes precipitation of the cytoplasm and thereby exerts a bactericidal effect. At low sublethal concentrations, CHX is bacteriostatic, causing low molecular weight substances, that is, potassium and phosphorus, to leak out without the cell being irreversibly damaged. It also can affect bacterial metabolism in several other ways such as abolishing the activity of the phosphotransferase system (PTS) sugar transport system and inhibiting acid production in some bacteria (60).

Substantivity

Owing to the cationic nature of its molecule, CHX can be absorbed by anionic substrates such as the

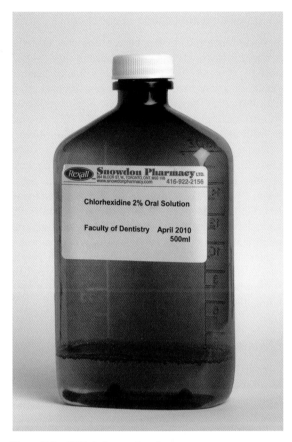

Figure 7.8   CHX dark container for storage.

Figure 7.9   CHX molecule.

oral mucosa (61, 62). CHX has the ability to bind to proteins such as albumin, which is present in serum or saliva, pellicle found on the tooth surface, salivary glycoproteins, and mucous membranes (63, 64). This reaction is reversible (65). CHX can also be adsorbed onto hydroxyapatite and teeth.

Studies have shown that the uptake of CHX onto teeth is also reversible. This reversible reaction of uptake and release of CHX leads to substantive antimicrobial activity and is referred to as *substantivity* (66). This effect depends on the concentration of CHX. At low concentrations of 0.005–0.01%, a stable monolayer of CHX is adsorbed and formed on the tooth surface, which might change the physical and chemical properties of the surface and may prevent or reduce bacterial colonization. At higher concentrations (>0.02%), a multilayer of CHX is formed on the surface providing a reservoir of CHX, which can rapidly release the excess into the environment as the concentration of the CHX in the surrounding environment decreases (67).

The antibacterial substantivity of three concentrations of CHX solution (4%, 2%, and 0.2%) after 5 min of application has been evaluated. Results revealed a direct relationship between the concentration of CHX and its substantivity (68). On the contrary, Lin *et al.* (69) attributed the substantivity of CHX to its ability to adsorb on to the dentin during the first hour. They stated that it is only after the saturation point is reached after the first hour that the antimicrobial capability of CHX increases with time. Furthermore, Komorowski *et al.* (70) revealed that 5 min application of CHX did not induce substantivity and that the dentin should be treated with CHX for 7 days. Taken together, it seems that residual antimicrobial activity of CHX in the root canal system remains for up to 12 weeks (68).

Cytotoxicity

In the medical field, CHX is normally used at concentrations between 0.12% and 2.0%. According to Löe (71), at these concentrations, CHX has a low level of tissue toxicity, both locally and systemically (71). Another report stated that when 2% CHX was used as a subgingival irrigant, no apparent toxicity was noted on gingival tissues (71, 72). Moreover, CHX rinse was reported to promote the healing of periodontal wounds (73). On the basis of these reports, Jeansonne and White (74) assumed that the apical tissues would be as tolerant to CHX as gingival tissues. In two studies it was found that when CHX and NaOCl were injected into the subcutaneous tissues of guinea pigs and rats, an inflammatory reaction was developed; however, the toxic reaction to CHX was less than that to NaOCl (75, 76). Furthermore, when CHX was applied as a rinse in the extraction sites of the third molars on the day of surgery and several days after, it was reported to reduce the incidence of alveolar osteitis (77). In addition, there are only a few allergic and anaphylactic reactions reported to CHX (78, 79).

Conversely, some studies have reported unfavorable effects of CHX on the tissues. Hidalgo (80) demonstrated that CHX is cytotoxic to some lines of cultured human skin fibroblasts. Recently, the behavior of osteoblastic human alveolar bone cells in the presence of CHX and povidone–iodine (PI) has been investigated. It has been reported that CHX has a higher cytotoxicity profile than PI (81). Faria *et al.* (82) also demonstrated that CHX injected into the hind paws of mice could induce severe toxic reactions. In addition, they reported that CHX induced apoptosis at lower concentrations and necrosis at higher concentrations when added to cultured L929 fibroblast cells.

Another interesting observation has been reported recently when CHX is in contact with other agents such as NaOCl. The by-product of the reaction of CHX with NaOCl is the formation of toxic breakdown products such as *para*-chloroaniline (PCA) that may have a negative impact on tissues (83). The toxicity level of CHX on apical tissues when applied in the root canals needs to be investigated further.

Chlorhexidine application in dentistry

CHX has several applications in dentistry. It has been used for the prevention of dental caries, plaque formation, and gingivitis, especially in the elderly and senile patients, as well as those with conditions such as cerebral palsy and patients with immune-compromising diseases. It has also been recommended for the prevention of alveolar osteitis after the extraction of third molars. Another application of CHX is in the treatment and management of periodontal diseases, as well as in the reduction of the incidence, severity, and duration of aphthous ulceration. In addition, it has been advocated as a denture disinfectant in patients susceptible to oral candidiasis. CHX can be prepared in the form of mouth rinses, gels, varnishes, and controlled-release devices (83).

Chlorhexidine application in endodontics

In endodontics, CHX has been studied as an irrigant and intracanal medication, both *in-vivo* (84–87) and *in-vitro* (88–91). *In-vitro*, CHX has at least as good, or even better, antimicrobial efficacy than Ca(OH)$_2$ (92). Notably, 2% CHX is very effective in eliminating a biofilm of *E. faecalis* (85). *In-vivo*, it inhibits experimentally induced inflammatory external root resorption when applied for 4 weeks (84). In infected root canals, it reduces bacteria as effectively as Ca(OH)$_2$ when applied for 1 week (93). Unlike Ca(OH)$_2$, CHX has substantive antimicrobial activity that, if imparted onto the root dentin, has the potential to prevent bacterial colonization of root canal walls for prolonged periods of time (70, 74). This effect depends on the concentration of CHX, not on its mode of application, which may be used either as liquid, gel, or a controlled-release device (89).

Chlorhexidine as an endodontic irrigant

CHX in liquid and gel form has been recommended as an irrigant solution, and its different properties have been tested in several studies, both *in-vitro* (9) and *in-vivo* (93–100).

Many investigations have been conducted to study the antibacterial effectiveness of CHX in different concentrations. It has been demonstrated that 2% CHX as an irrigant has a better antibacterial efficacy than 0.12% CHX *in-vitro*. Thus, it is concluded that the antibacterial efficacy of CHX depends on its concentration level (90). Because NaOCl is still the most commonly used irrigant, the antibacterial efficacy of CHX is tested against that of NaOCl. The results from these studies are not conclusive, but in general no significant difference between these two solutions has been reported. It is possible, however, that culture methods are not sensitive enough to detect differences in the antibacterial effectiveness of various antibacterial agents; that is, the methods may not be suitable to quantitate the killing of biofilm bacteria. Unlike NaOCl, CHX lacks the tissue-dissolving property. Therefore, NaOCl is still considered to be the primary irrigation solution used in endodontics.

The cleanliness of root canals using CHX in gel and liquid forms was evaluated with SEM in two separate experiments. In an *in-vitro* study, the canals treated with 2% CHX gel were cleaner than those treated with 2% CHX liquid or 5.25% NaOCl, and it was suggested that the mechanical action of the gel might have facilitated the cleansing of the canals. Another *in-vitro* study showed that the 2% CHX liquid was inferior to 2.5% NaOCl in cleaning the canals (101). However, *in-vitro* studies may not properly reflect the actual *in-vivo* situations, which are more clinically relevant.

The antibacterial effectiveness of CHX in the reduction of bacteria in infected root canals *in-vivo* has been investigated in several studies. Ringel *et al.* (102) reported that 2.5% sodium hypochlorite was significantly more effective than 0.2% CHX when the infected root canals were irrigated for 30 min by either of the solutions.

In a controlled and randomized clinical trial, the efficacy of 2% CHX liquid was tested against saline using a culture technique. All the teeth were initially instrumented and irrigated using 1% sodium hypochlorite. Then, either 2% CHX liquid or saline was applied as a final rinse. The authors reported a further reduction in the proportion of positive cultures in the CHX group. Their results showed a better disinfection of the root canals using chlorhexidine compared to saline as a final rinse (96).

In a recent study, the efficacy of 2% CHX gel was tested against 2.5% NaOCl in teeth with apical periodontitis and the bacterial load was assessed using real-time quantitative-polymerase chain reaction (RTQ-PCR) and colony forming units (CFU). The bacterial reduction in the NaOCl group was significantly greater than the CHX-group when measured by RTQ-PCR. On the basis of a culture technique, bacterial growth was detected in 50% of the CHX-group cases compared to 25% in the NaOCl group (103).

On the other hand, a more recent study also based on a culture technique revealed no significant difference between the antibacterial efficacy of 2.5% NaOCl and 0.12% CHX liquid when used as irrigants during the treatment of infected canals (99). It is important to point out one more time that culture techniques are not sensitive enough to detect bacterial growth.

CHX and dentin bonding

During the past two decades, chemical and technical advances have contributed to increases in resin–dentin bond strength. However, the premature loss of bond strength is one of the problems that still affects adhesive restorations (104) and markedly reduces their durability (105–108). Carrilho *et al.* (108) evaluated the effect of CHX on the resin–dentin bond stability *ex-vivo*. Results showed that with CHX, significantly better preservation of bond strength was observed after 6 months and protease inhibitors in the storage medium had no effect. Failure analysis showed significantly less failure in the hybrid layer with CHX, compared with controls after 6 months. Furthermore, they evaluated the effect of CHX on the preservation of the hybrid layer *in-vivo*. Findings showed that bond strength remained stable in the CHX-treated specimens, while bond strength decreased significantly in control teeth. Resin-infiltrated dentin in CHX-treated specimens exhibited normal structural integrity of the collagen network. Conversely, progressive disintegration of the fibrillar network was identified in control specimens. They concluded that autodegradation of collagen matrices can occur in resin-infiltrated dentin, but may be prevented by the application of a synthetic protease inhibitor, such as CHX (108). On the whole, because of its broad-spectrum matrix metalloproteinase (MMP)-inhibitory effect, CHX can significantly improve the resin–dentin bond stability.

Effect on biofilm

A dentin infection model was used to compare the antibacterial effect of different disinfecting solutions on young and old *E. faecalis* biofilms (Figure 7.10). High-concentration NaOCl (6%) showed the strongest antibacterial effect among the solutions tested for both young and old *E. faecalis* biofilms. QMiX, a product containing ethylenediaminetetraacetic acid (EDTA), CHX, and a detergent, was equally effective as 6% NaOCl in killing 1-day-old *E. faecalis* but slightly less effective against bacteria in 3-week-old biofilm. It is worth noting that 2% CHX and 2% NaOCl killed only 13–15% of the 3-week-old biofilm bacteria in dentin after 1 min of exposure. This result suggests that a quick final rinse with these two agents at the given concentration is not effective in reducing the number of viable bacteria in the tubules (109).

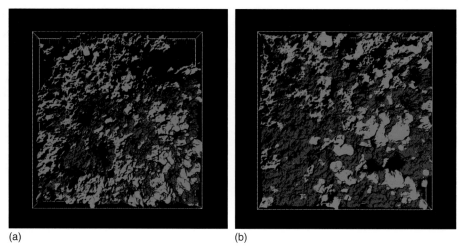

(a)   (b)

Figure 7.10   (a,b) Effect of CHX on biofilm.

Allergic reactions to CHX

CHX, although reported to be a relatively safe solution, may induce allergic reactions. The sensitization rate has been reported in several studies to be approximately 2% (110). One case of an anaphylactic shock after application of 0.6% CHX to intact skin, only showing signs of a rash following a minor accident, has been presented in the dermatological literature (111). Further allergic reactions such as anaphylaxis, contact dermatitis, and urticaria have been reported following direct contact with mucosal tissue or open wounds (112–115). There are no publications of allergic reactions following root canal irrigation with CHX (4). The main characteristics of CHX are summarized in Table 7.5.

Irrigant solutions with added detergent

Surface-active agents have been added to several newer irrigants to reduce surface tension and improve their wettability (5). Smear Clear (SybronEndo, Orange, CA), Chlor-Xtra (Vista Dental, Racine, WI), and CH plus (Vista Dental, Racine, WI), MTAD, and QMiX are examples of the EDTA, NaOCl, and CHX based irrigants that contain surface-active detergents (Figure 7.11) (116).

Several studies analyzed the antibacterial properties and wettability of these new irrigants with contrasting results: Williamson *et al.* (117) created a monoculture biofilm of a clinical isolate of *E. faecalis* and determined the susceptibility

Table 7.5   Characteristics of chlorhexidine.

(1)   CHX has a wide range of activity against both gram-positive and gram-negative bacteria.
(2)   CHX is an effective antifungal agent especially against *C. albicans*.
(3)   The effect of CHX on microbial biofilms is significantly less than that of NaOCl.
(4)   CHX has antibacterial substantivity in dentin for up to 12 weeks.
(5)   Dentin, dentin components (hyaluronic acid (HA) and collagen), microbial biomass, and inflammatory exudate in the root canal system may reduce or inhibit the antibacterial activity of CHX.
(6)   CHX has little to no ability to dissolve organic tissues.
(7)   Medication and/or irrigation with CHX may delay the contamination of root filled teeth by bacteria entering through the coronal restoration/tooth interface.
(8)   Medication and/or irrigation with CHX will not adversely affect the penetration of fluid through the root filled apical foramen.
(9)   Combination of NaOCl and CHX causes color changes and the formation of a precipitate, which may interfere with the seal of the root filling.
(10) CHX can significantly improve the integrity of the hybrid layer andresin–dentin bond stability.
(11) The biocompatibility of CHX is acceptable.

Mohammadi and Abbott (68). Reproduced with permission of John Wiley & Sons, Inc.

against four antimicrobial irrigants. Biofilms were subjected to 1-, 3-, and 5-min exposures to one of the following irrigants: 6% sodium hypochlorite (NaOCl), 2% chlorhexidine gluconate (CHX) or one

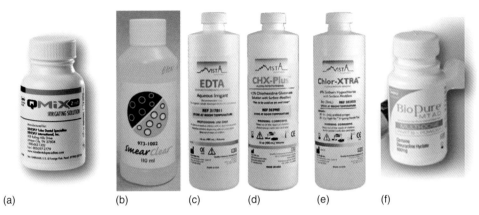

Figure 7.11   (a–f) Detergent additions to irrigants.

of the two new products, less than 6% NaOCl with surface modifiers (Chlor-XTRA) or 2% CHX with surface modifiers (CHX-Plus) (Vista Dental Products, Racine, WI). It was hypothesized that NaOCl and CHX would be equally effective and that the addition of surface modifiers would improve the bactericidal activity of the respective irrigants compared to the original formulations. Results indicate that 6% NaOCl and Chlor-EXTRA were superior against *E. faecalis* biofilms compared to 2% CHX and CHX-Plus at all-time points except 5 min.

On a similar line, Palazzi *et al.* (118) studied that the new 5.25% sodium hypochlorite solutions modified with surfactants, Hypoclean A and Hypoclean B, had surface tension values that were significantly lower ($P < 0.01$) than Chlor-Xtra and 5.25% NaOCl. Because of their low surface tension and increased contact with dentinal walls, these new irrigants have the potential to penetrate more readily into the uninstrumented areas of root canal system as well as allow a more rapid exchange with fresh solution, enabling greater antimicrobial effectiveness and enhanced pulp tissue dissolution ability.

In contrast, Jungbluth *et al.* (119) compared physicochemical features of these products and investigated their impact of 1% dilutions on bovine pulp tissue dissolution. No differences were detected between solutions with or without a detergent. It is not known at present whether the differences between the studies are at least partly affected by differences in experimental design such

as different dilutions (e.g., 6% vs. 1%) and different types of tissue tested.

Finally, Wang *et al.* (120) evaluated the effectiveness of dentin disinfection by different antibacterial solutions in the presence and absence of detergents using a novel dentin infection model and confocal laser scanning microscopy (CLSM). The addition of detergents in the disinfecting solutions used in the present study increased their antibacterial effects against *E. faecalis* in the dentinal tubules. When used alone as a single agent, cetrimide (CTR) showed antibacterial effectiveness comparable to 2% NaOCl, 2% CHX, and 2%/4% IPI.

Interaction NaOCl and CHX

A suggested clinical protocol by Zehnder (24) for treating the dentin before root canal filling consists of irrigation with NaOCl to dissolve the organic components, irrigation with EDTA to eliminate the smear layer, and irrigation with CHX to increase the antimicrobial spectrum of activity and impart substantivity. Although such a combination of irrigants may enhance the overall antimicrobial effectiveness (93), the possible chemical interactions among the irrigants have to be considered. Some studies have reported the occurrence of color change and precipitation when NaOCl and CHX are combined (Figure 7.12) (83, 121). Furthermore, concern has been raised that the color change may have some clinical relevance because of staining and that the precipitate might interfere with the seal of the root filling (121). The formation of a

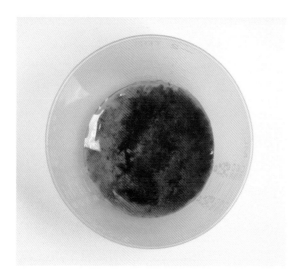

Figure 7.12   Interaction NaOCl and CHX.

precipitate could be explained by the acid–base reaction that occurs when NaOCl and CHX are mixed together. CHX, a dicationic acid, has the ability to donate protons while NaOCl is alkaline and can accept protons from the dicationic acid (122). This proton exchange results in the formation of a neutral and insoluble substance referred to as the *precipitate* (83). Basrani *et al.* (83) evaluated the chemical nature of this precipitate and reported that there was an immediate reaction when 2% CHX was combined with NaOCl, even at the low concentration (0.023%). Increasing the concentration of NaOCl to 0.19% (the sixth dilution in their series) resulted in the formation of a precipitate, which consisted mainly of PCA. This occurred through a substitution of the guanidine group in the CHX molecule. It was found that the amount of PCA directly increased with the increasing concentration of NaOCl. PCA has been shown to be toxic with short-term exposure of humans to PCA resulting in cyanosis, which is a manifestation of methemoglobin formation. In another study, Bui *et al.* (123) evaluated the effect of irrigating root canals with a combination of NaOCl and CHX on root dentin and dentinal tubules by using an environmental SEM and a computer program. Their findings indicated that there were no significant differences in the amount of debris remaining between the negative control group and the experimental groups although there were significantly

fewer patent tubules in the experimental groups when compared with the negative control group. They concluded that the NaOCl/CHX precipitate tends to occlude the dentinal tubules and suggested that until this precipitate is studied further, caution should be exercised when irrigating with both NaOCl and CHX.

Some studies have not corroborated this finding but the gas chromatography method of identification used in one of these studies may not have been sensitive enough to detect its presence (124). In the other study (125), the authors reported that only native CHX, *para*-chlorophenylurea (PCU), and *para*-chlorophenylguanidyl-1,6-diguanidyl-hexane (PCGH) present in the precipitate formed when CHX was mixed with NaOCl. However, it was shown later that PCU could be metabolized to form PCA and therefore still retained a risk (125).

A recent study aimed to determine if the formation of PCA can be avoided by using an alternative irrigant after sodium hypochlorite but before using CHX; however, none of the tested solutions used for intermittent irrigation prevented the formation of PCA. The investigators concluded that citric acid used as the intermediate irrigant resulted in the least amount of PCA formation in the canal system (122). When NaOCl and QMiX are mixed, there is no formation of a precipitate, but there is a change of color in the combination. This is the reason why the manufacturer recommends rinsing with saline solution before using QMiX.

Another study proposed that the precipitate could be prevented by using absolute alcohol or minimized by using saline and distilled water as intermediate flushes (126).

Taken together, the combination of NaOCl and CHX causes color changes and formation of a neutral and insoluble precipitate, which may interfere with the seal of the root filling. Alternatively, the canal can be dried using paper points before the final CHX rinse (24).

Decalcifying solutions

Until recently, decalcifying solutions in endodontics comprised only of chelators and acids, most commonly EDTA and citric acid. In the past few years, however, several combination products have appeared where the main function, decalcifying effect, has been combined with other characteristics thought to be helpful for the treatment. The added characteristics are reduced surface tension and perhaps, more importantly, antibacterial activity. The new combination products are based either on EDTA or citric acid. They are discussed at the end of this section after the "conventional" products.

A smear layer is formed during the preparation of the root canal. The smear layer consists of both an organic and an inorganic component. Both NaOCl and a decalcifying agent are required for the complete removal of the smear layer. No clear scientifically based understanding exists on whether this layer must be removed or can be left. However, a multitude of opinions have been offered on both sides of this question. In addition to weak acids, solutions for the removal of the smear layer include carbamide peroxide, aminoquinaldinium diacetate (i.e., Salvizol), and EDTA. In objective studies, carbamide peroxide and Salvizol appear to have little effect on smear layer buildup (127, 128). A 25% citric acid solution also failed to provide reliable smear layer removal (129).

EDTA

EDTA (Figure 7.13) is often suggested as an irrigation solution because it can chelate and remove the mineralized portion of smear layers.

EDTA is a widely used acronym for the chemical compound ethylenediaminetetraacetic acid. EDTA is a polyamino carboxylic acid with the formula $[CH_2N(CH_2CO_2H)_2]_2$. This colorless, water-soluble solid is produced on a large scale for many applications. Its prominence as a chelating agent arises from its ability to "sequester" di- and tricationic metal ions such as Ca^{2+} and Fe^{3+}. After being bound by EDTA, metal ions remain in solution but exhibit diminished reactivity. Its compounds and characteristics are shown in Table 7.6.

History

The compound was first described in 1935 by Munz, who prepared the compound from ethylenediamine and chloroacetic acid. Today, EDTA is mainly synthesized from ethylenediamine (1,2-diaminoethane), formaldehyde (methanal), and sodium cyanide.

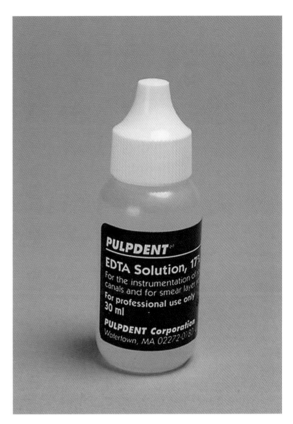

Figure 7.13   EDTA.

Table 7.6   Characteristics of the decalcifying solutions.

- Affecting the inorganic part of the smear layer
- Removal of the smear layer after NaOCl irrigation
- Contributing to the elimination of bacteria in the root canal
- Antifungal activity
- Demineralizing dentin (20–50 μm)
- Low toxicity

Mode of action

With direct exposure for extended time, EDTA extracts bacterial surface proteins by combining with metal ions from the cell envelope, which can eventually lead to bacterial death.

Applications in endodontics

EDTA alone normally cannot remove the smear layer effectively (Figure 7.14); a proteolytic component (e.g., NaOCl) must be added to remove

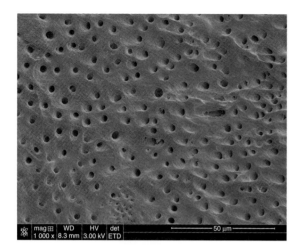

Figure 7.14   Dentin treated with NaOCl + EDTA.

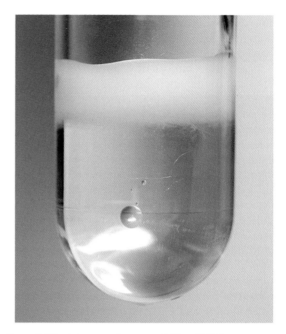

Figure 7.15   Interaction between CHX and EDTA.

the organic components of the smear layer (130). Commercial products with such combinations are available. EndoDilator N-Ø (Union Broach, York, PA) is a combination of EDTA and a quaternary ammonium compound. Such an irrigation fluid has a slight detergent effect in addition to the chelating effect. Several new irrigating solutions, MTAD (DENTSPLY Tulsa), QMiX, and Smear Clear (SybronEndo), have recently been studied. Smear clear, which is commercially available, is a clear, odorless, water-soluble solution containing water, 17% EDTA salts, a cationic surfactant (CTR), and anionic surfactants.

EDTA is normally used in a concentration of 17%. It removes smear layers in less than 1 min (Figure 7.15) if the fluid is able to reach the surface of the root canal wall. The decalcifying process is self-limiting because the chelator is used up. For root canal preparation, EDTA has limited value as an irrigation fluid. It may open up a hair-fine canal if given the time to soften the 50 μm it is capable of decalcifying. This amount, at two opposite canal walls, results in 100 μm. This is equivalent to the tip of a #010 file.

Although citric acid appears to be slightly more potent at similar concentration than EDTA, both agents show high efficiency in removing the smear layer. In addition to their cleaning ability, chelators may detach biofilms adhering to root canal walls (Gulabivala, K. personal communication). This may explain why an EDTA irrigant proved to be

highly superior to saline in reducing intracanal microbiota, despite the fact that its antiseptic capacity is relatively limited. Although never shown in a randomized clinical trial, an alternating irrigating regimen of NaOCl and EDTA may be more efficient in reducing bacterial loads in root canal systems than NaOCl alone. Antiseptics such as quaternary ammonium compounds (EDTAC, ethylenediaminetetraacetic acid plus Cetavlon) or tetracycline antibiotics (MTAD) have been added to EDTA and citric acid irrigants, respectively, to increase their antimicrobial capacity. EDTAC shows similar smear-removing efficacy as EDTA, but it is more caustic.

Chelating agents can be applied in liquid or paste-type form. The origin of paste-type preparations dates back to 1961, when Stewart devised a combination of urea peroxide with glycerol. Later, based on the results of that first preliminary study and the successful introduction of EDTA to endodontic practice, urea peroxide and EDTA were combined in a water-soluble carbowax (polyethylene glycol) vehicle. This product has since been commercially available. Similar paste-type chelators containing EDTA and peroxide have later been marketed by other manufacturers. However, none of these pastes should be used, as they are inefficient in preventing the formation of a smear layer. Furthermore, instead of lowering physical stress on rotary instruments as advocated, carbowax-based lubricants, depending on instrument geometry, have either no effect or are even counterproductive (131).

Interactions between EDTA, NaOCl, and CHX

Grawehr (132) studied the interactions of EDTA with sodium hypochlorite (NaOCl). Grawehr concluded that EDTA retained its calcium-complexing ability when mixed with NaOCl. However, EDTA caused NaOCl to lose its tissue-dissolving capacity, and virtually no free chlorine was detected in the combinations. Clinically, this suggests that EDTA and NaOCl should be used separately. In an alternating irrigating regimen, copious amounts of NaOCl should be administered to wash out remnants of the EDTA.

The combination of CHX and EDTA produces a white precipitate. Rasimick *et al.* (133) (Figure 7.15) determined if the precipitate involves the chemical degradation of CHX. The precipitate was produced and re-dissolved in a known amount of dilute trifluoroacetic acid. It was found that CHX forms a salt with EDTA rather than undergoing a chemical reaction.

Dentin erosion

Optimally, after irrigation, the root canal should be free of all organic debris, microorganisms, and smear layer (134). In addition, bacteria that have penetrated into the dentinal tubules should have been killed, while dentin characteristics (strength, composition, etc.) should not be affected in any negative manner. Recent studies showed that the sequence of use of the common endodontic irrigants, hypochlorite and demineralizing agents (EDTA), is a key factor in determining the level of erosion in root canal wall dentin. Although erosion occurred immediately after 1 min of hypochlorite exposure when done as the final rinse after the demineralizing agent and increased with the number of times of exposure to the irrigants, it is not known presently whether such erosion is harmful for the root dentin and the tooth. It is well known that the mineral component in hard connective

tissues contributes to strength and elastic modulus, whereas collagen is responsible for toughness (37, 109, 135). Theoretically, the observed erosion could be a contributing factor in vertical root fracture depending on the depth of erosion, thickness of the root, and the amount of sclerotic dentin in the root, for example, on the other hand, erosion may also help in achieving a maximally clean root canal wall surface, free of debris and bacteria.

On the basis of the available research, the following irrigation sequence is recommended during root canal treatment:

Full strength (5.25–6%) of NaOCl should be used during instrumentation. After instrumentation is over, final rinsing can be done following one of the following strategies: (i) 17% EDTA for 2 min, or (ii) EDTA followed by 2% CHX, or (iii) MTAD, SmearClear™, or QMiX. Constant agitation during irrigation is helpful to achieve a cleaner canal (Figure 7.16).

HEBP

HEBP (1-hydroxyethylidene-1,1-bisphosphonate; also called *etidronic acid*) is a chelator that can be used in combination with sodium hypochlorite (NaOCl) without affecting its proteolytic or antimicrobial properties (24). However, in contrast to EDTA, HEBP is a weak decalcifying agent and hence cannot be used as a mere final rinse. Therefore, it is recommended that HEBP be mixed with

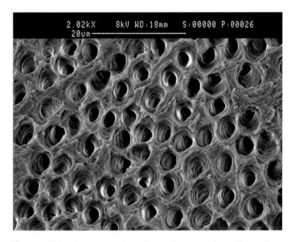

Figure 7.16 Strong erosion of root dentin surface after using NaOCl after EDTA. (Courtesy of Dr. Markus Haapasalo.)

NaOCl to be used as a more complete root canal irrigant. This combination is advantageous in that the solution keeps the hypochlorite–hypochlorous acid equilibrium toward hypochlorite, which has better tissue dissolution capacity than hypochlorous acid (136) and is also less cytotoxic (137). Furthermore, an irrigating protocol using the NaOCl + HEBP combination has been shown to be able to optimize the bonding by Resilon/Epiphany root fillings (138). HEBP is applied in pool water disinfection because of its compatibility with calcium hypochlorite (hypochlorite tablets in swimming pools). The HEBP prevents stain deriving from inorganic compounds at the water line. It is also used in many personal care products such as soaps. Systemically applied, it is known as *Didronel* (Norwich Pharmaceuticals, Inc., North Norwich, NY) and is used to treat Paget disease (139).

QMiX

QMiX was introduced in 2011. It is one of the new combination products introduced for root canal irrigation (Figure 7.17) (45, 140–142). It is recommended to be used at the end of instrumentation after NaOCl irrigation. QMiX contains EDTA, CHX, and a detergent; it comes as a ready-to-use clear solution.

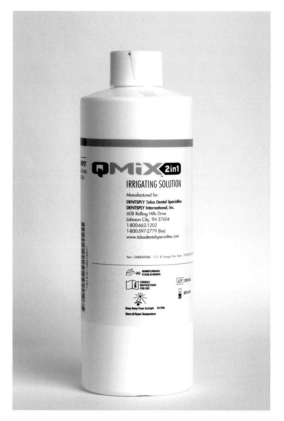

Figure 7.17   QMiX.

Protocol

QMiX is suggested to be used as a final rinse. If sodium hypochlorite was used throughout the cleaning and shaping, saline should be used to rinse out the NaOCl to prevent the formation of PCA, although no precipitate has been described when mixing QMiX and NaOCl (see interaction between NaOCl and CHX).

Surface tension

According to Grossman (5), low surface tension is one of the ideal characteristics of an irrigant. Lower surface tension may help in better penetration of the irrigating solutions into the dentinal tubules and inaccessible areas of the root canal system (143). In order to be more effective in debris removal and to penetrate more readily into the root canal system, irrigants must be in contact with the dentin walls.

The closeness of this contact is directly related to its surface tension (144). Irrigants with a low surface tension are more suitable as endodontic irrigants. QMiX incorporated a detergent in its formula to decrease the surface tension.

Smear layer removal

Stojicic *et al.* (45) investigated the effectiveness of smear layer removal by QMiX using SEM. QMiX removed smear layer equally well as EDTA ($P = 0.18$). They concluded that the ability to remove smear layer by QMiX was comparable to the ability of EDTA. Dai *et al.* examined the ability of two versions of QMiX on the removal of canal wall smear layers and debris using an open canal design. Within the limitations of an open canal design, the two experimental QMiX versions are as effective as 17% EDTA in removing canal wall smear layers after the use of 5.25% NaOCl as the initial rinse.

Antibacterial efficacy and effect on biofilms

Stojicic *et al.* (45) assessed in a laboratory experimental model the efficacy of QMiX, against *E. faecalis* and mixed plaque bacteria in planktonic phase and biofilms. QMiX and 1% NaOCl killed all planktonic *E. faecalis* and plaque bacteria in 5 s. QMiX and 2% NaOCl killed up to 12 times more biofilm bacteria than 1% NaOCl ($P < 0.01$) or 2% CHX ($P < 0.05$; $P < 0.001$). Wang *et al.* compared the antibacterial effects of different disinfecting solutions on young and old *E. faecalis* biofilms in dentin canals using a novel dentin infection model and CLSM. Six percent NaOCl and QMiX were the most effective disinfecting solutions against the young biofilm, whereas against the 3-week-old biofilm, 6% NaOCl was the most effective followed by QMiX. Both were more effective than 2% NaOCl and 2% CHX.

In-vivo clinical trials

The efficacy and biocompatibility of QMiX was demonstrated via nonclinical *in-vitro* and *ex-vivo* studies. Further clinical research from independent investigators is needed to corroborate the findings.

MTAD and Tetraclean

MTAD (6) and Tetraclean are two new irrigants based on a mixture of antibiotics, citric acid, and a detergent (Figure 7.18). MTAD (145) is the first irrigating solution capable of removing the smear layer and disinfecting the root canal system; also, it is a mixture of 3% doxycycline hyclate, 4.25% citric acid, and 0.5% polysorbate (Tween) 80 detergent (145). It has been commercialized as BioPure MTAD (BioPure, Dentsply, Tulsa Dental, Tulsa, OK, USA) and is available as a two-part set, in the form of a liquid in a syringe and powder in a bottle, which should be mixed before application. MTAD has been recommended in clinical practice as a final rinse after completion of a conventional chemomechanical preparation (145–149).

Tetraclean (Ogna Laboratori Farmaceutici, Muggio, Italy) is another combination product similar to MTAD. The two irrigants differ in the concentration of antibiotics (doxycycline 150 mg/5 ml for MTAD and 50 mg/5 ml for Tetraclean) and the kind

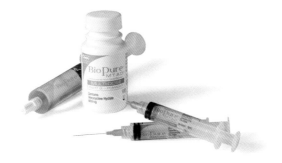

Figure 7.18   MTAD. (Courtesy of DENTSPLY Tulsa Dental Specialties.)

of detergent (Tween 80 for MTAD, polypropylene glycol for Tetraclean).

Mode of action

There is no detailed information on MTAD's exact mechanism of action in the removal of the smear layer and the killing of bacteria. In most studies, its effect on the smear layer is attributed to both doxycycline and citric acid. These two components of MTAD have been separately reported as effective smear layer removal solutions (150). Its antibacterial effect is mostly attributed to the doxycycline, which is an isomer of tetracycline. Tetracycline, including tetracycline HCl, minocycline, and doxycycline, are broad-spectrum antibiotics that are effective against a wide range of microorganisms. Tetracycline is a bacteriostatic antibiotic that exerts its effect through the inhibition of protein synthesis. According to Torabinejad *et al.* (145), this property may be advantageous because in the absence of bacterial cell lysis, antigenic by-products (i.e., endotoxin) are not released. In high concentrations, tetracycline may also have a bactericidal effect. The role of citric acid in killing bacteria is not well known. Tween 80 seems to have limited antibacterial activity, yet it may increase the antibacterial effect of some substances by directly affecting the bacterial cell membrane. It may facilitate the penetration of MTAD into dentin. On the other hand, Tween 80 may also be used as a nutrient by some bacteria, and it may inactivate the antibacterial properties of some disinfecting agents such as CHX and PI. Doxycycline, citric acid, and Tween 80 together might have a synergistic effect on the bacterial cell wall and on the cytoplasmic membrane.

Cytotoxicity of MTAD

Using a MMT-tetrazolium method, Zhang *et al.* (135) compared the cytotoxicity of MTAD to that of eugenol, 3% hydrogen peroxide, REDTA Aqueous Irrigant, Peridex (CHX 0.12%), Pulpdent Ca(OH)$_2$ paste, and four concentrations of NaOCl (5.25%, 2.63%, 1.31%, and 0.66%). They concluded that MTAD appeared to be less cytotoxic than eugenol, 3% H$_2$O$_2$, Ca(OH)$_2$ paste, 5.25% NaOCl, Peridex, and EDTA and more cytotoxic than 2.63%, 1.31%, and 0.66% NaOCl solutions (135). The authors suggested further investigation was needed to determine if the results from their *in-vitro* study could be applied to a clinical situation.

Surface tension

To decrease the surface tension, Tween 80 has been added to the MTAD solution. It is reported that MTAD has lower surface tension than 5.25% NaOCl, 17% EDTA, and water. Although it seems that lowering surface tension may help the penetration of the irrigants deeper into the dentinal tubules or other confined areas of the root canal system, and consequently improve the antibacterial effectiveness of the irrigants, there is no clinical evidence to support this possibility.

Smear layer removal

SEM has been used to determine the effectiveness of various irrigants to remove the smear layer. The paper that introduced MTAD addressed its potential in the removal of the smear layer in extracted human teeth (145). The authors reported that MTAD performed better than EDTA in cleaning dentinal tubules from debris and smear layer in the apical third of the root canals; however, there was no significant difference in the middle and coronal portions of the root canals. In the same study, the results also indicated that MTAD created less erosion than EDTA in the coronal and middle thirds of the root canals. The better efficacy of MTAD in the removal of the smear layer was attributed to the combination of citric acid, doxycycline, and Tween 80 in the MTAD solution. In two other studies, the efficacy of MTAD or EDTA in the removal of the smear layer was confirmed; however, no significant difference between these two solutions was reported (44, 151).

Antibacterial efficacy

Reported results regarding the antibacterial properties of MTAD are conflicting. The studies measuring zones of inhibition on agar plates have shown consistently that MTAD was an effective antibacterial agent against *E. faecalis* (145, 152, 153). Tay *et al.* (151) also found larger zones of bacterial inhibition using dentin cores irrigated with MTAD compared to NaOCl-irrigated dentin cores; however, when they applied MTAD to the dentin that was already irrigated with 1.3% NaOCl, they had a contradictory result. The diameters of zones of inhibition were significantly smaller than those of MTAD alone and comparable to those irrigated with 1.3% NaOCl alone. They concluded that the antimicrobial effect of MTAD was lost because of the oxidation of the MTAD by NaOCl (151). However, agar diffusion tests are no longer regarded as reliable, as there is no established link between the zone of inhibition on the agar plate and the true effectiveness of the endodontic disinfecting agents in the root canal.

A study using extracted human teeth contaminated with saliva showed that MTAD was more effective than 5.25% NaOCl in the disinfection of the teeth (146). In contrast, Krause *et al.* (153) using bovine tooth sections showed that 5.25% NaOCl was more effective than MTAD in the disinfection of the dentin discs inoculated with *E. faecalis*.

In another study performed on extracted human teeth inoculated with *E. faecalis*, a protocol of 1.3% NaOCl followed by 5 min MTAD, was more effective in the disinfection of canals than a protocol of 5.25% NaOCl followed by 1 min 17% EDTA and then 5 min 5.25% NaOCl as a final rinse (147).

Using a culture method and extracted human teeth inoculated with *E. faecalis*, the opposite was found, that is, the latter protocol was significantly superior to the 1.3% NaOCl/5 min MTAD protocol in the disinfection of the root canals (148).

In another study, the same investigators using the same model disinfected the canals with the same two protocols and then resected and pulverized the last 5 mm of the root ends in liquid nitrogen. After the inoculation of the samples on brain heart infusion (BHI) agar culture plates, the investigators found that there was no significant difference in the antimicrobial efficacy of those two protocols in the disinfection of the apical 5 mm of the infected canals (154).

In a series of studies, it was found that MTAD had failed to show a superior antibacterial efficacy against bacterial biofilms. Bacteria collected from the teeth of patients diagnosed with apical periodontitis were grown as a biofilm on hemisections of root apices. MTAD was shown to be an effective antibacterial agent in this model; however, it was not able to completely disrupt the bacterial biofilm compared to 6% NaOCl. NaOCl (5.25%) was the most effective irrigant against a biofilm of *E. faecalis* generated on cellulose nitrate membrane filters, while the bacterial load reduction using MTAD was not significant (155). MTAD was the least effective irrigant when compared to 6% and 1% NaOCl, SmearClear, 2% CHX, and REDTA, when tested in a flow cell generated biofilms of *E. faecalis* (156).

When the efficacy of four irrigants including MTAD was tested in teeth inoculated with *C. albicans*, it was demonstrated that 6% NaOCl and 2% CHX were equally effective and superior to MTAD and 17% EDTA. According to Portenier *et al.* (157), although the antibacterial effect of MTAD is comparable to that of CHX, calcium hydroxide, iodine potassium iodide, and sodium hypochlorite, the presence of dentin or bovine serum albumin causes a marked reduction in the antibacterial efficacy of MTAD against *E. faecalis*.

The results of the tests of antibacterial efficacy of medicaments, obtained from *in-vitro* studies, should be analyzed with caution, as they may be influenced by factors such as the test environment, bacterial susceptibility, and the different methodologies used to evaluate the results (15).

Pappen *et al.* (158) investigated the antibacterial effect of Tetraclean, MTAD, and five experimental irrigants using both direct exposure test with planktonic cultures and mixed-species *in-vitro* biofilm model. The results showed that Tetraclean was more effective than MTAD against *E. faecalis* in planktonic culture and in mixed-species *in-vitro* biofilm. CTR improved the antimicrobial properties of the solutions, whereas Tween 80 seemed to have a neutral or negative impact on their antimicrobial effectiveness.

In-vivo clinical trial

With the exception of the study (159) that evaluated the effect of MTAD on postoperative discomfort, there has been no other *in-vivo* study to address the other characteristics of MTAD. The results show that the removal of the smear layer and the disinfection of the root canal system using 1.3% NaOCl and MTAD does not lead to an increased incidence of postoperative pain compared to biomechanical instrumentation using 5.25% NaOCl and 17% EDTA. Malkhassian *et al.* (160) in a clinical controlled trial of 30 patients reported that the final rinse with MTAD did not reduce the bacterial counts in infected canals beyond levels achieved by chemomechanical preparation using NaOCl.

Protocol for use

The MTAD protocol was developed on the basis of a pilot project (146).

The results of this project showed that the consistent disinfection of the infected root canals could occur after chemomechanical preparation using 1.3% NaOCl as a root canal irrigant and a 5 min exposure time to MTAD as a final rinse.

Resistance to antibiotic

Resistance to tetracycline is not uncommon in bacteria isolated from root canals (146). The use of antibiotics instead of biocides such as hypochlorite or CHX appears unwarranted, as the former were developed for systemic use rather than local wound debridement, and have a far narrower spectrum than the latter.

The antimicrobial effect of MTAD has been largely attributed to the presence of doxycycline. In a recent study, CHX was added to or substituted for doxycycline to compare these three formulations in their ability to disinfect extracted human teeth infected with *E. faecalis*. Their results showed that although the addition of CHX did not negatively impact the efficacy of MTAD, the substitution of this antimicrobial agent for doxycycline significantly reduces the efficacy of the solution (146).

Hydrogen peroxide

Hydrogen peroxide has been used as an endodontic irrigant for a long period of time, mainly in concentrations ranging between 3% and 5%. It is active against bacteria, viruses, and yeasts. Hydroxy-free radicals (•OH) destroy proteins and DNA. The tissue-dissolving capacity of hydrogen peroxide is clearly lower than that of sodium hypochlorite; also, its antibacterial effect is considered weak. When used in combination with sodium hypochlorite, bubbling will occur as a result of evaporating oxygen. Although no longer recommended as a routine irrigant, its use is still not uncommon in some countries.

Iodine–potassium-iodide

IPI (161, 162) has been proposed and used as an endodontic disinfectant because of its excellent antibacterial properties and low cytotoxicity. It is used as a solution of 2% iodine in 4% potassium-iodide (163). Allergic reaction to iodine and staining of dentin are often mentioned as potential risks with the use of IPI; however, reports of such harmful side effects when IPI is used in endodontics seem to be extremely rare (164).

Green tea, Triphala

Natural products, especially food extracts, have been used in medicine and have been shown to be good alternatives to synthetic chemicals. The polyphenols of green tea (i.e., EGCg, epigallocatechin gallate) were found to be cost effective. They have inhibitory activity against the MMPs (−2, −9) found in saliva and dentin. Moreover, EGCg is also a broad-spectrum antibacterial, and studies have reported its effectiveness in inhibiting acid production in dental plaque bacteria as well as antimicrobial activity against *Streptococcus*

mutans. These findings open a new avenue for the prevention of caries and debonding. Triphala (165, 166) (IMPCOPS Ltd., Chennai, India) is an Indian ayurvedic herbal formulation consisting of dried and powdered fruits of three medicinal plants *Terminalia bellerica*, *Terminalia chebula*, and *Emblica officinalis* (green tea polyphenols (GTPs), Essence and Flavours (Mysore, India). Polyphenols found in green tea, the traditional drink of Japan and China, is prepared from the young shoots of the tea plant *Camellia sinensis*.

Japanese green teas (167) were found not to have an irritating potential and some results suggest that extracts of Japanese green tea (168) may be useful as a medicament for treatment of infected root canals. Herbal alternatives showed promising antibacterial efficacy on 3- and 6-week biofilm (163, 169–171). Presently, there is not enough evidence to support the use of antibacterial components of green tea or other herbs as endodontic disinfecting agents.

Conclusions

Irrigation has a key role in successful endodontic treatment. A suggested irrigation protocol is outlined in Figure 7.19. The main goal of root canal treatment is to completely eliminate the different components of pulpal tissue, bacteria, and biofilm and produce a hermetic seal to prevent infection or re-infection and promote the healing of the surrounding tissues. The extra time we gain by using rotary NiTi instruments should be used for abundant irrigation to achieve better cleaning of the root canal system, thereby contributing to improved success of the treatment.

The most commonly used irrigating solution is sodium hypochlorite. While sodium hypochlorite has many desirable qualities and properties, by itself it is not sufficient for the total cleaning of the root canal system of organic and inorganic debris and biofilm. For optimal irrigation, a combination of different irrigating solutions must be used. The dentist should be aware of the different interactions between the various chemicals used for irrigation, as they may weaken one another's activity and result in the development of reaction products that are harmful to the host. Developing a rational irrigation sequence, so that the chemicals are administered in a proper manner to release

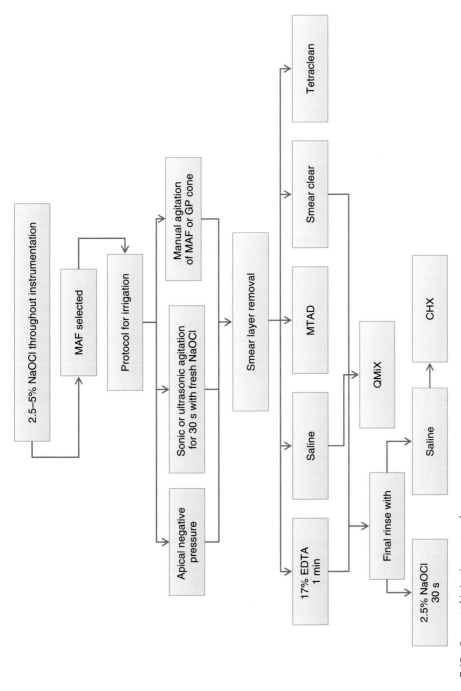

Figure 7.19 Suggested irrigation protocol.

their full potential, is imperative for successful endodontic treatments (172).

References

1. Kakehashi, S., Stanley, H. & Fitzgerald, R. (1965) The effects of surgical exposures of dental pulps in germ-free and conventional laboratory rats. *Oral Surgery, Oral Medicine, and Oral Pathology*, **20**, 340–349.
2. Bystrom, A. & Sundqvist, G. (1981) Bacteriologic evaluation of the efficacy of mechanical root canal instrumentation in endodontic therapy. *Scandinavian Journal of Dental Research*, **89**, 321–328.
3. *Collins English Dictionary – Complete and Unabridged*. © Harpercollins Publishers, Glasgow, 1991, 1994, 1998, 2000, 2003.
4. Hülsmann, M., Rödig, T. & Nordmeyer, S. (2007) Complications during root canal irrigation. *Endodontic Topics*, **16**, 27–63.
5. Grossman, L. & Meiman, B. (1941) Solution of pulp tissue by chemical agent. *The Journal of the American Dental Association*, **28**, 223–225.
6. Torabinejad, M. & Johnson, W.B. (2003) Irrigation solution and methods for use. Inventors; US patent 20030235804 and trademark office, assignee, USA.
7. Cheung, G. & Stock, C. (1993) In vitro cleaning ability of root canal irrigants with and without endosonics. *International Endodontic Journal*, **26**, 334–343.
8. Estrela, C., Barbin, E., Spanó, J., Marchesan, M. & Pécora, J. (2002) Mechanism of action of sodium hypochlorite. *Brazilian Dental Journal*, **13**, 113–117.
9. Gomes, B., Ferraz, C., Vianna, M., Berber, V., Teixeira, F. & Souza-Filho, F. (2001) In vitro antimicrobial activity of several concentrations of sodium hypochlorite and chlorhexidine gluconate in the elimination of enterococcus faecalis. *International Endodontic Journal*, **34**, 424–428.
10. Radcliffe, C., Potouridou, L., Qureshi, R., Habahbeh, N., Qualtrough, A. & Worthington, H. (2004) Antimicrobial activity of varying concentrations of sodium hypochlorite on the endodontic microorganisms Actinomyces israelii, A. naeslundii, Candida albicans and Enterococcus faecalis. *International Endodontic Journal*, **37**, 438–446.
11. Waltimo, T., Orstavik, D., Siren, E.K. & Haapasalo, M. (1999) In vitro susceptibility of candida albicans to four disinfectants and their combinations. *International Endodontic Journal*, **32**, 421–429.
12. Cvek, M., Nord, C.E. & Hollender, L. (1976) Antimicrobial effect of root canal debridement in teeth with immature root: a clinical and microbiological study. *Odontologisk Revy*, **27**, 1–13.

13. Hand, R.E., Smith, M.L. & Harrison, J.W. (1978) Analysis of the effect of dilution on the necrotic tissue dissolution property of sodium hypochlorite. *Journal of Endodontics*, **4**, 60–64.
14. Moorer, W. & Wesselink, P. (1982) Factors promoting the tissue dissolving capability of sodium hypochlorite. *International Endodontic Journal*, **15**, 187–196.
15. Siqueira, J., Rocas, I., Favieri, A. & Lima, K. (2000) Chemomechanical reduction of the bacterial population in the root canal after instrumentation and irrigation with 1%, 2.5%, and 5.25% sodium hypochlorite. *Journal of Endodontics*, **26**, 331–334.
16. Spangberg, L., Engström, B. & Langeland, K. (1973) Biologic effects of dental materials. 3. Toxicity and antimicrobial effect of endodontic antiseptics in vitro. *Oral Surgery, Oral Medicine, and Oral Pathology*, **36**, 856–864.
17. Shuping, G., Orstavik, D., Sigurdsson, A. & Trope, M. (2000) Reduction of intracanal bacteria using nickel–titanium rotary instrumentation and various medications. *Journal of Endodontics*, **26**, 751–755.
18. Mcgurkin-Smith, R., Trope, M., Caplan, D. & Sigurdsson, A. (2005) Reduction of intracanal bacteria using rotary instrumentation, 5.25% NaOCl, EDTA, and Ca(OH)$_2$. *Journal of Endodontics*, **3**, 359–363.
19. Peters, O.A. (2004) Current challenges and concepts in the preparation of root canal systems: a review. *Journal of Endodontics*, **30**, 559–567.
20. Grossman, L. & Meiman, B. (1941) Solution of pulp tissue by chemical agent. *The Journal of the American Dental Association*, **28**, 223–232.
21. Haapasalo, M., Shen, Y., Qian, W. & Gao, Y. (2010) Irrigation in endodontics. *Dental Clinics of North America*, **5**, 291–312.
22. Vianna, M.E., Gomes, B.P., Berber, V.B. *et al.* (2004) In vitro evaluation of the antimicrobial activity of chlorhexidine and sodium hypochlorite. *Oral Surgery, Oral Medicine, Oral Pathology, Oral Radiology, and Endodontics*, **97**, 79–84.
23. Portenier, I., Waltimo, T., Ørstavik, D. *et al.* (2005) The susceptibility of starved, stationary phase and growing cells of *Enterococcus faecalis* to endodontic medicaments. *Journal of Endodontics*, **31**, 380–386.
24. Zehnder, M. (2006) Root canal irrigants. Review. *Journal of Endodontics*, **32**, 389–398.
25. Clarkson, R.M. & Moule, A.J. (1998) Sodium hypochlorite and its use as an endodontic irrigant. *Australian Dental Journal*, **43**, 250–256.
26. Spencer, I., Ike, H. & Brennan, P.A. (2007) Review: the use of sodium hypochlorite in endodontics—potential complications and their management. *British Dental Journal*, **202**, 555–559.

27. Pashley, E., Birdsong, N., Bowman, K. & Pashley, D. (1985) Cytotoxic effects of NaOCl on vital tissue. *Journal of Endodontics*, **11**, 525–528.

28. Kleier, D., Averbach, R.E. & Mehdipour, O. (2008) The sodium hypochlorite accident: experience of diplomates of the American Board of Endodontics. *Journal of Endodontics*, **34**, 1346–1350.

29. Mehdipour, O., Kleier, D.J. & Averbach, R.E. (2007) Anatomy of sodium hypochlorite accidents. *Compendium of Continuing Education in Dentistry*, **28**, 544–546.

30. Kerbl, F., DeVilliers, P., Litaker, M. & Eleazer, P. (2012) Physical effects of sodium hypochlorite on bone: an ex vivo study. *Journal of Endodontics*, **38**, 357–359.

31. Currey, J., Brear, K. & Zioupos, P. (1994) Dependence of mechanical properties on fiber angle in narwhal tusk, a highly oriented biological composite. *Journal of Biomechanics*, **27**, 885–897.

32. Stoward, P.J. (1975) A histochemical study of the apparent deamination of proteins by sodium hypochlorite. *Histochemistry*, **45**, 213–226.

33. Oyarzun, A., Cordero, A.M. & Whittle, M. (2002) Immunohistochemical evaluation of the effects of sodium hypochlorite on dentin collagen and glycosaminoglycans. *Journal of Endodontics*, **28**, 152–156.

34. Slutzky-Goldberg, I., Maree, M., Liberman, R. & Heling, I. (2004) Effect of sodium hypochlorite on dentin microhardness. *Journal of Endodontics*, **3**, 880–882.

35. Grigoratos, D., Knowles, J., Ng, Y.L. & Gulabivala, K. (2001) Effect of exposing dentine to sodium hypochlorite and calcium hydroxide on its flexural strength and elastic modulus. *International Endodontic Journal*, **34**, 113–119.

36. Machnick, T., Torabinejad, M., Munoz, C.A. & Shabahang, S. (2003) Effect of MTAD on flexural strength and modulus of elasticity of dentin. *Journal of Endodontics*, **29**, 747–750.

37. Marending, M., Luder, H., Brunner, T., Knecht, S., Stark, W. & Zehnder, M. (2007) Effect of sodium hypochlorite on human root dentine—mechanical, chemical and structural evaluation. *International Endodontic Journal*, **40**, 786–793.

38. Zou, L., Shen, Y., Li, W. & Haapasalo, M. (2010) Penetration of sodium hypochlorite into dentin. *Journal of Endodontics*, **36**, 793–796.

39. Eun, H., Lee, A. & Lee, Y. (1984) Sodium hypochlorite dermatitis. *Contact Dermatitis*, **11**, 45–47.

40. Habets, J.M., Geursen-Reitsma, A.M., Stolz, E. & Van Joost, T. (1986) Sensitization to sodium hypochlorite causing hand dermatitis. *Contact Dermatitis*, **15**, 140–157.

41. Andersen, M., Lund, A., Andreasen, J. & Andreasen, F. (1992) In vitro solubility of human pulp tissue in calcium hydroxide and sodium hypochlorite. *Endodontics and Dental Traumatology*, **8**, 104–108.

42. Hasselgren, G., Olsson, B. & Cvek, M. (1988) Effects of calcium hydroxide and sodium hypochlorite on the dissolution of necrotic porcine muscle tissue. *Journal of Endodontics*, **14**, 125–128.

43. Noiri, Y., Ehara, A. & Kawahara, T. (2002) Participation of bacterial biofilms in refractory and chronic periapical periodontitis. *Journal of Endodontics*, **28**, 679–683.

44. Clegg, M.S., Vertucci, F.J., Walker, C., Belanger, M. & Britto, L.R. (2006) The effect of exposure to irrigant solutions on apical dentin biofilms in vitro. *Journal of Endodontics*, **32**, 434–437.

45. Stojicic, S., Shen, Y., Qian, W., Johnson, B. & Haapasalo, M. (2012) Antibacterial and smear layer removal ability of a novel irrigant, QMiX. *International Endodontic Journal*, **45**, 363–371.

46. Cunningham, W. & Joseph, S.W. (1980) Effect of temperature on the bactericidal action of sodium hypochlorite endodontic irritant. *Oral Surgery, Oral Medicine, and Oral Pathology*, **50**, 569–571.

47. Berutti, E., Marini, R. & Angeretti, A. (1997) Penetration ability of different irrigants into dentinal tubules. *Journal of Endodontics*, **23**, 725–727.

48. Kishen, A. (2005) What we leave behind in root canals after endodontic treatment: some issues and concerns. *Australian Endodontic Journal*, **3**, 1–7.

49. Fabiani, C., Mazzoni, A., Nato, F. *et al.* (2010) Final rinse optimization: influence of different agitation protocols. *Journal of Endodontics*, **36**, 282–285.

50. Al-Jadaa, A., Paqué, F., Attin, T. & Zehnder, M. (2009) Acoustic hypochlorite activation in simulated curved canals. *Journal of Endodontics*, **35**, 1408–1411.

51. Morris, M.D., Lee, K.W., Agee, K.A., Bouillaguet, S. & Pashley, D.H. (2001) Effects of sodium hypochlorite and RC-prep on bond strengths of resin cement to endodontic surfaces. *Journal of Endodontics*, **27**, 753–757.

52. Fardal, O. & Turnbull, R.S. (1986) A review of the literature on use of chlorhexidine in dentistry. *Journal of the American Dental Association*, **112**, 863–869.

53. Löe, H. (1973) Does chlorhexidine have a place in the prophylaxis of dental diseases? *Journal of Periodontal Research*, **12**, 93–99.

54. Greenstein, G., Berman, C. & Jaffin, R. (1986) Chlorhexidine. An adjunct to periodontal therapy. *Journal of Periodontology*, **57**, 370–375.

55. Denton, G. (1991) Chlorhexidine. In: Block, S.S. (ed), *Disinfection, Sterilization and Preservation*, 4 edn. Lea and Febiger, Philadelphia.

56. Davies, A. (1973) The mode of action of chlorhexidine. *Journal of Periodontal Research*, **12**, 68–69.

57. Hugo, W.B. & Longworth, A.R. (1966) The effect of chlorhexidine on the electrophoretic mobility, cytoplasmic constituents, dehydrogenase activity and cell walls of Escherichia coli and Staphylococcus aureus. *Journal of Pharmacy and Pharmacology*, **18**, 569–578.

58. Hugo, W. & Longworth, A. (1964) Some aspects of the mode of action of chlorhexidine. *Journal of Pharmacy and Pharmacology*, **16**, 751–758.

59. Hennessey, T.S. (1973) Some antibacterial properties of chlorhexidine. *Journal of Periodontal Research. Supplement*, **12**, 61–67.

60. Basrani, B. & Lemonie, C. (2005) Chlorhexidine gluconate. *Australian Endodontic Journal*, **31**, 48–52.

61. Winrow, M.J. (1973) Metabolic studies with radio-labelled chlorhexidine in animals and man. *Journal of Periodontal Research. Supplement*, 45–48.

62. Magnusson, B. & Heyden, G. (1973) Autoradiographic studies of 14c-chlorhexidine given orally in mice. *Journal of Periodontal Research. Supplement*, **12**, 49–54.

63. Rölla, G., Löe, H. & Schiott, C.R. (1970) The affinity of chlorhexidine for hydroxyapatite and salivary mucins. *Journal of Periodontal Research. Supplement*, **5**, 90–95.

64. Turesky, S., Warner, V., Lin, P.S. & Soloway, B. (1977) Prolongation of antibacterial activity of chlorhexidine adsorbed to teeth. Effect of sulfates. *Journal of Periodontology*, **48**, 646–649.

65. Hjeljord, L.G., Rolla, G. & Bonesvoll, P. (1973) Chlorhexidine–protein interactions. *Journal of Periodontal Research. Supplement*, **12**, 11–16.

66. Khademi, A.A., Mohammadi, Z. & Davari, A.R. (2008) Evaluation of the antibacterial substantivity of three concentrations of chlorhexidine in bovine root dentine. *Iranian Endodontic Journal*, **2**, 112–115.

67. Emilson, C.G., Ericson, T., Heyden, G. & Magnusson, B.C. (1973) Uptake of chlorhexidine to hydroxyapatite. *Journal of Periodontal Research. Supplement*, **17**, 17–21.

68. Mohammadi, Z. & Abbott, P.V. (2009) Antimicrobial substantivity of root canal irrigants and medicaments: a review. *Australian Endodontic Journal*, **35**, 131–139.

69. Lin, S., Zuckerman, O., Weiss, E.I. & Fuss, Z. (2003) Antibacterial efficacy of a new chlorhexidine slow-releasing device to disinfect dentinal tubules. *Journal of Endodontics*, **29**, 416–418.

70. Komorowski, R., Grad, H., Wu, X.Y. & Friedman, S. (2000) Antimicrobial substantivity of chlorhexidine-treated bovine root dentin. *Journal of Endodontics*, **26**, 315–317.

71. Löe, H. & Schiott, C.R. (1970) The effect of mouth rinses and topical application of chlorhexidine on the development of dental plaque and gingivitis in man. *Journal of Periodontal Research. Supplement*, **5**, 79–83.

72. Southard, S.R., Drisko, C.L., Killoy, W.J., Cobb, C.M. & Tira, D.E. (1989) The effect of 2% chlorhexidine digluconate irrigation on clinical parameters and the level of bacteroides gingivalis in periodontal pockets. *Journal of Periodontology*, **60**, 302–309.

73. Asboe-Jorgensen, V., Attstrom, R., Lang, N.P. & Löe, H. (1974) Effect of a chlorhexidine dressing on the healing after periodontal surgery. *Journal of Periodontology*, **45**, 13–17.

74. Jeansonne, M.J. & White, R.R. (1994) A comparison of 2.0% chlorhexidine gluconate and 5.25% sodium hypochlorite as antimicrobial endodontic irrigants. *Journal of Endodontics*, **20**, 276–278.

75. Yesilsoy, C., Whitaker, E., Cleveland, D., Phillips, E. & Trope, M. (1995) Antimicrobial and toxic effects of established and potential root canal irrigants. *Journal of Endodontics*, **21**, 513–515.

76. Oncag, O., Hosgor, M., Hilmioglu, S., Zekioglu, O., Eronat, C. & Burhanoglu, D. (2003) Comparison of antibacterial and toxic effects of various root canal irrigants. *International Endodontic Journal*, **36**, 423–432.

77. Caso, A., Hung, L.K. & Beirne, O.R. (2005) Prevention of alveolar osteitis with chlorhexidine: a meta-analytic review. *Oral Surgery, Oral Medicine, Oral Pathology, Oral Radiology, and Endodontics*, **99**, 155–159.

78. Okano, M., Nomura, M., Hata, S. *et al.* (1989) Anaphylactic symptoms due to chlorhexidine gluconate. *Archives of Dermatology*, **125**, 50–52.

79. Garvey, L.H., Roed-Petersen, J. & Husum, B. (2001) Anaphylactic reactions in anaesthetised patients – four cases of chlorhexidine allergy. *Acta Anaesthesiologica Scandinavica*, **45**, 1290–1294.

80. Hidalgo, E. & Dominguez, C. (2001) Mechanisms underlying chlorhexidine-induced cytotoxicity. *Toxicology in Vitro*, **15**, 271–276.

81. Cabral, C.T. & Fernandes, M.H. (2007) In vitro comparison of chlorhexidine and povidone–iodine on the long-term proliferation and functional activity of human alveolar bone cells. *Clinical Oral Investigations*, **11**, 155–164.

82. Faria, G., Celes, M.R., De Rossi, A., Silva, L.A., Silva, J.S. & Rossi, M.A. (2007) Evaluation of chlorhexidine toxicity injected in the paw of mice and added to cultured 1929 fibroblasts. *Journal of Endodontics*, **33**, 715–722.

83. Basrani, B., Manek, S., Sodhi, R., Fillery, E. & Manzur, A. (2007) Interaction between sodium hypochlorite and chlorhexidine gluconate. *Journal of Endodontics*, **33**, 966–969.

84. Barbosa, C.A., Goncalves, R.B., Siqueira, J.F. Jr. & De Uzeda, M. (1997) Evaluation of the antibacterial activities of calcium hydroxide, chlorhexidine, and camphorated paramonochlorophenol as intracanal medicament. A clinical and laboratory study. *Journal of Endodontics*, **23**, 297–300.

85. Lindskog, S., Pierce, A. & Blomlof, L. (1998) Chlorhexidine as a root canal medicament for treating inflammatory lesions in the periodontal space. *Endodontics and Dental Traumatology*, **14**, 181–190.

86. Manzur, A., Gonzalez, A.M., Pozos, A., Silva-Herzog, D. & Friedman, S. (2007) Bacterial quantification in teeth with apical periodontitis related to instrumentation and different intracanal medications: a randomized clinical trial. *Journal of Endodontics*, **33**, 114–118.

87. Paquette, L., Legner, M., Fillery, E.D. & Friedman, S. (2007) Antibacterial efficacy of chlorhexidine gluconate intracanal medication in vivo. *Journal of Endodontics*, **33**, 788–795.

88. Basrani, B., Ghanem, A. & Tjäderhane, L. (2004) Physical and chemical properties of chlorhexidine and calcium hydroxide-containing medications. *Journal of Endodontics*, **30**, 413–417.

89. Basrani, B., Santos, J.M., Tjäderhane, L. *et al.* (2002) substantive antimicrobial activity in chlorhexidine-treated human root dentin. *Oral Surgery, Oral Medicine, Oral Pathology, Oral Radiology, and Endodontics*, **94**, 240–245.

90. Basrani, B., Tjäderhane, L., Santos, J.M. *et al.* (2003) Efficacy of chlorhexidine- and calcium hydroxide-containing medicaments against enterococcus faecalis in vitro. *Oral Surgery, Oral Medicine, Oral Pathology, Oral Radiology, and Endodontics*, **96**, 618–624.

91. Siqueira, J.F. Jr. & De Uzeda, M. (1997) Intracanal medicaments: evaluation of the antibacterial effects of chlorhexidine, metronidazole, and calcium hydroxide associated with three vehicles. *Journal of Endodontics*, **23**, 167–169.

92. Lima, K.C., Fava, L.R. & Siqueira, J.F. Jr. (2001) Susceptibilities of enterococcus faecalis biofilms to some antimicrobial medications. *Journal of Endodontics*, **27**, 616–619.

93. Kuruvilla, J.R. & Kamath, M.P. (1998) Antimicrobial activity of 2.5% sodium hypochlorite and 0.2% chlorhexidine gluconate separately and combined, as endodontic irrigants. *Journal of Endodontics*, **24**, 472–476.

94. Leonardo, M.R., Tanomaru Filho, M., Silva, L.A., Nelson Filho, P., Bonifacio, K.C. & Ito, I.Y. (1999) In vivo antimicrobial activity of 2% chlorhexidine used as a root canal irrigating solution. *Journal of Endodontics*, **25**, 167–171.

95. Tanomaru Filho, M., Leonardo, M.R. & Da Silva, L.A. (2002) Effect of irrigating solution and calcium hydroxide root canal dressing on the repair of apical and periapical tissues of teeth with periapical lesion. *Journal of Endodontics*, **28**, 295–296.

96. Zamany, A., Safavi, K. & Spangberg, L.S.W. (2003) The effect of chlorhexidine as an endodontic disinfectant. *Oral Surgery, Oral Medicine, Oral Pathology, Oral Radiology, and Endodontics*, **96**, 578–581.

97. Ercan, E., Ozekinci, T., Atakul, F. & Gul, K. (2004) Antibacterial activity of 2% chlorhexidine gluconate and 5.25% sodium hypochlorite in infected root canal: in vivo study. *Journal of Endodontics*, **30**, 84–87.

98. Vianna, M.E., Horz, H.P., Gomes, B.P. & Conrads, G. (2006) In vivo evaluation of microbial reduction after chemo-mechanical preparation of human root canals containing necrotic pulp tissue. *Journal of Endodontics*, **39**, 484–492.

99. Siqueira, J.F. Jr., Paiva, S.S. & Rocas, I.N. (2007) Reduction in the cultivable bacterial populations in infected root canals by a chlorhexidine-based antimicrobial protocol. *Journal of Endodontics*, **33**, 541–547.

100. Siqueira, J.F. Jr., Rocas, I.N., Paiva, S.S., Guimaraes-Pinto, T., Magalhaes, K.M. & Lima, K.C. (2007) Bacteriologic investigation of the effects of sodium hypochlorite and chlorhexidine during the endodontic treatment of teeth with apical periodontitis. *Oral Surgery, Oral Medicine, Oral Pathology, Oral Radiology, and Endodontics*, **104**, 122–130.

101. Yamashita, J.C., Tanomaru Filho, M., Leonardo, M.R., Rossi, M.A. & Silva, L.A. (2003) Scanning electron microscopic study of the cleaning ability of chlorhexidine as a root-canal irrigant. *International Endodontic Journal*, **36**, 391–394.

102. Ringel, A.M., Patterson, S.S., Newton, C.W., Miller, C.H. & Mulhern, J.M. (1982) In vivo evaluation of chlorhexidine gluconate solution and sodium hypochlorite solution as root canal irrigants. *Journal of Endodontics*, **8**, 200–204.

103. Vianna, M.E., Horz, H.P., Gomes, B.P. & Conrads, G. (2006) In vivo evaluation of microbial reduction after chemo-mechanical preparation of human root canals containing necrotic pulp tissue. *International Endodontic Journal*, **39**, 484–492.

104. Mjör, I.A., Moorhead, J.E. & Dahl, J.E. (2000) Reasons for replacement of restorations in permanent teeth in general dental practice. *International Dental Journal*, **50**, 361–366.

105. Carrilho, M., Carvalho, R., De Goes, M.F. *et al.* (2007) Chlorhexidine preserves dentine bond in vitro. *Journal of Dental Research*, **86**, 90–94.

106. De Munck, J., Van Landuyt, K., Peumans, M. *et al.* (2005) A critical review of the durability of adhesion to tooth tissue: methods and results. *Journal of Dental Research,* **84,** 118–132.

107. Frankenberger, R., Pashley, D.H., Reich, S.M., Lohbauer, U., Petschelt, A. & Tay, F.R. (2005) Characterization of resin–dentine interfaces by compressive cyclic loading. *Biomaterials,* **26,** 2043–2045.

108. Carrilho, M.R., Carvalho, R.M., Tay, F.R., Yiu, C. & Pashley, D.H. (2005) Durability of resin–dentin bonds related to water and oil storage. *American Journal of Dentistry,* **8,** 315–317.

109. Wang, Z., Shen, Y. & Haapasalo, M. (2012) Effectiveness of endodontic disinfecting solutions against young and old Enterococcus faecalis biofilms in dentin canals. *Journal of Endodontics,* **38,** 1376–1379.

110. Krautheim, A.B., Jermann, T.H. & Bircher, A.J. (2004) Chlorhexidine anaphylaxis: case report and review of the literature. *Contact Dermatitis,* **50,** 113–115.

111. Autegarden, J.E., Pecquet, C., Huet, S., Bayrou, O. & Leynadier, F. (1999) Anaphylactic shock after application of chlorhexidine to unbroken skin. *Contact Dermatitis,* **40,** 215–217.

112. Ebo, D.G., Stevens, W.J., Bridts, C.H. & Matthieu, L. (1998) Contact allergic dermatitis and life-threatening anaphylaxis to chlorhexidine. *Journal of Allergy and Clinical Immunology,* **101,** 128–129.

113. Snellman, E. & Rantanen, T. (1999) Severe anaphylaxis after a chlorhexidine bath. *Journal of the American Academy of Dermatology,* **40,** 771–772.

114. Pham, N.H., Weiner, J.M., Reisner, G.S. & Baldo, B.A. (2000) Anaphylaxis to chlorhexidine. Case report. Implication of immunoglobulin e antibodies and identification of an allergenic determinant. *Clinical and Experimental Allergy,* **30,** 1001–1007.

115. Scully, C., Ng, Y.L. & Gulabivala, K. (2003) Systemic complications due to endodontic manipulations. *Endodontic Topics,* **4,** 60–68.

116. Haapasalo, M., Shen, Y., Qian, W. & Gao, Y. (2010) Irrigation in endodontics. *Dental Clinics of North America,* **54,** 291–312. Review.

117. Williamson, A.E., Cardon, J.W. & Drake, D.R. (2009) Antimicrobial susceptibility of monoculture biofilms of a clinical isolate of Enterococcus faecalis. *Journal of Endodontics,* **35,** 95–97.

118. Palazzi, F., Morra, M., Mohammadi, Z., Grandini, S. & Giardino, L. (2012) Comparison of the surface tension of 5.25% sodium hypochlorite solution with three new sodium hypochlorite-based endodontic irrigants. *International Endodontic Journal,* **45,** 129–135.

119. Jungbluth, H., Peters, C., Peters, O., Sener, B. & Zehnder, M. (2012) Physicochemical and pulp tissue dissolution properties of some household bleach brands compared with a dental sodium hypochlorite solution. *Journal of Endodontics,* **38,** 372–375.

120. Wang, Z., Shen, Y., Ma, J. & Haapasalo, M. (2012) The effect of detergents on the antibacterial activity of disinfecting solutions in dentin. *Journal of Endodontics,* **38,** 948–953.

121. Vivacqua-Gomes, N., Ferraz, C.C., Gomes, B.P., Zaia, A.A., Teixeira, F.B. & Souza-Filho, F.J. (2002) Influence of irrigants on the coronal microleakage of laterally condensed gutta-percha root fillings. *International Endodontic Journal,* **35,** 791–795.

122. Mortenson, D., Sadilek, M., Flake, N.M. *et al.* (2012) The effect of using an alternative irrigant between sodium hypochlorite and chlorhexidine to prevent the formation of para-chloroaniline within the root canal system. *International Endodontic Journal,* **45,** 878–882.

123. Bui, T.B., Baumgartner, J.C. & Mitchell, J.C. (2008) Evaluation of the interaction between sodium hypochlorite and chlorhexidine gluconate and its effect on root dentin. *Journal of Endodontics,* **34,** 181–185.

124. Thomas, J.E. & Sem, D.S. (2010) An in vitro spectroscopic analysis to determine whether para-chloroaniline is produced from mixing sodium hypochlorite and chlorhexidine. *Journal of Endodontics,* **36,** 315–317.

125. Nowicki, J.B. & Sem, D.S. (2011) An in vitro spectroscopic analysis to determine the chemical composition of the precipitate formed by mixing sodium hypochlorite and chlorhexidine. *Journal of Endodontics,* **37,** 983–988.

126. Krishnamurthy, S. & Sudhakaran, S. (2010) Evaluation and prevention of the precipitate formed on interaction between sodium hypochlorite and chlorhexidine. *Journal of Endodontics,* **36,** 1154–1157.

127. Berg, M.S., Jacobsen, E.L., Begole, E.A. & Remeikis, N.A. (1986) A comparison of five irrigating solutions: scanning electron microscopic study. *Journal of Endodontics,* **12,** 192–197.

128. Rome, W.J., Doran, J.E. & Walker, W.A. (1985) The effectiveness of glyoxide and sodium hypochlorite in preventing smear layer formation. *Journal of Endodontics,* **11,** 281–288.

129. Yamada, R.S., Armas, A. & Goldman, M. (1983) Sun Lin P: a scanning electron microscopic comparison of a high volume final flush with several irrigating solutions. Part 3. *Journal of Endodontics,* **9,** 137–142.

130. Goldman, M., Kronman, J.H., Goldman, L.B., Clausen, H. & Grady, J. (1976) New method of irrigation during endodontic treatment. *Journal of Endodontics,* **2,** 257–260.

131. Boessler, C., Peters, O.A. & Zehnder, M. (2007) Impact of lubricant parameters on rotary instrument torque and force. *Journal of Endodontics*, **33**, 280–283.

132. Grawehr, M., Sener, B., Waltimo, T. & Zehnder, M. (2003) Interactions of ethylenediamine tetraacetic acid with sodium hypochlorite in aqueous solutions. *International Endodontic Journal*, **36**, 411–417.

133. Rasimick, B.J., Nekich, M., Hladek, M.M., Musikant, B.L. & Deutsch, A.S. (2008) Interaction between chlorhexidine digluconate and EDTA. *Journal of Endodontics*, **34**, 1521–1523.

134. Qian, W., Shen, Y. & Haapasalo, M. (2011) Quantitative analysis of the effect of irrigant solution sequences on dentin erosion. *Journal of Endodontics*, **37**, 1437–1441.

135. Zhang, W., Torabinejad, M. & Li, Y. (2003) Evaluation of cytotoxicity of MTAD using the MTT-tetrazolium method. *Journal of Endodontics*, **29**, 654–657.

136. Christensen, C.E., McNeal, S.F. & Eleazer, P. (2008) Effect of lowering the pH of sodium hypochlorite on dissolving tissue in vitro. *Journal of Endodontics*, **4**, 449–452.

137. Aubut, V., Pommel, L., Verhille, B. *et al.* (2010) Biological properties of a neutralized 2.5% sodium hypochlorite solution. *Oral Surgery, Oral Medicine, Oral Pathology, Oral Radiology, and Endodontics*, **2**, 120–125.

138. De-Deus, G., Namen, F., Galan, J. Jr. & Zehnder, M. (2008) Soft chelating irrigation protocol optimizes bonding quality of Resilon/Epiphany root fillings. *Journal of Endodontics*, **6**, 703–705.

139. Paqué, F., Rechenberg, D.K. & Zehnder, M. (2012) Reduction of hard-tissue debris accumulation during rotary root canal instrumentation by etidronic acid in a sodium hypochlorite irrigant. *Journal of Endodontics*, **5**, 692–695.

140. Dai, L., Khechen, K., Khan, S. *et al.* (2011) The effects of QMiX, an experimental antibacterial root canal irrigant, on removal of canal wall smear layer and debris. *Journal of Endodontics*, **37**, 80–84.

141. Ma, J., Wang, Z., Shen, Y. & Haapasalo, M. (2011) A new noninvasive model to study the effectiveness of dentin disinfection by using confocal laser scanning microscopy. *Journal of Endodontics*, **37**, 1380–1385.

142. Eliot, C., Hatton, J.F., Stewart, G.P., Hildebolt, C.F., Jane Gillespie, M. & Gutmann, J.L. (2013) The effect of the irrigant QMix on removal of canal wall smear layer: an ex vivo study. *Odontology*, **19**, 1–19.

143. Tasman, F., Cehreli, Z.C., Ogan, C. & Etikan, I. (2000) Surface tension of root canal irrigants. *Journal of Endodontics*, **26**, 586–587.

144. Giardino, L., Ambu, E., Becce, C., Rimondini, L. & Morra, M. (2006) Surface tension comparison of four common root canal irrigants and two new irrigants containing antibiotic. *Journal of Endodontics*, **32**, 1091–1093.

145. Torabinejad, M., Shabahang, S., Aprecio, R.M. & Kettering, J.D. (2003) The antimicrobial effect of MTAD: an in vitro investigation. *Journal of Endodontics*, **29**, 400–403.

146. Shabahang, S. & Torabinejad, M. (2003) Effect of MTAD on Enterococcus faecalis-contaminated root canals of extracted human teeth. *Journal of Endodontics*, **29**, 576–579.

147. Shabahang, S., Pouresmail, M. & Torabinejad, M. (2003) In vitro antimicrobial efficacy of MTAD and sodium hypochlorite. *Journal of Endodontics*, **29 (7)**, 450–452.

148. Baumgartner, J.C., Johal, S. & Marshall, J.G. (2007) Comparison of the antimicrobial efficacy of 1.3% NaOCl/Biopure MTAD to 5.25% NaOCl/15% EDTA for root canal irrigation. *Journal of Endodontics*, **33**, 48–51.

149. Beltz, R.E., Torabinejad, M. & Pouresmail, M. (2003) Quantitative analysis of the solubilizing action of MTAD, sodium hypochlorite, and EDTA on bovine pulp and dentin. *Journal of Endodontics*, **29**, 334–337.

150. Haznedaroglu, F. & Ersev, H. (2001) Tetracycline HCl solution as a root canal irrigant. *Journal of Endodontics*, **27**, 738–740.

151. Tay, F.R., Pashley, D.H., Loushine, R.J. *et al.* (2006) Ultrastructure of smear layer-covered intraradicular dentin after irrigation with biopure MTAD. *Journal of Endodontics*, **32**, 218–221.

152. Davis, J.M., Maki, J. & Bahcall, J.K. (2007) An in vitro comparison of the antimicrobial effects of various endodontic medicaments on *Enterococcus faecalis*. *Journal of Endodontics*, **33**, 567–569.

153. Krause, T.A., Liewehr, F.R. & Hahn, C.L. (2007) The antimicrobial effect of MTAD, sodium hypochlorite, doxycycline, and citric acid on *Enterococcus faecalis*. *Journal of Endodontics*, **33**, 28–30.

154. Kho, P. & Baumgartner, J.C. (2006) A comparison of the antimicrobial efficacy of NaOCl/ BioPure MTAD versus NaOCl/EDTA against *Enterococcus faecalis*. *Journal of Endodontics*, **32**, 652–655.

155. Giardino, L., Ambu, E., Savoldi, E., Rimondini, R., Cassanelli, C. & Debbia, E.A. (2007) Comparative evaluation of antimicrobial efficacy of sodium hypochlorite, MTAD, and Tetraclean against *Enterococcus faecalis* biofilm. *Journal of Endodontics*, **33**, 852–855.

156. Dunavant, T.R., Regan, J.D., Glickman, G.N., Solomon, E.S. & Honeyman, A.L. (2006) Comparative evaluation of endodontic irrigants against *Enterococcus faecalis* biofilms. *Journal of Endodontics*, **32**, 527–531.

157. Portenier, I., Waltimo, T., Orstavik, D. & Haapasalo, M. (2006) Killing of Enterococcus faecalis by MTAD and chlorhexidine digluconate with or without cetrimide in the presence or absence of dentine powder or BSA. *Journal of Endodontics*, **32**, 138–141.

158. Pappen, F.G., Shen, Y., Qian, W., Leonardo, M.R., Giardino, L. & Haapasalo, M. (2010) In vitro antibacterial action of Tetraclean, MTAD and five experimental irrigation solutions. *International Endodontic Journal*, **43**, 528–535.

159. Torabinejad, M., Shabahang, S. & Bahjri, K. (2005) Effect of MTAD on postoperative discomfort: a randomized clinical trial. *Journal of Endodontics*, **31**, 171–176.

160. Malkhassian, G., Manzur, A.J., Legner, M. et al. (2009) Antibacterial efficacy of MTAD final rinse and two percent chlorhexidine gel medication in teeth with apical periodontitis: a randomized double-blinded clinical trial. *Journal of Endodontics*, **35**, 1483–1490.

161. Spångberg, L., Engström, B. & Langeland, K. (1973) Biologic effects of dental materials. 3. Toxicity and antimicrobial effect of endodontic antiseptics in vitro. *Oral Surgery, Oral Medicine, and Oral Pathology*, **36**, 856–871.

162. Spångberg, L., Rutberg, M. & Rydinge, E. (1979) Biological effects of endodontic antimicrobial agents. *Journal of Endodontics*, **5**, 166–175.

163. Sirén, E.K., Haapasalo, M.P.P., Waltimo, T.M.T. & Ørstavik, D. (2004) In vitro antibacterial effect of calcium hydroxide combined with chlorhexidine or iodine potassium iodide on Enterococcus faecalis. *European Journal of Oral Sciences*, **112**, 326–331.

164. Popescu, I., Popescu, M. & Man, D. (1984) Drug allergy: incidence in terms of age and some drug allergens. *Médecine Interne*, **22**, 195–202.

165. Prabhakar, J., Senthilkumar, M., Priya, M.S., Mahalakshmi, K., Sehgal, P.K. & Sukumaran, V.G. (2010) Evaluation of antimicrobial efficacy of herbal alternatives (Triphala and green tea polyphenols), MTAD, and 5% sodium hypochlorite against *Enterococcus faecalis* biofilm formed on tooth substrate: an in vitro study. *Journal of Endodontics*, **36**, 83–86.

166. Jagetia, G.C., Baliga, M.S., Malagi, K.J. et al. (2002) The evaluation of the radioprotective effect of Triphala (an Ayurvedic rejuvenating drug) in the mice exposed to radiation. *Phytomedicine*, **9**, 99–108.

167. Hamilton-Miller, J.M. (2001) Anti-cariogenic properties of tea (Camellia sinensis). *Journal of Medical Microbiology*, **50**, 299–302.

168. Xu, X., Zhou, X.D. & Wu, C.D. (2011) The tea catechin epigallatocatechin gallate suppresses cariogenic virulence factors of Streptococcus mutans. *Antimicrobial Agents and Chemotherapy*, **55**, 1229–1236.

169. Horiba, N., Maekawa, Y., Ito, M., Matsumoto, T. & Nakamura, H. (1991) A pilot study of Japanese green tea as a medicament: antibacterial and bactericidal effects. *Journal of Endodontics*, **17**, 122–124.

170. Mannello, F. (2006) Natural bio-drugs as matrix metalloproteinase inhibitors: new perspectives on the horizon? *Recent Patents on Anti-Cancer Drug Discovery*, **1**, 91–103.

171. Hirasawa, M., Takada, K. & Otake, S. (2006) Inhibition of acid production in dental plaque bacteria by green tea catechins. *Caries Research*, **40**, 265–270.

172. Basrani, B. & Haapasalo, M. (2012) Update on endodontic irrigation solutions. *Endodontic Topics*, **27**, 74–102.

8 Fluid Dynamics of Irrigation within the Root Canal System

Franklin R. Tay

Department of Endodontics, Georgia Regents University, Augusta, GA, USA

Introduction

The time-honored endodontic triad of debridement, disinfection, and obturation has been recognized for over a century (1). However, our discovery of the strategies for achieving these objectives has not followed a linear logic path, but has been sidetracked for decades by misunderstood scientific observations. Hunter's focal infection theory (2) was supported by the voluminous, yet specious, work of Price (3), but was challenged by clinicians like Grossman in the 1930s (4) who cultured materials taken from the root canals in a crude culturing incubator fabricated from nothing more than a lunch box and a light bulb. The culturing era basically ended in 1964 when Bender and Seltzer (5) published their seminal paper: "To culture or not to culture?" As it turned out, their work also was based on misunderstood and inaccurate scientific observations. Forty-two years later, Spånberg (6) criticized in an editorial that this paper began a 10-year "walk in the desert" until Byström

and Sundqvist (7) reestablished the importance of microorganisms in apical infections. Interestingly, Spånberg's editorial was written at about the same time as the discovery of endodontic biofilms. These biofilms were subsequently identified as the causative agents for apical periodontitis (8).

A thorough review of the fluid mechanics of root canal irrigation has already been performed by Gulabivala *et al.* (9). Readers are encouraged to read this excellent work. It cannot be denied that the subject of endodontic fluid dynamics is also wrought with myths, misunderstood observations, prejudices, biases, or often a simple lack of understanding. Accordingly, it is necessary to identify and explain these misconceptions, via evidence-based studies, that have unwittingly been embedded into this subject. These include (i) apical vapor lock effect, (ii) hydrolysis of organic components of the soft and hard pulp tissues and canal wall biofilms, (iii) technique misunderstandings, and (iv) patency safety issues. Following these demystifications, evidence-based studies should be used to identify

Disinfection of Root Canal Systems: The Treatment of Apical Periodontitis, First Edition. Edited by Nestor Cohenca.
© 2014 John Wiley & Sons, Inc. Published 2014 by John Wiley & Sons, Inc.

strategies for attaining safe and effective intra- and extracanal irrigant fluid dynamics.

Misconceptions

Apical vapor lock (AVL)

The AVL is a physical phenomenon wherein CO_2 and NH_3 arising from the hydrolysis of organic tissues mix and form a gas bubble in the apical portion of the root canal. This bubble cannot escape into the apical tissue if the apex is oriented in the upward position. When the apex is orientated downward, the gas bubble is trapped by the weight of the irrigant and its surface tension force resists the buoyancy force of the trapped gas (Figure 8.1). Furthermore, any attempt to "pop" the bubble in the latter orientation is counterproductive as explained in Figure 8.2. In 1983, Chow (10) observed air bubbles or columns *in-vitro* that could not be displaced or passed around except by placing a small needle very close to the apex without binding, a practice that would later prove to be

potentially dangerous (11). Recent findings have discovered that the interfacial force equilibrium at the dentin, gas, fluid interface can be disrupted only by the apical negative pressure or effective microstreaming (12).

History of discovery

The history of the discovery of AVL is important, because as recently as 2012, investigators were still failing to consider the AVL effect (13) during a protocol design involving endodontic irrigation systems and techniques believed to dissolve organic material in inaccessible areas. Although the use of sodium hypochlorite (NaOCl) as a tissue solvent had been documented as early as 1967 (14), it was not recognized widely until 1974 when Schilder (15) reported the use of an average of 39 ml of NaOCl per visit, combined with patency filing, to debride the instrumented root canal space. Schilder's irrigation protocol became the benchmark of excellent clinical treatment. Subjective radiographic inspection of his cases seemed to validate that intracanal irregularities and accessory canals were in fact

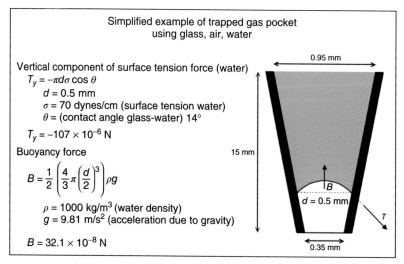

Figure 8.1   To explain how a gas pocket can be trapped under a fluid column, a simplified glass tube shaped as a 4% tapering cone with an apical diameter of 0.35 mm is filled with water, leaving a gas pocket at the bottom. The gas buoyancy acts vertically upward and will act only on the part of the pocket that is immersed in liquid, which is shown as a dotted line. The buoyancy force (B) is determined by the size of the immersed part that is determined by the shape of the meniscus, which can be calculated by the Young–Laplace equation. For simplicity, if the shape is considered to be spherical and of the diameter equal to that of the cone at that point, then B will be about 300 times smaller than the vertical component of the surface tension force (T_y). This means that the bubble is trapped. The surface tension force and the weight of the liquid are supported by the increase in pressure of the air pocket.

Effect of introducing a
"poping" device

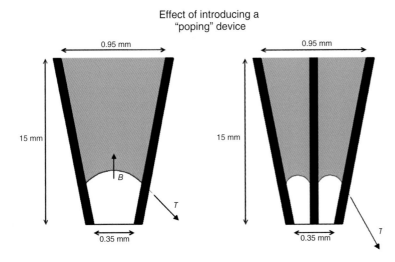

Figure 8.2 Elimination of the vapor lock via "popping" of the pocket is not an option, as inserting any object, such as a gutta-percha point, file, or needle into the hypothetical root canal space will only make the space smaller, with the effect of increasing the surface tension. In fact, when attempting to pop the bubble, the diameter of bubble ring that is formed is decreased and can be half of the initial diameter of the glass tube. The resulting surface tension to buoyancy ratio then can be roughly an entire order of magnitude higher, yielding a ratio of approximately 3000 to 1.

cleaned and obturated, an observation that was proven inaccurate 43 years later (16).

In 1971, Senia *et al.* (17) authored a classic paper in which he tested the efficacy of 5.25% NaOCl to dissolve intracanal pulp tissue in the mesial roots of lower molars. Briefly, the authors instrumented the mesial roots of lower molars to a size 30 instrument. Then, "the apex was sealed with green stick compound in order to retain the irrigating solutions within the canals, and the root was mounted upright on a glass slide." Final irrigation was accomplished by applying 5.25% NaOCl and stirring with a size 10 file for either 15 or 30 min. On histological examination, significant residual pulp tissue was found throughout the apical termination and the study concluded that "the value of sodium hypochlorite as an irrigating agent for dissolving pulp tissue in the apical 3 mm of narrow root canals is questionable."

Six years later, Salzgeber and Brilliant (18) conducted a clinical study to determine the flow characteristics of root canal irrigants in mandibular molars. The authors slightly altered the final shaping of the canal as described by Senia *et al.* (17), by enlarging the apical termination to a size 35 instrument. Also, they used a radiopaque dye (Hypaque) instead of NaOCl. This study observed that in spite of an extremely cautious irrigant delivery technique during treatment, Hypaque always reached the apical termination of the root canal, but also flowed into the apical tissue of infected

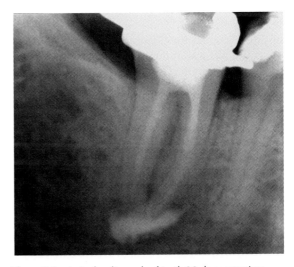

Figure 8.3 Apical radiograph of tooth 30 demonstrating excessive apical extrusion of Hypaque, a radiopaque contrasting medium, into the periapex, despite meticulous care in needle placement and clinical delivery, to ensure the delivery needle did not bind in the canal. Being biologically inert, Hypaque neither hydrolyzes organic material nor produces any gas. (Salzgeber and Brilliant (18). Reproduced with permission of Elsevier.)

teeth (Figure 8.3). The authors concluded that "the solution is not confined to the instrumented space in cases with necrotic pulps and may occupy random dimensions when extruded into the apical lesion. Salzgeber summarized that "The study by Senia *et al.* (17) showed that little or no sodium hypochlorite reached the apical 3 mm when the root canals were enlarged to a size 30 instrument. The current study showed that the irrigant reaches the apex when the canals are opened larger than a size 30 file." The flaw with the Salzgeber and Brilliant study was the use of Hypaque instead of NaOCl, because Hypaque is biologically inert while NaOCl hydrolyzes organic materials, releasing NH_3 and CO_2, and in a closed root canal system forms the AVL.

It would be impractical to review the list of irrigation-related articles that were published between the publications of Salzgeber and Brilliant [18] and O'Connell et al. [19], as investigators examined instrumentation/irrigation regimes, different irrigants and their concentrations, as well as time and temperature of exposure. However, the O'Connell article epitomized the furthest advancement in canal system preparation and irrigation techniques in that time period. Importantly, the authors adopted the "Baumgartner protocol" [20] of sealing the apical foramen during instrumentation and irrigation. They used NiTi rotary instrumentation to open the apical foramen to a size 40 at a 4% taper, while irrigating with copious quantities of 5.25% NaOCl and 15% ethylenediaminetetraaceticacid (EDTA). Even with such canal enlargement and the use of dual irrigants to dissolve the organic and inorganic components of the canal wall smear layer, the authors reported that canal walls along the apical 1/3 of the root canals were not clean and the dentinal tubules were covered with the smear layer. However, 3 years later, Torabinejad et al. [21] reported extremely clean walls and open dentinal tubules in the apical 1/3 of the canal space, even though the apical foramen of the root canals were instrumented to a size 30 instrument, the same size as Senia et al. [17] had used 32 years earlier. In the work by Torabinejad et al. [21], the most favorable results were achieved when the authors used a combination of MTAD (an antimicrobial irrigant containing doxycycline, citric acid, and a surfactant) and a low concentration of NaOCl.

When these findings were published, Schoeffel was developing the EndoVac system of apical negative pressure for safety purposes. As the protocol by Torabinejad et al. [21] called for lower and safer concentration of NaOCl, Schoeffel tested the commercially available BioPure® MTAD in early 2005 (Figure 8.4a,b), using the standard "Baumgartner

protocol" to seal the apical foramen. It was readily apparent that clean dentinal tubules could not be realized in the apical 1/3 of the canal space by using BioPure MTAD. This was in stark contrast to the results obtained when a root canal with a sealed apex was irrigated with apical negative pressure (Figure 8.4c,d). Careful rereading of the Torabinejad et al. [21] paper revealed the following: "Opening the apical foramen of each tooth to a size 30 file and free flow of irrigant through the apical end of the root canal may have allowed more cleaning of the apical portions of root canals in this experiment." Schoeffel immediately realized that Senia et al. [17] had inadvertently created the conditions necessary to form an AVL when the authors mounted the roots in greenstick compound. Salzgeber and Brilliant [18] could never have formed an AVL with the use of a biologically inactive irrigant. Torabinejad et al. [21] had a vague idea that a flaw existed in their protocol, because the authors further elaborated: "Studies are in progress to determine the efficacy of various other techniques to carry MTAD into the apical portion of the root canal systems with closed apexes." Schoeffel's theory was first publicized in 2008 [22]; was validated in-vitro in 2010 [23] and in-vivo in 2012 [24]. The AVL is apparent in-vivo (Figure 8.5) and can be broken by either acoustic microstreaming, apical negative pressure, or by placing the irrigation needle at or extremely close to full working length [10]. The last method produces very high apical extrusion pressures under normal clinical delivery rates [11], which is addressed in the safety section.

The significance of the AVL is that several studies have erroneously assumed that an irrigant is present throughout all phases of canal preparation and irrigation, thus leading to inaccurate observations. For example, Zehnder [25] demonstrated that two liquids (coronal and apical) can be mixed once the canal is instrumented to size 40; however, the apical liquid would be a gas and would not mix. Boutsioukis et al. [26] assumed that a canal was completely filled with irrigant, without giving considerations to the existence of the AVL, when the authors designed their computational fluid dynamic model. Vera et al. [27] recognized the vexing problem associated with the AVL in root canal irrigation: "Factors such as complex root canal anatomy and the vapor lock phenomenon have been shown to limit the penetration of irrigating

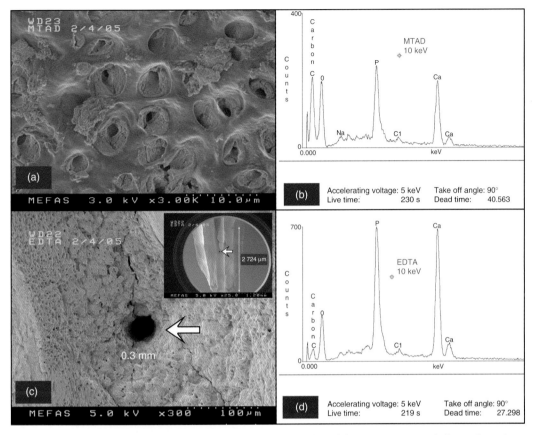

Figure 8.4 These two scanning electron microscopy (SEM) images were derived from noncarious teeth during the early stages of research and development of the EndoVac apical negative pressure irrigation system. (a) A representative SEM image of the dentin wall after treatment using BioPure MTAD according to manufacturer's instructions. The area is taken from the coronal portion of the apical 1/3 of the canal space where there is an abundance of dentinal tubules. The material in the tubules is undissolved pulpal debris. (b) Energy-dispersive spectroscopy (EDS) spectrum of the area shown in (a) that displays a wealth of carbon. The Ca, O, and P signals originate from hydroxyapatite. (c) A representative SEM image of the canal wall from the apical 1–3 mm of the canal space that was irrigated using apical negative pressure. A clean lateral canal (arrow), 0.3 mm in diameter, can be seen and is located at 2 mm from working length (Inset: arrow indicates the position of the lateral canal). (d) EDS spectrum of the area shown in (c) that reveals a very low carbon level, probably associated with collagen and noncollagenous proteins derived from the mineralized radicular dentin.

solutions into the apical third in both *in-vivo* and *in-vitro* studies involving small and wide canals." Jiang *et al.* (13) mixed dentin chips with 2% NaOCl for 5 min before placing the mixture in an apical canal groove model, mistakenly assuming that the groove was devoid of organic material (Figure 8.6a).

Dead water space or stagnation plane

As a matter of historical importance, prior to the *in-vitro* proof regarding the existence of the AVL

(23), a similar fluid dynamics problem was referred to as the *Dead Water Zone* (29), whereby irrigants are effectively exchanged only a short distance in front of the irrigation needle even though the entire root canal is completely filled with the irrigant. This phenomenon was first described by Chow (10) in 1983, who found that irrigation was strictly a function of the depth of the needle. In 2010, Gulabivala *et al.* (9) referred to the "Dead Water Zone" as the stagnation plane and devoted a comprehensive research paper attempting to identify a

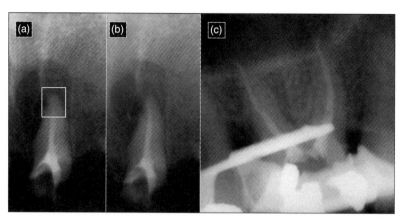

Figure 8.5 The radiopaque appearance in each radiograph is derived from a 1:1 mixture of omnipaque (Iohexol—an angiocardiography contrasting medium) and NaOCl. Because the radiopaque omnipaque is mixed with NaOCl, the exact location of the irrigant mixture can be determined. (a) A vapor lock (box) is present in the apical third of the canal space. (b) The irrigant flowed successfully to the apical termination after ultrasonic activation. (c) The mesial and distal roots of a maxillary molar after using the EndoVac microcannula to deliver the irrigant to full working length. The premolar was isolated with a rubber dam, cyanoacrylate, and a blockout resin. (Radiographs courtesy of Dr. Jorge Vera, Puebla, Mexico.)

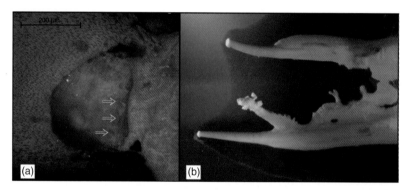

Figure 8.6 (a) Cross-section of a root canal at 5 mm coronal to the working length showing inaccessible amorphous organic mass with dentin shavings (red arrows) apparent at instrumentation interface. (De-Deus *et al.* (28). Reproduced with permission of Elsevier.) (b) Complex canal anatomy demonstrates several areas where biofilm may flourish in inaccessible areas, including the smallest fins, cul-de-sacs, and isthmus areas and the lateral canals that provide the portal to the apical area. Accordingly, debridement and disinfection via complete hydrolysis throughout the root canal system is essential to prevent biofilm recolonization, possibly from infected tubules. (Dr. G. John Schoeffel, Dana Point, California. Reproduced with permission of G.J. Schoeffel.)

mechanism to move the stagnation plane apically to be coincident with the canal terminus, without extruding beyond it. After a thorough investigation of needle designs, flow rates, and passive ultrasonic techniques, Gulabivala *et al.* concluded that "despite the significant advances in root canal treatment, there remains a lack of clarity about the mechanisms of irrigant delivery, replenishment, mixing, flushing, and wall erosion." It is important to realize that Gulabivala *et al.* (9) submitted their paper on June 17, 2009, almost a year before the work by Tay *et al.* (23) Regardless of AVL, dead water space, or stagnation plane, the resulting problem turned out to be the same always— lack of adequate irrigant exchange in the apical termination to effectively hydrolyze organic debris.

Hydrolysis of pulpal soft tissues and organic components of hard tissue debris

The subject of this chapter is fluid dynamics of irrigation within the root canal system. For effective debridement, there must be an exchange of irrigants throughout the root canal system including canal fins, cul-de-sacs, and isthmus areas. Thus, irrigants must be bioreactive chemicals in order to effectively dissolve, via hydrolysis, the variety of organic molecules encountered in the root canal system. It is interesting to note that sterilization is not part of the endodontic triad because that would require total eradication of every microbe in every tubule. In 1995, Peters *et al.* (30) reviewed the fate of bacteria in the dentinal tubules and concluded that "there is no evidence, however, that special measures should be taken to kill the bacteria in the dentinal tubules. Should time permit, a sound obturation technique immediately following the cleaning, shaping, and disinfection phases allows the remaining bacteria in the tubules to be either inactivated or prevented from repopulating the (former) canal space. In the vast majority of cases, those bacteria appear not to jeopardize the successful outcome of root canal treatment." Figure 8.6b exemplifies the concept proposed by Peters *et al.*,

wherein the very complex root canal system is fully obturated after successful chemical debridement via hydrolysis. Three-dimensional obturation of the root canal system deprives the space for biofilm to form. It should be further noted that complete obturation of the canal space is impossible if residual dead biofilm remains. This would leave behind spaces for repopulation by other biofilm colonies.

Irrigant concentration and exchange

Issues of irrigant type, concentration, activation, and delivery time must be considered. If one considers a biofilm simply as an organic material (similarly to pulp tissues) that must be hydrolyzed into gas, the disinfection problem then becomes one of simple debridement via hydrolysis (Figure 8.7). Hydrolysis via NaOCl is a simple equilibrium reaction, as demonstrated by the reaction of NaOCl with lysine: $18ClO^- + C_6H_{14}N_2O_2 \Rightarrow 18Cl^- + 8H_2O + 2NH_3 + 6CO_2$. As reported by Hand *et al.* (31), the speed of the dissolution of the organic material is a function of NaOCl concentration. These authors demonstrated that 0.5% NaOCl dissolved approximately 55,000% less necrotic tissues per unit time than 5.25% NaOCl. Although chlorhexidine has

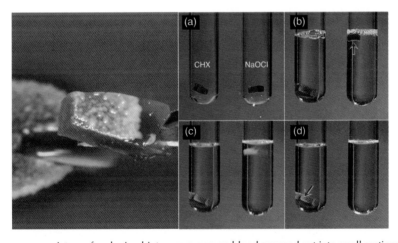

Figure 8.7 A heterogeneous mixture of oral microbiota was grown on blood agar and cut into small sections (left panel). (a) The agar and microbiota are placed in test tubes that will receive either 2% chlorhexidine (CHX) or 6% sodium hypochlorite (NaOCl). (b) Immediately after the solutions are added, the agar specimen in the NaOCl rises to the top as hydrolysis begins, indicated by the bubbles released on the bottom (red arrow). (c) A few minutes later, only a faint hint of the polysaccharide composing the agar is apparent. (d) Finally, both the agar and microbiota are completely reduced to carbon dioxide and ammonia, while both the agar and now dead microbiota in the CHX remain in their original state. In the root canal scenario, this debris would prevent adequate obturation.

Solution	SEM		Culture growth
	Presence of bacteria	Biofilm status	
6% NaOCl	−	Absent	0%
3% NaOCl	−	Absent	20%
1% NaOCl	+	Disrupted	90%
1% NaOCl/MTAD	+	Disrupted	0%
2% CHX	+	Intact	0%
+ Control	+	Intact	100%
− Control	−	Absent	0%

Figure 8.8   Only 6% NaOCl was able to completely remove biofilm and prevent growth.

also been advocated as an antimicrobial irrigant, its hydrolytic effect on oral biofilms is not as pronounced as NaOCl (Figure 8.7). Clegg *et al.* (32) examined several contemporary irrigants against oral biofilms using both scanning electron microscopy (SEM) and culturing methods (Figure 8.8). Their results are in agreement with what is shown in Figure 8.7, in that chlorhexidine has minimal effect in destroying biofilms. Likewise, Siqueira *et al.* (33) was unable to achieve 100% negative culture when chlorhexidine was employed as an irrigant clinically. Ercan *et al.* compared the antibacterial activity of chlorhexidine versus NaOCl (34) and concluded that "although it [NaOCl] is an effective antimicrobial agent and has excellent solvent properties for vital, necrotic, and fixed tissues, it is known to be highly irritating for apical tissues, especially at high concentrations. Because of the adverse effects of this irrigant, researchers have developed alternative irrigants."

The negative implication to NaOCl's aforementioned positive attributes is safety. It can cause severe tissue reaction (35), neurological complications (36), facial deformity (37), life-threatening situations (38), as well as litigation considerations (39). Accordingly, the dental profession has been looking for methods to safely deliver NaOCl in concentrations higher than 3% safely to full working length. As mentioned earlier, because of the existence of an AVL, there are three proven methods to deliver NaOCl to full working length. The safety consideration of using positive-pressure delivery close to full working length is discussed later. Munoz and Camacho-Cuadra (12) demonstrated that irrigants can be delivered high up in the canal and worked to the apical termination

with ultrasonic microstreaming. Alternatively, those irrigants may be pulled to the apical termination via apical negative pressure. Recently, three clinical studies tested both these methods. Cohenca *et al.* (40), using apical negative pressure irrigation (EndoVac), achieved 100% negative cultures both after final irrigation and 1 week recall. Paiva *et al.* (41), using passive ultrasonic instrumentation (PUI), failed to observe a significant difference in the bacteriologic status. The authors concluded that "although supplementary disinfection with either PUI or a final rinse with chlorhexidine can reduce the number of cases with positive culture and polymerase chain reaction results for bacteria, many cases still remain with detectable bacteria in the main root canal." In contrast to the clinical study by Cohenca *et al.* (40), Pawar and coworkers (42) failed to identify a significant difference when using the EndoVac. However, it must be pointed out that their study used only 0.5% NaOCl instead of the 5% concentration recommended by the EndoVac technique—a difference of 1000%. It must be recalled that Clegg *et al.* (32) demonstrated that less than 3% NaOCl produced approximately 90% culture growth and did not remove biofilm. Pawar *et al.* (42) stated that "the use of 0.5% NaOCl in this study could be considered responsible for the lack of significant differences in antimicrobial efficacy between EndoVac irrigation and standard irrigation." The Pawar study affirms the necessity to use NaOCl at concentrations higher than 3% during endodontic irrigation.

Irrigant activation via agitation

Proper instrument agitation in the amplitude range of 75 µm and driven at 30 kHz cavitation causes more effective intracanal debris removal than lower frequency and higher amplitude devices that are designed to operate in the range of 1.2 mm amplitude and 160 Hz (43). Furthermore, during ultrasonic activation, because the tip is smallest in diameter, it has the largest displacement thereby generating the largest shear stress. This is an important consideration once the NaOCl has been exhausted (9). However, microstreaming is dependent on the freedom of the instrument movement and, until recently, has not been evaluated for efficacy when its movement is restricted by a well-defined canal curvature. This point is addressed in detail later.

Chemical limitations of passive ultrasonic irrigation (PUI)

When the PUI technique is employed, the apical portion of the root canal is initially devoid of the irrigant (Figure 8.5a). Once PUI begins, acoustic microstreaming allows the irrigant to reach full working length (Figure 8.5b). Assuming all the irrigant delivered to the root canal system is circulated through the apical termination via microstreaming, the total volume would equal ≈0.0126 ml (Figure 8.9), as opposed to the ability of apical negative pressure (EndoVac) to circulate 1.8 ml at full working length (44). Thus, a difference of ≈14,000% volumetric exchange is realized between apical negative pressure irrigation and acoustic microstreaming via PUI, with the former providing a constant supply of NaOCl (>5%) that results in a consistent high-reaction velocity without irrigant depletion. Although the physical action of acoustic microstreaming is active during PUI, the ability of NaOCl to hydrolyze existing organic tissues is quickly exhausted, because less than a quarter of a drop of irrigant can be circulated to the apical termination per application. Accordingly, the problems with PUI are fluid exchange and concentration resulting from fluid dynamics encountered in a closed root canal system.

In concert with his clinical study, Cohenca and coworkers (45, 46) conducted two *in-vitro*

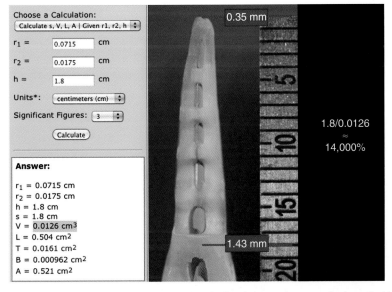

Figure 8.9 The volume of space in a root canal may be roughly calculated using a frustum calculator. In this example, a 1.8 cm long root canal instrumented to size 35, 0.06 taper would hold about 0.0126 ml of fluid. Assuming an irrigant delivery needle is not positioned closer than 4 mm from the working length, the apical vapor lock in the terminal 3 mm will not be filled until microstreaming is initiated. At that point, the clinician has only about 0.0126 ml of NaOCl to activate. The NaOCl will be quickly exhausted. However, apical negative pressure can draw approximately 1.8 ml of irrigant through the entire working length. That is approximately a 14,000% volumetric differential and helps to maintain the hydrolysis reaction at its fullest potential throughout the final irrigation phase.

studies using teeth infected with *Enterococcus faecalis* biofilms and examined the results of the final irrigation via culturing technique as well as SEM examination of the canal walls. Figure 8.10 demonstrates results from the Hockett study (45) comparing different preparation techniques and used a traditional irrigation technique or apical negative pressure for the final irrigation. Regardless of the preparation technique, all specimens treated with the EndoVac system tested negative, while 66% of the teeth treated with the traditional irrigation technique tested positive for microbial culturing. Figure 8.10a shows a thick biofilm at the apical termination. Figure 8.10b shows the biofilm completely removed; the absence of dentinal tubules is indicative that this section has been taken in the apical 2 mm of the root canal, wherein the tubules are obliterated by sclerotic mineral casts. Figure 8.10c shows dentinal tubules devoid of bacteria while the canal wall surface is devoid of bacteria or smear layer. SEM examination confirmed complete eradication of the canal wall biofilms. Figure 8.11 demonstrates results from the Saldivar study (46) that tested the efficacy of PUI in addition to apical negative pressure and traditional irrigation techniques. In this study, the EndoVac again produced 100% negative cultures, while the PUI group produced 53% positive cultures. The positive control (Figure 8.11a) demonstrates thick biofilms in the last apical 2 mm of the canal space. The PUI group (Figure 8.11b) shows canal walls covered by smear layers created during PUI as well as some intact clusters of *E. faecalis*. The EndoVac group (Figure 8.11c) demonstrates clean open tubules and complete eradication of bacteria. It is encouraging that the PUI technique had a profound effect on reducing the extent of biofilm, despite the fact that irrigant exchange at the apical termination was minimal following the fluid dynamics of irrigant exchange mentioned in the previous paragraph.

Increased temperature

As of the writing of this chapter, research on the efficacy of using warmed NaOCl for debridement of the canal space has basically stopped. However, after Abou-Rass and Oglesby (47) reported that 5.25% NaOCl heated to 140 °F could dissolve tissue up to nine times faster than 5.25% NaOCl at ambient temperature, many commercial NaOCl heating

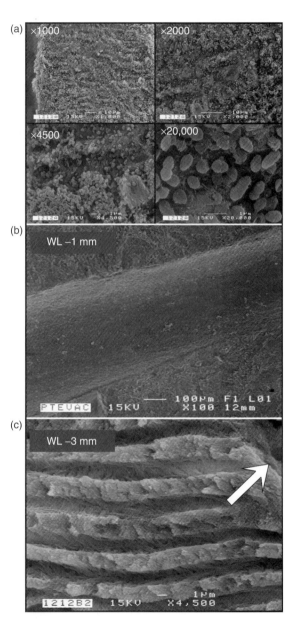

Figure 8.10   (a) A series of four SEM images taken with different magnifications from the positive control showing the presence of a thick biofilm in the apical 2 mm of the instrumented canal space. (b) SEM image of the instrumented canal wall at 1 mm from the working length. The canal wall is devoid of patent dentinal tubule orifices (sclerotic radicular dentin) and is completely devoid of bacteria biofilms. (c) SEM image of fractured radicular dentin at 3 mm from the working length. The surface of canal wall (arrow) is rendered smear-layer-free by the use of apical negative pressure irrigation and contains patent tubular orifices. No bacteria can be identified within the subsurface dentinal tubules. (Hockett *et al.* (45). Reproduced with permission of Elsevier.)

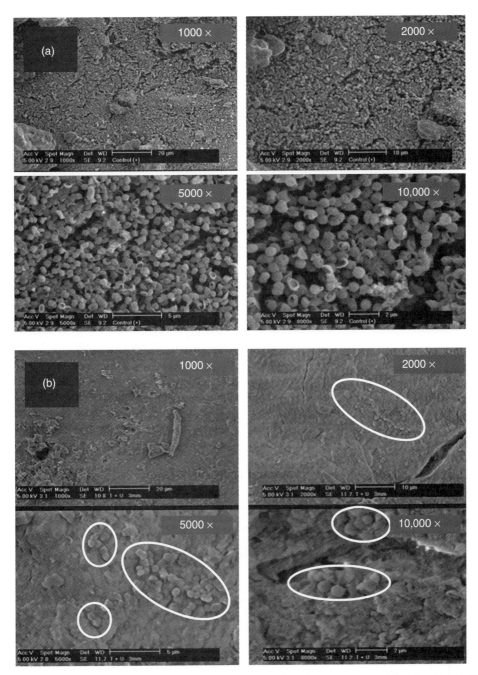

Figure 8.11 (a) A series of SEM images taken at different magnifications from the positive control showing thick biofilm formation in the apical 2 mm of the canal wall. (b) A series of SEM images taken at 3 mm coronal to the working length showing the conditions of the canal wall following irrigation with passive ultrasonic irrigation (PUI). Clusters of bacteria could be identified from the debrided canal wall (enclosed in ovals). (c) A series of SEM images taken at 3 mm coronal to the working length showing complete absence of smear layer, patent dentinal tubule orifices, and absence of bacteria after irrigation with 5.25% NaOCl and 17% EDTA with EndoVac negative apical pressure irrigation technique. (Images courtesy of Dr. Nestor Cohenca and Ana Maria González Amaro, San Luis Potosi, Mexico.)

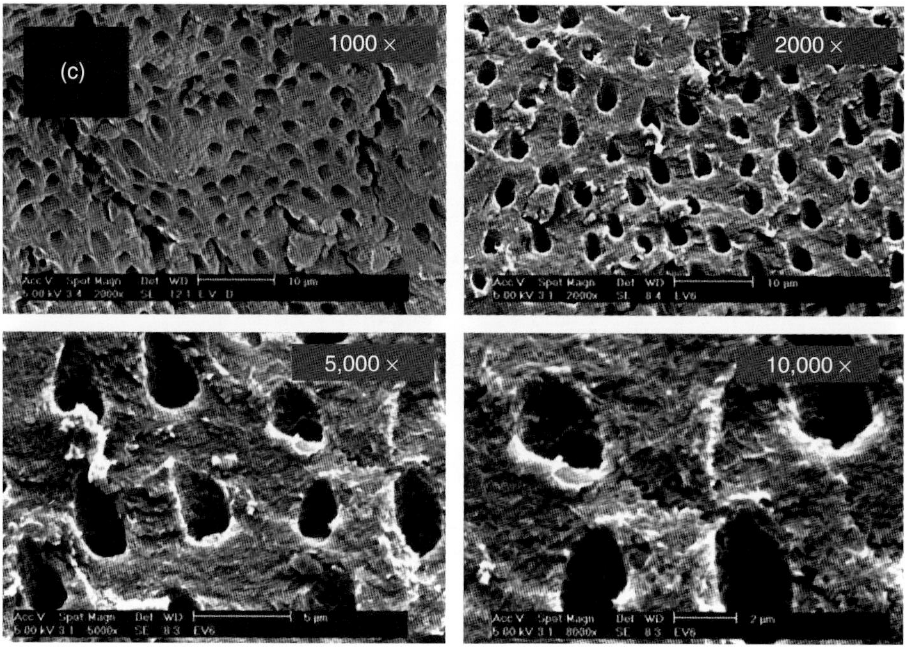

Figure 8.11   *(Continued)*.

devices became available (48). Interestingly, however, Berutti and Marini (49) reinvestigated the *in-vitro* parameters adopted by Abou-Rass and Oglesby using a wax-sealed, closed apex protocol. The authors reported that "unlike what was found in the middle third, no marked difference was seen between the two specimens in the structure of the smear layer in the apical third … this confirms that it is difficult to achieve proper irrigation of the apical third (of the canal wall)." In retrospect, this study also confirms the AVL theory.

Technical misunderstanding

Scientific research requires control and repeatability. This demands that investigators follow previously defined protocols unless otherwise stated for valid reasons. The apical negative pressure concept of root canal irrigation appeared suddenly in 2007, almost without any history of evolution. This has consequently created confusion, leading to misunderstandings regarding its method of operation and procedures to ensure proper control and repeatability.

Townsend study—an example

The study by Townsend and Maki (50) exemplifies this lack of understanding. The authors compared the ability of several irrigation systems to remove biofilm in a curved plastic canal and concluded that "in a plastic simulated canal, ultrasonic agitation was significantly more effective than needle irrigation and EndoVac." The investigators violated the repeatability standard by not using the essential agent required for the EndoVac system—NaOCl in concentrations higher than 5%. Instead, the authors justified their use of water as an irrigant by rationalizing that their study was designed "to assess only the mechanical effects of agitation and irrigation at removing *E. faecalis* from a canal." In addition, Townsend and Maki misquoted Hockett *et al.* (45) by stating "Hockett *et al.* showed that active or *'positive-pressure'* irrigation has the potential to achieve significantly better infection control…" What Hockett *et al.* actually wrote was "the results of this *in-vitro* study showed that *apical negative-pressure* irrigation has the potential to achieve better microbial control…." This cognitive dissonance contributed at large to the general misconception regarding apical negative pressure. For example, Torabinejad (51) unintentionally quoted Townsend study in a collegial publication and stated that "based on the results of this investigation, the authors conclude that ultrasonic agitation is significantly more effective than needle irrigation and EndoVac irrigations at removing intracanal bacteria."

Failure to follow established protocol

Jiang et al. (13) also compared canal irrigation with apical negative pressure with other methods of canal irrigation to examine the efficacy of debris removal efficacy. The failure of that study to follow the manufacturer's instructions produced erroneous observations that compounded the mistakes made by Townsend and Maki (50) and Pawar et al. (42). For the negative apical pressure (EndoVac) group, the authors inadvertently employed the microcannula only, as opposed to the combined use of the macro-/microcannulae. Not only is the combined use clearly part of the manufacturer's instructions, but it is a key element of the EndoVac's patented system (52). Irrigation with the microcannula without first using the macrocannula would have most certainly resulted in premature blockage of the filtration holes of the microcannula, causing either slowing or complete obstruction of irrigant flow. This created results that were skewed against the performance of the negative apical pressure irrigation system. Unlike other studies (53, 54), the irrigant flow rate through the EndoVac's evacuation tube was not reported by Jiang et al. (13).

Patient safety and intracanal fluid dynamics

Patient safety is paramount when considering intracanal fluid dynamics including irrigant delivery rate, agitation and exchange, needle design, pressure gradient management, wall shear stress and cleaning efficacy, and ultimately, treatment outcome. The endodontic literature is replete with case histories of NaOCl extrusion incidents (55), specific and serious examples of which have been previously mentioned (37–39). This axiom is best stated by Boutsioukis et al. (26): "from a clinical point of view, the prevention of extrusion should precede the requirement for adequate irrigant replacement and wall shear stress." Three types of NaOCl extrusion incidents have been reported: careless iatrogenic injection (56), extrusion into the maxillary sinus (57), and, finally, systemic extrusion or infusion via the root canal space. All three situations are avoidable by controlling the pressure gradient delivery differential.

Maxillary sinus

Extrusion of NaOCl into the maxillary sinus has been reported with complications varying from inconsequential (58) to severe facial pain requiring hospitalization and operative intervention under general anesthesia (38). Hauman et al. (59) describe these accidents in a review article and state that "the alveolar bone can become thinner with increasing age, particularly in the areas surrounding the apices of teeth, so that root tips projecting into the sinus are covered only by an extremely thin (sometimes absent) bony lamella and the sinus membrane." In such a case, there would be no resistance to the flow of irrigants into the maxillary sinus. Recently, Khan et al. (11) reported apically directed pressures of 2.6 mm of Hg using a nonbound side-vented needle with a flow rate of 1 ml/min positioned at 1 mm from working length. However, in the study by Jiang et al. (13) the authors used a flow rate of 6 ml with needles in the same position, in which case the apically direct pressure would have been 72 mm Hg (11). In either case, sufficient pressure would cause extrusion of NaOCl into the maxillary sinus if the Schneiderian membrane was missing, as described by Hauman et al. (59). Sleiman (60) reported the following case: on examination of a referred female patient for evaluation of her upper right first molar, the patient reported having experienced the sensation of chlorine in her throat arising from her nose. A panoramic radiograph (Figure 8.12) revealed a diffusion irregularity. After taking the history and examining the panoramic X-ray, cone beam computed tomography of the maxilla was taken. Figure 8.13 shows the right maxillary sinus filled with inflammatory tissues. Figure 8.14a–c shows that the posterior wall of the sinus was nonexistent in some places. It was concluded that the position of the patient during the root canal procedure could have resulted in the

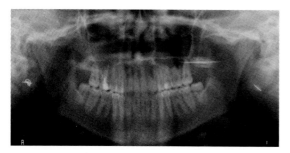

Figure 8.12 Panoramic radiograph showing irregular appearance of the right maxillary sinus. (Courtesy of Dr. Philippe Sleiman, Beirut, Lebanon.)

stagnation of NaOCl on the posterior wall of the sinus and aggravated the damage.

Intravenous infusion

When Sabala and Powell (35) reported one of the first remarkable NaOCl accidents in 1989, they mentioned that only 0.5 ml of NaOCl could have been extruded; yet the tissue reaction was out of proportion. The authors attributed the cause of the accident to angioneurotic edema with histamine release, without any further mention of any other physiological mechanisms responsible for the disproportionate event. They further recommended the use of a side-delivery orifice needle to prevent such accidents. These observations may have created a very myopic view of the mechanism causing a devastating NaOCl incident. Zairi and Lambrianidis (61) reported NaOCl extrusion into the maxillary sinus when a side port needle was used and opined that the malfunction was probably caused by "forceful injection." What is forceful injection? A review of the literature indicates that clinicians with a wide variety of clinical experience deliver NaOCl from at rates that vary from 1.2 to 48 ml/min via 30-gauge side-vented needles (62). Zairi and Lambrianidis opined that "needles with a side-delivery orifice and a rounded tip have been manufactured to prevent perforating the apex and allows safe irrigation of the entire length of the root canal. In the present case, such needles were used, and the fact that inadvertent extrusion of sodium hypochlorite occurred verifies the observation made by Bradford *et al.* (63) that no needle design

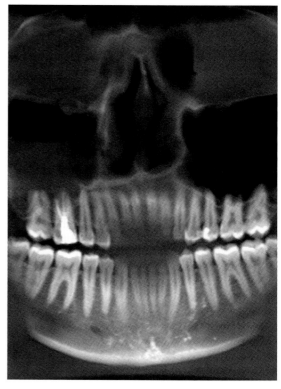

Figure 8.13 Cone beam computed tomography (CBCT) image of the clinical case presented in Figure 8.12 showing one-half of the right maxillary sinus filled with inflammatory tissues. (Courtesy of Dr. Philippe Sleiman, Beirut, Lebanon.)

seems to prevent high pressures delivered beyond the apex."

The paper by Bradford *et al.* (63) quoted that at least one case of human death has occurred because air was injected into a cuspid tooth causing a fatal intravenous air embolism (64). Further literature review has verified three additional cases of death attributed to intravenous air embolism fatalities during dental implants (65). Still further review outside the specific area of endodontic irrigation had suggested and implicated direct intravenous infusion of endodontic paste into the venous system (66–69). After determining the physiological possibility of infusing NaOCl into the venous system, a literature search (70–78) as well as cases reported by Hülsmann and Hahn (79) demonstrate consistent patterns. One example is identified in Figure 8.15a as reported by Witton and Brennan (36), in which the patient's upper right lateral

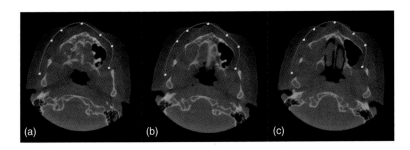

Figure 8.14 (a–c) CBCT sectional views of the posterior wall of the right maxillary sinus with areas of nonexistent osseous structure. (Courtesy of Dr. Philippe Sleiman, Beirut, Lebanon.)

incisor was irrigated with NaOCl. It is important to note that the area immediately above the involved tooth was not bruised, yet the patient's eye lid and the angle of her mouth were clearly affected. What causes this appearance? Figure 8.15b demonstrates bruising of the superficial palpebral (arrow)–angular–facial venous complex. However, a very short distance from this complex, the facial vein runs deep (Figure 8.15c) under the zygomatic muscles, and associated adipose tissue thus bleeding in this area is masked until the vein becomes superficial again at that angle of the mouth where it drains both the superior and inferior labial veins. In some rare situations, the maxillary anterior teeth drain directly into the tributaries of the facial vein (Figure 8.15d) (80). Furthermore, unlike peripheral veins, the intraosseous venous sinusoids do not collapse in response to pressure gradients (65) and they rapidly absorb infused substances, transporting them to the central veins (81). Thus, NaOCl infusion into and through the associated venous sinusoids can occur, depending on the intensity of the irrigation. A rare example demonstrating the full course of the anterior facial vein and its associated tributaries is illustrated in Figure 8.16.

Apical pressures developed by nonbinding irrigation needles at various irrigation delivery rates

A search of the current literature identified two studies that calculated apically directed pressure (26, 82). These two studies were conducted using similar needle placement (3 mm from working length), canal preparation size (size 45, 0.06 taper), canal length (19 mm), and flow rate (15 ml/min). Both studies calculated an apically

directed pressure of ≈75 mm Hg. Later, Jiang et al. (13) examined six different irrigation techniques using a model with slightly different parameters: needle placement (1 mm from working length); canal preparation size (first prepared to size 30, 0.06 taper, followed by preparation to size 40, 0.02 taper); canal length (15 mm); and flow rate (6 ml/min). It should be noted that in their study, Jiang et al. moved the irrigation needle 2 mm closer to the apical termination and slowed the delivery rate by more than half that was reported in the two aforementioned studies (26, 82). Jiang et al. did not report apically directed pressure. Realizing the potential for an intravenous infusion when apically directed pressures exceeding central venous pressure (CVP; ≈6 mm Hg), Khan et al. (11) measured apical pressures developed by nonbinding irrigation needles at various irrigant delivery rates using a polycarbonate model shaped according to the parameters described by Jiang et al. (13). The only difference between the two studies was that the canal length in the Khan study was 17 mm long. The root canal in the Khan study was a closed system, and the apex foramen was attached to a manometer via 1/16 inch internal diameter vinyl tubing. Flow rates varied from 0.5 to 8 ml/min and apical pressure was recorded (Figure 8.17). Except for the VPro™ EndoSafe™ (Vista Dental Products, Racne, WI; claimed by the manufacturer to be a negative pressure, simultaneous irrigation, and evacuation device), device delivery rates at 1 ml/min or less produced apically directed pressures less than the CVP. At 6 ml/min, both the Max-i-Probe® (Dentsply-Rinn, Elgin, IL; a 30-gauge side-venting needle) and the NaviTip (Ultradent Products Inc., South Jordan, WI; a 30-gauge non-beveled, open-ended needle) produced apically directed pressures 1000% greater than the CVP.

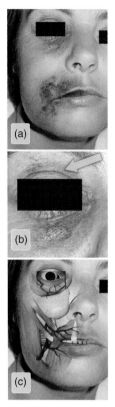
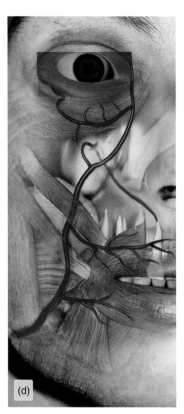

Figure 8.15   (a) This case history exemplifies the pathognomonic appearance of a classical NaOCl accident. Interestingly, the tooth treated was the patient's upper right lateral incisor and the tissue immediately superficial to its apical termination is not ecchymotic; yet the upper and lower eyelids and angle of the mouth clearly demonstrate bruising, with an unaffected area between both. Why? (b) The superior palpebral vein—note the very well-defined ecchymotic appearance of this vein (arrow)—connects to the angular vein near the margin of the eye. Then almost immediately, the angular vein merges with the inferior palbebral venous complex and facial vein where the facial vein proceeds down the midface. (c) Shortly after this confluence, the facial vein is covered by both zygomatic muscles, associated adipose tissue and the malar fat pad, and any hemorrhage in this deep area is masked by these different tissue layers. The facial vein becomes *very* superficial again at the angle of the mouth where it receives the superior and inferior labial veins, thus revealing the ecchymotic appearance at the angle of the mouth and both lips. (d) Normally, the blood from the maxillary teeth drains to the pterygoid plexus; however, sometimes drainage from the anterior teeth may be via tributaries of the anterior facial vein. If the apical foramen is patent and the apically directed irrigation pressure gradient exceeds CVP and the tooth's blood drains to the anterior facial vein, then irrigants can flow along the interconnecting venous complex as demonstrated in this and similar case histories. The ecchymotic appearance would vary depending on the amount and concentration of NaOCl entering the venous complex, as well as the specific location of the venous elements and associated tissues. (Witton and Brennan, Figure 1 (36). Adapted with permission of Macmillan Publishers Ltd.)

Debridement efficacy in inaccessible areas of the root canal system

As previously mentioned, sterilization of the root canal is not one of the tenets of root canal treatment. Countless studies have failed or succeeded in producing sterility results according to the culturing method. Miller and Baumgartner (83) inoculated sterilized roots with *E. faecalis* and debrided the canals with a 30-gauge side-vented needle or the EndoVac system. The authors then pulverized the apical 5 mm of the roots to test for vital bacteria within the tubules or other morphologic irregularities. They found live bacteria in the pulverized powder obtained from roots irrigated by both methods. Likewise, Brito *et al.* (84) and

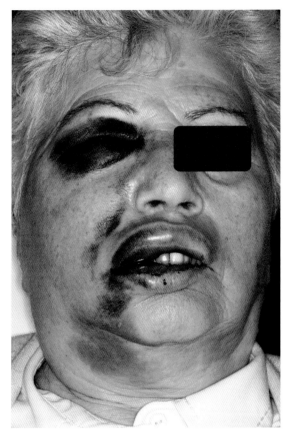

Figure 8.16 Patient experienced NaOCl extrusion through the upper right cuspid. As the anterior facial vein is located closer to the midline than usual and is not covered by the zygomatic muscles, adipose tissue, or malar fat pad, its complex tributaries, including the palpebral veins, the angular vein, tributaries of the superior and inferior labial veins, and the entire length of the anterior facial vein is apparent. Finally, the path of the ecchymosis crosses under the mandible and joins the common facial vein. (Hülsmann (2009), figure 13 (79). Reproduced with permission of John Wiley & Sons, Inc.)

Miranda *et al.* (85) produced positive cultures after final irrigation. Conversely, Hockett *et al.* (45) produced negative cultures using Trope's standard culturing technique (86, 87). Bacteria reduction is also relative; if proper debridement, disinfection, and obturation are inadequate, bacteria can survive a period of starvation and eventually repopulate intracanal voids (88). Accordingly, complete debridement and successful obturation of isthmus between roots and mechanically inaccessible fins

and grooves have recently risen to paramount importance.

Isthmus areas

In 1997, Siqueira *et al.* (89) used five different contemporary instrumentation techniques and determined that isthmus areas were virtually impossible to clean. This finding led to the invention of several different endodontic irrigation techniques after the turn of the 21st century to address the problem of cleaning inaccessible isthmus areas. Figure 8.18a demonstrates the problem previously described by Siqueira *et al.* where the area in between both mesial roots still harbors soft tissues that would interfere with any obturation technique, and when degeneration and liquefaction of those soft tissues would leave space to support a biofilm. A different and recently developed technique (Figure 8.18b) not only effectively cleaned the isthmus area at the apical termination, but also its associated isthmus area and uninstrumented canal. Gutarts *et al.* (90) published the first study that specifically addressed this problem by using continuous flow of irrigants and ultrasonic activation (i.e., active ultrasonic irrigation). This study was succeeded by the study of Klyn *et al.* (91), who tested the "F" file, EndoActivator, passive ultrasonics, and the Max-i-Probe, while Susin *et al.* (92) reported on the EndoVac apical negative pressure system and the manual dynamic agitation technique. All three studies were similar in that they used mandibular mesial roots and examined the last millimeter of the instrumented canal space for the efficacy of isthmus debridement. Unfortunately, endodontic research often lags behind current developments and none of the listed studies properly compared a control technique to the other. In the case of the EndoVac, Susin *et al.* followed the manufacturer's directions exactly, while Klyn *et al.* used an irrigation protocol similarly to the products' directions for use. Their results are summarized in Figure 8.19.

Wall shear stress

According to Gulabivala *et al.* (9), once the chemical effect of NaOCl is depleted, wall shear stress will be

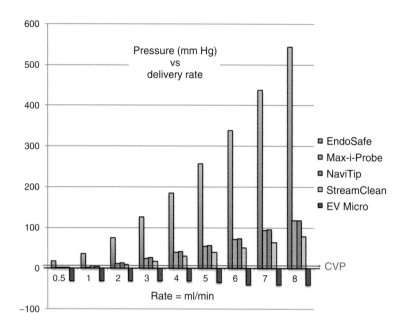

Figure 8.17   With the exception of the VPro™ EndoSafe™, all other tested delivery systems created an apically directed pressure gradient less than center venous pressure (CVP) at a delivery rate of 1 ml/min or less. It is noteworthy that the side-vented Max-i-Probe® produced only slightly less apically directed pressure than the open-ended NaviTip, while the EndoVac always created apical negative pressure.

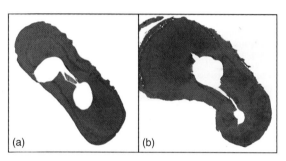

Figure 8.18   Light microscopy images of Masson trichrome-stained, demineralized root sections taken at 1 mm from the apical termination showing canal and isthmus cleanliness after the use of different irrigation techniques. (a) Typical results achieved with the manual dynamic agitation (MDA) irrigation technique showing tissue debris remaining within the canal isthmus. (b) Typical results achieved with the EndoVac apical negative pressure irrigation technique showing completely clean canals and isthmus. Note that although one canal was instrumented, the adjacent uninstrumented canal and the isthmus were completely clear of intracanal debris because of the intracanal fluid dynamics. (Courtesy of Dr. Lisiane Susin, Georgia, USA.)

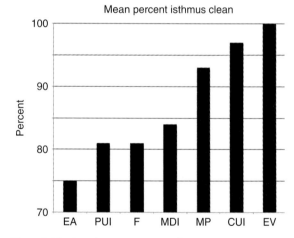

Figure 8.19   Bar chart summarizing the mean percentage isthmus cleanliness values derived from three studies. EA, EndoActivator™ (K); PUI, passive ultrasonic irrigation (K); F, "F" File (K); MDI, manual dynamic irrigation (S), MP, Max-i-Probe® (K); CUI, continuous ultrasonic irrigation (K); and EV, EndoVac (S). Investigators: K, Klyn *et al.* (91); G, Gutarts *et al.* (90); S, Susin *et al.* (92).

solely responsible for the mechanical debridement of the root canal space: "the streaming flow at the end of the instrument can penetrate into the region of spent resident irrigant located at the apical portion of the root canal system, and it is this that is likely to play an important role in debriding the biofilm-infected apical anatomy." Gulabivala *et al.* further stated that "if the instrument is constrained and confined in its oscillation, then it is unlikely that this process would occur." This is in keeping with the conclusion of van der Sluis *et al.* (93): " … acoustic microstreaming depends inversely on the surface area of the file touching the root canal wall." van der Sluis and coworkers have conducted several studies since 2004 using a unique model consisting of a split tooth and washed dentin (STWD). This model consists of a single-rooted tooth that can accurately be reassembled, with one side containing an inaccessible artificial groove extending 4 mm in length, starting from 2 mm coronal of the apical termination and having a width of 0.2 and 0.5 mm in depth. This groove is prefilled with dentin debris previously mixed with 2% NaOCl for 5 min to simulate a situation in which dentin debris is accumulated in uninstrumented canal extensions. The STWD model has tested the cleaning efficacy of sonic device versus ultrasonics (43), syringe versus ultrasonic irrigation (94), instruments of various tapers (95), volume, type of irrigant and flushing methods (96), removal of calcium hydroxide (97), pulsed ultrasound (98), oscillation direction (99), and different final irrigation techniques (13).

The STWD model contains several flaws. First, the investigators incorrectly assumed that after initial instrumentation, the NaOCl dissolves all organic debris in the inaccessible groove leaving only dentin shavings; hence the reason for precleaning the dentin shavings with NaOCl. Recently, Kirkpatrick's group (91, 100), using a closed apical termination model (Figure 8.20a,b), visually affirmed earlier findings by De-Deus *et al.* (28) using an open apical termination model (Figure 8.20c), that in either situation, undissolved pulp tissues remain in the inaccessible uninstrumented areas, and not just in the cleaned and isolated dentin chips. Second, van der Sluis *et al.* (93) has stated and proven with the STWD model (95) that freedom of the instrument's movement is essential to efficient acoustic microstreaming. Yet, no STWD test has been conducted in curved canals for reasons that are addressed shortly. Finally, needle position and the rate of irrigant delivery are important safety concerns as previously determined by Khan *et al.* (11).

Wall shear stress effects of different endodontic irrigation techniques and systems

Recently, the effect of wall shear stress was evaluated in a multicurved canal by Goode *et al.* (101). These authors employed most of the test groups and the inaccessible groove design as reported by

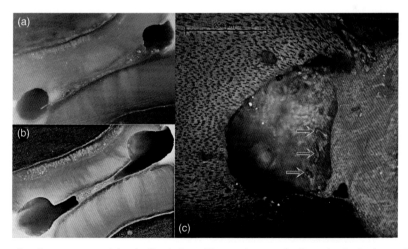

Figure 8.20   Two studies demonstrate partial pulp dissolution without existence of solitary dentin shavings at XS at 5 mm from WL. Left panel: Cleanliness of the canals and isthmus in the mesial roots of mandibular first molars. Irrigation was performed with the root apex sealed. (a) After the use of a guide file and irrigation with saline only. (b) Effect of instrumentation using 0.5 ml of 6% NaOCl in between instrument change. Right panel: (c) High contrast enhancement of Figure 8.6a showing dentin shavings (red arrows) embedded in the pulp tissue along the instrumentation interface. The specimen was subsequently irrigated with an unsealed root apex, using a total of 30 ml of 5.25% NaOCl during instrumentation. (Klyn *et al.* (91). Reproduced with permission of Elsevier.)

Jiang *et al.* (13), with several exceptions. First, a relatively safe flow rate of 1 ml/min was used, based on the results reported by Khan *et al.* (11). Second, in order to simulate a multicurved canal system, a model canal with primary, secondary, and tertiary curvatures of 17°, 24°, and 68°, respectively, and with a groove on one side of the canal was milled into mirrored medical-grade titanium (Figure 8.21). The milled groove replicated the groove in the study by Jiang *et al.* (13) starting at 2 mm from the apical termination, extending 4 mm coronally, and measuring 0.2 mm wide and 0.5 mm deep. Third, as the concept that only dentin shavings exist in uninstrumented areas is incorrect, calcium hydroxide was used because of its clinical relevancy, chemical inertness to NaOCl, and precedence of use in this model (97). Fourth, Goode *et al.* expanded their

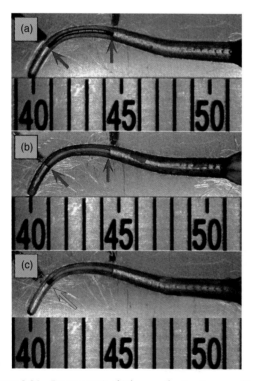

Figure 8.21   Representative high magnification images of the curved simulated canal fin milled in a titanium root canal mode, showing varying extents of calcium hydroxide paste removal. (a) Complete removal showing empty groove between red arrows; (b) completely filled groove between red arrows; (c) partially cleaned groove indicated by green arrow. (Goode *et al.* (101). Reproduced with permission of Elsevier.)

study to include the use of the EndoActivator and the Max-i-Probe. The study by Jiang *et al.* did not use classical passive ultrasonic irrigation (PUI) but employed continuous ultrasonic irrigation (CUI), which as shown by Castelo-Baz *et al.* (102) to be better than PUI in increasing the penetration of irrigating solutions into simulated lateral canals. Fifth, the EndoVac macrocannula was used in the study by Goode *et al.* in conjunction with the EndoVac microcannula, because the former is an integral part of the apical negative pressure irrigation technique. The irrigation needle in each group was placed at 1 mm coronal to the working length during irrigant delivery, except for the EndoVac microcannula, which was inserted to full working length. Each group received exactly 1 ml of irrigant over 1 min; the mechanical activation and EndoActivator groups each received an extra 30 s of activation time. After separating the titanium split blocks, the remaining $Ca(OH)_2$ was digitally evaluated. Figure 8.22 shows the results and statistical analysis. The EndoVac group consistently removed more than 99% of the $Ca(OH)_2$ from the lateral groove within the curved canal model. This was followed by the CUI group, which removed approximately 10% of the $Ca(OH)_2$ from the lateral groove. The results reported by Goode *et al.* demonstrated the immense wall shear stress effects produced by apical negative pressure.

Extracanal fluid dynamics and outcome results

Goode *et al.* (101) reported an unpublished result from the study by Khan *et al.* (11), that the EndoVac macrocannula produced apical directed aspiration (negative) pressure as high as −250 mm Hg. It indicates not only does the safety of the macrocannula, but also its ability to exert aspiration forces on apical and/or intracanal components such as purulent materials or foreign debris.

Apical aspiration

A typical example of this aspiration force is illustrated in Figure 8.23. The patient was suffering from pain on percussion of tooth 29 and the tooth

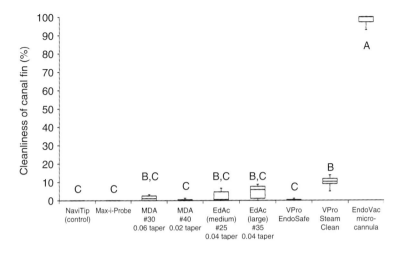

Figure 8.22 Boxplots showing the percentage cleanliness achieved by the nine groups within the curved simulated canal fin shown in Figure 8.21 (*N* = 10). Abbreviations: MDA, manual dynamic agitation; EdAc, EndoActivator™. For each group, the boxplot graphically depicts the sample minimum, lower quartile, median upper quartile, and the sample maximum. Groups labeled with the same upper case letter are not significantly different (*P* > 0.05). (Goode *et al.* (101). Reproduced with permission of Elsevier.)

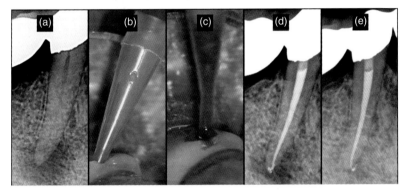

Figure 8.23 Emergency treatment combined with single-visit endodontics. (a) Preoperative radiograph of tooth 29. (b) (c) After patency was established, the EndoVac macrocannula was used to aspirate purulent exudate until the aspirant became hyperemic. (d) The canal was immediately obturated after canal instrumentation and debridement. (e) Apical radiograph taken at 6-month recall showing complete healing of the apical periodontitis. (Courtesy of Dr. Wyatt D. Simons, San Clemente, CA, USA.)

tested nonvital. Diagnosis of tooth 29 was pulp necrosis with acute apical abscess (Figure 8.23a). After gaining access, establishment of a glide path, and instrumentation of the canal space, the EndoVac macrocannula was used according to the manufacturer's instructions. Aspiration of the purulent exudate was noted immediately, being evacuated via the microcannula (Figure 8.23b). The clinician held the macrocannula in the apical most possible position until the purulent aspirant was replaced with a hemorrhagic exudate (Figure 8.23c). The microcannula was subsequently employed by insertion to full working length. The debrided canal space was obturated in a single visit without any incident (Figure 8.23d). Complete

resolution of the apical periodontitis was evident at 6-month recall (Figure 8.23e). Several objectives, supported by recent studies, were achieved in this case. First, it is apparent that the inflammatory mediators were aspirated successfully without resorting to a trephination-type procedure. Second, on the basis of the results reported by Goode *et al.* (101), it is likely that most of the inaccessible areas of the root canal system were successfully cleaned via chemical and wall shear stress debridement. From the recent *in-vitro* study by Hockett *et al.* (45) and the clinical study by Cohenca *et al.* (40), it is probable that the walls of the root canal system were effectively devoid of living or dead biofilms.

Single-visit treatment with apical periodontitis

In 2012, Paredes-Vieyra and Enriquez (103) published a 2-year success rate study of single- versus two-visit root canal treatment of teeth with apical periodontitis using a randomized controlled trial study design. The single-visit group consisted of 146 teeth. The reported successful result based on complete resolution of apical periodontitis was 97%. In contrast, Su *et al.* (104) published a review of similar studies a year earlier. In that study, the criteria for success was less stringent, and was based on relative radiographic size of the original apical radiolucency to the recall density, combined with signs and symptoms. The success outcome in the review by Su *et al.* (104) for single-visit teeth with apical periodontitis was 80%. Paredes-Vieyra and Enriquez (103) reported one tooth that did not heal in the single-visit group, while the prognosis of four additional teeth was uncertain. In the discussion, the authors opined that "mechanical instrumentation facilitates the removal of infected dentin. However, the apical portion of the root canal is especially difficult to clean with root canal instruments because of its complicated anatomy of apical deltas and narrow isthmuses. Disinfection depends on chemicals and effective irrigation. The ability of an irrigant to reach the most apical part of a canal depends on canal anatomy, the size of canal enlargement, the delivery system, and the depth of needle penetration."

Canal obstructions and serendipitous results

Almost 30 years have elapsed before the significance of endodontic biofilms became apparent. Chow (10) defined three simple parameters for successful endodontic debridement: "for the solution to be mechanically effective in removing all the particles, it has to (i) reach the apex; (ii) create a current (force); and (iii) carry the particles away. As demonstrated in isthmus cleaning (91) and other inaccessible areas (101), apical negative pressure can achieve these three objectives extremely effectively. This chapter has discussed myths, pressures, and wall shear force relative to natural intracanal materials such as pulp tissues,

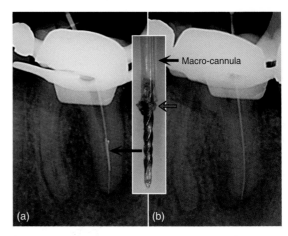

Figure 8.24   Serendipitous removable of separated instrument; retreatment debris is shown with the EndoVac macrocannula removed during retreatment. (a) The instrument (black arrow) is bypassed during retreatment. The macrocannula (inset) is shown capturing the fractured instrument as well as extraneous debris during evacuation (red arrow). (b) Radiograph taken after instrument removal. (Courtesy of Dr. Richard A. Rubinstein, Farmington, MI, USA.)

biofilms, dentin shavings, or intentionally placed intracanal medicaments. It has not discussed the beneficial effect of creating up to $-250\,mm\,Hg$ close to the apical termination for removing accidently embedded materials, such as broken instruments and treatment debris. Figure 8.24a illustrates a case in which a patient was referred for endodontic retreatment, with the canal space containing a separated instrument. The inserted photo shows aspiration of the separated instrument into the EndoVac's macrocannula. The arrows at the interface of the cannula and the separated instrument indicate old sealer that was being evacuated at the moment the instrument was captured. Figure 8.24b demonstrates successful instrument retrieval.

Conclusions

Endodontics has come a long way after Grossman's lunch box incubator. Intracanal fluid dynamics is a critical multifaceted treatment procedure that must be understood clearly. Biofilm has been proven to be the causative agent for apical periodontitis. This is both fortunate because it must have a place to exist, and a problem because many endodontic irrigation systems available today are incapable of completely eradicating organic and inorganic materials from the root canal system. It is important for manufacturers to design and improve their irrigation systems to achieve maximum safety and efficient cleanliness of the root canal system and also validate their results in carefully designed studies based on their directions for use. This will enable the profession to make the best decision regarding patient treatment.

The work of Pelka and Petschelt (39) cautions the profession of its duty to warn patients before using NaOCl. Rochelle (105), an American Board of Trial Advocates attorney, discusses the importance of the dentist's duty to be knowledgeable when making the best treatment decision for his/her patient and used the EndoVac as an example: "...that doctor has the affirmative duty to discuss that product with the patient. Alternatively, has medical science progressed to the degree of specialization that the doctor has the duty to simply select the new, lesser risk device? An example of such a newer medical device recently described in the peer review literature is the EndoVac delivery system for endodontic irrigation. Previously, the device utilized for irrigation in the root canal was a simple syringe to introduce sodium hypochlorite into the root canal for irrigation and debridement, an important and standard part of endodontic treatment. While the occurrence of sodium hypochlorite extrusion is uncommon, under any analysis of product liability law, the EndoVac would be the preferred alternative device. It is superior in that, for a minimal cost, it does not sacrifice treatment efficacy and eliminates the risk of severe debilitating injury that can occur from sodium hypochlorite extrusion from positive pressure."

References

1. Ingle, J.I. (1961) A standardized endodontic technique utilizing newly designed instruments and filling materials. *Oral Surgery, Oral Medicine, and Oral Pathology*, **14**, 83–91.
2. Hunter, W. (1911) The role of sepsis and antisepsis in medicine and the importance of oral sepsis as its chief cause. *Dental Register*, **44**, 579–611.
3. Price, W.A. (1925) Dental infections and related degenerative diseases. Some structural and biochemical factors. *The Journal of the American Medical Association*, **84**, 254–261.
4. Grossman, L.I. (1960) Focal infection: are oral foci of infection related to systemic disease? *Dental Clinics of North America*, **4**, 749–763.
5. Bender, I.B. & Seltzer, S. (1964) To culture or not to culture? *Oral Surgery, Oral Medicine, and Oral Pathology*, **18**, 527–540.
6. Spångberg, L.S.W. (2006) Editorial. *Oral Surgery, Oral Medicine, Oral Pathology, Oral Radiology, and Endodontics*, **102**, 577–578.
7. Byström, A. & Sundqvist, G. (1981) Bacteriologic evaluation of the efficacy of mechanical root canal instrumentation in endodontic therapy. *Scandinavian Journal of Dental Research*, **89**, 321–328.
8. Ricucci, D. & Siqueira, J.F. Jr. (2010) Biofilms and apical periodontitis: study of prevalence and association with clinical and histopathologic findings. *Journal of Endodontics*, **36**, 1277–1288.
9. Gulabivala, K., Ng, Y.L., Gilbertson, M. & Eames, I. (2010) The fluid mechanics of root canal irrigation. *Physiological Measurement*, **31** (**12**), R49–R84.
10. Chow, T.W. (1983) Mechanical effectiveness of root canal irrigation. *Journal of Endodontics*, **9**, 475–479.
11. Khan, S., Niu, L.N., Eid, A.A. *et al.* (2013) Periapical pressures developed by nonbinding irrigation needles at various irrigation delivery rates. *Journal of Endodontics*, **39**, 529–533.
12. Munoz, H.R. & Camacho-Cuadra, K. (2012) In vivo efficacy of three different endodontic irrigation systems for irrigant delivery to working length of mesial canals of mandibular molars. *Journal of Endodontics*, **38**, 445–448.
13. Jiang, L.M., Lak, B., Eijsvogels, L.M., Wesselink, P. & van der Sluis, L.W. (2012) Comparison of the cleaning efficacy of different final irrigation techniques. *Journal of Endodontics*, **38**, 838–841.
14. Luebke, R.C. (1967) Pulp cavity debridement and disinfection. *Dental Clinics of North America*, 603–663.
15. Schilder, H. (1974) Cleaning and shaping the root canal. *Dental Clinics of North America*, **18**, 269–296.
16. Ricucci, D. & Siqueira, J.F. Jr. (2010) Fate of the tissue in lateral canals and apical ramifications in response to pathologic conditions and treatment procedures. *Journal of Endodontics*, **36**, 1–15.
17. Senia, E.S., Marshall, F.J. & Rosen, S. (1971) The solvent action of sodium hypochlorite on pulp tissue of extracted teeth. *Oral Surgery, Oral Medicine, and Oral Pathology*, **31**, 96–103.
18. Salzgeber, R.M. & Brilliant, J.D. (1977) An in vivo evaluation of the penetration of an irrigating solution in root canals. *Journal of Endodontics*, **3**, 394–398.
19. O'Connell, M.S., Morgan, L.A., Beeler, W.J. & Baumgartner, J.C. (2000) A comparative study of smear layer removal using different salts of EDTA. *Journal of Endodontics*, **26**, 739–743.
20. Mader, C.L., Baumgartner, J.C. & Peters, D.D. (1984) Scanning electron microscopic investigation of the smeared layer on root canal walls. *Journal of Endodontics*, **10**, 477–483.

21. Torabinejad, M., Cho, Y., Khademi, A.A., Bakland, L.K. & Shabahang, S. (2003) The effect of various concentrations of sodium hypochlorite on the ability of MTAD to remove the smear layer. *Journal of Endodontics*, **29**, 233–239.

22. Schoeffel, G.J. (2008) The EndoVac method of endodontic irrigation: part 2—efficacy. *Dentistry Today*, **27**, 82, 84, 86, 87.

23. Tay, F.R., Gu, L.S., Schoeffel, G.J. *et al.* (2010) Effect of vapor lock on root canal debridement by using a side-vented needle for positive-pressure irrigant delivery. *Journal of Endodontics*, **36**, 745–750.

24. Vera, J., Arias, A. & Romero, M. (2012) Dynamic movement of intracanal gas bubbles during cleaning and shaping procedures: the effect of maintaining apical patency on their presence in the middle and cervical thirds of human root canals-an in vivo study. *Journal of Endodontics*, **38**, 200–203.

25. Zehnder, M. (2006) Root canal irrigants. *Journal of Endodontics*, **32**, 389–398.

26. Boutsioukis, C., Verhaagen, B., Versluis, M., Kastrinakis, E., Wesselink, P.R. & van der Sluis, P.R. (2010) Evaluation of irrigant flow in the root canal using different needle types by an unsteady computational fluid dynamics model. *Journal of Endodontics*, **36**, 875–897.

27. Vera, J., Hernández, E.M., Romero, M., Arias, A. & van der Sluis, L.W. (2012) Effect of maintaining apical patency on irrigant penetration into the apical two millimeters of large root canals: an in vivo study. *Journal of Endodontics*, **38**, 1340–1343.

28. De-Deus, G., Reis, C., Beznos, D., de Abranches, A.M., Coutinho-Filho, T. & Paciornik, S. (2008) Limited ability of three commonly used thermoplasticized gutta-percha techniques in filling oval-shaped canals. *Journal of Endodontics*, **34**, 1401–1405.

29. Shen, Y., Gao, Y., Qian, W. *et al.* (2010) Three-dimensional numeric simulation of root canal irrigant flow with different irrigation needles. *Journal of Endodontics*, **36**, 884–889.

30. Peters, L.B., Wesselink, P.R. & Moorer, W.R. (1995) The fate and the role of bacteria left in root dentinal tubules. *International Endodontic Journal*, **28**, 95–99.

31. Hand, R.E., Smith, M.L. & Harrison, J.W. (1978) Analysis of the effect of dilution on the necrotic tissue dissolution property of sodium hypochlorite. *Journal of Endodontics*, **4**, 60–64.

32. Clegg, M.S., Vertucci, F.J., Walker, C., Belanger, M. & Britto, L.R. (2006) The effect of exposure to irrigant solutions on apical dentin biofilms in vitro. *Journal of Endodontics*, **32**, 434–437.

33. Siqueira, J.F. Jr., Paiva, S.S. & Rôças, I.N. (2007) Reduction in the cultivable bacterial populations in infected root canals by a chlorhexidine-based antimicrobial protocol. *Journal of Endodontics*, **33**, 541–547.

34. Ercan, E., Ozekinci, T., Atakul, F. & Gül, K. (2004) Antibacterial activity of 2% chlorhexidine gluconate and 5.25% sodium hypochlorite in infected root canal: in vivo study. *Journal of Endodontics*, **30**, 84–87.

35. Sabala, C.L. & Powell, S.E. (1989) Sodium hypochlorite injection into periapical tissues. *Journal of Endodontics*, **15**, 490–492.

36. Witton, R. & Brennan, P.A. (2005) Severe tissue damage and neurological deficit following extravasation of sodium hypochlorite solution during routine endodontic treatment. *British Dental Journal*, **198**, 749–750.

37. Markose, G., Cotter, C.J. & Hislop, W.S. (2009) Facial atrophy following accidental subcutaneous extrusion of sodium hypochlorite. *British Dental Journal*, **206**, 263–264.

38. Bowden, J., Ethunandan, M. & Brennan, P. (2006) Life-threatening airway obstruction secondary to hypochlorite extrusion during root canal treatment. *Oral Surgery, Oral Medicine, Oral Pathology, Oral Radiology, and Endodontics*, **101**, 402–404.

39. Pelka, M. & Petschelt, A. (2008) Permanent mimic musculature and nerve damage caused by sodium hypochlorite: a case report. *Oral Surgery, Oral Medicine, Oral Pathology, Oral Radiology, and Endodontics*, **106**, e80–e83.

40. Cohenca, N., Paranjpe, A., Heilborn, C. & Johnson, J.D. (2013) Antimicrobial efficacy of two irrigation techniques in tapered and non-tapered canal preparations. A randomized controlled clinical trial. *Quintessence International*, **44**, 217–228.

41. Paiva, S.S., Siqueira, J.F. Jr., Rôças, I.N. *et al.* (2013) Molecular microbiological evaluation of passive ultrasonic activation as a supplementary disinfecting step: a clinical study. *Journal of Endodontics*, **39**, 190–194.

42. Pawar, R., Alqaied, A., Safavi, K., Boyko, J. & Kaufman, B. (2012) Influence of an apical negative pressure irrigation system on bacterial elimination during endodontic therapy: a prospective randomized clinical Study. *Journal of Endodontics*, **38**, 1177–1181.

43. Jiang, L.M., Verhaagen, B., Versluis, M. & van der Sluis, L.W. (2010) Evaluation of a sonic device designed to activate irrigant in the root canal. *Journal of Endodontics*, **36**, 143–146.

44. Desai, P. & Himel, V. (2009) Comparative safety of various intracanal irrigation systems. *Journal of Endodontics*, **35**, 545–549.

45. Hockett, J.L., Dommisch, J.K., Johnson, J.D. & Cohenca, N. (2008) Antimicrobial efficacy of two irrigation techniques in tapered and nontapered canal preparations: an in vitro study. *Journal of Endodontics*, **34**, 1374–1377.

46. Saldivar, F.P. (2010) Limpieza De Tercio Apical Por Medio De Presion Apical Negativa En Combinacion Con Ultrasoundio: Estudio in Vitro, Autor: Felix Palomares Saldivar. Tesis Presentada Para Obtener El Grado de: Mastero En Endodoncia, Co-Director De Tesis: Ana Maria Gonzalez Amaro, Co-Director De Tesis, Nestor Cohence, Universidad Autonoma De San Luis Potosi, Junio.

47. Abou-Rass, M. & Oglesby, S.W. (1981) The effects of temperature, concentration, and tissue type on the solvent ability of sodium hypochlorite. *Journal of Endodontics*, **7**, 376–377.

48. Castellucci, A. (2005) *Endodontics*. Vol. **II**. II Tridente. ISBN:88-89411-02-3.

49. Berutti, E. & Marini, R. (1996) A scanning electron microscopic evaluation of the debridement capability of sodium hypochlorite at different temperatures. *Journal of Endodontics*, **22**, 467–470.

50. Townsend, C. & Maki, J. (2009) An in vitro comparison of new irrigation and agitation techniques to ultrasonic agitation in removing bacteria from a simulated root canal. *Journal of Endodontics*, **35**, 1040–1043.

51. Torabinejad, M. (2011) *Endodontics: Colleagues for Excellence, Root Canal Irrigants and Disinfectants*. Winter Issue, p. 6.

52. Schoeffel GJ. Method and apparatus for evacuation of root canal. United States Patent Office 6,997,714, Feb 14, 2006.

53. Brunson, M., Heilborn, C., Johnson, D.J. & Cohenca, N. (2010) Effect of apical preparation size and preparation taper on irrigant volume delivered by using negative pressure irrigation system. *Journal of Endodontics*, **36**, 721–724.

54. Heilborn, C., Reynolds, K., Johnson, J.D. & Cohenca, N. (2010) Cleaning efficacy of an apical negative-pressure irrigation system at different exposure times. *Quintessence International*, **41**, 759–767.

55. Mehdipour, O., Kleier, D.J. & Averbach, R.E. (2007) Anatomy of sodium hypochlorite accidents. *Compendium of Continuing Education in Dentistry*, **28**, 544–546.

56. Gursoy, U.K., Bostanci, V. & Kosger, H.H. (2006) Palatal mucosa necrosis because of accidental sodium hypochlorite injection instead of anaesthetic solution. *International Endodontic Journal*, **39**, 157–161.

57. Ehrich, D.G., Brian, J.D. Jr. & Walker, W.A. (1993) Sodium hypochlorite accident: inadvertent injection into the maxillary sinus. *Journal of Endodontics*, **19**, 180–182.

58. Kavanagh, C.P. & Taylor, J. (1998) Inadvertent injection of sodium hypochlorite into the maxillary sinus. *British Dental Journal*, **185**, 336–337.

59. Hauman, C.H., Chandler, N.P. & Tong, D.C. (2002) Endodontic implications of the maxillary sinus: a review. *International Endodontic Journal*, **35**, 127–141.

60. Sleiman P. (2013) Irrigation for the root canal and nothing but the root canal. Dental Tribune Jan 30, 2013. http://www.dental-tribune.com/articles/specialities/endodontics/11609_irrigation_for_the_root_canal_and_nothing_but_the_root_canal.html.

61. Zairi, A. & Lambrianidis, T. (2008) Accidental extrusion of sodium hypochlorite into the maxillary sinus. *Quintessence International*, **39**, 745–748.

62. Boutsioukis, C., Lambrianidis, T., Kastrinakis, E. & Bekiaroglou, P. (2007) Measurement of pressure and flow rates during irrigation of a root canal ex vivo with three endodontic needles. *International Endodontic Journal*, **40**, 504–513.

63. Bradford, C.E., Eleazer, P.D., Downs, K.E. & Scheetz, J.P. (2002) Apical pressures developed by needles for canal irrigation. *Journal of Endodontics*, **28**, 333–335.

64. Rickles, N.H. & Joshi, B.A. (1963) A possible case in a human and an investigation in dogs of death from air embolism during root canal therapy. *Journal of the American Dental Association*, **67**, 397–404.

65. Davies, J.M. & Campbell, L.A. (1990) Fatal air embolism during dental implant surgery: a report of three cases. *Canadian Journal of Anaesthesia*, **37**, 112–121.

66. Ahonen, M. & Tjäderhane, L. (2011) Endodontic-related paresthesia: a case report and literature review. *Journal of Endodontics*, **37**, 1460–1464.

67. Poveda, R., Bagán, J.V., Fernández, J.M. & Sanchis, J.M. (2006) Mental nerve paresthesia associated with endodontic paste within the mandibular canal: report of a case. *Oral Surgery, Oral Medicine, Oral Pathology, Oral Radiology, and Endodontics*, **102**, e46–e49.

68. Alantar, A., Tarragano, H. & Lefèvre, B. (1994) Extrusion of endodontic filling material into the insertions of the mylohyoid muscle. A case report. *Oral Surgery, Oral Medicine, and Oral Pathology*, **78**, 646–649.

69. Manisali, Y., Yücel, T. & Erişen, R. (1989) Overfilling of the root. A case report. *Oral Surgery, Oral Medicine, and Oral Pathology*, **68**, 773–775.

70. Mehra, P., Clancy, C. & Wu, J. (2000) Formation of a facial hematoma during endodontic therapy. *Journal of the American Dental Association*, **131**, 67–71.

71. Bosch-Aranda, M.L., Vázquez-Delgado, E. & Gay-Escoda, C. (2011) Atypical odontalgia: a systematic review following the evidence-based principles of dentistry. *Cranio*, **29**, 219–226.

72. de Sermeño, R.F., da Silva, L.A., Herrera, H., Herrera, H., Silva, R.A. & Leonardo, M.R. (2009) Tissue damage after sodium hypochlorite extrusion during root canal treatment. *Oral Surgery, Oral Medicine, Oral Pathology, Oral Radiology, and Endodontics*, **108**, e46–e49.

73. Gernhardt, C.R., Eppendorf, K., Kozlowski, A. & Brandt, M. (2004) Toxicity of concentrated sodium hypochlorite used as an endodontic irrigant. *International Endodontic Journal*, **37**, 272–280.

74. Spencer, H.R., Ike, V. & Brennan, P.A. (2007) Review: the use of sodium hypochlorite in endodontics – potential complications and their management. *British Dental Journal*, **202**, 555–559.

75. van Hooft, E. & van Es, R.J. (2008) Injury following sodium hypochlorite irrigation during endodontic treatment. *Nederlands Tijdschrift voor Tandheelkunde*, **115**, 157–160. (Article in Dutch)..

76. Joffe, E. (1991) Complication during root canal therapy following accidental extrusion of sodium hypochlorite through the apical foramen. *General Dentistry*, **39**, 460–461.

77. Paschoalino Mde, A., Hanan, A.A., Marques, A.A., Garcia Lda, F., Garrido, A.B. & Sponchiado, E.C. Jr. (2012) Injection of sodium hypochlorite beyond the apical foramen—a case report. *General Dentistry*, **60**, 16–19.

78. Oreadi, D., Hendi, J. & Papageorge, M.B. (2010) A clinico-pathologic correlation. *Journal of the Massachusetts Dental Society*, **59**, 44–46.

79. Hülsmann (2009). *Endodontic Topics*, **16**, 27–63.

80. Drake, R.L., Vogl, A.W. & Mitchell, A.W.M. (eds) (2012) *Gray's Basic Anatomy*. Elsevier, Churchill Livingstone, Philadelphia PA.

81. Drinker, C.K., Drinker, K.R. & Lund, C.C. (1922) The circulation in the mammalian bone marrow. *American Journal of Physiology*, **62**, 1–92.

82. Boutsioukis, C., Gogos, C., Verhaagen, B., Versluis, M., Kastrinakis, E. & van der Sluis, L.W. (2010) The effect of apical preparation size on irrigant flow in root canals evaluated using an unsteady computational fluid dynamics model. *International Endodontic Journal*, **43**, 874–881.

83. Miller, T.A. & Baumgartner, J.C. (2010) Comparison of the antimicrobial efficacy of irrigation using the EndoVac to endodontic needle delivery. *Journal of Endodontics*, **36**, 509–511.

84. Brito, P.R., Souza, L.C., de Oliveira, J.C.M. *et al.* (2009) Comparison of the effectiveness of three irrigation techniques in reducing intracanal Enterococcus faecalis populations: an in vitro study. *Journal of Endodontics*, **35**, 1422–1427.

85. Miranda, R.G., Santos, E.B., Souto, R.M., Gusman, H. & Colombo, A.P. (2013) Ex vivo antimicrobial efficacy of the EndoVac system plus photodynamic therapy associated with calcium hydroxide against intracanal Enterococcus faecalis. *International Endodontic Journal*, **46**, 499–505.

86. McGurkin-Smith, R., Trope, M., Caplan, D. & Sigurdsson, A. (2005) Reduction of intracanal bacteria using GT rotary instrumentation, 5.25% NaOCl, EDTA, and Ca(OH)$_2$. *Journal of Endodontics*, **31**, 359–363.

87. Card, S.J., Sigurdsson, A., Orstavik, D. & Trope, M. (2002 Nov) The effectiveness of increased apical enlargement in reducing intracanal bacteria. *Journal of Endodontics*, **28** (**11**), 779–783.

88. Chávez de Paz, L.E., Hamilton, I.R. & Svensäter, G. (2008) Oral bacteria in biofilms exhibit slow reactivation from nutrient deprivation. *Microbiology*, **154** (**Pt 7**), 1927–1938.

89. Siqueira, J.F. Jr., Araújo, M.C., Garcia, P.F., Fraga, R.C. & Dantas, C.J. (1997) Histological evaluation of the effectiveness of five instrumentation techniques for cleaning the apical third of root canals. *Journal of Endodontics*, **23**, 499–502.

90. Gutarts, R., Nusstein, J., Reader, A. & Beck, M. (2005) In vivo debridement efficacy of ultrasonic irrigation following hand-rotary instrumentation in human mandibular molars. *Journal of Endodontics*, **31**, 166–170.

91. Klyn, S.L., Kirkpatrick, T.C. & Rutledge, R.E. (2010) In vitro comparisons of debris removal of the EndoActivator system, the F file, ultrasonic irrigation, and NaOCl irrigation alone after hand-rotary instrumentation in human mandibular molars. *Journal of Endodontics*, **36**, 1367–1371.

92. Susin, L., Liu, Y., Yoon, J.C. *et al.* (2010) Canal and isthmus debridement efficacies of two irrigant agitation techniques in a closed system. *International Endodontic Journal*, **43**, 1077–1090.

93. van der Sluis, L.W., Versluis, M., Wu, M.K. & Wesselink, P.R. (2007) Passive ultrasonic irrigation of the root canal: a review of the literature. *International Endodontic Journal*, **40**, 415–426.

94. Lee, S.J., Wu, M.K. & Wesselink, P.R. (2004) The effectiveness of syringe irrigation and ultrasonics to remove debris from simulated irregularities within prepared root canal walls. *International Endodontic Journal*, **37**, 672–678.

95. van der Sluis, L.W., Wu, M.K. & Wesselink, P.R. (2005) The efficacy of ultrasonic irrigation to remove artificially placed dentine debris from human root canals prepared using instruments of varying taper. *International Endodontic Journal*, **38**, 764–768.

96. van der Sluis, L.W., Gambarini, G., Wu, M.K. & Wesselink, P.R. (2006) The influence of volume, type of irrigant and flushing method on removing artificially placed dentine debris from the apical root

canal during passive ultrasonic irrigation. *International Endodontic Journal*, **39**, 472–476.

97. van der Sluis, L.W., Wu, M.K. & Wesselink, P.R. (2007) The evaluation of removal of calcium hydroxide paste from an artificial standardized groove in the apical root canal using different irrigation methodologies. *International Endodontic Journal*, **40**, 52–57.

98. Jiang, L.M., Verhaagen, B., Versluis, M., Zangrillo, C., Cuckovic, D. & van der Sluis, L.W. (2010) An evaluation of the effect of pulsed ultrasound on the cleaning efficacy of passive ultrasonic irrigation. *Journal of Endodontics*, **36**, 1887–1891.

99. Jiang, L.M., Verhaagen, B., Versluis, M. & van der Sluis, L.W. (2010) Influence of the oscillation direction of an ultrasonic file on the cleaning efficacy of passive ultrasonic irrigation. *Journal of Endodontics*, **36**, 1372–1376.

100. Dietrich, M.A., Kirkpatrick, T.C. & Yaccino, J.M. (2012) In vitro canal and isthmus debris removal of the self-adjusting file, K3, and WaveOne files in the mesial root of human mandibular molars. *Journal of Endodontics*, **38**, 1140–1144.

101. Goode, N., Khan, S., Eid, A.A. *et al.* (2013) Wall shear stress effects of different endodontic irrigation techniques and systems. *Journal of Dentistry*, **41**, 636–641.

102. Castelo-Baz, P., Martín-Biedma, B., Cantatore, G. *et al.* (2012) In vitro comparison of passive and continuous ultrasonic irrigation in simulated lateral canals of extracted teeth. *Journal of Endodontics*, **38**, 688–691.

103. Paredes-Vieyra, J. & Enriquez, F.J. (2012) Success rate of single- versus two-visit root canal treatment of teeth with apical periodontitis: a randomized controlled trial. *Journal of Endodontics*, **38**, 1164–1169.

104. Su, Y., Wang, C. & Ye, L. (2011) Healing rate and post-obturation pain of single- versus multiple-visit endodontic treatment for infected root canals: a systematic review. *Journal of Endodontics*, **37**, 125–132.

105. http://rochellegriffith.com/2009/11/02/has-the-doctors-duty-to-warn-been-replaced-by-the-need-to-simply-make-the-best-decision-for-the-patient-endovac-use-in-root-canals/.

9

Positive Pressure Irrigation

Cesar de Gregorio
Department of Endodontics, University of Washington, Seattle, WA, USA

Carlos Heilborn
Private Practice, Asunción, Paraguay

Nestor Cohenca
Department of Endodontics and Pediatric Dentistry, University of Washington, Seattle, WA, USA

Introduction

The foundation of endodontic therapy is the debridement and disinfection of the root canal system. These procedures would allow the clinician to achieve the ultimate endodontic goal: to preserve the health of apical tissues or to eliminate the apical inflammatory disease when it has already established as a consequence of bacterial colonization of the root canal system (1).

Our relentless pursuit to eliminate all irritants within a root canal system remains a committed objective. Unfortunately, our ultimate goal to completely disinfect every root canal system has not yet been practical. Predictable elimination of microorganisms remains our main challenge and

has not changed significantly since 1965 (2). The terminology of disinfection as opposed to sterilization is appropriate as a result of the shortcoming in our objective. Although *"cleaning and shaping"* are done concurrently, disinfection actually begins after the desired shape has been accomplished (3). Traditional endodontic techniques are based on the theory that files shape and irrigants clean (4). Said differently, there is greater potential to completely disinfect the root canal system after it has been cleaned and shaped. This statement highlights the knowledge that there are uninstrumentable areas of pulpal anatomy. Studies confirm that better microbial removal and more effective irrigation occur when canals are instrumented to larger apical sizes (5–7). However, even after cleaning and shaping,

Disinfection of Root Canal Systems: The Treatment of Apical Periodontitis, First Edition. Edited by Nestor Cohenca.
© 2014 John Wiley & Sons, Inc. Published 2014 by John Wiley & Sons, Inc.

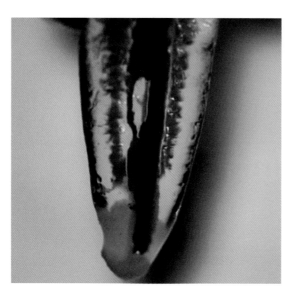

Figure 9.1 Irrigation of a complex anatomy. Presence of an accessory canal in middle third. Irrigation was performed in a cleared tooth using apical negative pressure.

microorganisms found in biofilm structures remain in the root canal system and dentinal tubules.

The efficacy of intracanal irrigation has been evaluated and reported extensively in the endodontic literature (8–13). Sodium hypochlorite (NaOCl) is considered to be the most effective irrigant solution because of its antimicrobial and tissue dissolution properties (10, 13–15). However, sodium hypochlorite must be in direct contact with the tissue to be disinfected in order to oxidize, hydrolyze, and to some extent osmotically draw fluids out of the tissues (16). This means enabling the sodium hypochlorite to contact the dentinal tubules throughout the complex root canal anatomy at working length (WL), as well as the anatomic variations like lateral canals and isthmuses (Figure 9.1).

From the early days of endodontics, the objective of achieving an aseptic root canal was pursued using disinfectants applied to the coronal portion of the canals. However, the persistence of apical pathoses demonstrated that the entire length of the root canal system required exposure and contact with the chemical irrigant in order to provide for adequate disinfection. The first delivery system into the root canal was a needle connected to a syringe, currently termed *positive pressure (PP) irrigation*. The basic concept and clinical aim is to

deliver the irrigant solution into the entire root canal, while generating a hydrodynamic flow to facilitate the removal of debris through the canal orifii. The latter is essentially aimed at avoiding accumulation and packing of debris produced during the instrumentation, particularly at the apical third, causing mechanical blockage and facilitating the growth of microorganisms and biofilm formation.

PP irrigation uses a syringe and a needle. The technique involves inserting the needle into the canal followed by the deposition of the irrigant solution. It is the most traditional technique and still considered the "gold standard" for endodontic irrigation (17–19), despite the questionable results reported in the current literature (15, 20–22).

Better understanding of fluid dynamics is required in order to understand the chemophysical properties directly correlated to the flow of irrigants in a closed-end canal system. By learning the physical limitations of fluid dynamics, we will realize that the delivery system is perhaps equal or even more important than the irrigant solution itself. This statement is supported by a number of *in-vitro* studies analyzing the efficacy of irrigants on dentin disks in which the solutions easily contacted the surface to be treated (23–25). Sodium hypochlorite has extraordinary qualities for disinfection and organic tissue dissolution. In combination with chelating substances such as ethylenediaminetetraacetic acid (EDTA), the disinfection should become more predictable, at least from a direct microbiological standpoint. Unfortunately, the clinical situation is very different and complex because of physical, chemical, and anatomical constraints. Therefore, it is unreasonable to extrapolate the results of *in-vitro* studies, when they do not replicate the clinical situation. Recently, the importance of using a closed-canal system was demonstrated by Parente *et al.* (26). We must realize and accept the fact that we are facing a challenging clinical situation ruled by physical principles. This challenge is further complicated by the chemical principles and limitations of irrigation solutions. The surface tension and viscosity of the irrigant produce a phenomenon known as *dead zone* or *stagnation zone* at the apical level in which the irrigant penetration is limited, making the renewal of the solutions virtually nonexistent.

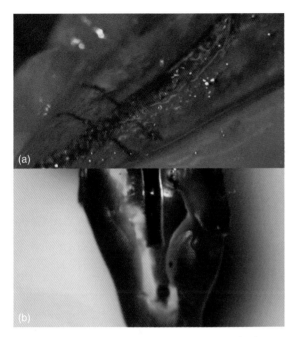

Figure 9.2   Penetration of sodium hypochlorite and a dye marker in a cleared tooth model where artificial lateral canals were created. Image (a) shows an open system with penetration into lateral canals and up to working length while image (b) shows a closed system with limited penetration at the tip of the needle.

The irrigant exchange achieved at the apical third when using PP irrigation is critical for the disinfection and removal of debris (11, 27, 28). Understanding fluid dynamics within a closed-canal system surrounded by apical tissues is extremely important when evaluating the goals of irrigation (Figure 9.2).

Positive pressure: the technique

PP irrigation basically consists of syringes and needles inserted into the canal while pressure is applied to distribute the irrigant solution to the entire canal system. The only difference between this procedure and injection is that during root canal irrigation, the solution should enter and exit via the same orifii. This technique is quite a different clinical reality than inserting an injection where the objective is the insertion of liquid into the body with a syringe.

The syringe comprises a piston and a cylinder and is connected to a needle on one end using Luer lock connection that twists onto the needle hub for secure attachment and a leak-free connection. The alternative is to use a simple friction connection that may leak following elevated pressure generated by the piston, resulting in the leakage of the irrigants over the patient and operator.

Taking into consideration that the needle is the most influential component in this delivery system, few studies have analyzed the dimensions and correlation with ISO standards. Although instruments used in endodontics had been the subject of several studies for decades (18–20), this correlation was not analyzed until recently when Boutsioukis *et al.* (29) concluded that units of the widely used "gauge" system cannot be directly extrapolated to clinical practice. Thus, knowledge of the tip's external diameter is crucial for the selection of the appropriate size irrigation probe during endodontic treatment.

The level of penetration of the needle is critical to the efficacy of PP irrigation. Wedging of the needle into the canal space should always be avoided in order to prevent accidental extrusion of the irrigants into the apical tissues (22, 23). A clinical dilemma is determining the apical preparation size required to match the needle's gauge allowing deeper and safer penetration.

Stainless steel needles ranging from 21 to 30 G were analyzed and found in compliance with that of ISO 9626:1991 and 9626:1991/Amd 1:2001 specifications (29). However, the only NiTi needle analyzed, the Stropko Flexi-Tip (Vista Dental Products, Racine, WI, USA), exceeded the external diameter limits. The researchers observed deficiencies on the internal surface in all needles, regardless of the material or the manufacturer. This factor could directly affect the irrigant flow. The main concern raised by the study was the discrepancy between the needles' gauge and the ISO standardized sizes in any specific point, probably because of the great variability of the particular designs. The variability identifies a lack of standardization in the manufacturing process. We must consider that the displayed gauge could be variable at different levels within the needle but not specifically in its most apical section.

Factors affecting efficacy of positive pressure irrigation

Closed systems: the physical challenge

In endodontics, a closed system means that the portal of exit of the root canal system, including lateral canals, apical foramen, and accessory foramina, is surrounded by vital apical tissues, creating a permeable but closed system. The clinical implication is that the irrigant solution must be delivered through the canal orifice, flow and exit back via the same orifice. The only way to overcome that "virtual barrier" would be to elevate the flux ratio and consequently the intracanal pressure (30). This will result in the extrusion of toxic irrigants to the apical tissues eliciting an inflammatory response with necrosis of the affected area and edema (31).

There are case reports in which the dissolution power of NaOCl produced severe effects on the medullar bone tissue (24), as well as permanent sequelae such as asymmetries and paresthesia (25). A recent publication (32) reports a clinical case in which a "sodium hypochlorite accident" was evaluated using 3D imaging (CBCT, cone beam computed tomography) to assess the degree of injury and possible anatomical reasons for the extrusion. This case illustrates once again that the risk of extrusion is real, even in cases in which low pressure is applied during PP irrigation. In this particular clinical case, the apex was fenestrated and not covered by buccal cortical bone. This anatomical variation demonstrates that the integrity of apical bone structures plays a decisive role on the containment of endodontic irrigants. Bone resorption is always expected, to a certain degree, in apical periodontitis and should be a concern for the clinician. This finding was highlighted by Salzgeber in 1977 (33), who demonstrated that the probability of irrigant extrusion was higher in cases with necrotic pulp and apical periodontitis. The loss of integrity of apical tissues and the fact that necrotic pulp tissue is less intact than a vital pulp, or even nonexistent in some cases, facilitates a free flow of irrigants to the apical end of the root canal. Recent studies by Vera *et al.* (34–36) using a similar methodology analyzed the dynamics of irrigants using the needle of smaller gauge. Their

result concluded that irrigant penetration is very limited during root canal treatment and it is also conditioned by the formation of gas bubbles that get trapped at the apical or even middle third. This gas bubbles, produced primarily by ammonia and carbon dioxide liberation during pulp tissue dissolution, are termed *vapor lock*.

Patency

In a series of studies, Vera *et al.* (34–36) analyzed the effect of patency files on NaOCl penetration using a radiopaque contrast media. The studies concluded that maintaining apical patency did not have a significant effect on irrigant penetration at the apical third, even when canals were prepared to a size 30/09. Passive ultrasonic irrigation (PUI) had a positive result with more irrigant flow at the apical third. This data is in accordance with the results obtained with cleared teeth (37), where PUI demonstrated significant better results than PP on irrigant penetration to WL. Figure 9.3 shows penetration of NaOCl mixed with a dye marker using PP followed by activation with PUI in cleared teeth (Figure 9.3). Conversely, there are studies demonstrating satisfactory action in teeth with very similar preparations (12). This could be the result of different methodologies.

The maintenance of patency in teeth with apical diameters greater than 30 was analyzed by Vera

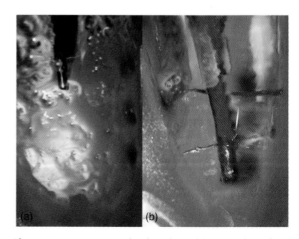

Figure 9.3 Penetration of sodium hypochlorite in cleared teeth: irrigant delivered using positive pressure (a) and activation of the solution with PUI (b).

et al. (34), and the results demonstrated that patency maintenance with an #10 ISO file improved apical penetration of irrigants but only with great apical preparations. Thus, further apical enlargement could play an effective role in irrigant penetration, but this comes at the expense of apical transportation in 56% of the cases, according to the results of Goldberg *et al.* (38).

Apical diameter and taper of preparation

In a classic histological study, Senia (39) demonstrated the limited efficacy of sodium hypochlorite on the dissolution of organic matter at the apical third and isthmus areas of mandibular molars. This study confirmed that the size of apical preparation is determinant and directly related with irrigant penetration, getting more irrigant penetration in large apical preparations. The main strength of this study is that despite not being a current study, the author performed the investigation using a complete closed system design in an attempt to reproduce the flow dynamics of the clinical environment.

Vera *et al.* (34) observed that when apical preparation reached 40/06, the use of small diameter (#10 ISO) allowed for a significant improvement in irrigant penetration to WL. The #10 hand file did not show any effect in smaller apical diameters.

Increasing apical size allows better apical penetration of the irrigant and a greater renewal rate. Chow (11) described the difficulties for PP to exert a flushing action beyond the tip of the needle and the lack of action at the apical third. In this study, using glass tubes and a gel simulating pulpal and dentinal debris produced during canal preparation, a clear correlation was observed between the insertion depth of the needle and the flushing action of the irrigant.

Healing of apical lesions has also been demonstrated to be significantly better when apical preparation was enlarged to 3 ISO sizes over anatomical apical diameter, determined by the first file to bind at length (40). Although the research was not aimed at analyzing possible correlation between apical size, irrigation, and healing, we can assume that removing more contaminated dentin and allowing better apical irrigation contributed to the positive outcome.

Taper also plays an important role when irrigating with PP (41), but not for apical negative pressure (ANP) (discussed later in this chapter), which depends more on the ability to place the micro cannula at WL (42).

The influence of patency on gas and air bubbles is discussed in the following section.

"Vapor lock" phenomenon

The physical phenomenon of vapor lock is caused by gas entrapment, especially at the apical third of the root canal, impairing the access of irrigants to the whole extent of the root canal system. It is caused by one of the principal properties of sodium hypochlorite, the dissolution capacity of the organic component. This process leads to the formation of carbon dioxide and ammonia in the root canals, producing small bubbles that prevent the penetration and renewal of irrigants at the most apical levels.

Currently there are many studies analyzing this phenomenon. The first group to study this physic-chemical challenge was Tay *et al.* (43). Using a closed system, they analyzed the penetration of the irrigation solution (combined with cesium chloride (CsCl) as contrast) using scanning electron microscopy (SEM). The study highlighted the limitation of PP irrigation to remove debris from the apical third, even when the irrigant was delivered at 1 mm from WL. The only delivery system that was not affected by the vapor lock was ANP (Figure 9.4) (26). Figure 9.5 shows the vapor lock phenomenon (see arrow) affecting the PP irrigation (Figure 9.5).

Recently, another study analyzed the presence of vapor lock in correlation with the apical diameter and needle design (44). The results were in agreement with other studies reporting the presence of apical gas entrapment in 48% of the cases while using PP irrigation. Increasing the apical size, using an open-ended needle, positioning the needle closer to WL, and delivering the irrigant at higher flow rate appeared to result in smaller vapor lock *in-vitro*. When this recommendation is extrapolated to the patients, increasing the flow rate at 1 mm from WL will elevate the apical pressure and expose the patients to irrigant extrusion, severe irritation of apical tissues, and consequently

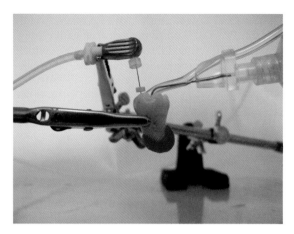

Figure 9.4 Apical negative pressure irrigation using microcannula of EndoVac at working length while the irrigant is delivered in the pulp chamber with the Master Delivery Tip.

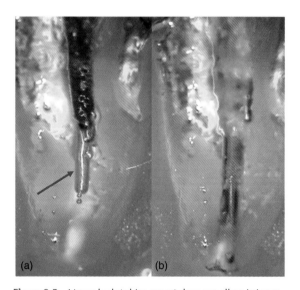

(a)   (b)

Figure 9.5 Vapor lock (white arrow) does not allow irrigant penetration up to working length when positive pressure is used (a) while apical negative pressure eliminates gas entrapment (b).

the efficacy of irrigation in curved canals is limited (45–47). The presence of slight curvatures, starting from 25°, represents a clinical challenge (48). Taking into consideration that the majority of clinical cases present with mild or greater curvatures, it is necessary to further study this major limitation and possible techniques to overcome.

In a microbiological study, the decreased effectiveness of PP in curved canals was demonstrated using bioluminescent bacteria (46). This study presented very relevant data concerning the physical limitations of the efficacy of needle irrigation. It was observed that in 24–28° curvatures, the differences obtained in the removal of the biological substrate were significant and correlated with the preparation size. Larger preparation sizes resulted in better apical irrigation.

When comparing PP with other activation systems or simultaneous combination of PP and activation, it was demonstrated that PP irrigation alone was not enough to obtain an adequate cleaning of the apical third (43). Conversely, when combined with activation systems like PUI, the results were significantly better, regardless of the curvature. A recent study confirmed that the action of PUI allows for irrigation at least 3 mm ahead of the ultrasonic file, even in curvatures greater than 50° and with 5 mm radius (49). Munoz and Camacho-Cuadra (50) evaluated irrigant penetration *in-vivo*, using a radiopaque contrast material. Mesial roots of mandibular molars were instrumented to 35/05 and a 27 G needle was positioned at 2 mm from WL. PP failed to irrigate at full WL while PUI and ANP obtained significantly better results.

Despite the available evidence regarding the advantage of using hybrid techniques for root canal irrigation (i.e., combining PP with PUI or sonic activation), Dutner *et al.* (51) reported that almost half of the clinicians do not use any coadjutant system while irrigating with PP.

Methods used in the analysis of irrigant penetration

Different methods have been employed for fluid dynamics and apical irrigation research, including the thermal image analysis proposed by Hsieh *et al.* (41), which employs a technology never used

pain. Safety, efficiency, and predictability must be the main factors to consider when selecting PP or a different irrigant delivery/activation system.

The degree of root canal curvatures directly affects the penetration of the irrigation needle and consequently restricts the irrigant flow at the apical portion. The number of studies analyzing before in endodontics. This method consists of a temperature distribution analysis among oral tissues and is commonly employed in oral pathology research (52). The energy emitted by an irrigant solution heated to 50 °C and placed into root canals of teeth previously cooled up to 10 °C was analyzed. With this method, the level of the solution extension is known with relative accuracy. It was observed that a minimum apical preparation to ISO size #30, along with the placement of a 27 G needle up to 3 mm from WL, was needed to detect temperature changes in the last millimeter of the samples. Contrary to what we might deduce for larger diameter preparations (over ISO #80), equivalent to teeth with immature apices, the efficacy of irrigation does not increase, but decreases because of the turbulence generated in the root canal during irrigation, which prevents the solution to reach the complete preparation length.

Between 2009 and 2011, various papers have been published (37, 53, 54) that reported analyses in an *in-vitro* model to evaluate irrigant penetration in real time with different devices, including PP. This model used cleared teeth with the external surface sealed with wax, creating closed systems in which contrast colored sodium hypochlorite was visualized. This model allowed visualization of the entire canal length and for standardization of noninstrumented, artificially created lateral canals of 60 μm in diameter.

The main conclusion from these studies is that PP, compared with different delivery and activation systems, does not accomplish the objective of delivery of the irrigant to WL and to difficult access areas as lateral canals. In the three papers published with this methodology, PP was not able to reach the results obtained with ANP (EndoVac®) for WL penetration, and the results obtained with PUI for noninstrumented areas.

Computed fluid dynamics (CFD)

In 2009, a new method for irrigation analysis was introduced. The computed fluid dynamics (CFD) has been used in engineering for many years, and more recently in medicine, to analyze blood flow patterns in circulatory pathologies (55) or breathing flow conditions (56). This technology overcomes limitations of previous methods used in the study of fluid dynamics (57–60), which provided only macroscopic assessment and very general information.

CFD allows one to obtain data about fluid speed, something inconceivable in an experimental model. Information about fluid speed, intracanal pressures, and stress over canal walls can be easily gathered with this technique. The first CFD analysis focused on the effect of irrigant fluid speed during final irrigation using a 30 G side-vented needle on the flow pattern produced in a root canal instrumented to 45/06.

In this computational analysis, the irrigation needles were measured to determine the internal and external diameter and the incidence and degree of deviation from ISO 9626:1991 and ISO 9626:1991/Amd 1:2001 specifications (29). Root canals were standardized to 19 mm length with continuous 6% taper and apical diameter ISO #45 (0.45 mm), based on the results of a final 45/06 K3 file (Sybron Endo). At the apical level, an apical constriction was tridimensional constructed as an inverted cone, to better simulate the clinical situation of a natural root canal. This anatomy design was based on a previous study by Ponce and Vilar Fernandez (61) that described a maxillary central incisor.

For the irrigation process, the irrigation needle was placed 3 mm from WL and centered in the root canal. For fluid speeds, data from the 2007 study were used (29). For the design of irrigant fluid, density, viscosity, and specific gravity of 1% NaOCl were applied, and the root canal was considered impermeable, closed at the apical end and full of fluid.

Fluid movements on delivery by the needle depended on the speed applied and marked a 30° angle trajectory from the side port exit surrounding the needle tip and forming a vortex into the apical zone. The current flowed laterally through the side port at the maximum speed producing reduced irrigant replacement at the apical zone of the root canal. Even when greater flow speeds were applied, the irrigant could not advance more than 1 mm ahead from the needle tip. Only with very intense flow speed rarely used in clinical procedures because of extrusion risk it was possible to achieve 1.5 mm ahead from the needle tip. Besides the intracanal irrigant speed data, relevant information was obtained relative to the mechanical efficacy of close-ended and side-vented needles, particularly related to the irrigant stress produced over the dentinal wall at the exit site level. The term *stress* is directly related to the "flushing" phenomenon, responsible for the debris removal effect. From this study, it was concluded that the removal of debris attached to the canal wall would be more efficient in the areas near the side port.

There are currently some disadvantages in this method of studying irrigation using computational models, for example, the absence of dentinal chips, pulp tissue. The friction between the fluid and dentinal walls is also absent. The simulated root canal is completely closed apically, without extrusion risk. From this first study by Boutsioukis *et al.* fluid dynamics acquires an important role in the field of irrigation. For this reason, six more studies were later published with similar methodology. We discuss two of these for methodology validation.

In a study by Gao *et al.* (62), the aim was to identify the turbulence mode that best reproduces the clinical situation, comparing the results obtained by CFD with the observation of *in-vitro* simulation. Instrumentation of a methacrylate resin block was used to simulate a prepared root canal *in-vitro* (Endo Training Block; Dentsply Maillefer, Ballaigues, Switzerland). The blocks were instrumented to an apical size of 30/09, corresponding to a ProTaper F3 file, and the foramen was sealed with modeling wax in order to create a closed system. The prepared root canal was reconstructed by computer to perform the CFD analysis using a micro-CT scanner in order to obtain an exact reproduction. Comparing this model with the one used by Boutsioukis *et al.*, we find that the main difference (besides root canal preparation) is the presence of curvature. The needle used by Gao *et al.* is also different, as the 28 G side-vented Max-I-Probe had a wider caliber.

The identification of the efficacy of this model was one of the objectives; considering that the flux of distilled water used as irrigant is considered laminar, it changes to turbulence following the lateral exit and collision with the canal wall. The second was to analyze if the model was able to correctly identify the "dead water" or "stagnation zone" area. After comparing CFD results with those recorded by a macro mode video camera during irrigation with water stained with a dye,

they concluded that from the different turbulence models applied, only one, SST k-u, corresponded with the *in-vitro* experiment.

One interesting finding in this study was the pressure against the wall of the root canal exerted by irrigation measured as 600 Pa, much higher than the intravascular pressure found in blood vessels, which could be in intimate relationship with the root foramen. In the event of irrigant extrusion, there would be no limitations for its penetration into blood vessels once the vascular wall had been damaged. This incident would permit the rapid dissemination of the irrigant. In the case of sodium hypochlorite this would provoke tissue destruction in a much more extensive area. This analysis could explain the exaggerated tissue reaction produced even in the opposite arch with a very extensive facial area (63). Because intracanal vessels are noncollapsible and these have the main quality of absorbing any fluid coming in contact with them, an irrigant extruded apically would be quickly transported to central veins (64).

Another study also compared the results obtained with CFD with a curved canal of a methacrylate cube (65). In this study, the irrigant flow data was evaluated using three different needles up to 3 and 5 mm from WL. The results for side-vented needles were similar to previous studies considering different apical preparations (40/06 for Shen *et al.* and 30/09 for Gao *et al.*), demonstrating a particularly marked apical stagnation zone when the needle was inserted at 5 mm from WL. The most elevated intracanal pressures were generated when needles were placed at 3 mm from WL and the notched and beveled ended needles generated more elevated pressures than side-vented.

The possibilities for this technology to evaluate irrigant extrusion are also important, something that was confirmed in the study by Boutsioukis *et al.* in which an *in-vitro* model was probably more precise than the one used by Gao *et al.*

Both studies employed polydimethylsiloxane (PDMS) for the construction of the *in-vitro* root canals, but the Greek group also used particle image velocity (PIV) technology instead of a dye. Besides the purpose of CFD results validation with *in-vitro* data, they analyzed the influence of the needle position in relation to the canal walls, from a centered position into the root canal to more close relation to the walls. The un-centered effect of the needle into the root canal demonstrated a limited influence, generating a slight increase in the irrigant speed. Another important change in relation to the first study in 2009 was that the root canal was created in all dimensions instead of using half of the canal and posterior symmetrical construction.

Besides PIV, a better control was applied in the reconstruction of the needle and the dimensions of the needle lumen. This was possible because the tridimensional reconstruction was supported by the 2007 exhaustive study about the standardization of irrigation needles (29).

Boutsioukis et al. (44) developed a new CFD analysis simulating the vapor lock phenomenon. This is the only attempt to create bubble gas entrapment in a CFD model and it could be considered an interesting way to create a physical situation closer to clinical environment. Although this technology has been used only to analyze PP irrigation, the research design allows for further investigation using other irrigation delivery systems.

CFD—influence of apical diameter and taper

Although several articles have been published that focus on the effect of apical preparation on irrigation, the vast majority have evaluated debris and bacteria elimination, or applied in-vitro models that permitted only a macroscopic analysis of fluid dynamics.

The only study to apply CFD to the apical diameter was published by Boutsioukis et al. (66) in which four different ISO diameters were evaluated: 25, 35, 45, and 55. In this virtual model, irrigation was applied with two different types of 30 G needles, flat and side-vented. The increase of apical diameter permitted more apical penetration of the irrigant, regardless of the type of needle used. For side-vented needles, the differences were smaller than for flat type. For ISO 25 apical preparation size, the side-vented needle produced an effective renewal of the irrigant up to 0.75 mm from the needle tip, whereas at ISO 55 apical preparation, the projection of the irrigant reached 1.5 mm.

When a flat needle was used with a larger 55/06 preparation, a complete renewal of irrigant was achieved. The risk of irrigant extrusion through

wide apical preparations should be considered, particularly when the needle tip is placed close to WL. Although the stress area of the root canal wall increased with the increase of apical preparation size, the stress over that area decreased when irrigation was applied to bigger apical preparations. This is because in wider preparation, the space between the needle and the wall is increased, and the reverse flux of irrigant escapes from the inside of the canal with less resistance toward the coronal access orifice.

The only study found in relation to taper preparation is again the one by Boutsioukis et al. (67) in which the influence of tapered preparations 30/02, 30/04, 30/06, 30/09, and a great diameter and minimum taper 60/02 were tested for irrigant flux with 30 G flat and side-vented needles. The apical exchange gradually increased as the canal size increased from 30/04, 30/06, and 30/09. The only preparation size that permitted exchange of irrigants 2 mm ahead from the tip of the needle was 60/02. The bigger the taper, the more intracanal pressure decreased and consequently the risk of irrigant extrusion.

CFD—influence of needle insertion depth

Along with the aforementioned publication by Shen et al. (65), in which different types of needles were evaluated at 3 and 5 mm from WL, another study reported data on the influence of irrigant penetration with different needle insertion depths (68). Although differences were reported for different insertion depths (side-vented and flat), the most important factor was the needle design. Also, the two factors that are modified when changing insertion depth, distance from WL and distance from canal walls, were also analyzed. These results are in accordance with the one obtained by Shen et al. at 3 and 6 mm. At 6 mm, the irrigant penetration observed by the thermal analysis of the image was very limited. This is explained by the data generated by CFD and by the multiple vortex generated in the flux when the distance with the canal walls is increased.

Considering the limitations of a computational simulation study, the authors concluded that the side-vented design could be used at 1 mm from WL and the flat design up to 3 mm from WL

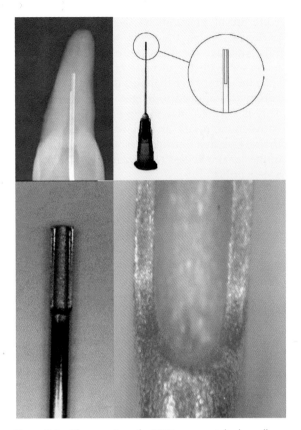

Figure 9.6   Close caption of a 30 G gauge notched needle.

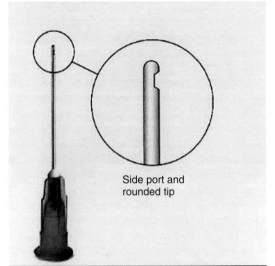

Side port and rounded tip

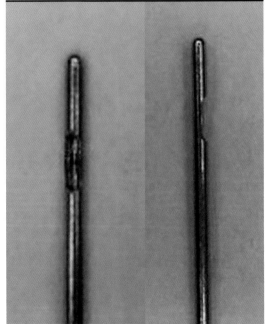

Figure 9.7   Close caption of a 30 G gauge side-vented and round (safe) tip needle.

using reasonable pressures. However, as there is no exact limit for extrusion risk and as the reference is established only on comparisons of needle design, particular clinical case considerations such as tooth type, pulpal and apical status, and apical diameter are critical for a safe irrigation procedure. Numerical data representations contribute valuable information but should not replace clinical information and judgment.

CFD—influence of needle design

Boutsioukis *et al.* (69) analyzed different needle designs using CFD technology. Along with the traditional side-vented and flat designs previously evaluated, this new study included four additional commercially available designs, all of them with 30 G gauge: side-vented, beveled, notched, and multivented (Figures 9.6 and 9.7). The multivented needle, as opposed to the other needle designs tested, is not manufactured for the purpose of irrigant delivery by means of PP, but corresponds to the EndoVac system microcannula, aimed to suction the irrigant from WL through negative pressure.

Data obtained from needle designs with multiple ports or orifices are particularly valuable, especially in the case of the double side-vented needle design, in which 93.5% of the total irrigant flux was delivered through the proximal port, the most distant from the needle tip and WL. In the multivented needle, 73% is delivered by the proximal orifices, but this data is less relevant because of those 100 μm orifices are very close to the needle tip and WL (0.2–0.7 mm), which is not the case for double side-vented needles.

Stress patterns over canal walls were similar for all designs although intensity was greater for beveled, notched, and double side-vented. Previous CFD demonstrated that stress on canal wall is greater at the side port level. This stress is related to the mechanical efficacy and dragging power as well as the capacity of these devices in the biofilm removal.

According to the results of this study, the needles that allowed greater penetration of irrigant also generated greater pressures at apical foramen. Safety should prevail over the possibility of high pressure generation that could easily remove debris and biofilms. The use of open-ended needles should be considered as a risk factor for extrusion when delivering irrigants apically.

Irrigant extrusion

Once we have studied the characteristics of the surgical field, it is necessary to understand the risks of irrigant extrusion from the closed system of root canals, which although hermetic in physiological conditions, may cease to be if the pressure applied during irrigation is elevated or favored by other factors, such as the needle design or the delivery system insertion depth.

The methods applied to this type of study have evolved enormously. In the past, the technology applied was limited to the use of radiopaque contrast and radiographic control. Currently, the use of computational technology seems to be the standard.

The effects of irrigant extrusion to apical tissues vary greatly depending on the irrigant solution extruded. Sodium hypochlorite has demonstrated the most harmful consequences because of its properties of organic matter dissolution. This property

of NaOCl is not selective, and when in contact with apical tissues, consequences could be devastating: producing inflammatory reaction and tissue necrosis.

A review case report (70–74) reveals that some clinical features predispose to this type of accident, such as vertical root fractures, resorptions, or immature apices. In other situations, this phenomenon appears randomly, but recent research offers some data that could alert the clinician. It is necessary to remember that the use of activation systems and negative pressure delivery systems has demonstrated safety in extrusion research models, and therefore seem an ideal complement for PP, mainly in situations in which the elevated extrusion risk precludes the penetration of the needle tip at the apical third.

The maxilla is the area of greater risk following its anatomical features: less density of medullar bone and intimate relationship of roots with the maxillary sinus. Even though the inflammatory reaction and tissue destruction depends on sodium hypochlorite concentration and on the amount of the extruded irrigant (63, 75–77), the use of low concentrations does not completely eliminate this risk.

The incidence, as was previously mentioned, has not been reliably determined, although a survey published by Kleier *et al*. (78) reported that 42% of endodontists that responded to the survey have had at least one case of apical extrusion of NaOCl.

Methods employed for extrusion analysis

Considering the relevance of this issue, many methods have been proposed for the analysis of irrigant extrusion, based mainly on the model by Fairbourn *et al*. (79), and later modified by Myers and Montgomery (80). This model consists of the quantification of extruded irrigant through the foramen by placing the tooth on an empty vial. The pressure in the vial is equal to atmospheric pressure, so the system is considered completely opened, and therefore the volume of irrigant recorded should be greater than if measured in clinical conditions where apical tissues present resistance to the fluids. Apical tissues play a fundamental role in *in-vivo* studies, such as that published by Salzgeber (33). This study was designed to evaluate the level of irrigant penetration in cases where tissue integrity was not complete and demonstrated that extrusion is relatively frequent. During clinical procedures, particular interest should be taken to identify the types of situations at higher risk in order to guarantee safe irrigation of the root canal system.

Simulation of apical tissues

Several attempts have been made to reproduce the anatomical and physiological situation in the most accurate model, using liquids in contact with the external root surface (81, 82) or gels that offer less resistance to irrigants (83, 84). The problem with this type of method is that the control of the amount of extrusion is severely compromised. In other situations, the sensitivity of the gels around the root to the irrigant contact at WL is so elevated that many false positives result, as in cases of ANP (85).

New analysis method

A recent study (86) proposed a new research model for the quantitative analysis of the extruded solution. The focus of this method is on real time quantification during irrigation instead of an accumulative result after the irrigation process is over. In addition, the degree of tissue simulation impact can be evaluated, along with the effects of needle design, apical preparation, and constriction diameters.

The real time measurement system consists of a device that analyzes the electrolyte concentration in the vial. The influence of apical tissues is proved using a completely closed system or one that simulates a bone lesion at the apical level, placing an additional vial on the last radicular millimeters.

The absence of simulated apical tissues confirmed a 60-fold overestimation of the amount of irrigant extrusion. Use of needles without a side port resulted in more extrusion. Curiously, greater preparation sizes did not correlate with more extrusion; therefore, it can be concluded that a determinant factor in irrigant extrusion is the maintenance of the apical constriction. In the present study, increasing the constriction diameter from 15 to 35 produced a progressive increase in the amount of the extruded irrigant, but this difference was not statistically significant. These results are in agreement with the outcome of the previous studies (87).

The influence of the constriction diameter on irrigant extrusion is more important than the influence of the preparation diameter; therefore, patency with files bigger than 10 should be avoided to maximize anatomy preservation (82, 88). Using a conductivity probe, Psimma et al. (31) showed that open-ended needles were not safe compared with side-vented needles and that when the tips were placed more coronally, the extrusion also decreased. The most innovative result of this study was that canal curvature did not influence irrigant extrusion, at least when curvatures between 0° and 30° were analyzed.

The determining factor: intracanal pressure

One of the decisive factors in the accidental extrusion of irrigants is the pressure generated into the root canal system. As described in this chapter, one of the desired effects of irrigation is the flushing of debris after instrumentation, and that efficacy is greater as the irrigant flow and the stress it produces over dentinal walls increases. The problem is that as pressure level increases, the possibility of apical extrusion of irrigants also increases.

A review of the literature shows the advantages and disadvantages of different delivery systems, as well as the capacity for apical delivery of irrigant and the renewal rate and efficacy at apical level. Also, it is not usual to find studies that analyze the pressure generated for the irrigants into the root canal space. In some cases, the pressure is mistaken for flux rate, and although correlated, the effects are different. If the small surface of the needle and the force applied by the clinician are considered, on many occasions, the pressure is elevated and out of control. Therefore, the knowledge of the pressures generated by different needle designs is essential for a secure irrigation procedure. Even though efficacy and flushing efficiency are pursued, safety of the patient should be the priority over other objectives.

These types of studies have been previously performed in neurosurgery (89). In our field, one of the studies analyzing this data and proposing to establish clinically useful guidelines is the one by Psimma et al. (86) in which this important information is registered using a differential pressure transducer.

Although it is difficult to standardize the PP irrigation procedure operated by a clinician, it could be concluded that male operators exerted higher pressures whereas female operators registered lower and longer sustained pressures. The type of needle was also important. For this study, 25 G side-vented, 27 G Monoject, and 30 G side-vented were used, and it was recommended that 3–5 ml syringes be used because the pressure applied by the clinician was not as elevated as the pressure recorded with 10 ml syringes.

In a literature review on irrigant extrusion (90), it was confirmed that there is a lack of clinical studies focusing on this accident. Published case reports offered very limited information on the factors affecting extrusion. Considering *ex-vivo* studies, it was found they were not conclusive because of important methodology limitations and the variability between the protocols used.

In-vivo studies on the consequences of irrigant extrusion and its effect on apical tissues have been performed in animal models. One such study by Pashley *et al.* attempted to reproduce a tissue reaction subsequent to accidental extrusion by injecting sodium hypochlorite into the subcutaneous tissue of rats. All specimens demonstrated a reaction similar to those described on clinical case reports. The outcome supports previous literature, demonstrating the discrepancy of the relative pressures as an argument for extrusion into the adjacent vessels and diffuses effect to more extended areas. Considering intracanal pressures generated during PP irrigation (600 Pa = 4.50 mm Hg) and the reduced pressure existent in a blood vessel (883.94 Pa = 5.88 mm Hg), this theory would explain the random appearance of the accident.

Recently, two different groups have taken an interesting approach to analyze the pressures generated during intracanal irrigation. One of these developed an artificial canal using a polycarbonate rod (91). Because the only way to prevent an accidental injection of the irrigant into the apical tissues has been the nonbinding position of the needle (31), the results of this *in-vitro* study provide us with pivotal information. Using a nanometer placed in the apical foramen of the artificial canal that was instrumented to 40/06, they observed that all the needles tested, including side-vented 30 G,

exceeded the CVP (central venous pressure) at flow rates higher than 1 ml/min.

The other group, Park *et al.* (30), analyzed *in-vitro* the intracanal pressure generated in the apical third of the root canals instrumented to a size 35/06. The authors concluded that apical pressure at high irrigation flow rates was several times higher than at low flow rates. When the 30 G needles (open-ended and side-vented) were placed at the critical level of 1 mm from WL, the design was also a significant factor. The mesiobuccal canals of mandibular molars were used but the canal curvature was not measured in the study. This factor could influence the results obtained, specifically affecting the side-vented needles because the side window could be blocked against the dentinal walls in the case of moderate curvatures. However, the study demonstrated that delivery of irrigants through PP at 1 mm from WL was never safe with any of the needles tested. Taking in consideration all these studies, the practitioner should have control of the needle penetration using rubber stoppers, preferable placed 2 mm shorter of WL. Moreover, an up and down motion is recommended to avoid wedging and intracanal pressure during the delivery of the irrigant.

Influence of irrigation on postoperative pain

Gondim *et al.* (92) studied the issue of the influence of irrigation on postoperative pain. A precise standardized instrumentation protocol was followed to instrument root canals with the exclusion of teeth with apical pathology. Evaluation of postoperative pain was performed after the root canals had been irrigated with the Max-i-Probe (Dentsply Rinn, Elgin, IL) or with ANP irrigation using the EndoVac (SybronEndo, Orange, CA). Results demonstrated that PP as a delivery system produced a statistically significant higher occurrence of cases with postoperative pain when compared to ANP. Data were recorded at 4, 24, and 48 h. The need for analgesic medication (200 mg Ibuprofen) during the first 24 h also increased in the PP group.

The only possibility that would explain the most elevated number of cases that presented postoperative pain when irrigating with 30 G side-vented needle is the contact of the sodium hypochlorite within the apical tissues. Even in the absence of a NaOCl accident, the use of PP could, considering these results, be related with more postoperative pain.

The use of systems that ensure chemical preparation confining its action to the root canal systems should be considered. Without the occurrence of extrusion, the irritation produced by the contact of the irrigant with apical tissues could be responsible for this type of complications, which although not severe, could be avoided. These results confirm the findings of Camoes *et al.* (73), which confirmed the minimum extrusion of irrigants in teeth treated with and without patency.

Similarly, a study by Parirokh *et al.* (93) analyzed the influence of the type of irrigant used during instrumentation on the amount of debris extruded. The results confirmed that 5.25% NaOCl produced greater debris extrusion than at lower concentrations and compared to chlorhexidine.

Devices combining positive pressure and activation of irrigants

Considering that PP is applied only as a delivery system, the effort of the industry for introducing activation to the irrigation procedure has been constant. During the past years, new devices combining PP and activation have been released to the market. Although these devices are activation systems, which are reviewed in this book, a preliminary revision would be performed over studies that have demonstrated efficacy under specific conditions, considering that the delivery system employed is PP. A classification could be presented considering the type and intensity of activation.

PP and ultrasonic activation: continuous ultrasonic irrigation (CUI)

Different devices have been proposed to combine delivery and PUI; some of them are the PiezoFlow (Dentsply, Tulsa Dental Specialties, Tulsa, OK) and the VPro StreamClean System (VSS) (Vista Dental Products, Racine, WI). Some scientific publications have reported increased efficacy while using PP, mainly because of the synergistic effect of delivery and activation (94).

While it is true that in some cases the caliber of ultrasonic needles is similar to those employed with PP irrigation as the 30 G of VSS system, in other cases could be wider, as de 25 G of the PiezoFlow. Therefore, the possibilities of generating high pressures and of canal wall instrumentation increase considerably (91). The needle material could also be different being NiTi for the VSS and stainless steel for the PiezoFlow. Another factor to be considered is related to the extrusion risk as the position of the port is frontal and not lateral.

Considering the fact that these devices present an ultrasonic needle instead of an ultrasonic file, it could be concluded that the stream generated along the needle could be different from the one produced by specific activation files, and particularly taking into account the minor volume of metal, the amplitude and frequency of movement could differ from a wire or file and the effect of the irrigant flowing inside the needle during activation.

PP and sonic activation

In this category of delivery and activation combination, the Vibringe® (Cavex Holland BV, The Netherlands) system consists of a syringe with a device transmitting sonic activation attached to the piston so that the needle transmits the activation to the irrigant in the root canal. This device permits the use of different needle gauges.

Continuous irrigation during instrumentation

Recently, the system self-adjusting file (SAF) (ReDent, Raanana, Israel) has been released into the market. The system incorporates an intracanal device that adapts to the shape of the canal while delivering the irrigant throughout the "brushing" procedure. The irrigant is delivered in the coronal portion of the canal, due to the intention of flowing within the mesh of the instrument. It must be pointed out that SAF does not produce intracanal PP thanks to this coronal delivery. The main advantage of this contemporary system is the use of great amounts of irrigant, but the disadvantage is that the irrigant delivered is limited to the coronal third of the instrument, although pecking motion allows

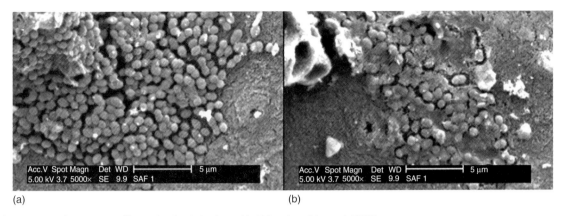

(a)   (b)

Figure 9.8   (a,b) Presence of bacteria after irrigation with SAF at 1 and 3 mm (×5000).

for more apical penetration of the irrigant (54). The system does not provide any activation device attached, but some studies have proposed that the SAF, which is formed by a compressible NiTi mesh and performs an apical–coronal movement of 0.4 mm amplitude at high rpm (4000–5000), produces activation because of an ineffective piston effect (95). Some authors had even described it as a sonic system, considering the intensity of movement (96), and good results have been obtained regarding debridement and disinfection of oval canals (97).

The literature reports that SAF was not efficient in mature biofilm elimination, particularly in the last apical millimeters. One of these reports (98) analyzed the residual bacterial load by means of microbiological sampling and SEM of the last apical millimeters where the results are deficient (Figure 9.8). These data support the findings of de Gregorio *et al.* (54) (Figure 9.9), which through fluid dynamics analysis on cleared teeth confirm minimal penetration of irrigant at apical level, without improving the results obtained with PP.

PP and hydrodynamic activation

The only device using this technology is the Rinsendo (Dürr Dental, Bietigheim, Germany). This device is connected to the dental unit, and once the syringe is connected to the hand piece containing the irrigant solution, it generates a high pressure intermittent delivery (1.6 Hz). Even though it has been proved to be more efficient

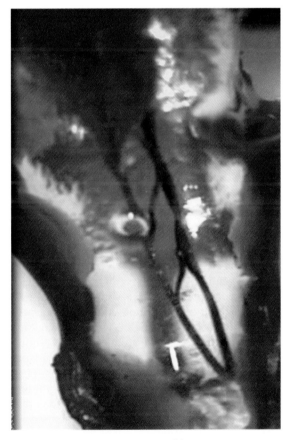

Figure 9.9   Activation using SAF unable to promote irrigant penetration up to WL and into artificial lateral canals.

than PP in the elimination of debris from noninstrumented areas (99) as well as better removal of collagen membranes (100), representing biofilm presence, the Rinsendo has demonstrated an elevated risk of extrusion because of the high pressure during delivery (101). This is a consequence not only of the pressure generated by the device but also by the ISO 55 needle diameter that produces a very small reflux space between the needle and the root canal space.

Conclusions

From this literature review, it can be concluded that PP delivery system represents the most used method for irrigation during root canal treatment. In addition, the delivery of the irrigating solution exerts a flushing effect that removes particles from the root canal as dentinal chips and pulp tissue. From the analysis of the studies published comparing PP with other devices, it can also be concluded that the ability of PP to deliver the irrigants at WL and the replacing rate are limited to the level of needle penetration and physical rules that were not full considered till recently. The only procedure that ensures that objective consists of placing the needle tip at 1 mm from WL, but considering the high risk of extrusion of the system when placed close to the apical limit, studies recommend positioning the tip at 3 mm from WL, where it has demonstrated more safety. The use of side-vented and small gauge is recommended in order to reduce the extrusion risk and to permit the flow of the irrigant toward the coronal direction of the root canal.

The effect of this system in noninstrumented areas is limited. Therefore, the use of complementary devices should be considered in order to improve efficacy, flushing effect, and to facilitate the contact of the irrigant with the root canal system surface. All the aforementioned should be performed while maintaining safety and preventing extrusion of toxic irrigant solutions. These factors combined would permit a longitudinal (WL) and transversal (noninstrumented areas) extension of irrigation, which could be defined as a *tridimensional irrigation* of the root canal system.

References

1. Strindberg, L. (1956) The dependence of the results of pulp therapy on certain factors. An analytic study based on radiographic and clinical follow-up examinations. *Acta Odontologica Scandinavica*, **14**, 1–175.

2. Kakehashi, S., Stanley, H.R. & Fitzgerald, R.J. (1965) The effects of surgical exposures of dental pulps in germ-free and conventional laboratory rats. *Oral Surgery, Oral Medicine, and Oral Pathology*, **20**, 340–349.

3. Machtou, P. (1980) *Irrigation Investigation in Endodontics*. Paris VII, Paris.

4. Schilder, H. (1976) Canal debridement and disinfection. In: Cohen, S. & Burns, R.C. (eds), *Pathways of the Pulp*. Mosby, St. Louis, pp. 111–133.

5. Siqueira, J.F. Jr., Lima, K.C., Magalhaes, F.A., Lopes, H.P. & de Uzeda, M. (1999) Mechanical reduction of the bacterial population in the root canal by three instrumentation techniques. *Journal of Endodontics*, **25 (5)**, 332–335.

6. Shuping, G.B., Orstavik, D., Sigurdsson, A. & Trope, M. (2000) Reduction of intracanal bacteria using nickel-titanium rotary instrumentation and various medications. *Journal of Endodontics*, **26 (12)**, 751–755.

7. Dalton, B.C., Orstavik, D., Phillips, C., Pettiette, M. & Trope, M. (1998) Bacterial reduction with nickel–titanium rotary instrumentation. *Journal of Endodontics*, **24 (11)**, 763–767.

8. Cameron, J.A. (1987) The use of 4 per cent sodium hypochlorite, with or without ultrasound, in cleansing of uninstrumented immature root canals; SEM study. *Australian Dental Journal*, **32 (3)**, 204–213.

9. Cheung, G.S. & Stock, C.J. (1993) In vitro cleaning ability of root canal irrigants with and without endosonics. *International Endodontic Journal*, **26 (6)**, 334–343.

10. Bystrom, A. & Sundqvist, G. (1985) The antibacterial action of sodium hypochlorite and EDTA in 60 cases of endodontic therapy. *International Endodontic Journal*, **18 (1)**, 35–40.

11. Chow, T.W. (1983) Mechanical effectiveness of root canal irrigation. *Journal of Endodontics*, **9 (11)**, 475–479.

12. Brito, P.R., Souza, L.C., Machado de Oliveira, J.C. *et al.* (2009) Comparison of the effectiveness of three irrigation techniques in reducing intracanal Enterococcus faecalis populations: an in vitro study. *Journal of Endodontics*, **35 (10)**, 1422–1427.

13. Harrison, J.W. (1984) Irrigation of the root canal system. *Dental Clinics of North America*, **28 (4)**, 797–808.

14. Senia, E.S., Marshall, F.J. & Rosen, S. (1971) The solvent action of sodium hypochlorite on pulp tissue of extracted teeth. *Oral Surgery, Oral Medicine, and Oral Pathology*, **31 (1)**, 96–103.

15. Baumgartner, J.C. & Cuenin, P.R. (1992) Efficacy of several concentrations of sodium hypochlorite for root canal irrigation. *Journal of Endodontics*, **18** (**12**), 605–612.

16. Pashley, E.L., Birdsong, N.L., Bowman, K. & Pashley, D.H. (1985) Cytotoxic effects of NaOCl on vital tissue. *Journal of Endodontics*, **11** (**12**), 525–528.

17. Torabinejad, M., Khademi, A.A., Babagoli, J. *et al.* (2003) A new solution for the removal of the smear layer. *Journal of Endodontics*, **29** (**3**), 170–175.

18. Khademi, A., Yazdizadeh, M. & Feizianfard, M. (2006) Determination of the minimum instrumentation size for penetration of irrigants to the apical third of root canal systems. *Journal of Endodontics*, **32** (**5**), 417–420.

19. Grandini, S., Balleri, P. & Ferrari, M. (2002) Evaluation of Glyde File Prep in combination with sodium hypochlorite as a root canal irrigant. *Journal of Endodontics*, **28** (**4**), 300–303.

20. Usman, N., Baumgartner, J.C. & Marshall, J.G. (2004) Influence of instrument size on root canal debridement. *Journal of Endodontics*, **30** (**2**), 110–112.

21. O'Connell, M.S., Morgan, L.A., Beeler, W.J. & Baumgartner, J.C. (2000) A comparative study of smear layer removal using different salts of EDTA. *Journal of Endodontics*, **26** (**12**), 739–743.

22. Albrecht, L.J., Baumgartner, J.C. & Marshall, J.G. (2004) Evaluation of apical debris removal using various sizes and tapers of ProFile GT files. *Journal of Endodontics*, **30** (**6**), 425–428.

23. Qian, W., Shen, Y. & Haapasalo, M. (2011) Quantitative analysis of the effect of irrigant solution sequences on dentin erosion. *Journal of Endodontics*, **37** (**10**), 1437–1441.

24. Marending, M., Luder, H.U., Brunner, T.J., Knecht, S., Stark, W.J. & Zehnder, M. (2007) Effect of sodium hypochlorite on human root dentine—mechanical, chemical and structural evaluation. *International Endodontic Journal*, **40** (**10**), 786–793.

25. Del Carpio-Perochena, A.E., Bramante, C.M., Duarte, M.A. *et al.* (2011) Biofilm dissolution and cleaning ability of different irrigant solutions on intraorally infected dentin. *Journal of Endodontics*, **37** (**8**), 1134–1138.

26. Parente, J.M., Loushine, R.J., Susin, L. *et al.* (2010) Root canal debridement using manual dynamic agitation or the EndoVac for final irrigation in a closed system and an open system. *International Endodontic Journal*, **43** (**11**), 1001–1012.

27. Jiang, L.M., Verhaagen, B., Versluis, M. & van der Sluis, L.W. (2010) Evaluation of a sonic device designed to activate irrigant in the root canal. *Journal of Endodontics*, **36** (**1**), 143–146.

28. van der Sluis, L.W., Vogels, M.P., Verhaagen, B., Macedo, R. & Wesselink, P.R. (2010) Study on the influence of refreshment/activation cycles and irrigants on mechanical cleaning efficiency during ultrasonic activation of the irrigant. *Journal of Endodontics*, **36** (**4**), 737–740.

29. Boutsioukis, C., Lambrianidis, T. & Vasiliadis, L. (2007) Clinical relevance of standardization of endodontic irrigation needle dimensions according to the ISO 9,626:1991 and 9,626:1991/Amd 1:2001 specification. *International Endodontic Journal*, **40** (**9**), 700–706.

30. Park, E., Shen, Y., Khakpour, M. & Haapasalo, M. (2013) Apical pressure and extent of irrigant flow beyond the needle tip during positive pressure irrigation in an in vitro root canal model. *Journal of Endodontics*, **39** (**4**), 511–515.

31. Psimma, Z., Boutsioukis, C., Kastrinakis, E. & Vasiliadis, L. (2013) Effect of needle insertion depth and root canal curvature on irrigant extrusion ex vivo. *Journal of Endodontics*, **39** (**4**), 521–524.

32. Behrents, K.T., Speer, M.L. & Noujeim, M. (2012) Sodium hypochlorite accident with evaluation by cone beam computed tomography. *International Endodontic Journal*, **45** (**5**), 492–498.

33. Salzgeber, R.M. & Brilliant, J.D. (1977) An in vivo evaluation of the penetration of an irrigating solution in root canals. *Journal of Endodontics*, **3** (**10**), 394–398.

34. Vera, J., Hernandez, E.M., Romero, M., Arias, A. & van der Sluis, L.W. (2012) Effect of maintaining apical patency on irrigant penetration into the apical two millimeters of large root canals: an in vivo study. *Journal of Endodontics*, **38** (**10**), 1340–1343.

35. Vera, J., Arias, A. & Romero, M. (2012) Dynamic movement of intracanal gas bubbles during cleaning and shaping procedures: the effect of maintaining apical patency on their presence in the middle and cervical thirds of human root canals–an in vivo study. *Journal of Endodontics*, **38** (**2**), 200–203.

36. Vera, J., Arias, A. & Romero, M. (2011) Effect of maintaining apical patency on irrigant penetration into the apical third of root canals when using passive ultrasonic irrigation: an in vivo study. *Journal of Endodontics*, **37** (**9**), 1276–1278.

37. de Gregorio, C., Estevez, R., Cisneros, R., Paranjpe, A. & Cohenca, N. (2010) Efficacy of different irrigation and activation systems on the penetration of sodium hypochlorite into simulated lateral canals and up to working length: an in vitro study. *Journal of Endodontics*, **36** (**7**), 1216–1221.

38. Goldberg, F., Alfie, D. & Roitman, M. (2004) Evaluation of the incidence of transportation after placement and removal of calcium hydroxide. *Journal of Endodontics*, **30** (**9**), 646–648.

39. Senia, E.S., Marshall, F.J. & Rosen, S. (1971) The solvent action of sodium hypochlorite on pulp tissue of extracted teeth. *Oral Surgery, Oral Medicine, and Oral Pathology*, **31** (**1**), 96–103.

40. Saini, H.R., Tewari, S., Sangwan, P., Duhan, J. & Gupta, A. (2012) Effect of different apical preparation sizes on outcome of primary endodontic treatment: a randomized controlled trial. *Journal of Endodontics*, **38** (**10**), 1309–1315.

41. Hsieh, Y.D., Gau, C.H., Kung Wu, S.F., Shen, E.C., Hsu, P.W. & Fu, E. (2007) Dynamic recording of irrigating fluid distribution in root canals using thermal image analysis. *International Endodontic Journal*, **40** (**1**), 11–17.

42. Hockett, J.L., Dommisch, J.K., Johnson, J.D. & Cohenca, N. (2008) Antimicrobial efficacy of two irrigation techniques in tapered and nontapered canal preparations: an in vitro study. *Journal of Endodontics*, **34** (**11**), 1374–1377.

43. Tay, F.R., Gu, L.S., Schoeffel, G.J. *et al.* (2010) Effect of vapor lock on root canal debridement by using a side-vented needle for positive-pressure irrigant delivery. *Journal of Endodontics*, **36** (**4**), 745–750.

44. Boutsioukis, C., Kastrinakis, E., Lambrianidis, T., Verhaagen, B., Versluis, M. & van der Sluis, L.W.M. (2013) Formation and removal of apical vapor lock during syringe irrigation: a combined experimental and computational fluid dynamics approach. *International Endodontic Journal*, **47** (**2**), 191–201.

45. Rodig, T., Dollmann, S., Konietschke, F., Drebenstedt, S. & Hulsmann, M. (2010) Effectiveness of different irrigant agitation techniques on debris and smear layer removal in curved root canals: a scanning electron microscopy study. *Journal of Endodontics*, **36** (**12**), 1983–1987.

46. Nguy, D. & Sedgley, C. (2006) The influence of canal curvature on the mechanical efficacy of root canal irrigation in vitro using real-time imaging of bioluminescent bacteria. *Journal of Endodontics*, **32** (**11**), 1077–1080.

47. Caron, G., Nham, K., Bronnec, F. & Machtou, P. (2010) Effectiveness of different final irrigant activation protocols on smear layer removal in curved canals. *Journal of Endodontics*, **36** (**8**), 1361–1366.

48. Zmener, O., Pameijer, C.H., Serrano, S.A., Palo, R.M. & Iglesias, E.F. (2009) Efficacy of the NaviTip FX irrigation needle in removing post instrumentation canal smear layer and debris in curved root canals. *Journal of Endodontics*, **35** (**9**), 1270–1273.

49. Malki, M., Verhaagen, B., Jiang, L.M. *et al.* (2012) Irrigant flow beyond the insertion depth of an ultrasonically oscillating file in straight and curved root canals: visualization and cleaning efficacy. *Journal of Endodontics*, **38** (**5**), 657–661.

50. Munoz, H.R. & Camacho-Cuadra, K. (2012) In vivo efficacy of three different endodontic irrigation systems for irrigant delivery to working length of mesial canals of mandibular molars. *Journal of Endodontics*, **38** (**4**), 445–448.

51. Dutner, J., Mines, P. & Anderson, A. (2012) Irrigation trends among American Association of Endodontists members: a web-based survey. *Journal of Endodontics*, **38** (**1**), 37–40.

52. Komoriyama, M., Nomoto, R., Tanaka, R. *et al.* (2003) Application of thermography in dentistry—visualization of temperature distribution on oral tissues. *Dental Materials Journal*, **22** (**4**), 436–443.

53. de Gregorio, C., Estevez, R., Cisneros, R., Heilborn, C. & Cohenca, N. (2009) Effect of EDTA, sonic, and ultrasonic activation on the penetration of sodium hypochlorite into simulated lateral canals: an in vitro study. *Journal of Endodontics*, **35** (**6**), 891–895.

54. de Gregorio, C., Paranjpe, A., Garcia, A. *et al.* (2012) Efficacy of irrigation systems on penetration of sodium hypochlorite to working length and to simulated uninstrumented areas in oval shaped root canals. *International Endodontic Journal*, **45** (**5**), 475–481.

55. Pekkan, K., de Zelicourt, D., Ge, L. *et al.* (2005) Physics-driven CFD modeling of complex anatomical cardiovascular flows–a TCPC case study. *Annals of Biomedical Engineering*, **33** (**3**), 284–300.

56. Xu, C., Sin, S., McDonough, J.M. *et al.* (2006) Computational fluid dynamics modeling of the upper airway of children with obstructive sleep apnea syndrome in steady flow. *Journal of Biomechanics*, **39** (**11**), 2043–2054.

57. Goldman, M., Kronman, J.H., Goldman, L.B., Clausen, H. & Grady, J. (1976) New method of irrigation during endodontic treatment. *Journal of Endodontics*, **2** (**9**), 257–260.

58. Krell, K.V., Johnson, R.J. & Madison, S. (1988) Irrigation patterns during ultrasonic canal instrumentation. Part I. K-type files. *Journal of Endodontics*, **14** (**2**), 65–68.

59. Kahn, F.H., Rosenberg, P.A. & Gliksberg, J. (1995) An in vitro evaluation of the irrigating characteristics of ultrasonic and subsonic handpieces and irrigating needles and probes. *Journal of Endodontics*, **21** (**5**), 277–280.

60. Zehnder, M. (2006) Root canal irrigants. *Journal of Endodontics*, **32** (**5**), 389–398.

61. Ponce, E.H. & Vilar Fernandez, J.A. (2003) The cemento-dentino-canal junction, the apical foramen, and the apical constriction: evaluation by optical microscopy. *Journal of Endodontics*, **29** (**3**), 214–219.

62. Gao, Y., Haapasalo, M., Shen, Y. *et al.* (2009) Development and validation of a three-dimensional computational fluid dynamics model of root canal irrigation. *Journal of Endodontics*, **35** (9), 1282–1287.

63. Hulsmann, M. & Hahn, W. (2000) Complications during root canal irrigation—literature review and case reports. *International Endodontic Journal*, **33** (3), 186–193.

64. Drinker, C.K., Drinker, K.R. & Lund, C.C. (1922) The circulation in the mammalian bone marrow. *American Journal of Physiology*, **62**, 1–92.

65. Shen, Y., Gao, Y., Qian, W. *et al.* (2010) Three-dimensional numeric simulation of root canal irrigant flow with different irrigation needles. *Journal of Endodontics*, **36** (5), 884–889.

66. Boutsioukis, C., Gogos, C., Verhaagen, B., Versluis, M., Kastrinakis, E. & Van der Sluis, L.W. (2010) The effect of apical preparation size on irrigant flow in root canals evaluated using an unsteady computational fluid dynamics model. *International Endodontic Journal*, **43** (10), 874–881.

67. Boutsioukis, C., Gogos, C., Verhaagen, B., Versluis, M., Kastrinakis, E. & Van der Sluis, L.W. (2010) The effect of root canal taper on the irrigant flow: evaluation using an unsteady computational fluid dynamics model. *International Endodontic Journal*, **43** (10), 909–916.

68. Boutsioukis, C., Lambrianidis, T., Verhaagen, B. *et al.* (2010) The effect of needle-insertion depth on the irrigant flow in the root canal: evaluation using an unsteady computational fluid dynamics model. *Journal of Endodontics*, **36** (10), 1664–1668.

69. Boutsioukis, C., Verhaagen, B., Versluis, M., Kastrinakis, E., Wesselink, P.R. & van der Sluis, L.W. (2010) Evaluation of irrigant flow in the root canal using different needle types by an unsteady computational fluid dynamics model. *Journal of Endodontics*, **36** (5), 875–879.

70. Mehdipour, O., Kleier, D.J. & Averbach, R.E. (2007) Anatomy of sodium hypochlorite accidents. *Compendium of Continuing Education in Dentistry*, **28** (10), 544–546, 548, 550.

71. Zairi, A. & Lambrianidis, T. (2008) Accidental extrusion of sodium hypochlorite into the maxillary sinus. *Quintessence International*, **39** (9), 745–748.

72. de Sermeno, R.F., da Silva, L.A., Herrera, H., Silva, R.A. & Leonardo, M.R. (2009) Tissue damage after sodium hypochlorite extrusion during root canal treatment. *Oral Surgery, Oral Medicine, Oral Pathology, Oral Radiology, and Endodontics*, **108** (1), e46–e49.

73. Camoes, I.C., Salles, M.R., Fernando, M.V., Freitas, L.F. & Gomes, C.C. (2009) Relationship between the size of patency file and apical extrusion of sodium hypochlorite. *Indian Journal of Dental Research: Official Publication of Indian Society for Dental Research*, **20** (4), 426–430.

74. Lee, J., Lorenzo, D., Rawlins, T. & Cardo, V.A. Jr. (2011) Sodium hypochlorite extrusion: an atypical case of massive soft tissue necrosis. *Journal of Oral and Maxillofacial Surgery: Official Journal of the American Association of Oral and Maxillofacial Surgeons*, **69** (6), 1776–1781.

75. Gallas-Torreira, M.M., Reboiras-Lopez, M.D., Garcia-Garcia, A. & Gandara-Rey, J. (2003) Mandibular nerve paresthesia caused by endodontic treatment. *Medicina Oral: organo oficial de la Sociedad Espanola de Medicina Oral y de la Academia Iberoamericana de Patologia y Medicina Bucal*, **8** (4), 299–303.

76. Ehrich, D.G., Brian, J.D. Jr. & Walker, W.A. (1993) Sodium hypochlorite accident: inadvertent injection into the maxillary sinus. *Journal of Endodontics*, **19** (4), 180–182.

77. Ferraz, C.C., Gomes, N.V., Gomes, B.P., Zaia, A.A., Teixeira, F.B. & Souza-Filho, F.J. (2001) Apical extrusion of debris and irrigants using two hand and three engine-driven instrumentation techniques. *International Endodontic Journal*, **34** (5), 354–358.

78. Kleier, D.J., Averbach, R.E. & Mehdipour, O. (2008) The sodium hypochlorite accident: experience of diplomates of the American Board of Endodontics. *Journal of Endodontics*, **34** (11), 1346–1350.

79. Fairbourn, D.R., McWalter, G.M. & Montgomery, S. (1987) The effect of four preparation techniques on the amount of apically extruded debris. *Journal of Endodontics*, **13** (3), 102–108.

80. Myers, G.L. & Montgomery, S. (1991) A comparison of weights of debris extruded apically by conventional filing and canal master techniques. *Journal of Endodontics*, **17** (6), 275–279.

81. Kustarci, A., Akpinar, K.E. & Er, K. (2008) Apical extrusion of intracanal debris and irrigant following use of various instrumentation techniques. *Oral Surgery, Oral Medicine, Oral Pathology, Oral Radiology, and Endodontics*, **105** (2), 257–262.

82. Tinaz, A.C., Alacam, T., Uzun, O., Maden, M. & Kayaoglu, G. (2005) The effect of disruption of apical constriction on periapical extrusion. *Journal of Endodontics*, **31** (7), 533–535.

83. Mitchell, R.P., Baumgartner, J.C. & Sedgley, C.M. (2011) Apical extrusion of sodium hypochlorite using different root canal irrigation systems. *Journal of Endodontics*, **37** (12), 1677–1681.

84. Fukumoto, Y., Kikuchi, I., Yoshioka, T., Kobayashi, C. & Suda, H. (2006) An ex vivo evaluation of a new root canal irrigation technique with intracanal aspiration. *International Endodontic Journal*, **39** (2), 93–99.

85. Mitchell, R.P., Yang, S.E. & Baumgartner, J.C. (2010) Comparison of apical extrusion of NaOCl using the EndoVac or needle irrigation of root canals. *Journal of Endodontics*, **36** (2), 338–341.

86. Psimma, Z., Boutsioukis, C., Vasiliadis, L. & Kastrinakis, E. (2013) A new method for real-time quantification of irrigant extrusion during root canal irrigation ex vivo. *International Endodontic Journal*, **46** (7), 619–631.

87. George, R. & Walsh, L.J. (2008) Apical extrusion of root canal irrigants when using Er:YAG and Er,Cr:YSGG lasers with optical fibers: an in vitro dye study. *Journal of Endodontics*, **34** (6), 706–708.

88. Lambrianidis, T., Tosounidou, E. & Tzoanopoulou, M. (2001) The effect of maintaining apical patency on periapical extrusion. *Journal of Endodontics*, **27** (11), 696–698.

89. Krebs, J., Ferguson, S.J., Bohner, M., Baroud, G., Steffen, T. & Heini, P.F. (2005) Clinical measurements of cement injection pressure during vertebroplasty. *Spine*, **30** (5), E118–E122.

90. Boutsioukis, C., Psimma, Z. & van der Sluis, L.W. (2013) Factors affecting irrigant extrusion during root canal irrigation: a systematic review. *International Endodontic Journal*, **46** (7), 599–618.

91. Khan, S., Niu, L.N., Eid, A.A. *et al.* (2013) Periapical pressures developed by nonbinding irrigation needles at various irrigation delivery rates. *Journal of Endodontics*, **39** (4), 529–533.

92. Gondim, E. Jr., Setzer, F.C., Dos Carmo, C.B. & Kim, S. (2010) Postoperative pain after the application of two different irrigation devices in a prospective randomized clinical trial. *Journal of Endodontics*, **36** (8), 1295–1301.

93. Parirokh, M., Jalali, S., Haghdoost, A.A. & Abbott, P.V. (2012) Comparison of the effect of various irrigants on apically extruded debris after root canal preparation. *Journal of Endodontics*, **38** (2), 196–199.

94. Curtis, T.O. & Sedgley, C.M. (2012) Comparison of a continuous ultrasonic irrigation device and conventional needle irrigation in the removal of root canal debris. *Journal of Endodontics*, **38** (9), 1261–1264.

95. Hof, R., Perevalov, V., Eltanani, M., Zary, R. & Metzger, Z. (2010) The self-adjusting file (SAF). Part 2: mechanical analysis. *Journal of Endodontics*, **36** (4), 691–696.

96. De-Deus, G., Souza, E.M., Barino, B. *et al.* (2011) The self-adjusting file optimizes debridement quality in oval-shaped root canals. *Journal of Endodontics*, **37** (5), 701–705.

97. Metzger, Z., Teperovich, E., Cohen, R., Zary, R., Paque, F. & Hulsmann, M. (2010) The self-adjusting file (SAF). Part 3: removal of debris and smear layer—a scanning electron microscope study. *Journal of Endodontics*, **36** (4), 697–702.

98. Paranjpe, A., de Gregorio, C., Gonzalez, A.M. *et al.* (2012) Efficacy of the self-adjusting file system on cleaning and shaping oval canals: a microbiological and microscopic evaluation. *Journal of Endodontics*, **38** (2), 226–231.

99. Rodig, T., Sedghi, M., Konietschke, F., Lange, K., Ziebolz, D. & Hulsmann, M. (2010) Efficacy of syringe irrigation, RinsEndo and passive ultrasonic irrigation in removing debris from irregularities in root canals with different apical sizes. *International Endodontic Journal*, **43** (7), 581–589.

100. McGill, S., Gulabivala, K., Mordan, N. & Ng, Y.L. (2008) The efficacy of dynamic irrigation using a commercially available system (RinsEndo) determined by removal of a collagen 'bio-molecular film' from an ex vivo model. *International Endodontic Journal*, **41** (7), 602–608.

101. Desai, P. & Himel, V. (2009) Comparative safety of various intracanal irrigation systems. *Journal of Endodontics*, **35** (4), 545–549.

10 Apical Negative Pressure Irrigation (ANP)

Nestor Cohenca

Department of Endodontics and Pediatric Dentistry, University of Washington, Seattle, WA, USA

Cesar de Gregorio and Avina Paranjpe

Department of Endodontics, University of Washington, Seattle, WA, USA

Introduction

It has been well established for the past several years that the etiology for endodontic disease is microbial pathogens. Toxic metabolites and by-products released from microorganisms within the canal diffuse into apical tissues and elicit inflammatory responses and bone resorption (1, 2). The host immune response plays an important role at this time by preventing the infection from spreading into the various parts of the body. However, because of the lack of blood supply in a necrotic tooth, the host response cannot affect the bacteria that are present in the root canal system. Hence it is necessary to mechanically and chemically remove these microorganisms during root canal treatment procedures. Irrigation along with the instrumentation of the canal can help achieve the goal of disinfection of the root canals. Irrigation supports mechanical instrumentation along with

killing and removing any residual microbes left back in the canal. Currently, there are numerous irrigation solutions and irrigation techniques available and many of them have showed improvement even in the most complex canal systems. This chapter focuses on the apical negative pressure (ANP) irrigation system's unique abilities, advantages, and benefits, one of which is exemplified in Figure 10.1.

Positive pressure (PP) irrigation is still widely used by many clinicians. However, a review of the literature shows that PP irrigation systems have their limitations—inadequate debridement and disinfection in the apical area. Previous studies have demonstrated that PP irrigation had virtually no effect on the orifice of the needle (3). Furthermore, some more recent studies have demonstrated the effectiveness of other irrigation systems over the traditional PP systems (4–6). In addition to debridement and disinfection, safety is another

---

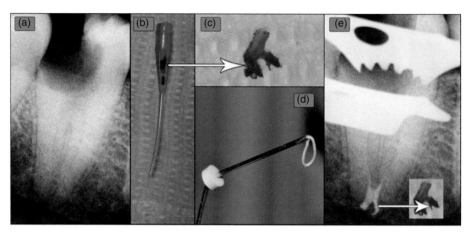

Figure 10.1   (a) An obviously infected root canal space demonstrating apical rarefaction and condensing osteitis. After instrumentation, the (b) macrocannula component of the EndoVac (ANP) system aspirated unexpected material (dark matter in cannula) that was in fact the (c) terminal portion (arrow) of the still vital, yet infected pulp tissue. *Notice the lateral portion facing to the right.* Injectable gutta-percha (d) was the method of obturation. (e) The lateral canal was obviously obturated and matches the shape of the recovered pulp tissue. (Case courtesy: Dr. Filippo Santarcangelo.)

concern with PP irrigation. Sodium hypochlorite (NaOCl) accidents have been described in the literature previously with some being more severe than others (7, 8). The main cause for this seems to be attributed to the amount of pressure created during PP irrigation in comparison to the capillary blood pressure (9, 10). More recent studies have also demonstrated the dangers of PP irrigation in relation to central venous pressure (11, 12).

ANP overview

Whatever irrigation procedure is used during a root canal treatment, it must be performed bearing in mind that effectiveness cannot supersede the safety of the patients. The main problem with PP and NaOCl accidents is the randomness of its nature. This unpredictability seems to be related to the apical status (13) and anatomical factors (14). Clinically, we cannot immediately diagnose when a significant amount of irrigant has been extruded to the apical tissues, and it is virtually impossible to predict these undesirable NaOCl accidents (15). Another drawback of PP irrigation is the apical stagnation plane (16, 17). This barrier allows for gas entrapment, produced by the decomposition of organic tissue. This physical phenomenon is called *vapor lock* making it difficult to adequately debride

the canal's apical termination (18, 19). In order to overcome all these drawbacks, the ANP technique for irrigation was introduced and is discussed in detail in this chapter.

The effectiveness of an irrigating solution is dependent mainly on its adequate diffusion into the root canal system and its volume. The depth of needle placement conditions, the irrigant penetration, and delivering of large amounts of irrigants have been related to high pressures (20). This is one of the main reasons why traditional irrigation systems fail to completely debride the root canal especially because they are placed in a safety depth of 2–3 mm of the working length (WL) to avoid the hypochlorite accident (3). This is not the case with the ANP systems, which because of its philosophy, has the ability to deliver irrigants up to the WL and eliminating any risk of apical extrusion (21). In addition, studies have demonstrated the effectiveness of the ANP systems to deliver irrigants to the WL in comparison with traditional irrigation, which also relates to the apical vapor lock phenomenon (18, 22).

The most significant advantage is its safety considerations. Studies have compared other irrigation systems to ANP, specifically the EndoVac, currently marketed by SybronEndo (SybronEndo, Orange, CA). Desai and Himel (21) in an *in-vitro* study demonstrated that the ANP did not extrude any irrigant while the groups including the Max-i-Probe (Dentsply Rinn, Elgin, IL), Rinsendo (Dürr Dental GmbH & Co. KG, Bietigheim-Bissingen, Germany), and the continuous ultrasonic irrigation (CUI) needle extruded significant amounts of irrigant that could irritant and be toxic to the apical tissues. This extrusion of irrigant could lead to significant postoperative pain. This parameter was examined by Gondim *et al.* (23) who reported significant reduction in postoperative pain levels when patients were treated using ANP as compared to traditional needle irrigation.

Orientation: This and the next paragraphs are presented as a precursor to more detailed discussions in this chapter. First, as ANP systems can be safely taken to WL, microbiological studies have demonstrated a statistically significant difference between ANP and PP irrigation *in-vitro*. The ANP groups have shown no positive cultures compared with the PP groups, and no significant differences between types of preparations and apical sizes have been noted (24). A recent randomized clinical study involving patients with apical apical periodontitis in lower molars confirmed these results (25). However, an increase in the apical size preparation from #35 to #40 and an increase in taper from 0.02 to 0.04 did demonstrate an increased volume of irrigant being delivered to WL, which in turn could contribute to the microbiological success when using this system (26, 27). Yet, some conflicting studies have been published and the reason for their different findings are thoroughly explained. For example, Pawar *et al.* (28) demonstrated the importance of following the manufacturer's instructions when that study failed to demonstrate differences in efficacy between PP needle irrigation and ANP, greater than or equal to 5% NaOCl was not used. Six years earlier Clegg *et al.* (29) proved that 1% would not prevent culture growth.

In addition to its antimicrobial efficacy, there are many studies that have demonstrated the effectiveness of the ANP system for tissue dissolution, debris removal, and smear-layer removal. The classic study by Nielsen and Craig Baumgartner (30) performed in extracted teeth demonstrated significantly less debris with the ANP group at 1 mm from WL in comparison with conventional needle irrigation. Other *in-vitro* studies done in different teeth types and using different methodologies such as scanning electron microscopy (SEM) have

demonstrated and supported Nielsen results using different methods (6, 31–34).

Besides being used in teeth with closed apices and for routine root canal treatment procedures, ANP irrigation has also been studied in regenerative endodontic procedures. The use of the ANP irrigation in dogs during regenerative endodontic procedures has proved to be a promising disinfection protocol suggesting that the use of the triple antibiotic paste may not be necessary (35, 36).

Rational

For years, numerous *in-vitro* studies using an open canal system, where the apical tissues were not simulated, have shown good irrigation results using PP irrigation (37). However, in the clinical situation, the root canal system is closed because of apical tissues. Tay *et al.* (38) conclusively demonstrated the importance of using a closed system when evaluating irrigation results. Efficient debridement of the root canal system and isthmuses was recently tested using two irrigant agitation techniques in a closed system and confirmed that the correct simulation of a closed system is essential to re-create the fluid dynamics occurring during the endodontic irrigation (31). The challenge is to predictably create a direct contact between the chemical substance and the complexity of the canal system plus a continuous renewal of the irrigant, thus allowing disinfection and removing debris, all this with no or minimal apical extrusion. These objectives are difficult to achieve by any system. It is a unique physical and anatomical situation that must be understood in order to find a solution toward a better endodontic outcome.

We can categorize irrigation devices into two major groups: activation and delivery systems. Activation systems aim to improve the movement of the irrigant within a complex space. Delivery systems, such as ANP, were developed to overcome the physical facts existing into a semipermeable canal system, thus allowing full penetration of the irrigant with no risk of extrusion. This is a new philosophy and actually contradicts the needle irrigation we have been using for more than 50 years.

Fukumoto *et al.* (39, 40) published the first articles explaining the rationale, and, in 2007, the first commercial ANP system, the EndoVac system (SybronEndo, Orange, CA), was introduced. Recently, another ANP system, INP (ASI Medical, Englewood, CO), has been introduced using materials and methods vastly different from the EndoVac system and it lacks research to provide evidence based on its efficacy. Fukumoto's specimens were placed in a container colored salt agar with 1% of a dye (Caries Detector, Kuraray Co., Ltd., Osaka, Japan) with the aim of analyzing the irrigant and subsequent extrusion. This log samples were analyzed by SEM to observe the cleanliness produced by NaOCl, and ethylenediaminetetraaceticacid (EDTA), in the apical 3 mm of PP and ANP irrigation. The groups irrigated with ANP demonstrated better cleanliness in the apical millimeter. Extrusion results demonstrated that ANP system was significantly safer than PP, extruding a minimum amount of irrigant during the entire process. Irrigant extrusion was the same for ANP groups while the cannula, that is, at two different depths, not for PP, where the greater proximity of the needle to WL (3 mm) caused a greater extrusion, corresponding to previous

studies (10). The findings of the study confirmed the effectiveness of intracanal aspiration system in clearing the last few millimeters of the preparations, as well as greater security of this system compared to irrigation with PP.

Basically, the ANP system includes four major components: a multiport adapter (MPA), master delivery tip (MDT), macrocannulas, and microcannulas. The MDT was designed to deposit the solution at the access and pulp chamber and autoevacuate any excess. The macro- and microcannulas are aimed at aspirating the irrigant solution into the canal creating dynamic flow with constant renewal of the solution, thus decreasing the loss of effectiveness of our irrigants to contact organic and inorganic residues. This allows us to employ large volumes of irrigants without the danger of causing damage to the apical area.

The device and clinical technique

EndoVac (SybronEndo, Orange, CA) was the first ANP system available commercially (Figure 10.2).

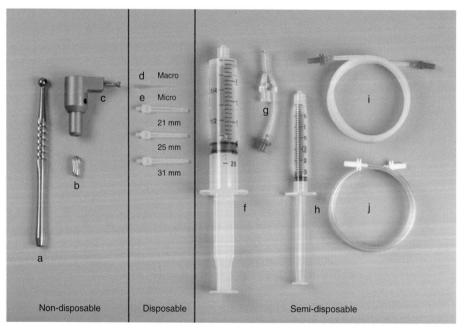

Figure 10.2 (a) Handpiece; (b) fingerpiece; (c) multiport adapter; (d) macrocannula; (e) microcannula (21, 25, 31 mm); (f) syringe 20 cc (for NaOCl); (g) master delivery tip (MDT); (h) syringe 3 cc (for EDTA); (i) MDT evacuation tubing (blue); and (j) handpiece/fingerpiece evacuation tubing (white).

It has been thoroughly investigated since 2007 and, as mentioned above, it is based on four main components: the hand and finger pieces, the macro- and microcannula, the MPA, and the MDT.

1. The multiport adapter (MPA): The MPA plugs directly into Hi-Vac and serves as a caddy for the EndoVac tubing, and other components are easily removed and reattached to the Hi-Vac system for maximum portability between operatories (Figure 10.3).
2. The master delivery tip (MDT): The MDT plugs directly into the blue port of the MPA and provides a constant flow of the irrigant without the risk of overflow. The MDT is used during coronal flaring and after each instrument change to remove gross debris arising from instrumentation (Figure 10.4c).
3. The macrocannula is an ISO 55 plastic cannula used to remove coarse debris inside the canal after all instrumentation is completed. In this step, the macrocannula and the MDT are used at the same time. It is helpful to have a dental assistant delivering the irrigant with the MDT while the clinician works the macrocannula up and down each canal (Figure 10.4. The macrocannula is designed for single use and should be discarded after each treatment.
4. The microcannula is a 30-gauge needle (0.32 mm) with 12 laser-drilled, microscopic evacuation holes—each less than 100 μm in size—all of them placed within the last 0.7 mm of the needle (Figure 10.4b,d). Fluid is drawn to the apical termination through these holes, creating a vortex-like cleaning of the apical third. The microcannula is designed for single use and should be discarded after each treatment.

Clinical technique

The EndoVac irrigation procedure uses two different cannulas of different materials size and configuration in each canal, already described as the macro- and microcannula. They are attached to Hi-Vac to create vacuum pressure, thus allowing them to pull the irrigants to their tips, thereby preventing apical extrusion while concurrently and omnidirectionally aspirating debris from the root canal system. The irrigants are delivered passively at the lip of the access opening via the MDT.

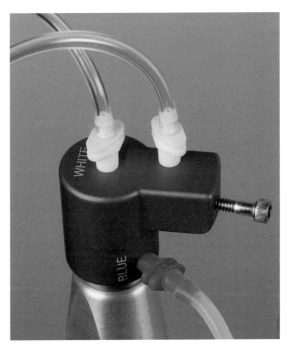

Figure 10.3   The multiport adapter.

Canal instrumentation

During the entire instrumentation process, the MDT is used to supply 1 ml of 5–6% NaOCl before and after every instrument change. This replenishment process evacuates the instrumented debris drawn into the pulp chamber by the preparation instruments while concurrently providing fresh irrigant that will be worked down the canal by the next instrument. In a randomized clinical study, Cohenca et al. (25) determined that instrumentation strategies or types did not affect the efficacy of the EndoVac irrigation procedure. However, the minimum apical preparation size to accommodate the microcannula is 0.32 mm, being necessary an instrumentation with at least a #35/0.02 hand instrument to WL after smaller sizes of NiTi instrumentation is complete.

Macroevacuation

A macro is used to evacuate the gross debris from the root canal cavity after instrumentation. It is used for 30 s in each canal after instrumentation by rapidly moving it from a point where it stopped its apical progression to just below the pulpal floor as

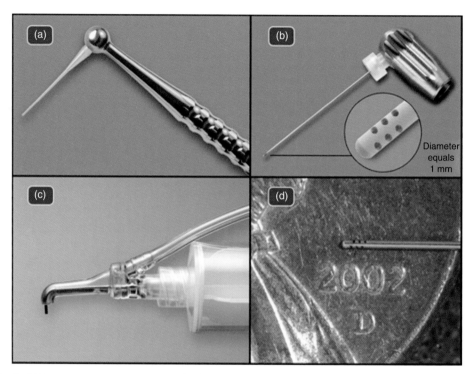

Figure 10.4   EndoVac components: (a) macrocannula; (b) microcannula demonstrating the evacuation holes in the apical 0.7 mm; (c) master delivery tip; and (d) microcannula.

5–6% NaOCl is passively delivered via the MDT at approximately 6–8 ml/min. Current flow is constantly monitored through the Macro's transparent polypropylene wall to ensure blockage has not occurred. After 30 s of rapid irrigant exchange, the canal is left "Charged" with NaOCl by quickly withdrawing the macrocannula from the canal while continuing to deliver 5–6% NaOCl via the MDT. The canal is left undisturbed for 60 s (the "passive wait") while the other canals are treated in the same method. In the case of a single-rooted tooth, the canal is left undisturbed for these 60 s.

Microevacuation

Micro irrigation begins immediately following the macro irrigation's passive wait. *Note—there is a definite learning curve to acquiring this technique—the most frequent mistake made by clinicians when learning this technique is the improper use of the Macrocannula as described above, resulting in unnecessary clogging of the Microcannula's filtration holes*. Once the micro

is in place at full WL, the MDT delivers an uninterrupted flow of irrigant into the pulp chamber. During this irrigant application, the microcannula's exhaust tube is observed to confirm irrigant flow.

Microcycles

Three irrigant "microcycles" (NaOCl, EDTA, and NaOCl) comprise microevacuation. The first microcycle clears the most apically positioned walls of debris and/or biofilm, as 6% NaOCl is delivered to the pulp chamber. After 6 s, the irrigant flow is stopped allowing the canal to be sucked dry (the "purge") thereby evacuating the bubbles formed from hydrolysis; this is repeated four more times for a total of 30 s; then the microcannula is quickly withdrawn from the canal like the macrocannula before, leaving it charged for 60 s while the other canals are treated. After the NaOCl-charged passive wait, the second microirrigation cycle incorporating 17% EDTA was initiated to clear the smear layer. The microcannula is replaced at full WL and 17% EDTA is added for 10 s and the microcannula is again removed leaving the canal charged for an additional 60 s while the other canals are treated. As gas bubbles are not formed by the EDTA, purging is not necessary. Finally, with the gross debris and/or biofilm and smear layer removed from the canal walls, the tubules and the neighboring lateral and associated irregularities are treated via a second round of 5–6% NaOCl, as previously described, thus allowing NaOCl to diffuse into these areas. In the end, the canals are purged of all irrigant and one or two paper points are used to dry the canals. A representative clinical case is showed in Figure 10.5, demonstrating the different steps of ANP (Figure 10.5).

Efficacy

The EndoVac's effectiveness is based on its ability to create negative pressure ranging from approximately −30 to −260 mm Hg throughout

the root canal system extending from the coronal access opening and terminating at the apical extent of the major diameter (41). This allows irrigants to be safely and effectively drawn in abundant quantities down and/or across the canal walls and/or through intracanal irregularities like isthmus areas and wall fins as they are added coronally and evacuated apically. Depending on the type of the irrigant used, organic and inorganic debris is hydrolyzed, chelated, and/or mechanically dislodged from the canal system and subsequently evacuated. Furthermore, this constant irrigant exchange extends beyond the fluid dynamics of delivery and evacuation by allowing the establishment of a diffusion gradient whereby hyperconcentrated solutions like 5% NaOCl diffuse into dead-end spaces (42).

Penetration

Regardless of the analytical method used, various studies evaluating the penetration of irrigants into

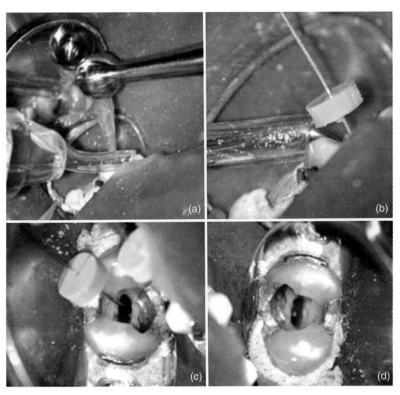

Figure 10.5   (a) Irrigation with macrocannula; (b) rubber stop of the microcannula placed at WL; (c) irrigation with the microcannula; and (d) canals after ANP.

the canal irregularities when delivered via ANP are in unanimous agreement. The first study that evaluated EndoVac's ability to introduce the irrigant into main canal and canal irregularities was conducted by de Gregorio *et al.* in 2010 (43). This study used an *in-vitro* model consisting of cleared teeth embedded in wax to create a closed system, the irrigant solution used was a mix of 5.25% NaOCl and a dye in equal amounts. The irrigant was delivered short of the apical termination via PP and activated by either sonic or passive ultrasonic irrigation (PUI) or complemented with ANP irrigation (EndoVac). The importance of this model is that it could simultaneously measure the depth of the irrigant into the main canal and its penetration into the simulated noninstrumented lateral canals measuring 60 μm in diameter and placed at 2, 4, and 6 mm from the apical termination. Evaluation of these cleared teeth provided information about the penetration up to WL and the ability of the irrigant to be moved into the artificial lateral canals.

The root canals that were instrumented to an ISO #40 demonstrated complete penetration of the irrigant to the apical termination in all EndoVac samples; this was statistically significant compared to the other groups. This validated the microcannula's ability to produce adequate ANP to resolve the vexing physical barrier problem, described in a "stagnation zone" (16) or the "vapor lock" (38). Regarding the penetration of artificial lateral canals, the EndoVac system, designed primarily to safely place abundant irrigant flow to the canal's full length and not as an activation mechanism, was not as effective at filling the lateral canals as PUI. However, this limitation can be balanced by the diffusion effect described by Pashley *et al.* (44) even though this effect was not analyzed in cleared teeth. However, throughout the history, PUI has proved its efficacy cleaning noninstrumented areas and removing debris in relatively straight canals (45–48). However, van der Sluis *et al.* (49) stated that the resultant acoustic microstreaming depends inversely on the surface area of the file touching the root canal wall. Furthermore, Goode *et al.* in 2013 (41) demonstrated that ultrasonic activation could not effectively clean debris from a multiplaner canal; but the EndoVac produced significantly better debris removal than PP, manual dynamic, sonic, and ultrasonic activation.

Cohenca's research team evaluated different irrigation systems in oval canals: EndoVac, PP, and self-adjusting file (SAF) system (50, 51). Results again confirmed the advantages of EndoVac, which delivered a full and constant irrigation at WL, showing significant differences compared to the other two systems. The conclusions of these two studies were confirmed by Spoorthy *et al.* (52) who tested the de Gregorio model but added a new experimental group: ANP + PUI. This new group of PUI + ANP showed better results in the most apical termination, demonstrating the synergistic effect of both techniques, and not affected by root canal curvature (53).

Munoz and Camacho-Cuadra (22) clinically evaluated the irrigant penetration *in-vivo* using a radiopaque contrast solution in mesial curved canals of mandibular molars. Because of the flexibility of microcannula, the effectiveness of EndoVac was confirmed, showing a statistically significant difference in the irrigation at full canal length in comparison with PP and similar results to PUI. However, it is important to realize the limitation of this study because Munoz and Camacho-Cuadra determined only the apical placement of the irrigant and not the critical volume of irrigant delivered or aspirated at the apical termination.

Debridement

Debridement is one of the basic three objectives of endodontic treatment. NaOCl's solvent action dissolves and facilitates removing pulp remnants. As many studies have shown that chemomechanical preparation does not eliminate all the remnants, a proper delivery of NaOCl is needed to maximize its action (54, 55). With PP delivery, the debridement action of NaOCl is directly related to the flow rate of the irrigant and its apical pressure. This is emphasized at the end of this section. The higher intracanal pressure, the greater the cleaning effect is, but unfortunately the extrusion risk is higher; therefore, is important to rely on proper irrigation systems. Traditionally, to enhance debridement, increase of the diameter and taper apical preparation has been proposed (56, 57); however, the EndoVac's safe delivery design enables abundant and safe irrigant delivery when the apical preparation is as small as a #35 ISO (21). Hockett *et al.*

(24) concluded that ANP is crucial in the cleaning and disinfection of the canals than the use of bigger tapers.

Several recent studies have unanimously demonstrated positive proof regarding EndoVac's debridement abilities within the root canal system. Susin *et al.* (31) selected 20 teeth with narrow isthmuses using micro-computed tomography (micro-CT); these samples were analyzed under light microscopy for the presence of debris in the canals of both, instrumented areas and isthmuses. For the analysis of this study, 10 slides were obtained and analyzed between 1 and 2.8 mm from WL. The groups included a manual dynamic activation (MDA) group with a fitted gutta-percha cone. Results did not show a significant difference between groups in the main canal; however, in the isthmuses areas, ANP was more effective removing organic debris (Figure 10.6).

The results of this study are consistent with the outcome of the research by Siu and Baumgartner (5) who achieved better debridement in the very last millimeters when using ANP than PP group. According to the results of this study and that of Susin and Baumgartner, MDA showed a better cleaning than PP. PP and ANP showed similar results at coronal thirds; these can be explained as an effect at the level where the tip needle was placed, in concordance with the results obtained by Boutsioukis *et al.* (58, 59) using computational fluid dynamics (CFD), as higher stress was observed on dentinal walls, which could be influenced by the level, depth, and orientation of the tip needle.

In closed systems, debridement by PP is adversely affected by the presence of apical tissues (38). Parente *et al.* (32) showed that ANP is not affected by a closed system, while MDA had poor results in the same clinical conditions. Nielsen and Craig Baumgartner (30) used a very similar methodology and concluded that at the 1 mm level, significantly less debris was found in the EndoVac group ($P \leq 0.0347$). Relevant data provided by this study are the volume of irrigants used and its influence on tissue dissolution. Within the same period of time, EndoVac allows the use of 42 ml of irrigant in comparison with 15 ml used in PP group.

It is interesting to note that Howard *et al.* (60) obtained different results than the previously discussed studies. They found no significant differences between ANP, PP, and CUI by PiezoFlow device (ProUltra, Dentsply, Tulsa, OK) in the mesial roots of the mandibular molars. However, a close examination of their materials and methods reveals a disturbing fact—the flow rate used during the CUI irrigation was set at 15 ml/min. Two years subsequent to this study, Khan *et al.* (11) tested the apical pressure generated by different irrigation techniques using nonbound needles placed at WL—1 mm up to a maximum delivery rate of 8 ml/min. At 8 ml/min, the CUI group produced 78 mm Hg apically directed pressure. Following this study, Zhu *et al.* (61), in a review manuscript, determined that a maximum flow rate of 3.5 ml/min for an unbound needle would produce 30 mm Hg apically directed pressure—the maximum limit for preventing an intravenous

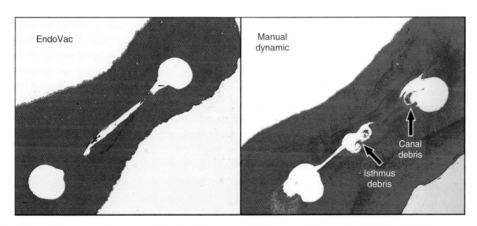

Figure 10.6 Both sections were taken at working length—1 mm. In the manual dynamic activation (MDA) group, greater isthmus debris was apparent and statistically significant at $P = 0.001$.

injection of an endodontic irrigant. Endodontic irrigation is a function of both safety and efficacy.

Smear layer

Effectiveness of ANP is based on a deeper penetration of the irrigant solutions, exposure time, and volume of irrigant. In the previous section, we reviewed the debridement efficacy of ANP, which has showed similar results removing smear layer. Currently, only a few studies have analyzed the effects of ANP on the smear layer. Saber Sel and Hashem (62) found that the activation of 17% EDTA either by MDA or ANP showed a statistically better smear-layer removal than with PP or PUI. However, at approximately the same time as Tay was validating the vapor lock theory (38) in a separate study, his team was investigating smear-layer removal in open and closed root canal systems using two different groups: MDA and ANP (32). The study concluded that the ability of manual dynamic agitation to remove smear layer and debris in a closed canal system was significantly less effective than in an open canal system and significantly less effective than the EndoVac ($P < 0.001$). Thus, they not only established the efficacy of the EndoVac to remove at the most apical depths of a closed canal system; they also reproved the vapor lock theory and called into question all former irrigation studies performed in open-ended samples.

In 2003, Torabinejad et al. (63) defined a scoring method for determining smear-layer removal. This method relies on analyzing the amount of smear layer covering the tubules. However, the tubules are scarce, inherently smaller, and look sclerotic in the walls in the very apical portion of the root canal (64). In 2006, Fukumoto et al. (40) devised a unique method to overcome this problem by amputating the apical 3 mm thereby assuring plentiful tubules at the apical extent of the modified canal. This study was the first reported use of ANP, and the SEM results demonstrated more effective removal of the smear layer than traditional irrigation. Gómez-Pérez (65) repeated Fukumoto's study using the EndoVac system obtaining the same positive results (Figure 10.7).

Antimicrobial effect

The primary factor that determines the treatment outcome of well-treated and restored teeth is the biological status of the root canal system at the time of treatment. The success rate for noninfected root canal systems is about 92% (66, 67) while infected canal systems are generally only 80% successful (68). Since the early part of this century, the scientific community began to suspect the pathogenic role of biofilm within the root canal system as opposed to a solitary organism like Enterococci (69). Finally, in 2010, Ricucci and Siqueira (70) concluded that overall findings are consistent with acceptable criteria to include apical periodontitis in the set of biofilm-induced diseases. In short, biofilm is a community of all different types of microorganisms that adhere to surfaces frequently embedded in a self-produced matrix of extracellular polymeric substance (EPS). This type of infection is extremely difficult to destroy with antibiotics because of the EPS, but it can be totally destroyed with NaOCl at the proper concentration and volume.

In 2006, Clegg et al. (29) demonstrated that wild biofilm grown in-vitro could be completely hydrolyzed in a concentration of 5% NaOCl. In

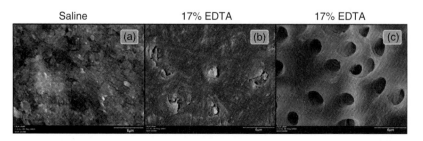

Figure 10.7   SEM examination at WL—1 mm. (a) Saline control; (b) traditional irrigation; and (c) EndoVac irrigation. (Dr. Arianna Gomez-Perez.)

2011, Del Carpio-Perochena *et al.* (71) demonstrated a similar finding when the biofilm was grown *in-vivo*. Both studies agreed that chlorhexidine did not destroy the biofilm. Accordingly, the objective to obtaining biofilm destruction is to flow an adequate volume of greater than 5% NaOCl to the apical termination. This has proven difficult with various types of endodontic irrigation systems. For example, the SAF system is designed to concurrently deliver the irrigant during instrumentation. In a recent study by Paranjpe *et al.* (51) using the SAF system demonstrated that after instrumentation, which included a final irrigation, biofilm still remained at both the 1 and 3 mm—WL level (Figure 10.8).

It is necessary to further emphasize that biofilms have developed *several other* mechanisms against disinfecting methods; at mature stages of biofilm growth, these mechanisms are stronger. Shen *et al.* (72) demonstrated the importance of this factor and according to their analysis, at day 21 of growth, biofilms develop certain defense characteristics and observed differences in their architecture between young and old stages. Results cannot be extrapolated to a clinical environment, because the methodology of these studies compare the disinfecting power of irrigation or activation systems against planktonic or immature biofilms. Therefore, studies where biofilms can be analyzed at longer periods of time are encouraged.

In a precursor study to a randomized clinical study, Hockett *et al.* (24) analyzed the effectiveness of ANP and PP irrigation in eliminating biofilms of *Enterococcus faecalis* in previously instrumented canals, this being the first study evaluating mature biofilms (30 days) (Figure 10.9). The influence of the taper in both techniques was evaluated as well.

ANP was effective in both groups: with variable taper (ProTaper, Tulsa Endodontics, Tulsa, OK) and without taper (Lightspeed LSX, Discus Dental, Culver City, CA). Sampling was aggressive in that a #30 file was used to scrape shavings from the walls to ensure capture of residual biofilm. The culture results demonstrated 100% negative cultures from the ANP groups versus 33% negative in the same groups (Figure 10.10).

A randomized clinical trial based on mandibular first and second molars with separate mesiobuccal (MB) and mesiolingual (ML) canals was conducted by Cohenca *et al.* (25). Inclusion criteria were radiographic evidence of a apical radiolucent lesion associated with tooth (any sex, ethnicity, or race), necrotic pulp as indicated by thermal or electric pulp testing, no history of previous endodontic treatment of the tooth, healthy patients (ASA I, ASA II) consent to participate in this study, compliance with the treatment schedule. Exclusion criteria included teeth with unfavorable conditions for rubber-dam application, if vital pulp tissue was observed during the treatment, immature teeth with open apices, patients younger than 14, pregnant women, medically compromised patients with conditions that were contraindicated to the dental treatment (ASA III), severely curved canals in which apical instrumentation is not predictable, and patients who received systemic antibiotic treatment 3 months prior to treatment. The results were virtually identical to the *in-vitro* study. No positive cultures were obtained from the EndoVac group after final irrigation while the PP group produced 33% positive cultures. The results were statistically significant ($P = 0.03$).

Pawar *et al.* (28) also clinically tested the EndoVac and found no significant differences between ANP

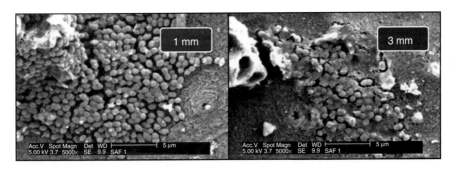

Figure 10.8   After SAF instrumentation and irrigation, biofilm still remained vital and apparent on the walls of the test group.

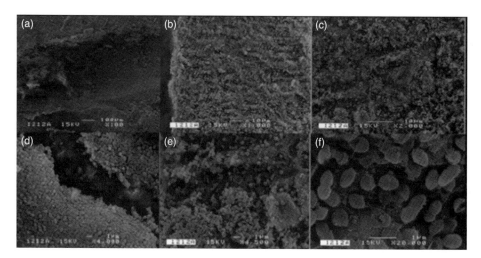

Figure 10.9   Positive control. SEM analysis. (a) At 100×, the presence of bacteria over the root canal surface is shown. (b–d) At 1000×, 2000×, and 4000×, respectively, the bacterial arrangement as biofilms is observed. (e). At 4500×, note the cell aggregations of bacteria covering the dentinal tubules. (f). *E. faecalis* colonization of the root canal and dentinal tubules is confirmed at 20,000×.

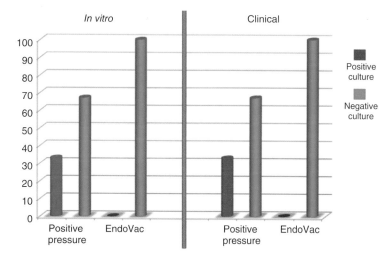

Figure 10.10   *In-vitro*: 33% of the positive pressure irrigation groups rendered positive culture at the end of the incubation period. A significant statistical difference was evident when comparing the apical negative pressure irrigation versus positive pressure irrigation that failed to produce a single positive culture ($P = 0.004$). Clinical: The clinical results mirrored the *in-vitro* with 33% positive cultures in the positive pressure group versus no positive cultures in the apical negative pressure group ($P = 0.03$).

and traditional irrigation. As readers, we must be critical and take into consideration the weaknesses and limitations of all studies. In Pawar *et al.*, the researchers did not follow manufacturer's instructions and used 0.5% NaOCl, a 1000% dilution from the recommended dose. This contradicts the existing evidence presented by Clegg 6 years earlier. In their discussion, the authors recognize that the use of 0.5% NaOCl in this study could be considered responsible for the lack of significant differences in antimicrobial efficacy between EndoVac irrigation and standard.

Brito *et al.* (73) formed biofilm in extracted teeth and this group also did not follow manufacturer's directions because they used 2.5% NaOCl. Furthermore, prior to sampling the canals after the final irrigation, a Hedstrom was used to aggressively file the walls thereby obtaining microbes within the dentinal tubules. This study failed to obtain negative cultures. In a similar study, Miller and Baumgartner (27) inoculated extracted teeth and followed the manufacturer's instructions. Then the research team pulverized the teeth after final irrigation. This study determined that the bacterial reduction was 99.7% in the EndoVac group. It is important to note that they recovered bacteria and not biofilms from the dentinal tubules. This leads to the important question: What is the significance of bacteria trapped in dentinal tubules? In a review paper by Peters *et al.* (74), the authors presented a conflictive statement claiming that there is no evidence that special measures should be taken to kill the bacteria in the dentinal tubules. Should time permit, a sound obturation technique immediately following the cleaning, shaping, and disinfection phases allows the remaining bacteria in the tubules to be either inactivated or prevented from repopulating the (former) canal space. In the vast majority of cases, those bacteria appear not to jeopardize the successful outcome of root canal treatment. However, microorganisms remaining in lateral canal and dentinal tubules might regrow and serve as a source reinfection (75), and hence the critical importance on keep searching for the best and most reliable root canal disinfection, as previously mentioned.

Safety: the NaOCl accident

This chapter has explored several delivery irrigation techniques and or systems in endodontics and their efficacy including penetration of canal irregularities, intracanal debridement, smear-layer removal, and the antimicrobial effects, through the use of greater than 5% NaOCl. However, the extrusion of NaOCl beyond the canal's termination is sometimes the source of morbid consequences including permanent facial disfigurement (76), loss of sensory perception (77), loss of facial muscular control (78), and life-threatening consequences (79). Furthermore, until just recently, the dental profession was mystified regarding the exact consequences of such a small quantity of NaOCl escaping the root canal space. One of the first reported NaOCl accidents reported that less than 0.5 cc of NaOCl could have escaped the confines of the root canal system and yet half the patient's face became inordinately swollen and demonstrated a strange pattern of ecchymosis (80). Sabala hypothesized that this reaction could be the result of an angioneurotic edema response. However, this type of reaction was not classically observed in a comprehensive study regarding the toxicity

of NaOCl by Pashley *et al.* (44). This classic study provides interesting facts about NaOCl toxicity when injected directly into vital tissue. Interestingly, Pashley *et al.* failed to produce the clinical signs and symptoms of a hypochlorite accident as reported in the Sabala and similar cases. In the Pashley finding, tissue reactions were confined to the area of injection while in the Sabala case report, the accidental injection of NaOCl in a second upper premolar triggered tissue reactions around the facial bones and even the patient's neck.

Could it be possible that the Sabala case was not a case of angioneurotic edema, but an intravenous injection of a small amount of NaOCl into the anterior facial vein complex? To refer to Chapter 8 Figure 15A, it is clearly apparent that the superior palpebral vein is well defined. Furthermore, the superior palpebral vein is part of the anterior facial venous complex that sometimes extends from the maxillary anterior and also directly to the heart (81). With that anatomical information, it is understandable how at least one patient died from air injected into a bicuspid tooth that resulted in a cardiac air embolism (82). How much pressure would be required to cause an intravenous injection via the root canal system? In a recent review study published by Gyamfi, it has been determined that 30 mm Hg of apically directed pressure is sufficient to produce an intravenous injection, if anatomical and mechanical conditions, like a patent apex and a rogue vein, are present in the area (61).

Using CFD technology, Boutsioukis (58) irrigated at a flow rate of 15.6 ml/min with the irrigant delivery needle placed 3 mm short of WL and realized an apically directed pressure of approximately 9 kPa or about 65 mm Hg. Certainly, more than enough apical pressure to cause an intravenous injection if the other conditions defined by Gyamfi (61) were present. In a more recent *in-vitro* study, Jiang *et al.* (83) moved the needle to 1 mm from WL, but reduced the delivery rate to 6 ml/s. Khan *et al.* (11) reproduced the Jiang's model, placing a wide variety of nonbinding needles at 1 mm from WL. That study determined that a delivery rate of 3 ml/min (half the Jiang rate) is the absolute safety limit for PP irrigant delivery with a nonbound needle placed at 1 mm from WL. Khan determined that the EndoVac microcannula produced an average of −30 mm Hg across all flow rates.

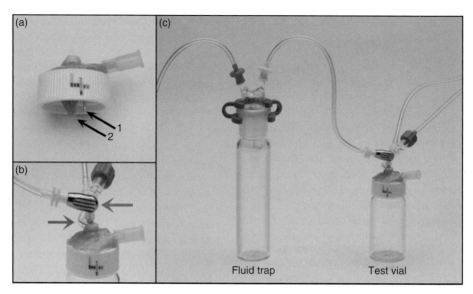

Figure 10.11 The Desai testing apparatus consisted of (a) mounting and sealing a single-rooted tooth (arrow 2) and an 18-gauge atmospheric balancing needle (arrow 1) to the cap of a hermetically sealed collection vial; (b) a finger piece (red arrow) was positioned such that its attached microcannula extended to full working length, while the MDT was positioned to deliver and aspirate the irrigant at the access opening; (c) any irrigant that escaped the test specimen would be trapped in the test vial while all irrigants that passed through the microcannula was trapped and measured in the fluid trap.

The first study to analyze *in-vitro* the extrusion of ANP was done by Desai and Himel (21) (Figure 10.11) and demonstrated that the EndoVac (both macro and micro cannula) failed to extrude any material from a tooth suspended inside a neutral atmospheric chamber, like an apex in a maxillary sinus not covered by bone or even a Schneiderian membrane, while all PP delivery systems did extrude irrigant. Mitchell *et al.* (84) attempted to mimic the clinical situation via an *in-vitro* study in which a water soluble pH sensitive gel was used to simulate apical tissue. The PP pressure samples demonstrated large areas of irrigant extrusion beyond the apical termination, while the EndoVac group demonstrated the outline of the tooth with no apical extrusion.

Irrigation and postoperative pain

Pain associated with root canal treatment is a serious subjective and objective issue. In fact, just the term *root canal* is linked with word "nerve," which for the lay population is a synonymous with pain. It is impossible to determine how many patients have opted for extraction rather than endodontic treatment based on the perception of pain. Accordingly, it is the duty of the profession to mitigate or eliminate the pain associated with endodontic treatment without compromising treatment outcome.

Objectively endodontic pain can be categorized into (i) pain arising from reversible or irreversible pulpitis; (ii) preoperative pain arising from the apical area as a direct result of the inflammation process including hyperemia and accumulation of white blood cells—pus; and (iii) postoperative pain initiated by the root canal procedure often referred to as a *flare-up*. In the case of pulpitis, a simple pulpotomy almost certainly relieves the pain and virtually immediately. In the second category, when the patient reports intrapulpal and/or apical pain resulting from the inflammation process, the treatment must address two problems, elimination of microbial agents and, if possible, the drainage of any apical exudate and/or hyperemia. Figure 10.12 demonstrates spontaneous discharge of both hyperemia and purulent exudate. However, sometimes, this serendipitous event fails to happen, leaving the apical area in a state of inflammation characterized by varying degrees of

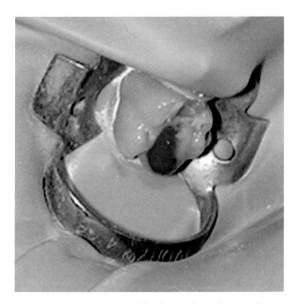

Figure 10.12 Spontaneous bleeding and purulent exudate on access opening.

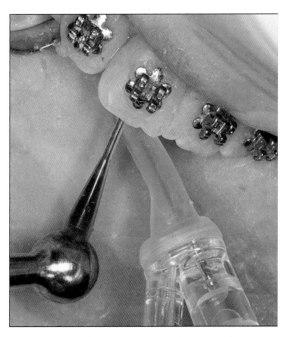

Figure 10.13 EndoVac's macro-cannula proactively aspirating hemorrhagic exudate.

both hyperemia and accumulated exudate. Until recently, the clinician did not have a proactive methodology to aspirate the inflammatory products from the apical area; however, of late, it has been realized that the EndoVac's macrocannula could produce apical ANPs in the area of −250 mm Hg (almost twice systolic blood pressure) (41). This significant apically directed negative pressure has been clinically demonstrated to aspirate both purulent exudate (Figure 10.13).

Once the clinician has eliminated the inflammatory exudates resulting from the root canal space infection, the root canal system must be properly disinfected prior to obturation. Studies already mentioned have proven that it is possible to obtain a high percentage of negative cultures in the initial treatment (24, 25). Furthermore, there is more high-level evidence-based literature showing that there is no statistical success/failure difference between a single- or two-visit treatment (68, 85–90). Accordingly, with the use of the EndoVac system, it is possible to adequately disinfect the root canal without resorting to a calcium hydroxide treatment in a single visit without compromising the outcome. Note that the clinician must maintain a patent apical termination to enable apical aspiration.

This leaves the third category of endodontic pain—the flare-up. In an attempt to determine the frequency of flare-ups and to evaluate correlated factors, Tsesis *et al.* (91) used a meta-analysis study of six cohort studies between 1989 and 2006. He determined that the flair-up frequency was 8.4% following endodontic treatment, but failed to identify a specific common denominator for cause. With the advent of the EndoVac system, Gondim *et al.* (23) conducted a 2-year study prospective of randomized clinical trial. This studied 110 single-rooted teeth that were asymptomatic with irreversible pulpitis caused by carious exposures or normal pulps if the patient had been referred for prosthetic reasons. Although this study did not include symptomatic teeth, its narrow inclusion offered the opportunity to study only the specific effects of different irrigation protocols. The patients were monitored by questionnaire at 4, 24, and 48 h as well as the amount of analgesic taken during this time period. The results demonstrated that the pain experience within those patients randomly assigned to the negative apical pressure group was significantly lower than when using the needle irrigation ($P < 0.0001$ [4, 24, 48 h]). Between 0 and 4 and 4 and 24 h, the intake of analgesics was significantly lower in the group treated by the negative apical pressure device ($P < 0.0001$ [0–4 h], $P = 0.001$ [4–24 h]). The difference for the 24 to 48-h period was not statistically different ($P = 0.08$). Gondim *et al.* concluded: "the negative apical pressure irrigation system EndoVac resulted in significantly less postoperative pain and necessity for analgesic medication than a conventional needle irrigation protocol using the Max-i-Probe." From the results of this study, it may be assumed that it is safe to use a negative apical pressure irrigation protocol for antimicrobial debridement up to the full WL.

Although Gondim's research was very specific and with minimum variables, it gives a broader understanding of treating infected root canal systems. The safety offered by the EndoVac system (last section) provides the efficacy required to obtain the required degree of canal debridement and disinfection, while at the same time offering the ancillary benefit of frequently eliminating the results of apical inflammation via apically directed negative pressure.

Factors affecting ANP/exposure time and volume

Heilborn *et al.* (33) published the only study that compare the cleaning efficacy in the last millimeters of straight canals using ANP and PP as test groups, at different exposure times and volumes (Figure 10.14). Histological analysis failed to demonstrate any significant difference in canal cleanliness at the 3 mm level, whereas at 1 mm from WL with ANP produced a better debris removal even with less exposure time than PP (Figure 10.15).

Regarding the volume of irrigants aspirated by the microcannula, results were different from those published by Nielsen and Craig Baumgartner (30), in which the authors measured the volume of irrigant aspirated by the MDT instead of the microcannula, whether or not the solution reached WL.

It is important to notice that most of the solution release by the MDT is aspirated by the same syringe, which incorporates a suction at its tip before it reaches WL. Thus, Heilborn *et al.* reported a volume aspirated by the micro at WL of 1.8 ml/min, while for the macro (because of its larger diameter) was 34 ml/min. In contrast, the volume released with PP was 3 ml/min, a greater amount than the one generated with the micro. However, a large volume of irrigant used with PP did not result in a better cleaning effect, because a portion of the debris is ejected and traveled apically and not coronally. The main conclusion of this study was that the fluid dynamics has a greater importance in the canals cleaning than the volume of the irrigant and exposure time. Desai and Himel (21) evaluated the volume of the irrigant aspirated by ANP, expressing the volume in percentages. Results for the macrocannula were 82–99% of solution aspirated and for the microcannula, 51–54%.

Total volume (ml) of NaOCl exchanged apically per group upon completion of apical instrumentation.				
	Control or measured flow †	Group 1	Group 2	Group 3
EndoVac Macro	34.0	17.0	5.67	NA
EndoVac Micro*	1.8	1.8	0.54	NA
Maxi-i-Probe	3.0	NA	NA	4.50

* The volume flowing through the microcannula is the actual volume reaching and flowing through full working length.

† These data represent the positive control expressed as the maximum volume of NaOCl aspirated and measured by the micro-and microcannulae and by the 30G Max-i-Probe

Figure 10.14   Measurement volume of irrigant through the aspiration cannula at different times.

Proportion achieving a clean canal (0% debris)				
	n	Canals with no debris	% Clean	P*
Clean canal at 1 mm				
Group 1: EndoVac, 210 s	14	14	100.0	0.03
Group 2: EndoVac, 150 s	15	15	100.0	
Group 3: PP, 210 s	15	11	73.3	
Clean canal at 3 mm				
Group 1: EndoVac, 210 s	15	15	100.0	0.32
Group 2: EndoVac, 150 s	15	15	100.0	
Group 3: PP, 210 s	15	13	86.7	

P* value from Fisher exact test for an overall difference across the three study groups.

Figure 10.15   Despite less volume and time, between Groups 1 and 2 call canals, both EndoVac group were judged 100% clean, while debris remained at both the 1 and 3 mm from WL levels. This was significant at the 1 mm level and not significant at 3 mm, which agrees with Nielsen and Baumgartner.

Factors affecting ANP/synergy with other systems

Recent studies by de Gregorio *et al.* (43) have demonstrated that PP (Figure 10.16a), the most common method currently used for endodontic irrigation, is incapable of delivering irrigants to full WL because of the previously discussed vapor lock. ANP does deliver irrigants to full WL (Figure 10.16b), but does not mechanically force irrigants into small irregularities that is accomplished by diffusion as stated earlier in this chapter. This fact was conclusively proven by Malentacca *et al.* (42) and is discussed later. Sonic irrigation, the EndoActivator (Advanced Endodontics, Santa Barbara, CA), has shown its ability to force irrigants into artificial irregularities in the apical area (Figure 10.16c), but it cannot deliver irrigants to full WL. Not shown are the results of PUI activation that effectively forced irrigants into virtually every artificial lateral canal in all of de Gregorio's studies.

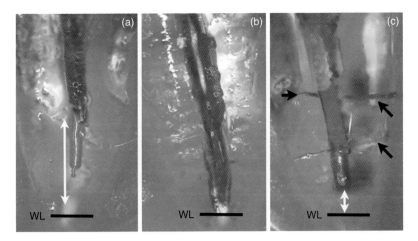

Figure 10.16   Irrigant penetration using different devices in cleared teeth. (a) Positive pressure at 2 mm from WL showing the result of a vapor lock phenomenon. (b) EndoVac (ANP) delivers irrigation to full WL. (c) Although PUI activation does not permit movement of irritant to full working length, it allows penetration into simulated lateral canals (black arrows), which represent uninstrumented areas.

PUI activation has been proven to be very effective at forcing irrigants into artificial canals 0.60 mm in diameter (43). Accordingly, it is important to examine the physics of PUI irrigation versus diffusion. In 2004, Lee et al. (46) working at the University of Amsterdam developed a model for testing PUI efficacy in inaccessible areas of plastic blocks and eventually refined the model to include extracted teeth. Briefly, this model involves instrumenting a single-rooted straight canal to predetermined sizes and tapers and longitudinally splitting the block/teeth and cutting a groove measuring 0.2 mm wide, 0.5 mm deep, and 4.0 mm long extending up from WL −2 mm on one side. This groove would be filled with debris like dentin dust, then the block/teeth was/were reassembled and PUI irrigation was used according to specific parameters. After the PUI irrigation was performed, the blocks were dissembled, and the debris remaining in the groove was quantified via a digital camera attached to a digital microscope. From 2005, this model was used exclusively to test instruments of varying taper (45); in 2006, it tested volume, type of irrigant, and flushing (92); in 2007, it was tested using $Ca(OH)_2$ in the groove (93); in 2010, it tested sonic versus ultrasonic activation (94); in 2010, it was used to test pulsed ultrasound (95); and, in 2012, it was used to test several different irrigation techniques including CUI (83). It is important to note that all of these tests were done in straight canals while we know that the resultant acoustic microstreaming (from PUI) depends inversely on the surface area of the file touching the root canal wall (49).

Realizing that molar teeth are usually multiplaner, Goode et al. (41) devised a reusable titanium model based exactly on the geometry described by Jiang et al. in 2012 (83) including the exact groove feature, except that the canal contained three curves in order to simulate a multiplaner situation. The canal had a primary curvature of 17°, a secondary curvature of 24°, and a tertiary curvature of 68° (Figure 9.19). In earlier Jiang studies, PUI was always tested, but in the 2012 study, Jiang et al. introduced the CUI based on a study by Castelo-Baz et al. (96) in which CUI was equally effective as PUI in the placement of the irrigant in the apical root canal but more effective in the irrigant placement in lateral canals. Instead of using dentin chips, the Goode team used the same type of $Ca(OH)_2$ employed by van der Sluis et al. in 2007 and tested each of the devices described by Jiang et al. in 2012 including the CUI delivery system. There were two other differences between Jiang (2012) and Goode (2013): the delivery rate and the inclusion of the EndoVac's macrocannula per manufacturer's instructions. Earlier, Khan et al. (11) demonstrated that a flow rate of greater than 1 ml/min using a nonbound needle 1 from WL could produce apically directed pressures in excess of central venous pressure and possibly produce an intravenous injection of the irrigant, which is to be proven later to be the root cause of the devastating NaOCl accident (61). The results using a curved canal model demonstrated a dramatic decrease in the efficacy of ultrasonic activation. EndoVac was the only technique that removed more than 99% calcium hydroxide debris from the canal fin at the destined flow rate. This group was significantly different ($P < 0.05$) from the other groups that exhibited incomplete $Ca(OH)_2$ removal.

The Goode et al. model tested the statement about microstreaming being inversely dependent on the surface area of the file touching the root canal wall (41). This begs two questions. First, what is the clinical relevancy of all the studies using straight canals to multiplanner root canal systems where the microstreaming effect is inversely reduced by the instrument touching the walls? Second, could the movement of the irrigant into lateral canals be enhanced if the EndoVac is combined with either PUI or converted to CUI system?

The answer to the latter question has been provided by Malentacca et al. (42) who used a straight transparent block to create root canal model prepared with an F5 ProTaper. Lateral canals (0.20 mm diameter holes) were drilled into the main canal at 2, 5, 8, and 11 mm from WL and a 0.3 ml apical chamber was created to simulate an apical lesion. The lateral canals and apical chamber were filled with prepared bovine pulp. Efficacy and safety were tested PP, EndoVac, and an ultrasonically activated needle in both the PP mode (IUNI-irrigation ultrasonic needle in injection mode) and in the ANP mode (IUNA Irrigation ultrasonic needle in aspiration mode). Regarding their safety findings, the apical lesion all demonstrated various extrusions of NaOCl, except the EndoVac. The study by Gyamfi et al. (61) must be kept in mind because there was no noncollapsing vascularity in the apical chamber

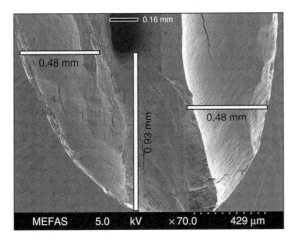

Figure 10.17 Apex of a maxillary cuspid showing a 0.16 mm lateral canal deeply cleaned using the EndoVac technique. The lateral canal is located 0.93 mm from the apical termination and is devoid of pulpal tissue despite the fact that the tooth was vital at the time of extraction. Notice that approximately 0.5 mm represents the distance from the canal wall to the outer limit of the root canal.

of NaOCl that would facilitate movement via diffusion areas of lower concentration. Malentacca et al. (42) proved this is true. Thus maintaining a higher concentration of NaOCl via constant fluid exchange is critical. Furthermore, a 0.5 mm movement into a lateral canal (or other irregularity) represents a practical clinical expectation. The SEM shown on Figure 10.17 was obtained from one of the pilot tests evaluating ANP. The apparent lateral canal is completely devoid of tissue despite the tooth having been vital at the time of extraction. Owing to the presence of smear layer, it is apparent that the second and third microcycles had not yet been applied, yet the lateral canal is clear of tissue as deep as the limit of the SEM can image. Finally, this is a maxillary cuspid, one of the largest single-rooted teeth in the mouth, and 0.5 mm represents the distance required to go from the canal wall to the outermost limit of the root canal. In the other types of teeth, this distance would be expected to be less than or approximately the same (Figure 10.18).

and there is no way to determine the venous extent of travel possible. Regarding the hydrolysis of the tissue in the lateral canals, the ultrasonic groups demonstrated hydrolysis as far as 2–4 mm from the central canal wall while the EndoVac demonstrated hydrolysis as far as 0.5 mm. Earlier in this chapter, it was mentioned that the abundant exchange via the EndoVac would maintain a high concentration

Regarding the synergistic effects of combining the EndoVac with other activation systems, the clinician must always consider safety. The Malentacca study proved that the EndoVac produces the necessary diffusion of NaOCl into pulp tissue located in adjacent lateral canals without the danger of any apical diffusion or extrusion; conversely, it also proved that ultrasonic activation via passive, continuous positive, always caused some

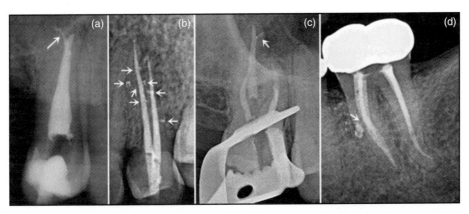

Figure 10.18 (a–d) Each tooth shown in this graphic had a vital intact pulp on access opening. The apparent obturation of the various sizes of lateral canals could be possible only if the tissue had been chemically removed. (Cases (a) by Dr. Filippo Santarcangelo. (b–d) by Dr. Dan Boehne.)

apical diffusion or extrusion in addition to lateral movement.

Factors affecting ANP/canal size, taper, and curvature

As the ANP system is based on the aspiration of the irrigant through their intracanal cannulas, clinicians must consider the factors that influence its suction capacity. Given that the microcannula, given its small size and standing to full WL, is the most difficult aspect, we focus on studies examining suction capacity under different clinical situations. These factors are mainly the size of the preparation and the degree of curvature of the canal. That said, it is important to consider that the following two studies were published before Goode et al. (41) findings in which only 1 ml/min was applied to the root canal system and yet the inassessible groove feature was 99.8% or 1000% cleaner than the next closest group (Table 9.3). The measurement of irrigant flow was accomplished via a fluid trap (Figure 10.19).

Brunson et al. (26) examined the following instrument sizes and tapers #35/0.06, #40/0.06, #45/0.06, #40/0.02, #40/0.04, #40/0.06, and #40/0.08 by placing the microcannula at full WL and delivering an interrupted flow of irritant at the access opening. Results are presented in Figure 10.20.

Following this study, de Gregorio et al. (97) examined various curvatures, tapers, and sizes. The results are presented in Figure 10.21.

It is interesting to note that in the Goode et al. (41) study, the canal preparation was exactly the same as the one used by Jiang et al. (83). In both studies, the apical preparation was 30.06 to WL and a final reaming with a #40/0.02 to create the apical seat. Furthermore, there were three curvatures introduced into the canal system 17°, 24°, 68°, and the inassessable groove was 99.8% clean. It is apparent that in terms of wall shear stress effects, a high flow rate is not required to create effective physical cleansing. This brings the discussion back to the last section. How much irrigant flow over what period of time is required to realize the outstanding results demonstrated by Malentacca et al. (42) and the case histories presented in Figure 10.18. Accordingly, until this question is positively answered, the authors suggest adhering to the manufacturer's directions for use that exceed the parameters of Goode et al.

Revascularization

Immature teeth with apical periodontitis are a challenge; the chemical and mechanical preparation of these anatomies are really difficult because of the difficulties to treat the whole area of the RCS

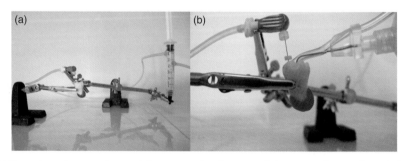

Figure 10.19   (a,b) The syringe shown at the top right recovered and measured the irrigant flowing through the microcannula.

Flow rate according to size and taper							
	#35/0.06	#40/0.06	#45/0.06	#40/0.02	#40/0.04	#40/0.06	#40/0.08
Average flow rate in ml/min	2.00	2.86	2.98	1.58	2.74	2.88	2.96

Figure 10.20   Flow rate according to size and taper.

Flow rate according to curvature			
	Curvature in degrees		
Apical preparation	0–10	11–30	31–65
#35/0.06	0.98	0.92	0.70
#40/0.04	1.38	1.20	0.98
#40/0.06	1.48	1.34	1.14
#45/0.04	1.42	1.32	1.04
#45/0.06	1.46	1.36	1.10
Flow rate is ml/min			

Figure 10.21   It should be noted that there was a difference between the Hi-Vac pressures in these two studies; Brunson *et al.* used 7.5 mm Hg versus 4.42 mm Hg in de Gregorio *et al.*

and the risk of apical extrusion. In those teeth, the microflora is really large and the maturity of the biofilms present in the canal leads to a great resistance to some irrigants and even to very effective solutions when these are used at low concentrations. The apex walls are parallels and sometimes even divergent (98, 99) making easier the apical extrusion. Also, the thin walls make the teeth very fragile, making worse the long-term prognosis.

Therefore, some authors have proposed the use of antibiotic pastes with the aim of eliminating the intracanal microflora. Unfortunately, there are marked disadvantages using this technique because of coronal discoloration (100), bacterial resistance (101, 102), and allergies (103–106). Hence, the ANP technology has recently been

applied with the objective of taking advantage of the disinfection (24), debridement (30), and certain elimination of apical extrusion (21, 42).

In an *in-vivo* study, Cohenca *et al.* (36) compared the efficacy of PP plus TRIMIX antibiotic paste against ANP to disinfect necrotic immature teeth in dogs. The bacterial reduction obtained by EndoVac was comparable to that provided by PP plus antibiotic paste. In a follow-up study, using the same animals and treated teeth, da Silva *et al.* (35) applied MDT to the disinfected pulp chambers and examined them histologically after the application. The EndoVac group showed more mineralized formations (Figure 10.22), more well-structured apical connective tissue as well as more advanced regenerative processes than when the teeth were treated with triantibiotic paste (TRIMIX). The only

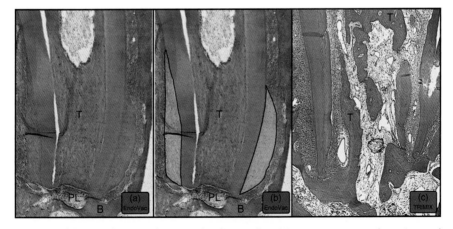

Figure 10.22   (a) Closure of the apical opening by mineralized tissue deposition, new cementum formation, and normal periodontal ligament and alveolar bone. HE—Zeiss—×5 magnification. (b) Note the new cementum formed after treatment (same image as (a)). (c) Absence of a newly formed mineralized tissue in the root apex and the beginning of the repair process, with a connective tissue rich in cells and vessels. HE—Zeiss—×10 magnification.

difference in this protocol when EndoVac was used, compared with the standard protocol, is the use of NaOCl at lower concentration, of 2.5%, in order to avoid the damage into the apical cells responsible for starting the revascularization process and the invagination of the apical tissues into the canal.

Together, the results of these two studies conclude that the disinfection protocol using ANP with the aim to revascularize necrotic immature teeth is, at least, comparable to that protocol used previously with PP and TRIMIX. Moreover, the ANP protocol is done in only one session, and the risk of irrigant extrusion is enormously decreased and discoloration as well as allergic reactions are eliminated, as antibiotics are not used.

Outcome

A careful reading of Peters' opinion demonstrates a simple rearticulation of the endodontic triad: debridement, disinfection (not sterilization), and obturation of the root canal system. Accordingly, the studies of Brito and Miller that determined that root canals are extremely well disinfected after the EndoVac was used, and the studies by Hockett and Cohenca that demonstrated an apparent absence of microbes as remnants of biofilm on dentinal walls, these findings beg the question: "What degree of intracanal disinfection is required to improve clinical success, at least, if not better, than vital results?" In a systematic review, Su et al. stated that success rate for non-vital endodontically treated teeth were 80% (68). It is important to identify that Su's favorable outcome after 1 year was determined by the radiographic assessment of the size of the apical radiolucency, combined with

clinical examinations of signs and symptoms. In 2012, Paredes-Vieyra and Enriquez (90) published an extensive (282 cases) 2-year success/failure of nonvital teeth treated with the EndoVac system. This study examined single- and multiple-visit treatments and found no statistical difference. Accordingly, the combined findings are presented in Figure 10.23.

Paredes et al.'s criterion for healed teeth was very strict. According to them, teeth with complete restitution of the periodontal contours were judged as healed. They classified "Uncertain healing" as teeth with a reduced apical rarefaction. Teeth with symptoms or unchanged radiolucencies were judged as failure. Similar outcome studies like the one by Penesis et al. (107) judged "successful" using the PAI (periapical index) score ≤ 2 (small changes in bone structure). Furthermore, the number of patients in Paredes' study was almost three times higher when comparing to the systematic review published by Su et al. Paredes' strict criteria for success and higher statistical power, demonstrated non-statistical differences on outcome rate when comparing non-vital to vital teeth irrigated with the ANP system (Figure 10.24).

Conclusions

The vacuum pressure created by ANP not only permits evacuation of apical exudate, but also allows abundant full-strength NaOCl to be used *SAFELY* at full WL, thus assuring eradication of biofilm as proven by the cited *in-vitro* and clinical studies in this chapter. We could assume that highest efficiency and reliability on root canal disinfection will positively affect the treatment outcome.

Distribution of teeth according to outcome classification		
Total	282	
Healed	262	92.90%
Uncertain healing	15	5.31%
Not healed	5	1.77%

Figure 10.23 Paredes followed 282 nonvital cases treated with the EndoVac system for 2 years. Ninety-three percent (93%) were judged successful and about two percent (2%) were judged as failures. It is important to realize that the "Uncertain healing" could have been judged as "Healed" by other examiners.

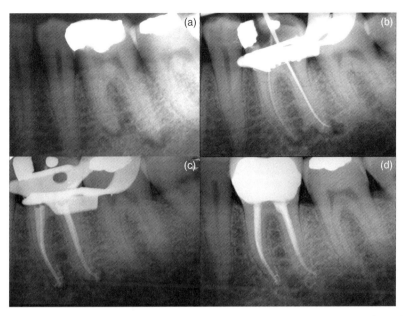

Figure 10.24   (a) Nonvital case with apical periodontitis. (b) Working X-ray with microcannula in distal canal and guide file in mesial. (c) Immediate postoperative. (d) Six-month recall with complete restitution of periodontal contours matching Paredes's *et al.* criteria for success. (Dr. Filippo Santarcangelo.)

References

1. Kakehashi, S., Stanley, H.R. & Fitzgerald, R. (1969) The exposed germ-free pulp: effects of topical corticosteroid medication and restoration. *Oral Surgery, Oral Medicine, and Oral Pathology*, **27 (1)**, 60–67.
2. Moller, A.J., Fabricius, L., Dahlen, G., Ohman, A.E. & Heyden, G. (1981) Influence on periapical tissues of indigenous oral bacteria and necrotic pulp tissue in monkeys. *Scandinavian Journal of Dental Research*, **89 (6)**, 475–484.
3. Chow, T.W. (1983) Mechanical effectiveness of root canal irrigation. *Journal of Endodontics*, **9 (11)**, 475–479.
4. Abarajithan, M., Dham, S., Velmurugan, N., Valerian-Albuquerque, D., Ballal, S. & Senthilkumar, H. (2011) Comparison of Endovac irrigation system with conventional irrigation for removal of intracanal smear layer: an in vitro study. *Oral Surgery, Oral Medicine, Oral Pathology, Oral Radiology, and Endodontics*, **112 (3)**, 407–411.
5. Siu, C. & Baumgartner, J.C. (2010) Comparison of the debridement efficacy of the EndoVac irrigation system and conventional needle root canal irrigation in vivo. *Journal of Endodontics*, **36 (11)**, 1782–1785.
6. Shin, S.J., Kim, H.K., Jung, I.Y., Lee, C.Y., Lee, S.J. & Kim, E. (2010) Comparison of the cleaning efficacy of a new apical negative pressure irrigating system with conventional irrigation needles in the root canals. *Oral Surgery, Oral Medicine, Oral Pathology, Oral Radiology, and Endodontics*, **109 (3)**, 479–484.
7. Kavanagh, C.P. & Taylor, J. (1998) Inadvertent injection of sodium hypochlorite into the maxillary sinus. *British Dental Journal*, **185 (7)**, 336–337.
8. Doherty, M.A., Thomas, M.B. & Dummer, P.M. (2009) Sodium hypochlorite accident—a complication of poor access cavity design. *Dental Update*, **36 (1)**, 7–8, 10–12.
9. Chien, S. (1985) Hemodynamics of the dental pulp. *Journal of Dental Research*, **64**(Spec No), 602–606.
10. Bradford, C.E., Eleazer, P.D., Downs, K.E. & Scheetz, J.P. (2002) Apical pressures developed by needles for canal irrigation. *Journal of Endodontics*, **28 (4)**, 333–335.
11. Khan, S., Niu, L.N., Eid, A.A. *et al.* (2013) Periapical pressures developed by nonbinding irrigation

needles at various irrigation delivery rates. *Journal of Endodontics*, **39 (4)**, 529–533.

12. Park, E., Shen, Y., Khakpour, M. & Haapasalo, M. (2013) apical pressure and extent of irrigant flow beyond the needle tip during positive-pressure irrigation in an in vitro root canal model. *Journal of Endodontics*, **39 (4)**, 511–515.

13. Salzgeber, R.M. & Brilliant, J.D. (1977) An in vivo evaluation of the penetration of an irrigating solution in root canals. *Journal of Endodontics*, **3 (10)**, 394–398.

14. Behrents, K.T., Speer, M.L. & Noujeim, M. (2012) Sodium hypochlorite accident with evaluation by cone beam computed tomography. *International Endodontic Journal*, **45 (5)**, 492–498.

15. Oreadi, D., Hendi, J. & Papageorge, M.B. (2010) A clinico-pathologic correlation. *Journal of the Massachusetts Dental Society*, **59 (3)**, 44–46.

16. Boutsioukis, C., Lambrianidis, T. & Kastrinakis, E. (2009) Irrigant flow within a prepared root canal using various flow rates: a computational fluid dynamics study. *International Endodontic Journal*, **42 (2)**, 144–155.

17. Gulabivala, K., Ng, Y.L., Gilbertson, M. & Eames, I. (2010) The fluid mechanics of root canal irrigation. *Physiological Measurement*, **31 (12)**, R49–R84.

18. Schoeffel, G.J. (2008) The EndoVac method of endodontic irrigation, part 2—efficacy. *Dentistry Today*, **27 (1**, 82, 84, 86, 87).

19. Vera, J., Arias, A. & Romero, M. (2012) Dynamic movement of intracanal gas bubbles during cleaning and shaping procedures: the effect of maintaining apical patency on their presence in the middle and cervical thirds of human root canals-an in vivo study. *Journal of Endodontics*, **38 (2)**, 200–203.

20. Abou-Rass, M. & Piccinino, M.V. (1982) The effectiveness of four clinical irrigation methods on the removal of root canal debris. *Oral Surgery, Oral Medicine, and Oral Pathology*, **54 (3)**, 323–328.

21. Desai, P. & Himel, V. (2009) Comparative safety of various intracanal irrigation systems. *Journal of Endodontics*, **35 (4)**, 545–549.

22. Munoz, H.R. & Camacho-Cuadra, K. (2012) In vivo efficacy of three different endodontic irrigation systems for irrigant delivery to working length of mesial canals of mandibular molars. *Journal of Endodontics*, **38 (4)**, 445–448.

23. Gondim, E. Jr., Setzer, F.C., Dos Carmo, C.B. & Kim, S. (2010) Postoperative pain after the application of two different irrigation devices in a prospective randomized clinical trial. *Journal of Endodontics*, **36 (8)**, 1295–1301.

24. Hockett, J.L., Dommisch, J.K., Johnson, J.D. & Cohenca, N. (2008) Antimicrobial efficacy of two irrigation techniques in tapered and nontapered

canal preparations: an in vitro study. *Journal of Endodontics*, **34 (11)**, 1374–1377.

25. Cohenca, N., Paranjpe, A., Heilborn, C. & Johnson, J.D. (2013) Antimicrobial efficacy of two irrigation techniques in tapered and non-tapered canal preparations. A randomized controlled clinical trial. *Quintessence International*, **44 (3)**, 217–228.

26. Brunson, M., Heilborn, C., Johnson, D.J. & Cohenca, N. (2010) Effect of apical preparation size and preparation taper on irrigant volume delivered by using negative pressure irrigation system. *Journal of Endodontics*, **36 (4)**, 721–724.

27. Miller, T.A. & Baumgartner, J.C. (2010) Comparison of the antimicrobial efficacy of irrigation using the EndoVac to endodontic needle delivery. *Journal of Endodontics*, **36 (3)**, 509–511.

28. Pawar, R., Alqaied, A., Safavi, K., Boyko, J. & Kaufman, B. (2012) Influence of an apical negative pressure irrigation system on bacterial elimination during endodontic therapy: a prospective randomized clinical study. *Journal of Endodontics*, **38 (9)**, 1177–1181.

29. Clegg, M.S., Vertucci, F.J., Walker, C., Belanger, M. & Britto, L.R. (2006) The effect of exposure to irrigant solutions on apical dentin biofilms in vitro. *Journal of Endodontics*, **32 (5)**, 434–437.

30. Nielsen, B.A. & Craig Baumgartner, J. (2007) Comparison of the EndoVac system to needle irrigation of root canals. *Journal of Endodontics*, **33 (5)**, 611–615.

31. Susin, L., Liu, Y., Yoon, J.C. et al. (2010) Canal and isthmus debridement efficacies of two irrigant agitation techniques in a closed system. *International Endodontic Journal*, **43 (12)**, 1077–1090.

32. Parente, J.M., Loushine, R.J., Susin, L. et al. (2010) Root canal debridement using manual dynamic agitation or the EndoVac for final irrigation in a closed system and an open system. *International Endodontic Journal*, **43 (11)**, 1001–1012.

33. Heilborn, C., Reynolds, K., Johnson, J.D. & Cohenca, N. (2010) Cleaning efficacy of an apical negative-pressure irrigation system at different exposure times. *Quintessence International*, **41 (9)**, 759–767.

34. Ribeiro, E.M., Silva-Sousa, Y.T., Souza-Gabriel, A.E., Sousa-Neto, M.D., Lorencetti, K.T. & Silva, S.R. (2012) Debris and smear removal in flattened root canals after use of different irrigant agitation protocols. *Microscopy Research and Technique*, **75 (6)**, 781–790.

35. da Silva, L.A., Nelson-Filho, P., da Silva, R.A. et al. (2010) Revascularization and periapical repair after endodontic treatment using apical negative pressure irrigation versus conventional irrigation plus triantibiotic intracanal dressing in dogs' teeth with apical periodontitis. *Oral Surgery, Oral Medicine,*

Oral Pathology, Oral Radiology, and Endodontics, **109 (5)**, 779–787.

36. Cohenca, N., Heilborn, C., Johnson, J.D., Flores, D.S., Ito, I.Y. & da Silva, L.A. (2010) Apical negative pressure irrigation versus conventional irrigation plus triantibiotic intracanal dressing on root canal disinfection in dog teeth. *Oral Surgery, Oral Medicine, Oral Pathology, Oral Radiology, and Endodontics*, **109 (1)**, e42–e46.

37. Torabinejad, M., Cho, Y., Khademi, A.A., Bakland, L.K. & Shabahang, S. (2003) The effect of various concentrations of sodium hypochlorite on the ability of MTAD to remove the smear layer. *Journal of Endodontics*, **29 (4)**, 233–239.

38. Tay, F.R., Gu, L.S., Schoeffel, G.J. *et al.* (2010) Effect of vapor lock on root canal debridement by using a side-vented needle for positive-pressure irrigant delivery. *Journal of Endodontics*, **36 (4)**, 745–750.

39. Fukumoto, Y. (2005) Intracanal aspiration technique for root canal irrigation: evaluation of smear layer removal. *Kōkūbyō Gakkai Zasshi*, **72 (1)**, 13–18.

40. Fukumoto, Y., Kikuchi, I., Yoshioka, T., Kobayashi, C. & Suda, H. (2006) An ex vivo evaluation of a new root canal irrigation technique with intracanal aspiration. *International Endodontic Journal*, **39 (2)**, 93–99.

41. Goode, N., Khan, S., Eid, A.A. *et al.* (2013) Wall shear stress effects of different endodontic irrigation techniques and systems. *Journal of Dentistry*, **41 (7)**, 636–641.

42. Malentacca, A., Uccioli, U., Zangari, D., Lajolo, C. & Fabiani, C. (2012) Efficacy and safety of various active irrigation devices when used with either positive or negative pressure: an in vitro study. *Journal of Endodontics*, **38 (12)**, 1622–1626.

43. de Gregorio, C., Estevez, R., Cisneros, R., Paranjpe, A. & Cohenca, N. (2010) Efficacy of different irrigation and activation systems on the penetration of sodium hypochlorite into simulated lateral canals and up to working length: an in vitro study. *Journal of Endodontics*, **36 (7)**, 1216–1221.

44. Pashley, E.L., Birdsong, N.L., Bowman, K. & Pashley, D.H. (1985) Cytotoxic effects of NaOCl on vital tissue. *Journal of Endodontics*, **11 (12)**, 525–528.

45. van der Sluis, L.W., Wu, M.K. & Wesselink, P.R. (2005) The efficacy of ultrasonic irrigation to remove artificially placed dentine debris from human root canals prepared using instruments of varying taper. *International Endodontic Journal*, **38 (10)**, 764–768.

46. Lee, S.J., Wu, M.K. & Wesselink, P.R. (2004) The efficacy of ultrasonic irrigation to remove artificially placed dentine debris from different-sized simulated plastic root canals. *International Endodontic Journal*, **37 (9)**, 607–612.

47. Al-Jadaa, A., Paque, F., Attin, T. & Zehnder, M. (2009) Necrotic pulp tissue dissolution by passive ultrasonic irrigation in simulated accessory canals: impact of canal location and angulation. *International Endodontic Journal*, **42 (1)**, 59–65.

48. Al-Jadaa, A., Paque, F., Attin, T. & Zehnder, M. (2009) Acoustic hypochlorite activation in simulated curved canals. *Journal of Endodontics*, **35 (10)**, 1408–1411.

49. van der Sluis, L.W., Versluis, M., Wu, M.K. & Wesselink, P.R. (2007) Passive ultrasonic irrigation of the root canal: a review of the literature. *International Endodontic Journal*, **40 (6)**, 415–426.

50. de Gregorio, C., Paranjpe, A., Garcia, A. *et al.* (2012) Efficacy of irrigation systems on penetration of sodium hypochlorite to working length and to simulated uninstrumented areas in oval shaped root canals. *International Endodontic Journal*, **45 (5)**, 475–481.

51. Paranjpe, A., de Gregorio, C., Gonzalez, A.M. *et al.* (2012) Efficacy of the self-adjusting file system on cleaning and shaping oval canals: a microbiological and microscopic evaluation. *Journal of Endodontics*, **38 (2)**, 226–231.

52. Spoorthy, E., Velmurugan, N., Ballal, S. & Nandini, S. (2013) Comparison of irrigant penetration up to working length and into simulated lateral canals using various irrigating techniques. *International Endodontic Journal*, **46 (9)**, 815–822.

53. Malki, M., Verhaagen, B., Jiang, L.M. *et al.* (2012) Irrigant flow beyond the insertion depth of an ultrasonically oscillating file in straight and curved root canals: visualization and cleaning efficacy. *Journal of Endodontics*, **38 (5)**, 657–661.

54. Senia, E.S., Marshall, F.J. & Rosen, S. (1971) The solvent action of sodium hypochlorite on pulp tissue of extracted teeth. *Oral Surgery, Oral Medicine, and Oral Pathology*, **31 (1)**, 96–103.

55. Svec, T.A. & Harrison, J.W. (1977) Chemomechanical removal of pulpal and dentinal debris with sodium hypochlorite and hydrogen peroxide vs normal saline solution. *Journal of Endodontics*, **3 (2)**, 49–53.

56. Albrecht, L.J., Baumgartner, J.C. & Marshall, J.G. (2004) Evaluation of apical debris removal using various sizes and tapers of ProFile GT files. *Journal of Endodontics*, **30 (6)**, 425–428.

57. Usman, N., Baumgartner, J.C. & Marshall, J.G. (2004) Influence of instrument size on root canal debridement. *Journal of Endodontics*, **30 (2)**, 110–112.

58. Boutsioukis, C., Verhaagen, B., Versluis, M., Kastrinakis, E., Wesselink, P.R. & van der Sluis, L.W. (2010) Evaluation of irrigant flow in the root canal using different needle types by an unsteady computational fluid dynamics model. *Journal of Endodontics*, **36 (5)**, 875–879.

59. Boutsioukis, C., Lambrianidis, T., Verhaagen, B. *et al.* (2010) The effect of needle-insertion depth on the irrigant flow in the root canal: evaluation using an unsteady computational fluid dynamics model. *Journal of Endodontics*, **36 (10)**, 1664–1668.

60. Howard, R.K., Kirkpatrick, T.C., Rutledge, R.E. & Yaccino, J.M. (2011) Comparison of debris removal with three different irrigation techniques. *Journal of Endodontics*, **37 (9)**, 1301–1305.

61. Zhu, W.C., Gyamfi, J., Niu, L.N. *et al.* (2013) Anatomy of sodium hypochlorite accidents involving facial ecchymosis – a review. *Journal of Dentistry*, **41 (11)**, 935–948.

62. Saber Sel, D. & Hashem, A.A. (2011) Efficacy of different final irrigation activation techniques on smear layer removal. *Journal of Endodontics*, **37 (9)**, 1272–1275.

63. Torabinejad, M., Khademi, A.A., Babagoli, J. *et al.* (2003) A new solution for the removal of the smear layer. *Journal of Endodontics*, **29 (3)**, 170–175.

64. Carrigan, P.J., Morse, D.R., Furst, M.L. & Sinai, I.H. (1984) A scanning electron microscopic evaluation of human dentinal tubules according to age and location. *Journal of Endodontics*, **10 (8)**, 359–363.

65. Gómez-Pérez, A. (2009) *Remoción De Barro Dentinario En Tercio Apical Por Medio De Presión Apical Negativa*. Universidad Autónoma De San Luis Potos, San Luis Potosi.

66. Friedman, S., Abitbol, S. & Lawrence, H.P. (2003) Treatment outcome in endodontics: the Toronto Study. Phase 1: initial treatment. *Journal of Endodontics*, **29 (12)**, 787–793.

67. Ricucci, D., Russo, J., Rutberg, M., Burleson, J.A. & Spangberg, L.S. (2011) A prospective cohort study of endodontic treatments of 1,369 root canals: results after 5 years. *Oral Surgery, Oral Medicine, Oral Pathology, Oral Radiology, and Endodontics*, **112 (6)**, 825–842.

68. Su, Y., Wang, C. & Ye, L. (2011) Healing rate and post-obturation pain of single- versus multiple-visit endodontic treatment for infected root canals: a systematic review. *Journal of Endodontics*, **37 (2)**, 125–132.

69. Spangberg, L.S. (2006) Infatuated by Enterococci. *Oral Surgery, Oral Medicine, Oral Pathology, Oral Radiology, and Endodontics*, **102 (5)**, 577–578.

70. Ricucci, D. & Siqueira, J.F. Jr. (2010) Biofilms and apical periodontitis: study of prevalence and association with clinical and histopathologic findings. *Journal of Endodontics*, **36 (8)**, 1277–1288.

71. Del Carpio-Perochena, A.E., Bramante, C.M., Duarte, M.A. *et al.* (2011) Biofilm dissolution and cleaning ability of different irrigant solutions on intraorally infected dentin. *Journal of Endodontics*, **37 (8)**, 1134–1138.

72. Shen, Y., Stojicic, S. & Haapasalo, M. (2011) Antimicrobial efficacy of chlorhexidine against bacteria in biofilms at different stages of development. *Journal of Endodontics*, **37 (5)**, 657–661.

73. Brito, P.R., Souza, L.C., Machado de Oliveira, J.C. *et al.* (2009) Comparison of the effectiveness of three irrigation techniques in reducing intracanal Enterococcus faecalis populations: an in vitro study. *Journal of Endodontics*, **35 (10)**, 1422–1427.

74. Peters, L.B., Wesselink, P.R. & Moorer, W.R. (1995) The fate and the role of bacteria left in root dentinal tubules. *International Endodontic Journal*, **28 (2)**, 95–99.

75. Ricucci, D. & Siqueira, J.F. Jr. (2010) Fate of the tissue in lateral canals and apical ramifications in response to pathologic conditions and treatment procedures. *Journal of Endodontics*, **36 (1)**, 1–15.

76. Markose, G., Cotter, C.J. & Hislop, W.S. (2009) Facial atrophy following accidental subcutaneous extrusion of sodium hypochlorite. *British Dental Journal*, **206 (5)**, 263–264.

77. Witton, R. & Brennan, P.A. (2005) Severe tissue damage and neurological deficit following extravasation of sodium hypochlorite solution during routine endodontic treatment. *British Dental Journal*, **198 (12)**, 749–750.

78. Pelka, M. & Petschelt, A. (2008) Permanent mimic musculature and nerve damage caused by sodium hypochlorite: a case report. *Oral Surgery, Oral Medicine, Oral Pathology, Oral Radiology, and Endodontics*, **106 (3)**, e80–e83.

79. Bowden, J.R., Ethunandan, M. & Brennan, P.A. (2006) Life-threatening airway obstruction secondary to hypochlorite extrusion during root canal treatment. *Oral Surgery, Oral Medicine, Oral Pathology, Oral Radiology, and Endodontics*, **101 (3)**, 402–404.

80. Sabala, C.L. & Powell, S.E. (1989) Sodium hypochlorite injection into periapical tissues. *Journal of Endodontics*, **15 (10)**, 490–492.

81. Drake, R., Vogl, A.W. & Mitchell, A.W.M. (2009) Imaging. In: Drake, R., Vogl, A.W. & Mitchell, A.W.M. (eds), *Gray's Anatomy for Students*. Elsevier, London.

82. Rickles, N.H. & Joshi, B.A. (1963) A possible case in a human and an investigation in dogs of death from air embolism during root canal therapy. *Journal of the American Dental Association*, **67**, 397–404.

83. Jiang, L.M., Lak, B., Eijsvogels, L.M., Wesselink, P. & van der Sluis, L.W. (2012) Comparison of the cleaning efficacy of different final irrigation techniques. *Journal of Endodontics*, **38 (6)**, 838–841.

84. Mitchell, R.P., Yang, S.E. & Baumgartner, J.C. (2010) Comparison of apical extrusion of NaOCl using the EndoVac or needle irrigation of root canals. *Journal of Endodontics*, **36 (2)**, 338–341.

85. Waltimo, T., Trope, M., Haapasalo, M. & Orstavik, D. (2005) Clinical efficacy of treatment procedures in endodontic infection control and one year follow-up of periapical healing. *Journal of Endodontics*, **31 (12)**, 863–866.

86. Kvist, T., Molander, A., Dahlen, G. & Reit, C. (2004) Microbiological evaluation of one- and two-visit endodontic treatment of teeth with apical periodontitis: a randomized, clinical trial. *Journal of Endodontics*, **30 (8)**, 572–576.

87. Gesi, A., Hakeberg, M., Warfvinge, J. & Bergenholtz, G. (2006) Incidence of periapical lesions and clinical symptoms after pulpectomy—a clinical and radiographic evaluation of 1- versus 2-session treatment. *Oral Surgery, Oral Medicine, Oral Pathology, Oral Radiology, and Endodontics*, **101 (3)**, 379–388.

88. Molander, A., Warfvinge, J., Reit, C. & Kvist, T. (2007) Clinical and radiographic evaluation of one- and two-visit endodontic treatment of asymptomatic necrotic teeth with apical periodontitis: a randomized clinical trial. *Journal of Endodontics*, **33 (10)**, 1145–1148.

89. Figini, L., Lodi, G., Gorni, F. & Gagliani, M. (2008) Single versus multiple visits for endodontic treatment of permanent teeth: a Cochrane systematic review. *Journal of Endodontics*, **34 (9)**, 1041–1047.

90. Paredes-Vieyra, J. & Enriquez, F.J. (2012) Success rate of single- versus two-visit root canal treatment of teeth with apical periodontitis: a randomized controlled trial. *Journal of Endodontics*, **38 (9)**, 1164–1169.

91. Tsesis, I., Faivishevsky, V., Fuss, Z. & Zukerman, O. (2008) Flare-ups after endodontic treatment: a meta-analysis of literature. *Journal of Endodontics*, **34 (10)**, 1177–1181.

92. van der Sluis, L.W., Gambarini, G., Wu, M.K. & Wesselink, P.R. (2006) The influence of volume, type of irrigant and flushing method on removing artificially placed dentine debris from the apical root canal during passive ultrasonic irrigation. *International Endodontic Journal*, **39 (6)**, 472–476.

93. van der Sluis, L.W., Wu, M.K. & Wesselink, P.R. (2007) The evaluation of removal of calcium hydroxide paste from an artificial standardized groove in the apical root canal using different irrigation methodologies. *International Endodontic Journal*, **40 (1)**, 52–57.

94. Jiang, L.M., Verhaagen, B., Versluis, M. & van der Sluis, L.W. (2010) Evaluation of a sonic device designed to activate irrigant in the root canal. *Journal of Endodontics*, **36 (1)**, 143–146.

95. Jiang, L.M., Verhaagen, B., Versluis, M., Zangrillo, C., Cuckovic, D. & van der Sluis, L.W. (2010) An evaluation of the effect of pulsed ultrasound on the cleaning efficacy of passive ultrasonic irrigation. *Journal of Endodontics*, **36 (11)**, 1887–1891.

96. Castelo-Baz, P., Martin-Biedma, B., Cantatore, G. et al. (2012) In vitro comparison of passive and continuous ultrasonic irrigation in simulated lateral canals of extracted teeth. *Journal of Endodontics*, **38 (5)**, 688–691.

97. de Gregorio, C., Arias, A., Navarrete, N., Del Rio, V., Oltra, E. & Cohenca, N. (2013) Effect of apical size and taper on volume of irrigant delivered at working length with apical negative pressure at different root curvatures. *Journal of Endodontics*, **39 (1)**, 119–124.

98. Banchs, F. & Trope, M. (2004) Revascularization of immature permanent teeth with apical periodontitis: new treatment protocol? *Journal of Endodontics*, **30 (4)**, 196–200.

99. Shabahang, S. & Torabinejad, M. (2000) Treatment of teeth with open apices using mineral trioxide aggregate. *Practical Periodontics and Aesthetic Dentistry*, **12 (3)**, 315–320, quiz 322.

100. Windley, W. 3rd, Teixeira, F., Levin, L., Sigurdsson, A. & Trope, M. (2005) Disinfection of immature teeth with a triple antibiotic paste. *Journal of Endodontics*, **31 (6)**, 439–443.

101. Eickholz, P., Kim, T.S., Burklin, T. et al. (2002) Non-surgical periodontal therapy with adjunctive topical doxycycline: a double-blind randomized controlled multicenter study. *Journal of Clinical Periodontology*, **29 (2)**, 108–117.

102. Greenstein, G. & Polson, A. (1998) The role of local drug delivery in the management of periodontal diseases: a comprehensive review. *Journal of Periodontology*, **69 (5)**, 507–520.

103. Bhalla, M., Thami, G.P. & Singh, N. (2007) Ciprofloxacin-induced erythema nodosum. *Clinical and Experimental Dermatology*, **32 (1)**, 115–116.

104. de Paz, S., Perez, A., Gomez, M., Trampal, A. & Dominguez Lazaro, A. (1999) Severe hypersensitivity reaction to minocycline. *Journal of Investigational Allergology and Clinical Immunology*, **9 (6)**, 403–404.

105. Hausermann, P., Scherer, K., Weber, M. & Bircher, A.J. (2005) Ciprofloxacin-induced acute generalized exanthematous pustulosis mimicking bullous drug eruption confirmed by a positive patch test. *Dermatology*, **211 (3)**, 277–280.

106. Isik, S.R., Karakaya, G., Erkin, G. & Kalyoncu, A.F. (2007) Multidrug-induced erythema multiforme. *Journal of Investigational Allergology and Clinical Immunology*, **17 (3)**, 196–198.

107. Penesis, V.A., Fitzgerald, P.I., Fayad, M.I., Wenckus, C.S., BeGole, E.A. & Johnson, B.R. (2008) Outcome of one-visit and two-visit endodontic treatment of necrotic teeth with apical periodontitis: a randomized controlled trial with one-year evaluation. *Journal of Endodontics*, **34 (3)**, 251–257.

11 Disinfection of the Root Canal System by Sonic, Ultrasonic, and Laser Activated Irrigation

Luc van der Sluis

Department of Conservative Dentistry, Center for Dentistry and Oral Hygiene, University Medical Center, Groningen, The Netherlands

Bram Verhaagen

MIRA Institute for Biomedical Technology and Technical Medicine en MESA+ Institute for Nanotechnology, University of Twente, Enschede, The Netherlands

Ricardo G. Macedo

The Academic Centre for Dentistry in Amsterdam (ACTA), University of Amsterdam, Amsterdam, The Netherlands

Michel Versluis

MIRA Institute for Biomedical Technology and Technical Medicine en MESA+ Institute for Nanotechnology, University of Twente, Enschede, The Netherlands

Introduction

Apical periodontitis (AP) is defined as an oral inflammatory disease caused by a reaction of the host immune system to the presence of microorganisms (planktonic state or biofilm) or their products that are close to or in the root canal system or at the outside around the root apex (1). The goal of a root canal treatment is to prevent or heal AP; therefore, the microorganisms in both planktonic and biofilm state should be removed from the root canal system. Unfortunately, because of the complexity of the root canal system containing isthmuses, oval extensions, and lateral canals, a complete removal of biofilm from the root canal system is not feasible during a root canal treatment (1). Furthermore, the tooth and root structure consist of dentin, a porous material containing tubules with a typical

Disinfection of Root Canal Systems: The Treatment of Apical Periodontitis, First Edition. Edited by Nestor Cohenca.
© 2014 John Wiley & Sons, Inc. Published 2014 by John Wiley & Sons, Inc.

diameter of 0.6–3.2 μm and length of 1–2 mm and are accessible for microorganisms (1). Therefore, minimization of the number of microorganisms after treatment should be attempted.

A noninstrumentation technique to clean the root canal system would be ideal. This would avoid instrumentation-related disadvantages like smear layer and dentin debris production, iatrogenic errors, weakening of the root structure, and apical crack formation (2–5). This was recognized by Lussi and coworkers (6) who introduced an irrigation device for root canal cleaning without instrumentation. Promising results (*in-vitro* and *in-vivo*) were published; however, it was found that further improvements were needed and hence the system is currently not commercially available (7). Establishing an alternating negative and positive pressure that would enable an effective irrigation procedure without instrumentation and extrusion of the irrigant seems, for the moment, not to be possible. Therefore, it is still necessary to create space in the root canal system with instruments to be able to apply disinfection solutions or medicaments.

When the root canal system is infected, dentin debris and the smear layer also are infected, unfortunately. The smear layer can be defined as a mixture of dentin debris, remnants of pulp tissue, odontoblastic processes, and microorganisms (if present), which are strongly attached to the root canal wall and can penetrate up to 40 μm into the dentinal tubules (2, 8). Dentin debris may be defined as dentin chips, tissue remnants, and particles attached to the root canal wall or present in the root canal. Both dentin debris and smear layer can inactivate the root canal medicaments and irrigants and block their access to the biofilm (9). Recently, it was shown that the production of dentin debris and the subsequent blockage of isthmuses may be a larger problem than anticipated (10). After the first instrument is used in the root canal, the wall is covered with an infected smear layer at the sites where the file touches the canal wall. At these sites, the biofilm is mechanically disrupted but also merges with the smear layer. At the sites where the files do not touch the walls, biofilm is present, possibly covered with or blocked by dentin debris. This typical situation hinders disinfection procedures, and consequently the removal of dentin debris and smear layer plays a crucial role in the disinfection process.

Smear layer, dentin debris, and untouched biofilm can be removed only by irrigation. For an effective irrigation procedure, both the *mechanical* detachment of pulp tissue, dentin debris and smear layer (instrumentation products), microorganisms (planktonic or biofilm) and their products (now on referred to as *substrate*) from the root canal wall, their removal out of the root canal system, and the *chemical* dissolution or disruption are important. Both these mechanical and chemical aspects are related to the flow of the irrigant. Furthermore, irrigants are chemically inactivated after their reaction with the biofilm and therefore need to be mixed with fresh irrigants. Consequently, insight in the flow of the irrigant during a root canal treatment is crucial to understand the importance of the disinfection of the root canal system.

The objectives of irrigation are to create a flow that

- goes to the full extent of the root canal system, in order to come in close contact with the substrate, carry away the substrate, and provide lubrication for the instruments.
- ensures an adequate delivery throughout the root canal system, refreshment, and mixing of the irrigant, in order to retain an effective concentration of the active chemical component(s) and compensate for its rapid inactivation.
- ensures a force on the root canal wall (wall shear and normal stress), in order to detach/disrupt the substrate.
- is restricted within the constraints of the root canal, thus preventing irrigant extrusion toward the apical tissues.

During the irrigation procedure, two phases can be distinguished: a flow phase, during which the irrigant is delivered and flows in and out of the root canal, and a rest phase, where the irrigant is at rest in the root canal. As syringe irrigation alone has control concerning the flow produced (11), activation of the irrigant could help to improve irrigant delivery throughout the root canal system and also enhance the mixing, refreshment, and the chemical properties of the irrigant. Irrigant activation systems introduce an additional activation phase, enhancing the streaming of the irrigant by an energy source. This chapter discusses the operational characteristics, fluid dynamics, and mechanical and chemical interactions involved with sonic, ultrasonic, and laser activated irrigation (LAI).

Research evaluating the smear layer of the root canal wall is not discussed in this chapter because the reliability of the methodology is not fully developed (12).

Mechanical properties of biofilms in relation to fluid dynamics

As described in another chapter, biofilm consists of a substantial extracellular matrix of mainly proteins and polysaccharides (EPS, extracellular polymeric substance), which effectively protects microorganisms (13). The EPS can make up more than 80% of the biofilm content, which makes the biofilm a viscoelastic fluid (14), causing it to exhibit elastic behavior at low stress and viscous flow behavior at high stress (15), thereby protecting the contained bacteria. Therefore, in order to obtain an effective disinfection, disintegration of the matrix structure is essential. Its specific constitution depends mainly on the type of the microbial species (e.g., in one root canal, around 600 bacterial species have been found (16)) and the environmental conditions during growth such as nutrition and typical substances present (17). For example, metal ions like Ca^{++} can be incorporated in the matrix, causing cross-links of the negative binding sides of polysaccharides thus reinforcing the matrix (18).

Forces on the biofilm exerted by irrigant flow could disrupt the top layers of biofilm, or its EPS matrix (cohesive failure), or could completely remove the biofilm (adhesive failure). Disruption of the top layers or EPS matrix facilitates irrigant penetration in the biofilm and could therefore enhance the chemical effect of the irrigants. However, not much information is available in the literature on the effect of fluid flow on a biofilm, mainly because of a large variety in constituents and associated physical properties, which makes it a difficult multidisciplinary subject. Furthermore, measurement of the mechanical properties should take place on a short time scale (within minutes), because the biofilm is a living organism and will adapt to its environment (19). Critical loads necessary to disrupt biofilms by a variety of different techniques have recently been reviewed

(20). It was found that the sensitivity to certain loading modes, such as normal or shear stresses, varies extensively among biofilms. Furthermore, the reported values of adhesion strength depend greatly on the testing technique, which range from coarse macroscale measurements down to atomic force microscopy (AFM) operating on a nanoscale (20). Typical values found in the literature give an elastic modulus of the order of 10^{-1} to 10^2 Pa and a cohesive shear strength of 10^1 to 10^3 Pa (19–21). Pressures and shear stresses produced by different irrigation techniques show that some techniques are able to remove biofilm completely (Table 11.1). Unfortunately, the mechanical properties of an endodontic biofilm are not known; therefore, a prediction of the effect of fluidic stresses on biofilm removal in the root canal is not yet possible.

Recently, a 3D numerical study on the effect of fluid flow on biofilm has shown that for high EPS matrix stability, only exposed structures at the surface of the biofilm are detached. Low EPS matrix stabilities might lead to the detachment of large portions from the top of the biofilm (Figure 11.1). Interestingly, it has been observed that a smooth basal biofilm surface structure remains after detachment (26). This is confirmed by another study where smooth base biofilms remain after the biofilm had been subjected to high shear stresses using the fluid dynamic gauging (FDG) technique (27). These observations can be explained by the stratification of biofilms, which leaves older, stronger layers at the base of the biofilm, typically adhering strongly to the substrate (27, 28). Therefore, complete removal of biofilm from the root canal wall could be a difficult task and a combination of mechanical *and* chemical stress on the biofilm remains crucial. Figure 11.2 shows the possible biofilm removal mechanisms related to irrigant flow.

Sonic, ultrasonic, and laser activated irrigation systems

Sonic activation: operational characteristics

Sonic activation makes use of instruments that have an enforced vibration at one end (at the handpiece) and are allowed to vibrate freely at the other end. Sonic devices operate at audible frequencies

Table 11.1 Characteristics of irrigation and irrigant activation techniques, assuming a root canal of size #35/0.06 filled with water.

Technique	Characteristics	Fluid velocity	Shear stress	Pressure
Positive pressure syringe irrigation *Flow through a needle*	Needle size: 27–31 G Flow rate: 0.2 ml/s (Boutsioukis et al. (11))	*Inside the needle:* 10 m/s (Boutsioukis et al. (11)) *Outside the needle:* depends strongly on needle type and location in the root canal Limited flow into lateral canals	Up to 500 N/m² Shear stress distribution depends on needle type, but highest near outlet (Boutsioukis et al. (11))	*Apical pressure:* ca. 10 kPa (Boutsioukis et al. (11))
Negative-pressure syringe irrigation *Flow aspirated through a needle*	Flow rate: 0.05 ml/s (Brunson et al. (29)) Needle size: 30 G	*Inside needle:* 1 m/s *Outside needle:* 0.2 m/s between the needle and the walls; apical area unknown Limited flow into lateral canals	Up to 100 N/m² Highest near the tip of the microcannula	*Apical pressure:* Unknown, but expected to be small
Sonic activated irrigation *Oscillation of a plastic tip*	Frequency: ca. 100 Hz Amplitude: ca. 1 mm File diameter: 200 µm (Data for EndoActivator) (Jiang et al. (22)) Oscillating file has one node and one antinode	Steady: (does not exist) Oscillating: 1 m/s, only near the free end of the plastic tip	Steady: (does not exist) Oscillating: 8 N/m² (if it could oscillate unconstrained) Highest shear stress near the tip	*Next to tip:* Steady: (does not exist) Oscillatory: 7 Pa *Apical pressure:* Unknown, but expected to be small
Ultrasonic activated irrigation *Oscillation of a file*	Frequency: 30 kHz Amplitude: 50 µm File diameter: 200 µm Oscillating file has around 6 nodes and 6 antinodes, with a spacing of ca. 5 mm (Verhaagen et al. (23))	Steady: 2.5 m/s Oscillating: 10 m/s Maximum velocities at each antinode; decreasing toward the nodes Jets in the direction of oscillation	Steady: 3000 N/m² Oscillating: 2 N/m² Highest shear stresses at each antinode	*Next to oscillating file:* Steady: 3 kPa Oscillating: 9 kPa *Apical pressure:* Unknown, but expected to be small
Laser activated irrigation *Transmission of laser energy into the irrigant*	Laser type: Er:YAG Laser energy: <250 ml/pulse Pulse repetition rate: 1–25 Hz (De Groot et al. (24))	Bubble collapse with velocities of 1–10 m/s (Blanken and Verdaasdonk (25), De Groot et al. (24))	1000 N/m² (De Groot et al. (24))	*Apical pressure:* Unknown, but irrigant extrusion is reported (George et al. 30)

220

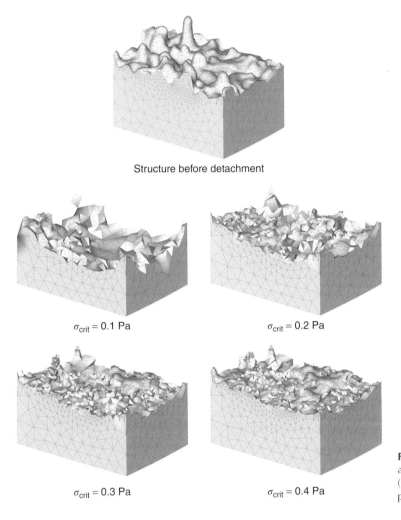

Structure before detachment

σ_{crit} = 0.1 Pa

σ_{crit} = 0.2 Pa

σ_{crit} = 0.3 Pa

σ_{crit} = 0.4 Pa

Figure 11.1 Biofilm structure before and after detachment at different strengths σ_{crit}. (Böl *et al.* (26) Figure 7. Reproduced with permission of John Wiley and Sons, Inc.)

(below 20 kHz) and have file oscillation amplitudes up to 1 mm (22). The sonically driven instruments exhibit a simple bending pattern, consisting of a large amplitude at the tip (antinode) and a small amplitude at the driven end (node) where the piezo-actuation takes place (31) (Figure 11.3). Because the amplitude at the antinode may be as large as 1 mm, which is larger than the diameter of a root canal, frequent wall contact occurs resulting in reduced effectiveness (22).

Ultrasonic activation: operational characteristics

Like sonic activation, the instruments used during ultrasonic activation have an enforced vibration at one end (at the handpiece) and are allowed to vibrate freely at the other end. Ultrasonic devices operate at higher frequencies (typically 20–200 kHz) and have amplitudes less than 100 μm (23, 32, 33). The higher frequency employed by ultrasonic activation leads to a more complex pattern of nodes and antinodes than those of sonic devices. Instruments driven by a piezo-electric element near 30 kHz exhibit a pattern of approximately three wavelengths, or six nodes and antinodes spaced approximately 5 mm apart (23) (Figure 11.3). The exact oscillation pattern depends on the instrument geometry and material. The oscillation amplitude of the tip of such instruments is on the order of 10–100 μm in the direction of oscillation; there is also an oscillation

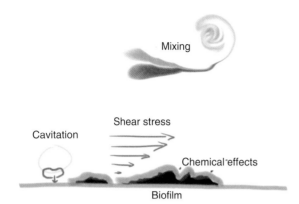

Figure 11.2 Sketch of the removed mechanisms of a biofilm from a surface. The biofilm may be attacked chemically, after which the consumed irrigant has to be replaced by mixing with fresh irrigant. Refreshment of the irrigant involves a flow that exerts shear stress on the wall. Finally, cavitation (formation and collapse of bubbles) may enhance the biofilm removal locally.

perpendicular to the main oscillation direction with a relative amplitude of approximately 10% (23, 34).

The cross-section of instruments available for ultrasonic activation is circular or square. Instruments with a square cross-section are mostly cutting because they are originally used for instrumentation of the root canal and consequently have an associated risk of damage to the root canal wall when used for irrigation purposes. In 1980, Weller *et al.* (35) proposed a smooth instrument and intentional wall contact; however, it was shown later that when intentional contact was prevented, irrigant streaming improved (36). Recently, it has been demonstrated in an *in-vitro* study involving 30 endodontists that contact with a root canal wall nearly always takes place, albeit unintentional. The amount of contact depends not only on the power setting used, but also on the instrument stiffness and on the force with which the instrument is pushed against the root canal wall. But light contact should not affect its cleaning mechanisms of streaming and cavitation, as the file oscillation is not damped out. Instead, it builds up a secondary oscillation at audible frequencies during which the file displaces away from the wall and keeps oscillating at the driving ultrasonic frequency (37). The term *ultrasonic activated irrigation* (*UAI*) has been suggested to replace *passive ultrasonic irrigation* (*PUI*) in order to avoid confusion.

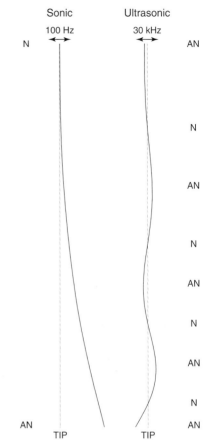

Figure 11.3 The sonically and ultrasonically driven instruments exhibit distinct patterns of nodes (N) and antinodes (AN). The exact pattern depends on the file geometry and material properties. The displacement is largest at the tip.

Laser activation: operational characteristics

Another technique for cleaning the root canal system is LAI, which employs laser energy to agitate the irrigant. These lasers are typically of the type Er:YAG or ErCrYSGG, with a wavelength in the infrared region (2796–2940 nm) that is absorbed well in water (38). The dynamics of LAI have been studied using high-speed imaging (24, 25) showing the generation and implosion of a large vapor bubble at the tip of the fiber, generated by the absorption of laser energy and fast heating of the irrigant. The collapse of this bubble may induce a shock wave and additional bubbles throughout the root canal system. The laser fiber tip may be placed near the apex of the root canal, or in the pulp chamber with normal fibers or specially developed fibers (photon-initiated photoacoustic streaming, PIPS) (39, 40).

Laser activated irrigation is an indirect technique, not relying on direct ablation of the biomaterial.

Flow characterization during sonic, ultrasonic, and laser activated irrigation

Sonic and ultrasonic activation

The sonic or ultrasonic oscillation of an instrument induces streaming of the fluid around it, which leads to alternating pressures and shear stresses on the root canal wall. The streaming also gives rise to the mixing of the irrigant, so that irrigant consumed during its reaction with biomaterial is replaced by fresh irrigant. When ultrasonically activated needles or a continuous flow in the pulp chamber is used, the irrigant will also be refreshed.

The pattern of nodes and antinodes along the instrument determines the flow around the file in the axial direction (Figure 11.4). The single antinode and node displayed by instruments driven sonically can induce a flow from the tip to the driven end of the file. The multitude of antinodes and nodes on an ultrasonically driven instrument leads to a more complex pattern of microstreaming along the instrument. The lateral flow induced by both instruments is advantageous for cleaning lateral extensions (lateral canals, isthmuses, oval extensions) of the root canal (41), which are difficult to clean with a flow created by positive (syringe) or negative pressure irrigation (41).

Neither sonic nor ultrasonic activation introduces a large fluid velocity into the apical direction (42), making extrusion of the irrigant unlikely. On the other hand, it necessitates the placement of these files near the apex. Nevertheless, the mixing and refreshment of irrigants and dentin debris removal take place when the ultrasonically activated instrument is inserted until 3 mm from working length (43).

The curvature of a root canal may affect the cleaning of the apical area (44), mostly because of the limited access for the instrument. When an

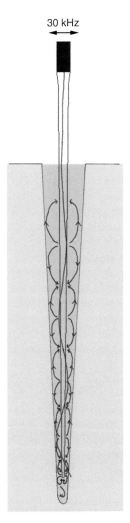

30 kHz

Figure 11.4 Microstreaming (blue arrows) induced inside a root canal model by an ultrasonically oscillating file that exhibits a pattern of nodes and antinodes (red line).

instrument is inserted to or near working length, its oscillation may be affected by severe contact or binding of the instrument with the root canal wall (45). Therefore, it is advised to insert the ultrasonically driven instrument just in the beginning of the curvature without bending the instrument. The flow itself should not be affected by the curvature, because the radius of curvature is typically much larger than the scale on which the streaming takes place (43).

Increasing the intensity of the ultrasound will result in more effective cleaning (46).

Acoustic streaming

Lateral streaming is induced at each of the antinodes along the file; this lateral component of the flow is typically much stronger than the axial component. Acoustic streaming is a phenomenon already introduced in 1884 by Rayleigh (47) and extended to the case of a cylinder oscillating with high amplitude (48) inside another cylinder (49, 50). Ultrasonic cleaning with acoustic streaming induced by an oscillating cylindrical object was already described by Williams and Nyborg in 1970 (51, 52), who used a thin, oscillating capillary or tungsten wire to remove biomaterial from a surface.

Typically, acoustic streaming is a superposition of two flows, one being an oscillatory component and the other a steady component whose strengths depend on the oscillation amplitude. A simple theory of acoustic streaming was used by Ahmad and coworkers (53) to support ultrasonic activation in endodontics; however, only the steady part of the flow was considered. It was shown recently that it is crucial to also include the oscillatory component (54) (Figure 11.5).

The oscillatory part of the acoustic streaming makes the flow oscillate forward and backward together with the file. In doing so, the fluid exerts an alternating pressure and shear stress on (the material on) the root canal wall. The fluid near the file oscillates with the same velocity (u_o) as the file

$$u_0 = A\omega, \qquad (11.1)$$

where A is the oscillation amplitude (in m) and ω the oscillation frequency (in Hz). This velocity decreases rapidly with the distance from the file. The pressure and shear stress on a nearby wall can be of the order of 100 and 1 kPa, respectively (54), which is larger than the typical biofilm attachment strengths as reported earlier. The values for the pressure and the shear stress are similar to those reported for syringe irrigation using a very high flow rate (0.26 ml/s) (11); however, for syringe irrigation these forces occur only near the outlet of the needle, whereas for ultrasonic activation these forces are present near every nodal section of the instrument. The oscillatory nature of the pressure and the shear stress may furthermore induce fatigue to the material that needs to be removed from the root canal wall (19). However, as the oscillatory component decreases rapidly with

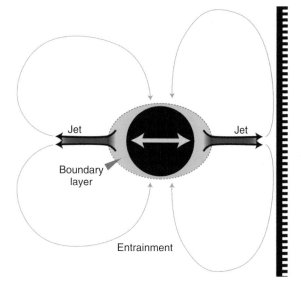

Figure 11.5   Schematic representation of the acoustic streaming that is induced by an ultrasonically oscillating instrument (black circle). Near the instrument there is a boundary layer in which the fluid oscillates together with the file (oscillatory component). In the direction of oscillation, jets are formed (steady component) that may impact on a nearby root canal wall and flow back toward the file (steady component) (entrainment).

distance from the oscillating file, this effect is most pronounced when the file is close to the wall.

Nonlinear effects of the fluid lead to a steady (nonoscillatory) streaming (jets) in the direction of oscillation (55), with a velocity u_s:

$$u_s = \frac{3}{4}\frac{\omega y^2}{R} \qquad (11.2)$$

where ω is the oscillation frequency (in Hz), y the oscillation amplitude (in m), and R the radius of the file (in m). The jet velocity is typically 1 m/s and increases with increasing amplitude or power setting (46).

This steady part of the flow is doing the actual transport and mixing of the fluid. The jets also exert a pressure (1 kPa) and shear stress (10 Pa) onto (the material on) the wall (54) even at relatively large distances from the instrument as the velocity of the jet decreases only slowly with increasing distance from the file. These values can be one or two orders of magnitude lower than the oscillatory components, depending on the proximity of the root canal wall, which has a significant effect on the streaming. The pressure is highest in the center of the jet; the shear stress is highest off-center, at a distance of 0.1 times the distance between the oscillating file and the wall (56, 57). Because of these jets, the direction of oscillation of the file should be taken into account in particular when cleaning oval canals, isthmuses, and lateral canals (55).

Acoustic streaming is induced for all of the cross-sectional designs of the current instruments, although the details of the streaming may change (58). Acoustic streaming or cavitation (see "Cavitation" section) is not possible for sonic activation because its frequency and associated oscillatory velocity are too low (22).

Cavitation

During the high-amplitude oscillation of the instrument during ultrasonic activation, *cavitation* may be induced. Cavitation is defined as the nucleation, the growth, and collapse of bubbles within a liquid (59, 60).

In order to create a vapor bubble, the stress within the liquid has to be larger than the tensile strength of the liquid, which is of the order of 10^7 Pa for pure water (61). However, in nonpure water (tap water, distilled water), there are often tiny pockets (*cavitation nuclei*) with entrapped gas on surfaces of walls or particles, from which it is much easier to grow bubbles (a process called *heterogeneous cavitation*), as only the ambient pressure of 10^5 Pa (plus the vapor pressure of 10^3 Pa) has to be overcome (59). The typical velocity u necessary to generate this negative pressure ΔP in a liquid of density ρ can be estimated from the Bernoulli relation:

$$\Delta P = \frac{1}{2}\rho u^2 \qquad (11.3)$$

In water, the velocity threshold is around 15 m/s, which is feasible with the current endodontic ultrasonic devices, but not with sonic devices (62).

Bubbles grow during the negative phase of a pressure wave and collapse when the pressure becomes positive. Near a solid hard wall, bubbles tend to collapse in the direction of the wall. Alternatively, during bubble collapse next to a soft wall (like a biofilm covering a wall), the soft material might be pulled from the wall toward the bubble (63). High-velocity jets (hundreds of meters per second), with associated local pressures of 1 GPa and shear stresses of 1 MPa (64) and shock waves, are reported to accompany the bubble collapse a.k.a. *the water hammer effect* (59, 65).

The bubble collapse can also trigger a couple of consecutive bubble growths and collapses, until it is damped out. The violent inertial bubble collapse is called *transient cavitation* and is associated with surface cleaning (66–68), medical therapy, surface erosion (64, 69), and other mechanical effects of ultrasonic cleaning (67). Severe cavitation damage to ship propellers was in fact the phenomenon that led Rayleigh to start investigating bubble dynamics (70).

Cavitation on or very close to endodontic instruments has been observed in a number of studies (46, 71–73), especially at regions with high-velocity gradients, such as near the sharp edges of files with a square cross-section (cutting files) (Figure 11.6). However, its contribution to cleaning in endodontics is not yet clear (71). Earlier studies have ruled out cavitation as a significant contribution to root canal cleaning (71, 72) whereas recent articles with newer ultrasound systems show otherwise (74, 62). High-speed imaging has revealed that a cloud of cavitation bubbles is generated around the tip of the instrument and that small, single bubbles occur around other antinodes on the instrument. The latter have been demonstrated to be sonochemically active. Parallel shaped instruments generate more cavitation around the antinodes alongside the instrument (62). A smaller confinement (i.e., a narrower root canal) increases the amount of cavitation. Irrigants with surface-active properties, such as NaOCl, may affect the bubble formation and collapse and therefore lead to a larger bubble cloud consisting of much smaller bubbles (62). In *in-vitro* models, the bubble cloud, however, collapses only onto the file and not onto a neighboring wall. Therefore, its contribution to root canal cleaning is still under debate. The cleaning efficacy mechanism could be different when the wall consists purely of dentin or when it is covered with a biofilm.

Bubbles do not necessarily need to collapse. Gas-filled bubbles may be stable for a relatively long time and oscillate together with the oscillating pressure field induced by the oscillating file. Even if this pressure field by itself is too low to induce any cleaning, this stable cavitation can enhance the streaming and consequently the cleaning locally

30 kHz

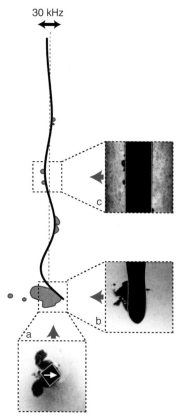

Figure 11.6 Sketch and short-exposure photos of the occurrence of cavitation (in red) along an ultrasonically oscillating file. At the tip there is a large bubble cloud ((a) viewed toward the tip, (b) viewed from the side; at other antinodes there are single, smaller bubbles (c).

significantly, through unsteady oscillations of the bubble shape (59, 75). Assistance in cleaning by a stable cavitation bubble was described already in 1958 by Jackson and Nyborg (76) and was recently also observed near an ultrasonically oscillating endodontic file near a layer of viscoelastic hydrogel (77). These stable gas bubbles may be introduced via entrainment through file-induced instabilities at the irrigant-air interface (62) or during gas-forming reactions of the irrigant with organic material (77, 78).

Stable bubbles oscillate optimally when they are at resonance with the ultrasound, which in water may be approximated with (59):

$$R_{bubble} = \frac{3.3 \text{ mmkHz}}{f} \qquad (11.4)$$

For ultrasound with a frequency of $f = 30$ kHz, bubbles are driven optimally when they have a radius of $R = 100$ μm. As stable bubbles dissolve slowly over time, their behavior is time-dependent, which is why the resting time between ultrasonic activations (or pulsations) may be important (79).

Laser activation irrigation

The dynamics of LAI have been studied using high-speed imaging (24, 25) that shows the generation and implosion of a large vapor bubble at the tip of the fiber, generated by the absorption of laser energy and fast heating of the irrigant (Figure 11.7). The size of the laser-generated bubble depends on the output energy, pulse duration, and frequency of the laser and absorption cross-section of the irrigant for the wavelength of the laser. The collapse of the laser-induced bubble pulls fluid from the coronal and the apical part toward the bubble center and thereby induces fluid velocities of several meters per second. This flow is associated with a strong shear stress (on the order of 1 kPa) on the wall, which is favorable for cleaning (24). The last stage of the bubble collapse was also observed to induce a shock wave that causes cavitation throughout the root canal, which may further enhance the cleaning of the root canal walls. Furthermore, stable bubbles that are already present in the root canal are driven by the pressure changes from the growth and collapse of the laser-induced bubble and may thereby enhance locally the streaming and associated cleaning. The exact cleaning mechanisms during LAI or PIPS are not fully clarified.

The bubble growth and collapse may again be affected by surface-active irrigants such as NaOCl, which has been demonstrated to lead to more and smaller bubbles as compared to water (24).

Irrigant flow in lateral canals, oval extensions, isthmuses, and tubules

Extensions of the main root canal, such as lateral canals, ramifications in the apical delta, isthmuses, and dentinal tubules are generally difficult to clean, because the irrigant does not easily penetrate those regions (42, 80, 81). Irrigation systems producing an irrigant flow parallel to the root canal wall,

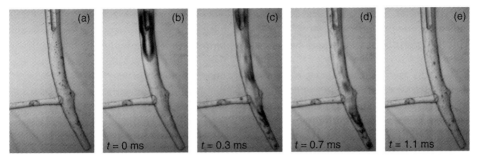

Figure 11.7   (a) High-speed visualization of the activity around a Er: YAG laser tip inside a curved root canal model with a lateral canal. The laser generated a large bubble that rapidly expands (b) and collapses (c). The collapse of this laser-induced bubble induces bubbles near the apex and inside the lateral canal (d, e), which may enhance cleaning in those areas. Recording speed of 9000 fps, laser energy of 80 mJ (KaVo KEY3 laser).

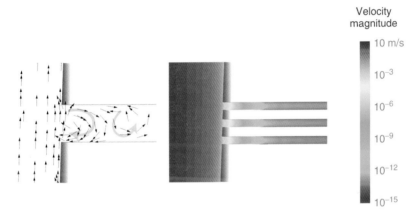

Figure 11.8   Flow pattern around the entrance of lateral canals (or tubules) because of a flow along the wall. Inside the lateral canal there are vortices generated (left), of which the velocity decreases rapidly (right). After two vortices, the velocity has become so small that diffusion becomes dominant.

such as syringe and negative pressure systems, only generate convection into the lateral canal within a distance twice the diameter of its entrance (Figure 11.8). Irrigant transport beyond this point is diffusion-driven and therefore slow (82, 83). Diffusion of the irrigant into a lateral canal may be improved by increasing the concentration or temperature of the irrigant (83).

The transport of irrigant into a lateral canal may also be enhanced by improving the convection, for which there has to be a flow toward the lateral canal (55, 83–85). Lateral flows may be induced by the sonic, ultrasonic, or laser activated systems, thereby enhancing tissue dissolution in lateral canals (86, 85, 87, 88), tissue dissolution or partial debris removal from isthmuses (89–92), or dentin

debris removal from oval extensions (24, 79, 93, 94). Furthermore, the microscale streaming induced by ultrasonic activation and by bubbles generated by ultrasonic and laser activation can enhance the convection near the lateral canal entrance and thereby increase irrigant transport within such canals (83).

Physical properties of irrigants

The flow of irrigants is affected by the physical properties of the irrigants, namely density, viscosity, contact angle, wetting behavior, and surface tension (95). The properties of endodontic irrigants are very similar to those of distilled water (96, 97), which can be explained by the fact that irrigants are mainly aqueous solutions. The surface tension of endodontic irrigants has been studied more extensively than the other two properties, under the assumption that it may have a significant effect on irrigant penetration in dentinal tubules and accessory root canals (98, 99) and on the dissolution of pulp tissue (100). Addition of wetting agents (surfactants) to commonly used irrigation solutions has also been suggested to reduce their surface tension (98, 99), although their exact concentration in the solutions is rarely reported (as they are extremely difficult to quantify) and mixing of NaOCl with other chemicals, like alcohol, in order to reduce the surface tensions that will reduce its effect (101). While density and viscosity always affect the flow, the effect of surface tension is important only where two immiscible fluids are present (e.g., irrigant and air) (95, 102). However, dentin is hydrophilic and the dentinal tubules are likely to contain dentinal fluid with fluidic properties similar to that of water (103), which will probably soak the root canal wall directly, limiting the effect of surfactants because the two fluids are miscible. Recent studies have also reported that surfactants did not enhance the ability of NaOCl to dissolve pulp tissue (104) or the ability of common chelators to remove calcium from dentin (105) or the smear layer (106, 107). On the contrary, it appears that the use of irrigants with a reduced surface tension *in-vitro* may result in deeper penetration of the smear layer into the dentinal tubules (108). The presence of an air bubble occupying the apical part of the root canal has been partially demonstrated *in-vitro* (86, 109) and *in-vivo* (110, 111). In such a case, surface tension could be important for the irrigant flow.

Vapor lock and apical penetration or irrigant

An air bubble may be trapped in the apical part of the root canal, which is also termed *vapor lock*. Such a bubble could be entrapped during irrigant delivery in an empty root canal by the advancing irrigant front (112) or during the coalescence of gas bubbles produced in the root canal during reaction between NaOCl and organic material (110, 112). A vapor lock could potentially obstruct irrigant penetration into the apical area.

Air entrapment has already been demonstrated and studied in top-filled conical capillaries

(49, 113–115) and has been shown that this air bubble disappears automatically, albeit after a relatively long time (116). However, in the case of root canal irrigation, the method of filling is different, as root canals are filled from the inside out and not from the top. Nevertheless a bubble may disappear over time. The results of a recently published experimental and computational fluid dynamics (CFD) study show that the occurrence of a vapor lock is decreased by using an open-ended needle, increasing the apical size, positioning the needle closer to working length, and delivering the irrigant at a higher flow rate (0.260 ml/s). Also, the brief insertion of the needle to working length could effectively remove an established vapor lock (117).

Negative pressure irrigation, ultrasonic activation of the irrigant, or application of the patency file can deliver irrigant solutions more efficiently into the apical third than syringe irrigation (86, 88, 110, 111). A recent *in-vivo* study demonstrated that both ultrasonic activation and negative pressure were equally effective in apical irrigant delivery in root canals of mesial roots of lower mandibular molars (118).

Interaction between a biofilm and the flow created by sonic, ultrasonic, or laser activation

Weak forces (low pressures and shear stresses) or a high EPS matrix stability cause only an elastic deformation of the biofilm that reverses as soon as the stress is removed. Repeated loading of the biofilm structure with a periodic stress, as is the case with sonic, ultrasonic, and laser activation, may result in the fatigue of the biofilm (19); however, the threshold (force and number of loading cycles) for damage following fatigue is unknown.

At increased force (or lower EPS matrix stability), viscous deformation of the biofilm may occur. The biofilm deforms and displaces in order to distribute and minimize the applied stresses (119). When a steady force is applied, for example, in the case of a steady flow, the biofilm will attain a steady state and no further deformation or removal will take place. Therefore, it may be advantageous to generate a nonsteady flow, for example, by unsteady oscillations of the ultrasonic file or by generating pulsations with ultrasound (79) or laser (24).

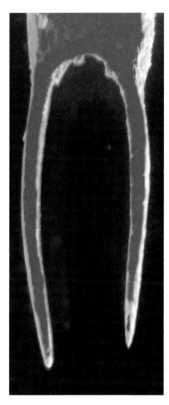

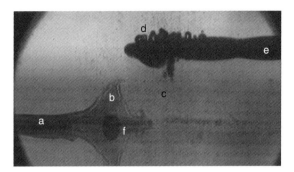

Figure 11.10 A biofilm-mimicking hydrogel (a) being removed (b) by streaming (c) and cavitation (d) generated by an ultrasonically oscillating file (e). There is also a stable bubble (f) that enhances the removal of the hydrogel.

For transient cavitation, velocities of 100 m/s are feasible at micron scales (63). The oscillation velocity of stable bubbles that are driven by the applied ultrasound field can be much higher than the oscillations induced by the ultrasound itself and typically occurs on a smaller scale (75).

Chemical effects enhanced by sonic, ultrasonic, and laser activated irrigation

Irrigants are chemically inactivated after their reaction with dentin, microorganisms or biofilm, tissue remnants (122, 123) or irrigants themselves (124), and therefore need to be mixed with fresh irrigant. Mixing of the irrigant involves transport of the irrigant, which may take place by either diffusion or convection (flow). Diffusion is the result of the random movement of individual particles (molecules/ions) in the fluid. This process is slow and depends (among others) on the temperature and concentration gradients present. Convection, on the other hand, is a faster and more efficient transport mechanism in which molecules are transported by the motion of the fluid (125). Convection contributes to effective delivery, refreshment, and mixing of the irrigant. The flow and activation phase of irrigant activation techniques therefore assist the chemical activity through convection and diffusion of the molecules/ions of the irrigant; during the resting phase, diffusion is dominant.

To obtain an optimal chemical effect of irrigants, they should be delivered throughout the root canal system and be refreshed and mixed as effectively

Figure 11.9 Illustration of a vapor lock, located at the apex of the root canal on the right. Blue color represents the irrigant, the white area represents air.

At stresses exceeding the cohesive or adhesive strength of the biofilm, parts of the biofilm may detach from the bulk biofilm (mechanical failure of the biofilm, a process called *sloughing* (21, 120, 121)) or from the substrate, respectively. Detached biofilm parts may reattach at a different location where the mechanical and chemical conditions are more favorable (19) (Figure 11.9).

Interaction with cavitation bubbles created by ultrasonic or laser activation

The gradients associated with the time scales and length scales of the exerted stress are important with regard to the behavior of a viscoelastic material. Cavitation bubbles, both transient and stable, typically exhibit large velocities and accelerations on a small time scale, making them efficient in plastic deformation of the biofilm (59, 77) (Figure 11.10).

as possible. This process can be characterized with the (second) Damköhler number, which is defined as the ratio of the typical irrigant transport time to the reaction time.[1]

It was shown recently that the Damköhler number in the apical area during syringe irrigation with a side-vented needle was higher than 1, suggesting that the fluid transport was too slow to ensure adequate refreshment of irrigants (126). Irrigant activation systems can improve the delivery throughout the root canal system (irrigant transportation time) and the refreshment/mixing of the irrigant by inducing additional convection.

The reaction rate of an irrigant with biofilm, pulp tissue, or the root canal wall (dentin and smear layer) is important to predict its chemical effect. Unfortunately, for the typical endodontic irrigants, only the reaction rate of NaOCl with dentin is known. In the literature, no influence of sonic activation on the chemical effect of irrigants has been reported. Laser or ultrasonic activation, on the other hand, does enhance the reaction rate of NaOCl with dentin, as does an increase in the concentration (127). The influence of activation was also observed in the resting phase (127). Such an increase will reduce over time during the reaction. A similar synergistic effect of NaOCl and ultrasound in the dissolution of tissue (122) or the removal of dentin debris from root canals has been reported in the literature (97). The influence of irrigant activation can be attributed to a sonochemical effect and/or refreshment/mixing of the irrigant (74), or because of the formation of small bubbles when NaOCl comes into contact with organic tissue. However, the exact cleaning mechanisms are not yet known.

pH may also contribute to the reaction rate (104), although the buffering effect of dentin may compensate this effect (127).

With ethylenediaminetetraaceticacid (EDTA), an improved penetration into dentinal tubules in the pulp chamber after ultrasonic activation has been reported (128), but the cause has not yet been elucidated. Sonochemical reactions can be ruled out because they are not easily achieved as high-energy input is needed to drive sonochemical reactions in EDTA (129).

Suggestions for clinical procedures

Irrigation activation protocols

An easily applicable irrigation protocol for sonic, ultrasonic, or LAI is the "Intermittent Flush Technique" first described by Cameron (130). First, the irrigant is delivered into the root canal by syringe irrigation. Then, the irrigant is activated inside the root canal, allowing the disruption of the substrate from the root canal wall. After activation, the root canal is rinsed using syringe irrigation thereby removing the substrate loosened from the root canal wall.

Another protocol comprises a continuous flow of the irrigant through or alongside the hand piece or fiber into the pulp chamber. The irrigant then has to flow from the pulp chamber or coronal root canal to the apical root canal by the activation of the instrument, thereby enhancing irrigant delivery into the (apical) root canal.

There are also needles (23–30 gauge) on the market that allow a continuous flow of the irrigant through the needle in the root canal during (ultra)sonic activation of the needle. These needles allow irrigant delivery, refreshment, and activation at the same time.

The irrigation protocols are most effective when the root canal has been shaped until the master apical file, because there is more space in the root canal for the fluid dynamical effects. However, this does not imply that the protocols cannot be used otherwise or will not be effective during the root canal treatment.

Sonic activation

Sonic activated irrigation can be performed using sonic hand pieces that can drive instruments at sonic frequencies. Traditionally, only cutting files are available. Nowadays, there are several new sonic activation systems available on the market like the EndoActivator® System or the Vibringe®.

---

[1]The second Damköhler number is defined as

$$Da = \frac{\text{irrigant transport time}}{\text{reaction time}} = \frac{L/(U_{\text{flow}} + \Omega_{\text{flow}}L + (D/L^2))}{\tau_{\text{reaction}}}$$

(11.5)

in which U is the velocity, Ω is the vorticity (rotation) of the irrigant, and D is the diffusion coefficient. The length scale L is a typical length over which the reaction between irrigant and biofilm takes place near the surface.

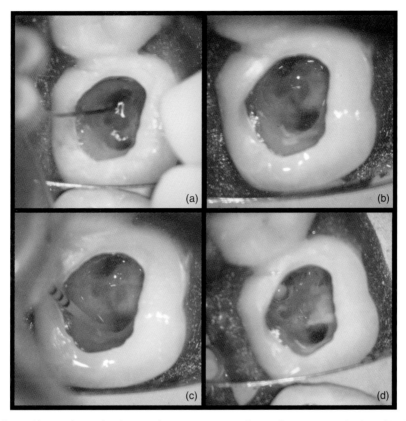

Figure 11.11   (a–d) a and b: canal rinsed with NaOCl using a syringe and a needle. c: sonic activation of NaOCl d: NaOCl after sonic activation.

The EndoActivator System allows a variation of the driving power and frequency and the size of polymer tips that will not cut in the root canal wall. The manufacturer advises to deliver the irrigant into the root canal by syringe irrigation after creating a "fully tapered shape." The irrigant is activated for 30–60 s using a pumping action in short 2–3 mm strokes (Figure 11.11).

Vibringe is an irrigant delivery system that uses a sonically oscillating needle to deliver the irrigant into the root canal. The Vibringe can be used throughout the complete root canal treatment procedure.

Ultrasonic activation

For ultrasonic activation, most of the ultrasonic devices already present in the clinic can be used, combined with a variety of instruments. Sometimes, special chucks or irrigation systems are needed. Instruments for all of the abovementioned activation protocols are available. They can be applied until 1–2 mm from working length (with the exception of some of the ultrasonically activated needles) or at the beginning of a strong curvature in order to prevent strong wall contact (43). For the "Intermittent Flush Technique" a sequence of three times 10 s seems to be favorable for dentin debris removal (79, 97). For a continuous flush, mostly 1 min is advised. For optimal cleaning efficacy of oval extensions and isthmuses and lateral canals of which the position is known, the instrument should be made to oscillate toward these areas if possible (55) (Figure 11.12).

At the moment, low intensity settings of the ultrasonic energy are advised to be used to prevent fracture of the instruments. Normally, fractured instruments will easily flow out of the root canal. Noncutting instruments are available that can be

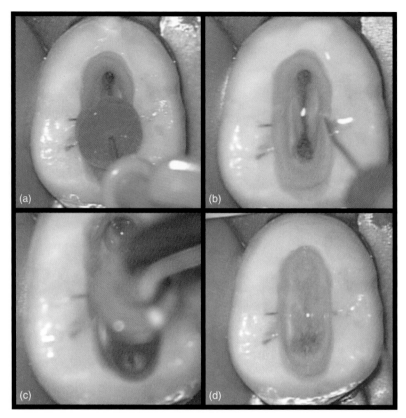

Figure 11.12   (a–d) a and b: canal rinsed with NaOCl using a syringe and a needle. c: ultrasonic activation of NaOCl d: NaOCl after ultrasonic activation.

used safely in the root canal. Strong contact of the file with the root canal walls should be avoided (37).

Laser activation

For LAI, Er:YAG or ErCrYSGG laser systems are available on the market. The "Intermittent Flush Technique" or a continuous flow into the pulp chamber can be used. The laser fiber can be inserted 1–2 mm short of working length and vertically moved within the apical third (24). It can also be placed in the pulp chamber just above the root canal orifice. The latter has been prescribed for conventional fibers (39) and for specially designed fibers (PIPS) (40) (Figure 11.13).

The commercially available laser devices allow for a variation of the size and type of the optic fibers, pulse repetition frequencies (PRFs), pulsation energy, and pulse length. De Groot *et al.* (24) reported as optimal settings a combination of

low power (80 mJ) per pulse and a PRF of 15 Hz. Significant loss of irrigant from the pulp chamber was reported for energy settings higher than 120 mJ per pulse, reducing the efficacy of the irrigation procedure.

For the PIPS technique, the recommended energy setting is even lower: 10 mJ. The PIPS fiber is placed at the coronal opening of the root canal after filling the root canal system and pulp chamber with the irrigant. There is severe irrigant loss during activation; therefore, a continuous flow of irrigant in the pulp chamber during activation is required.

Effect of the activation systems on the disinfection procedure

To conclude, ultrasonic and laser activation contribute positively to both the mechanical and the

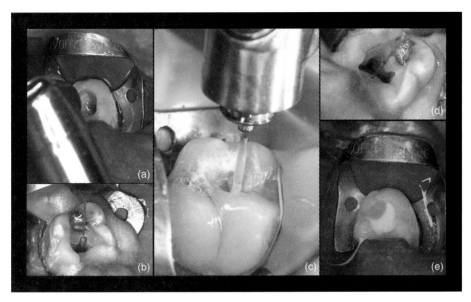

Figure 11.13   (a–e) a - d: placement of the laser fiber (PIPS) in the pulp chamber e: NaOCl after PIPS.

chemical aspects of the irrigation procedure. How- ever, it is not exactly known to what extent this will contribute to the disinfection procedure and if this eventually will improve the outcome of the treatment. Both systems have the potential to disrupt or remove biofilm, but to what extent they can remove biofilm from the root canal wall and from more remote regions such as oval extensions, lateral canals, and tubules is not known. No reliable endodontic biofilm models are currently available for research. AP is a multifactorial disease, and, therefore, its healing depends on a range of aspects, not only on the irrigation during the endodontic treatment. From clinical research, it is clear that the length and the quality of the root canal filling are two of the few risk factors that are obvious. However, the influence of the irrigation procedure, complex canal anatomy (apical delta and dentinal tubules), structure of the biofilm, external biofilm around the root apex on the endodontic outcome are not known because data from randomized controlled trials (RCTs) are lacking. Recently, it was demonstrated in a RCT that an ultrasonic assisted irrigation protocol did not result in a significant better endodontic outcome compared to syringe irrigation (131). This could indicate that we need to enhance even more the mechanical and chemical aspects of the irrigation procedures to influence

endodontic outcome or that other influential fac- tors are more important in determining endodontic outcome. More RCTs are necessary to answer these questions.

References

1. Haapasalo, M., Shen, Y. & Ricucci, D. (2011) Rea- sons for persistent and emerging post-treatment endodontic disease. *Endodontic Topics*, **18**, 31–50.

2. Sen, B.H., Wesselink, P.R. & Türkün, M. (1995) The smear layer: a phenomenon in root canal therapy. *International Endodontic Journal*, **28**, 141–148.

3. Gorni, F.G. & Gagliani, M.M. (2004) The outcome of endodontic retreatment: a 2-yr follow-up. *Journal of Endodontics*, **30**, 1–4.

4. Wu, M.K., van der Sluis, L.W. & Wesselink, P.R. (2004) Comparison of mandibular premolars and canines with respect to their resistance to vertical root fracture. *Journal of Dentistry*, **32**, 265–268.

5. Shemesh, H., Wesselink, P.R. & Wu, M.K. (2010) Incidence of dentinal defects after root canal fill- ing procedures. *International Endodontic Journal*, **43**, 995–1000.

6. Lussi, A., Nussbächer, U. & Grosrey, J. (1993) A novel noninstrumented technique for cleansing the root canal system. *Journal of Endodontics*, **19**, 549–553.

7. Attin, T., Buchalla, W., Zirkel, C. & Lussi, A. (2002) Clinical evaluation of the cleansing properties of the noninstrumental technique for cleaning root canals. *International Endodontic Journal*, **35**, 929–933.

8. Mader, C., Baumgartner, J. & Peters, D. (1984) Scanning electron microscopic investigation of the smeared layer on root canal walls. *Journal of Endodontics*, **10**, 477–483.

9. Haapasalo, M., Qian, W., Portenier, I. & Waltimo, T. (2007) Effects of dentin on the antimicrobial properties of endodontic medicaments. *Journal of Endodontics*, **33**, 917–925.

10. Paqué, F., Boessler, C. & Zehnder, M. (2011) Accumulated hard tissue debris levels in mesial roots of mandibular molars after sequential irrigation steps. *International Endodontic Journal*, **44**, 148–153.

11. Boutsioukis, C., Verhaagen, B., Versluis, M., Kastrinakis, E., Wesselink, P.R. & van der Sluis, L.W.M. (2010) Evaluation of irrigant flow in the root canal using different needle types by an unsteady computational fluid dynamics model. *Journal of Endodontics*, **36**, 875–879.

12. Zehnder, M. (2012) Research that matters—irrigants and disinfectants. *International Endodontic Journal*, **45**, 961–962.

13. Flemming, H.-C., Neu, T.R. & Wozniak, D.J. (2007) The EPS matrix: The "house of biofilm cells". *Journal of Bacteriology*, **189**, 7945–7947.

14. Wilking, J.N., Angelini, T.E., Seminara, A., Brenner, M.P. & Weitz, D.A. (2011) Biofilms as complex fluids. *Materials Research Society Bulletin*, **36**, 385–391.

15. Körstgens, V., Flemming, H.-C., Wingender, J. & Borchard, W. (2001) Uniaxial compression measurement device for investigation of the mechanical stability of biofilms. *Journal of Microbiological Methods*, **46**, 9–17.

16. Ozok, A.R., Persoon, I.F., Huse, S.M. *et al.* (2012) *International Endodontic Journal*, **45**, 530–541.

17. Marty, N., Dournes, J.L., Chabanon, G. & Montrozier, H. (1992) Influence of nutrient media on the chemical composition of the exopolysaccharide from mucoid and non-mucoid Pseudomonas aeruginosa. *FEMS Microbiology Letters*, **98**, 35–44.

18. van der Waal, S.V. & van der Sluis, L.W.M. (2012) Potential of calcium to scaffold an endodontic biofilm, thus protecting the micro-organisms from disinfection. *Medical Hypotheses*, **79**, 1–4.

19. Flemming, H.-C., Wingender, J. & Szewzyk, U. (2011) *Biofilm Highlights*. Springer Series on Biofilms, 1 edn. Springer, Berlin, Heidelberg, Germany.

20. Böl, M., Ehret, A.E., Albero, A.B., Hellriegel, J. & Krull, R. (2012) Recent advances in mechanical characterization of biofilm and their significance for material modeling. *Critical Reviews in Biotechnology*, **33**, 145–171.

21. Picioreanu, C., Van Loosdrecht, M. & Heijnen, J. (2001) Two-dimensional model of biofilm detachment caused by internal stress from liquid flow. *Biotechnology and Bioengineering*, **72**, 205–218.

22. Jiang, L.-M., Verhaagen, B., Versluis, M. & van der Sluis, L.W.M. (2010a) Evaluation of a sonic device designed to activate irrigant in the root canal. *Journal of Endodontics*, **36**, 143–146.

23. Verhaagen, B., Lea, S.C., van der Sluis, L.W.M., Walmsley, A.D. & Versluis, M. (2012b) Oscillation characteristics of endodontic files: numerical model and its validation. *IEEE Transactions on Ultrasonics, Ferroelectrics, and Frequency Control*, **59**, 2448–2459.

24. De Groot, S.D., Verhaagen, B., Versluis, M., Wu, M.-K., Wesselink, P.R. & van der Sluis, L.W.M. (2009) Laser activated irrigation within root canals: cleaning efficacy and flow visualization. *International Endodontic Journal*, **42**, 1077–1083.

25. Blanken, J.W. & Verdaasdonk, R.M. (2007) Cavitation as a working mechanism of the Er,Cr:YSGG Laser in endodontics: a visualization study. *Journal of Oral Laser Applications*, **7**, 97–106.

26. Böl, M., Möhle, R.B., Haesner, M., Neu, T.R., Horn, H. & Krull, R. (2009) 3D finite element model of biofilm detachment using real biofilm structures from CLSM data. *Biotechnology and Bioengineering*, **103**, 177–186.

27. Möhle, R.B., Langemann, T., Haesner, M. *et al.* (2007) Structure and shear strength of microbial biofilms as determined with confocal laser scanning microscopy and fluid dynamic gauging using a novel rotating disc biofilm reactor. *Biotechnology and Bioengineering*, **98**, 747–755.

28. Derlon, N., Massé, A., Escudié, R., Bernet, N. & Paul, E. (2008) Stratification in the cohesion of biofilms grown under various environmental conditions. *Water Research*, **42**, 2102–2110.

29. Brunson, M., Heilborn, C., Johnson, J.D., Cohenca, N. (2010) Effect of apical preparation size and preparation taper on irrigant volume delivered by using negative pressure irrigation system. *J Endod*, **36**, 721–724.

30. George, R., Walsh, L.J. (2008) Apical extrusion of root canal irrigants when using Er:YAG and Er,CR:YSGG with optical fibers: an in vitro dye study. *J Endod*, **34**, 706–708.

31. Lumley, P.J., Walmsley, A.D. & Laird, W.R.E. (1991) Streaming patterns produced around endosonic files. *International Endodontic Journal*, **24**, 290–297.

32. Ahmad, M., Roy, R.A., Kamarudin, A.G. & Safar, M. (1993) The vibratory pattern of ultrasonic files driven piezoelectrically. *International Endodontic Journal*, **26**, 120–124.

33. Lea, S.C., Walmsley, A.D., Lumley, P.J. & Landini, G. (2004) A new insight into the oscillation characteristics of endosonic files used in dentistry. *Physics in Medicine and Biology*, **49**, 2095–2102.

34. Lea, S.C., Walmsley, D. & Lumley, P.J. (2010) Analyzing endosonic root canal file oscillations: an *in vitro* evaluation. *Journal of Endodontics*, **36**, 880–883.

35. Weller, R.N., Brady, J.M. & Bernier, W.E. (1980) Efficacy of ultrasonic cleaning. *Journal of Endodontics*, **6**, 740–743.

36. van der Sluis, L.W.M., Versluis, M., Wu, M.-K. & Wesselink, P.R. (2007) Passive ultrasonic irrigation of the root canal: a review of the literature. *International Endodontic Journal*, **40**, 415–426.

37. Boutsioukis, C., Verhaagen, B., Walmsley, A.D., Versluis, M. & van der Sluis, L.W.M. (2013a) Measurement and visualization of file-wall contact during passive ultrasonic irrigation *in vitro*. *International Endodontic Journal*, **46 (11)**, 1046–1055.

38. Robertson, C.W. & Williams, D. (1971) Lambert absorption coefficients of water in the infrared. *Journal of the Optical Society of America*, **61**, 1316–1320.

39. Peeters, H.H. & Suardita, K. (2011) Efficacy of smear layer removal at the root tip by using ethylenediaminetetraacetic acid and erbium, chromium: yttrium, scandium, gallium garnet laser. *Journal of Endodontics*, **37**, 1585–1589.

40. Peters, O.A., Bardsley, S., Fong, J., Pandher, G. & Divito, E. (2011) Disinfection of root canals with photon-initiated photoacoustic streaming. *Journal of Endodontics*, **37**, 1008–1012.

41. Jiang, L.-M., Lak, B., Eijsvogel, E., Wesselink, P.R. & van der Sluis, L.W.M. (2012) A cleaning efficacy comparison of different irrigation techniques as final irrigation. *Journal of Endodontics*, **38**, 838–841.

42. Nanzer, J., Langlois, S. & Coeuret, F. (1989) Electrochemical engineering approach to the irrigation of tooth canals under the influence of a vibrating file. *Journal of Biomedical Engineering*, **11**, 157–163.

43. Malki, M., Verhaagen, B., Jiang, L.-M. *et al.* (2012) Irrigant flow beyond the insertion depth of an ultrasonically oscillating file in straight and curved root canals: visualization and cleaning efficacy. *Journal of Endodontics*, **38**, 657–661.

44. Amato, M., Vanoni-Heineken, I., Hecker, H. & Weiger, R. (2011) Curved versus straight root canals: the benefit of activated irrigation techniques on dentin debris removal. *Oral Surgery, Oral Medicine, Oral Pathology, Oral Radiology, and Endodontics*, **111**, 529–534.

45. Walmsley, A.D. & Williams, A.R. (1999) Effects of constraints on the oscillatory pattern of endosonic files. *Journal of Endodontics*, **15**, 189–194.

46. Jiang, L.-M., Verhaagen, B., Versluis, M., Langedijk, J., Wesselink, P.R. & van der Sluis, L.W.M. (2011) The influence of the ultrasonic intensity on the cleaning efficacy of passive ultrasonic irrigation. *Journal of Endodontics*, **37**, 688–692.

47. Rayleigh, L. (1884) On the circulation of air observed in Kundt's tubes and on some allied acoustical problems. *Philosophical Transactions of the Royal Society of London*, **175**, 1–21.

48. Stuart, J.T. (1966) Double boundary layers in oscillatory viscous flow. *Journal of Fluid Mechanics*, **24**, 673–687.

49. Duck, P.W. & Smith, F.T. (1979) Steady streaming induced between oscillating cylinders. *Journal of Fluid Mechanics*, **91**, 93–110.

50. Haddon, E.W. & Riley, N. (1979) The steady streaming induced between oscillating circular cylinders. *Quarterly Journal of Mechanics & Applied Mathematics*, **32**, 265–282.

51. Williams, A.R. & Nyborg, W.L. (1970) Microsonation using a transversely oscillating capillary. *Ultrasonics*, **8**, 36–38.

52. Williams, A.R. & Slade, J.S. (1971) Ultrasonic dispersal of aggregates of sarcina lutea. *Ultrasonics*, **8**, 85–87.

53. Ahmad, M., Pitt Ford, T.R. & Crum, L.A. (1987) Ultrasonic debridement of root canals: acoustic streaming and its possible role. *Journal of Endodontics*, **13**, 490–499.

54. Verhaagen, B., Boutsioukis, C., van der Sluis, L.W.M. & Versluis, M. (2014, in press) Acoustic streaming induced by an ultrasonically oscillating endodontic file. *Journal of the Acoustical Society of America*.

55. Jiang, L.-M., Verhaagen, B., Versluis, M. & van der Sluis, L.W.M. (2010b) The influence of the oscillation direction of an ultrasonic file on the cleaning efficacy of passive ultrasonic irrigation. *Journal of Endodontics*, **36**, 1372–1376.

56. Deshpande, M.D. & Vaishnav, R.N. (1982) Submerged laminar jet impingement on a plane. *Journal of Fluid Mechanics*, **114**, 213–236.

57. Phares, D.J., Smedley, G.T. & Flagan, R.C. (2000) The wall shear stress produced by the normal impingement of a jet on a flat surface. *Journal of Fluid Mechanics*, **418**, 351–375.

58. Kim, S.K. & Troesch, A.W. (1989) Streaming flows generated by high-frequency small-amplitude oscillations of arbitrary cylinders. *Physics of Fluids A*, **6**, 975–985.

59. Brennen, C.E. (1995) *Cavitation and Bubble Dynamics*. Oxford University Press, Oxford, UK.

60. Prosperetti, A. (2004) Bubbles. *Physics of Fluids*, **16**, 1852–1865.

61. Sedgewick, S.A. & Trevena, D.H. (1976) An estimate of the ultimate tensile strength of water. *Journal of Physics D: Applied Physics*, **9**, L203–L205.

62. Macedo, R.G., Verhaagen, B., Fernandez Rivas, D. *et al.* (2014) Sonochemical and high-speed optical characterization of cavitation generated by an ultrasonically oscillating dental file in root canal models. *Ultrasonics Sonochemistry*, Ultrason Sonochem. 2014 Jan;**21**(1): 324–335. doi: 10.1016/j.ultsonch.2013.03.001.

63. Brujan, E.-A., Nahen, K., Schmidt, P. & Vogel, A. (2001) Dynamics of laser-induced cavitation bubbles near an elastic boundary. *Journal of Fluid Mechanics*, **433**, 251–281.

64. Fernandez Rivas, D., Betjes, J., Verhaagen, B. *et al.* (2013) Erosion evolution in mono-crystalline silicon surfaces caused by acoustic cavitation bubbles. *Applied Physics Letters*, **113**, 064902.

65. Versluis, M., Schmitz, B., Von der Heydt, A. & Lohse, D. (2000) How snapping shrimp snap: through cavitating bubbles. *Science*, **289**, 2114–2117.

66. Fernandez Rivas, D., Verhaagen, B., Seddon, J. *et al.* (2012) Localized removal of layers of metal, polymer or biomaterial by ultrasound cavitation microbubbles. *Biomicrofluidics*, **6**, 034114.

67. Mason, T.J. & Peters, D. (2002) Practical Sonochemistry: Power Ultrasound Uses and Applications. Chemical Science Series (Horwood).

68. Junge, L., Ohl, C.-D., Wolfrum, B., Arora, M. & Ikink, R. (2003) Cell detachment method using shockwave-induced cavitation. *Ultrasound in Medicine and Biology*, **29**, 1769–1776.

69. Terwisga, W.J.C., Fitzsimmons, P.A., Ziru, L. & Foeth, E.J. (2009) Cavitation erosion—a review of physical mechanisms and erosion risk models. *Proceedings of the 7th International Symposium on Cavitation CAV2009*.

70. Lohse, D. (2003) Bubble puzzles. *Physics Today*, **56**, 36–41.

71. Ahmad, M., Pitt Ford, T.R., Crum, L.A. & Walton, A.J. (1988) Ultrasonic debridement of root canals: acoustic cavitation and its relevance. *Journal of Endodontics*, **14**, 486–493.

72. Lumley, P.J., Walmsley, A.D. & Laird, W.R.E. (1988) An investigation into cavitational activity occurring in endosonic instrumentation. *Journal of Dentistry*, **16**, 120–122.

73. Felver, B., King, D.V., Lea, S.C., Price, G.J. & Walmsley, A.D. (2009) Cavitation occurrence around ultrasonic dental scalers. *Ultrasonics Sonochemistry*, **16**, 692–697.

74. Tiong, J. & Price, G.J. (2012) Ultrasound promoted reaction of Rhodamine B with sodium hypochlorite using sonochemical and dental ultrasonic instruments. *Ultrasonics Sonochemistry*, **19**, 358–364.

75. Marmottant, P., Versluis, M., De Jong, N., Hilgenfeldt, S. & Lohse, D. (2006) High-speed imaging of an ultrasound-driven bubble in contact with a wall: "Narcissus" effect and resolved acoustic streaming. *Experiments in Fluids*, **41**, 147–153.

76. Jackson, F.J. & Nyborg, W.L. (1958) Small scale acoustic streaming near a locally excited membrane. *Journal of the Acoustical Society of America*, **30**, 614–619.

77. Verhaagen, B. (2012a) Root canal cleaning through cavitation and microstreaming. PhD thesis, University of Twente, The Netherlands.

78. Gmelin (1969) Chlor. In: *Handbuch der anorganische chemie*, 8 edn. German Chemical Society, Verlag Chemie Gmbh.

79. Jiang, L.-M., Verhaagen, B., Versluis, M., Zangrillo, C., Cuckovic, D. & van der Sluis, L.W.M. (2010c) An evaluation of the effect of pulsed ultrasound on the cleaning efficacy of passive ultrasonic irrigation. *Journal of Endodontics*, **36**, 1887–1891.

80. Orstavik, D. & Haapasalo, M. (1990) Disinfection by endodontic irrigants and dressings of experimentally infected dentinal tubules. *Endodontics and Dental Traumatology*, **6**, 142–149.

81. Nair, P.N.R. (2004) Pathogenesis of apical periodontitis and the cause of endodontic failures. *Critical Reviews in Oral Biology and Medicine*, **15**, 348–381.

82. Shankar, P.N. & Deshpande, M.D. (2000) Fluid mechanics in the driven cavity. *Annual Review of Fluid Mechanics*, **32**, 93–136.

83. Verhaagen, B., Boutsioukis, C., Sleutel, C.P., Kastrinakis, E., Versluis, M. & van der Sluis, L.W.M. (2014, in press) Irrigant transport into dental microchannels. *Microfluidics and Nanofluidics*.

84. Lumley, P.J., Walmsley, A.D., Walton, R.E. & Rippin, J.W. (1993) Cleaning of oval canals using ultrasonic or sonic instrumentation. *Journal of Endodontics*, **19**, 453–457.

85. Al-Jadaa, A., Paque, F., Attin, T. & Zehnder, M. (2009) Necrotic pulp tissue dissolution by passive ultrasonic irrigation in simulated accessory canals: impact of canal location and angulation. *International Endodontic Journal*, **42**, 59–65.

86. De Gregorio, C., Estevez, R., Cisneros, R., Heilborn, C. & Cohenca, N. (2009) Effect of EDTA, sonic, and ultrasonic activation on the penetration of sodium hypochlorite into simulated lateral canals: an in vitro study. *Journal of Endodontics*, **35**, 891–895.

87. De Gregorio, C., Estevez, R., Cisneros, R., Paranjpe, A. & Cohenca, N. (2010) Efficacy of different irrigation and activation systems on the penetration of sodium hypochlorite into simulated lateral canals and up to working length: an in vitro study. *Journal of Endodontics*, **36**, 1216–1221.

88. Castelo-Baz, P., Martín-Biedma, B., Cantatore, G. et al. (2012) In vitro comparison of passive and continuous ultrasonic irrigation in simulated lateral canals of extracted teeth. *Journal of Endodontics*, **38**, 688–691.

89. Goodman, A., Reader, A., Beck, M., Melfi, R. & Meyers, W. (1985) An in vitro comparison of the efficacy of the step-back technique versus a step-back/ultrasonic technique in human mandibular molars. *Journal of Endodontics*, **11**, 249–256.

90. Burleson, A., Nusstein, J., Reader, A. & Beck, M. (2007) The in vivo evaluation of hand/rotary/ultrasound instrumentation in necrotic, human mandibular molars. *Journal of Endodontics*, **33**, 782–787.

91. Paqué, F., Rechenberg, D.-K. & Zehnder, M. (2012) Reduction of hard-tissue debris accumulation during rotary root canal instrumentation by etidronic acid in a sodium hypochlorite irrigant. *Journal of Endodontics*, **38**, 692–695.

92. Adcock, J.M., Sidow, S.J., Looney, S.W. et al. (2011) Histologic evaluation of canal and isthmus debridement efficacies of two different irrigant delivery techniques in a closed system. *Journal of Endodontics*, **37**, 544–548.

93. De Moor, R.J., Meire, M., Goharkhay, K., Moritz, A. & Vanobbergen, J. (2010) Efficacy of ultrasonic versus laser-activated irrigation to remove artificially placed dentin debris plugs. *Journal of Endodontics*, **36**, 1580–1583.

94. Rödig, T., Bozkurt, M., Konietschke, F. & Hülsmann, M. (2010) Comparison of the Vibringe system with syringe and passive ultrasonic irrigation in removing debris from simulated root canal irregularities. *Journal of Endodontics*, **36**, 1410–1413.

95. White, F.M. (1999) *Fluid Mechanics*, 4 edn. McGraw-Hill, Boston, USA, pp. 1–56, 541.

96. Guerisoli, D.M.Z., Silva, R.S. & Pecora, J.D. (1998) Evaluation of some physico-chemical properties of different concentrations of sodium hypochlorite solutions. *Brazilian Endodontic Journal*, **3**, 21–23.

97. van der Sluis, L.W.M., Vogels, M.P., Verhaagen, B., Macedo, R. & Wesselink, P.R. (2010) Study on the influence of refreshment/activation cycles and irrigants on mechanical cleaning efficiency during ultrasonic activation of the irrigant. *Journal of Endodontics*, **36**, 737–740.

98. Abou-Rass, M. & Oglesby, S.W. (1981) The effects of temperature, concentration, and tissue type on the solvent ability of sodium hypochlorite. *Journal of Endodontics*, **7**, 376–377.

99. Taşman, F., Cehreli, Z.C., Oğan, C. & Etikan, I. (2000) Surface tension of root canal irrigants. *Journal of Endodontics*, **26**, 586–587.

100. Stojicic, S., Zivkovic, S., Qian, W., Zhang, H. & Haapasalo, M. (2010) Tissue dissolution by sodium hypochlorite: effect of concentration, temperature, agitation, and surfactant. *Journal of Endodontics*, **36**, 1558–1562.

101. Cunningham, W.T., Cole, J.S. & Balekjian, A.Y. (1982) Effect of alcohol on the spreading ability of sodium hypochlorite endodontic irrigant. *Oral Surgery, Oral Medicine, and Oral Pathology*, **54**, 333–335.

102. Kundu, P.K. & Cohen, I.M. (2004) *Fluid Mechanics*, 3 edn. Elsevier Academic Press, San Diego, CA, USA, pp. 1–23, 271–377.

103. Berggren, G. & Brännström, M. (1965) The rate of flow in dentinal tubules due to capillary attraction. *Journal of Dental Research*, **44**, 408–415.

104. Jungbluth, H., Marending, M., De-Deus, G., Sener, B. & Zehnder, M. (2011) Stabilizing sodium hypochlorite at high pH: effects on soft tissue and dentin. *Journal of Endodontics*, **37**, 693–696.

105. Zehnder, M., Schmidlin, P., Sener, B. & Waltimo, T. (2005) Chelation in root canal therapy reconsidered. *Journal of Endodontics*, **31**, 817–820.

106. Lui, J.N., Kuah, H.G. & Chen, N.N. (2007) Effect of EDTA with and without surfactants or ultrasonics on removal of smear layer. *Journal of Endodontics*, **33**, 472–475.

107. De-Deus, G., Namen, F., Galan, J.J. & Zehnder, M. (2008) Soft chelating irrigation protocol optimizes bonding quality of Resilon/Epiphany root fillings. *Journal of Endodontics*, **34**, 703–705.

108. Aktener, B.O., Cengiz, T. & Pişkin, B. (1989) The penetration of smear material into dentinal tubules during instrumentation with surface-active reagents: a scanning electron microscopic study. *Journal of Endodontics*, **15**, 588–590.

109. Tay, F.R., Gu, L.S., Schoeffel, G.J. et al. (2010) Effect of vapor lock on root canal debridement by using a side-vented needle for positive-pressure irrigant delivery. *Journal of Endodontics*, **36**, 745–750.

110. Vera, J., Arias, A. & Romero, M. (2011) Effect of maintaining apical patency on irrigant penetration into the apical third of root canals when using passive ultrasonic irrigation: an in vivo study. *Journal of Endodontics*, **37**, 1276–1278.

111. Vera, J., Arias, A. & Romero, M. (2012) Dynamic movement of intracanal gas bubbles during cleaning and shaping procedures: the effect of maintaining apical patency on their presence in the middle and cervical thirds of human root canals-an in vivo study. *Journal of Endodontics*, **38**, 200–203.

112. Gu, L., Kim, J.R., Ling, J., Choi, K.K., Pashley, D.H. & Tay, F.R. (2009) Review of contemporary irrigant agitation techniques and devices. *Journal of Endodontics*, **35**, 791–804.

113. Dovgyallo, G.I., Migun, N.P. & Prokhorenko, P.P. (1989) The complete filling of dead-end conical capillaries with liquid. *Journal of Engineering Physics and Thermophysics*, **56**, 395–397.

114. Migoun, N.P. & Azouni, M.A. (1996) Filling of one-side-closed capillaries immersed in liquids. *Journal of Colloid and Interface Science*, **181**, 337–340.

115. Migun, N.P. & Shnip, A.I. (2002) Model of film flow in a dead-end conic capillary. *Journal of Engineering Physics and Thermophysics*, **75**, 1422–1428.

116. Pesse, A.V., Warrier, G.R. & Dhir, V.K. (2005) An experimental study of the gas entrapment process in closed-end microchannels. *International Journal of Heat and Mass Transfer*, **48**, 5150–5165.

117. Boutsioukis, C., Kastrinakis, E., Verhaagen, B., Versluis, M. & van der Sluis, L.W.M. (2014) Apical vapor lock in root canals: a combined experimental and computational fluid dynamics approach. *International Endodontic Journal*, **47** (**2**), 191–201.

118. Munoz, H.R. & Camacho-Cuadra, K. (2012) In vivo efficacy of three different endodontic irrigation techniques for irrigant delivery to working length of mesial canals of mandibular molars. *Journal of Endodontics*, **38**, 445–448.

119. Klapper, I., Rupp, C.J., Cargo, R., Purvedorj, B. & Stoodley, P. (2002) Viscoelastic fluid description of bacterial biofilm material properties. *Biotechnology and Bioengineering*, **80**, 289–296.

120. Stoodley, P., Lewandowski, Z., Boyle, J.D. & Lappin-Scott, H.M. (1999) Structural deformation of bacterial biofilms caused by short-term fluctuations in fluid shear: an in situ investigation of biofilm rheology. *Biotechnology and Bioengineering*, **65**, 83–92.

121. Stoodley, P., Wilson, S., Cargo, R., Piscitteli, C. & Rupp, C.J. (2001) Detachment and other dynamic processes in bacterial biofilms. *Surfaces in Biomaterials 2001 Symposium Proceedings*, pp. 189–192.

122. Moorer, W.R. & Wesselink, P.R. (1982) Factors promoting the tissue dissolving capability of sodium hypochlorite. *International Endodontic Journal*, **15**, 187–196.

123. Haapasalo, M., Endal, U., Zandi, H. & Coil, J.M. (2005) Eradication of endodontic infection by instrumentation and irrigation solutions. *Endodontic Topics*, **10**, 77–102.

124. Rossi-Fedele, G., Doğramaci, E.J., Guastalli, A.R., Steier, L. & Poli de Figueiredo, J.A. (2012) Antagonistic interactions between sodium hypochlorite, chlorhexidine, EDTA, and citric acid. *Journal of Endodontics*, **38**, 426–431.

125. Incropera, F.P. & de Witt, D.P. (1990) *Fundamentals of Heat and Mass Transfer*, 3 edn. John Wiley & Sons, NJ, USA.

126. Verhaagen, B., Boutsioukis, C., Heijnen, G.L., van der Sluis, L.W.M. & Versluis, M. (2012c) Role of the confinement of a root canal on jet impingement during endodontic irrigation. *Experiments in Fluids*, **53**, 1841–1853.

127. Macedo, R.G., Wesselink, P.R., Zaccheo, F., Fanali, D. & van der Sluis, L.W. (2010) Reaction rate of NaOCl in contact with bovine dentine: effect of activation, exposure time, concentration and pH. *International Endodontic Journal*, **43**, 1108–1115.

128. Carrasco, L.D., Pécora, J.D. & Fröner, I.C. (2004) In vitro assessment of dentinal permeability after the use of ultrasonic-activated irrigants in the pulp chamber before internal dental bleaching. *Dental Traumatology*, **20**, 164–168.

129. Wang, J., Wang, X., Li, G., Guo, P. & Luo, Z. (2010) Degradation of EDTA in aqueous solution by using ozonolysis and ozonolysis combined with sonolysis. *Journal of Hazardous materials*, **176**, 333–338.

130. Cameron, J.A. (1988) The effect of ultrasonic endodontics on the temperature of the root canal wall. *Journal of Endodontics*, **14**, 554–558.

131. Liang, Y.-H., Jiang, L.-M., Jiang, L. *et al.* Radiographic healing following root canal treatments performed in single-rooted teeth with and without ultrasonic activation of the irrigant: a randomized controlled trial, *J. Endodont.* **39**, 1218–1225 (2013).

12 Ozonization and Electrochemical Root Canal Disinfection

Roberta Pileggi

Department of Endodontics, University of Florida, Gainesville, FL, USA

The importance of the use of irrigants in root canal therapy is well established. Several solutions and methods have been advocated to better eradicate bacteria and tissue remnants from the root canal system. This chapter focuses on two methods that have gained popularity for the past few years: ozonofication and electrochemical activation (ECA).

Ozone therapy

Ozone was introduced to medicine, food, and chemical industries several years ago following its antibactericidal, antiviral, and antifungal properties. It is recommended in the treatment of vascular, orthopedic, and infection diseases. Structurally, ozone is a molecule composed of three oxygen atoms, commonly delivered as gas or dissolved in water, where it forms oxidate radicals (1–5). It is 1.6-fold denser and 10-fold more soluble in water (49.0 ml in 100 ml water at 0°C) than oxygen (4).

The antimicrobial property of ozone is due to oxidation, which destroys the cell wall and the cytoplasmic membrane of microorganisms affecting osmotic stability. In a recent study where the effect of ozone on the membrane permeability and ultrastructure of *Pseudomonas aeruginosa* was examined, it was demonstrated that the cell inactivation was because of an increased membrane permeability and cytoplasm agglutination rather than cell lysis (6). Even with controversies related to ozone application following its toxicity, it is well established that depending on its dosage, it exhibits therapeutic properties. In medicine, it is mainly delivered as a mixture with oxygen (5). In an animal study, ozone therapy proved to be antimicrobial in infected sternal and mediastinal tissues of experimental methicillin-resistant *Staphylococcus aureus* animals (7).

In dentistry, ozone is applied mostly as an oxygen/ozone gas or as ozonated water. The antimicrobial effect of ozone in dentistry is controversial because of variability in the concentration of ozone and methodology utilized (8, 9).

In dentistry

In relation to caries, when *Streptococcus mutans* and *Streptococcus sobrinus* were examined following the use of an ozone-generating device for 10 s (Heolozone, USA), a reduction of both microorganisms was observed (10). In a well-controlled clinical trial, when ozone was applied on primary root carious lesions, it resulted in the arrest of lesions up to 1.5 years following initial treatment (11).

In a prospective clinical study, ozone improved noncavitated initial fissure caries in patients of high risk over a period of 3 months (12).

Polydorou *et al.* (13) examined the potential of ozone as an antimicrobial agent on two bonding agents to decrease the incidence of recurrent decay. They concluded that the use of ozone for 80 s in an *in-vitro* infected cavity model significantly reduced the presence of *S. mutans*. Muller *et al.* (14) evaluated the antimicrobial efficacy of ozone gas with photodynamic therapy *in-vitro*. In this study, 0.2% and 2% chlorhexidine and 0.5% and 5% sodium hypochlorite solutions were used on multispecies oral biofilm-coated discs with *Actinomyces naeslundii*, *Veillonella dispar*, *Fusobacterium nucleatum*, *S. sobrinus*, *Streptococcus orali*, and *Candida albicans*. Notably, only 5% sodium hypochlorite solution was effective in eliminating all the bacteria.

As ozone has been indicated as an antimicrobial agent, the effect of gaseous ozone application on enamel and dentin bond strength has been of interest, and several studies have demonstrated no negative influence on the bonding of the enamel and dentin bond strength (15–17). Azarpazhooh *et al.* (18) examined the effect of ozone treatment on tooth hypersensitivity and concluded that even though a reduction of sensitivity in the ozone group was present, this percentage of reduction was not different from the placebo. This is in agreement with the study by Elgalaid (19), who also showed that ozone was not significantly more successful than the placebo group.

In endodontics

In endodontics, most studies were focused primarily on the antimicrobial activity of ozone. These studies resulted in controversial findings depending on the microorganisms evaluated, type and concentration of ozone, and time of contact (Table 12.1).

Nagayoshi *et al.* (20) examined the antimicrobial effects of ozonated water in the dentinal tubules against *Enterococcus faecalis* and *S. mutans*. Their results suggested that ozonated water when used with sonication had approximately the same reduction of bacteria as 2.25% sodium hypochlorite and also noted that ozonated water is less cytotoxic than 2.25% sodium hypochlorite on L-929 mouse fibroblasts. Their results suggest that ozonated water not only killed the microorganisms invading the dentinal tubules but was also less cytotoxic.

Virtej *et al.* (21) demonstrated ozone (HealOzone®, Kavo, Biberach, Germany) to be as efficient as 3% sodium hypochlorite and Biopure MTAD (Dentsply Tulsa Dental, Tulsa, OK) on the elimination of bacteria. Lynch (26) recommend the use of high concentrations of ozone as the final step in the instrumentation of the canal system.

When the antimicrobial effect against *E. faecalis* of ozonated water, gaseous ozone, 2.5% sodium hypochlorite, or 2% chlorhexidine were evaluated in maxillary anterior extracted teeth, none of the irrigants completely eliminated the bacteria following 20 min of contact; however, the concentrations of ozone used were not specified (23). This result is in agreement with the finding of Case *et al.* (25), who demonstrated that ozone failed to eliminate more *E. faecalis* biofilm compared to sodium hypochlorite, even with a concentration as low as 1%.

Hems *et al.* (22) demonstrated that when a monobiofilm specie of *E. faecalis* was evaluated, ozonated water was not effective unless the sample was agitated. However, when planktonic *E. faecalis* cells were evaluated, ozone demonstrated antimicrobial activity following 240 s of contact.

When *C. albicans* was evaluated, in addition to *E. faecalis*, ozonated water applied for 20 min reduced the counts for both microorganisms. However, when a second sampling was taken from the root canal system, microbial counts had increased, demonstrating a lack of residual effect of ozonated water. In the same study, ozonated water was unable to neutralize *Escherichia coli* endotoxin in root canals (24).

Table 12.1 Summary of Studies Focused Primarily on the Action of Ozone in Endodontics

Study	Type of ozone gas/water	Concentration	Time	Microorganisms	Effectiveness
Nagayoshi et al. (20)	Ozonated water	4 mg/ml	10 min	Enterococcus faecalis and Streptococcus mutans on dentinal tubules	With sonication, comparable results with 2.5% NaOCl. Less cytotoxicity
Virtej et al. (21)	HealOzone®	Ozone gas	Not specified	Aerobic and anaerobic bacteria	As effective as 3% NaOCl and MTAD
Hems et al. (22)	Ozonated gas sparged through a broth and ozonated water and ozone gas on biofilm	Ozonated gas	Not specified	Enterococcus faecalis planktonic and biofilm	Effective on planktonic but not on biofilm
Estrela et al. (23)	Ozonated water and gaseous ozone	Not specified	20 min	Enterococcus faecalis	Not effective
Cardoso et al. (24)	Ozonated water	24 mg/l	20 min	Candida albicans, Enterococcus faecalis, and endotoxins	Effective immediately following application; however, not effective at later sampling Ineffective against endotoxin
Case et al. (25)	Ozone gas and passive ultrasound	Not specified	Not specified	Enterococcus faecalis	

Summary of studies focused primarily on the action of ozone in endodontics (by author).

Electrochemical activation

ECA is produced by applying an electric current (electrolysis) to a diluted salt solution—typically a sodium chloride solution. Direct electric current is impressed on an anode (positive charge) and a cathode (negative charge) separated by a permeable membrane. As salt solution (electrolyte) flows across the anode and cathode, the bonds of a portion of the solution constituents, H_2O and NaCl, are rearranged. The solution leaving the anode chamber is known as the *anolyte*, and may contain oxygen gas (O_2), chlorine gas (Cl_2), hypochlorite ion (OCl^-), hypochlorous acid (HOCl), hydrochloric acid (HCl), and unreacted NaCl. The solution leaving the cathode chamber is known as the *catholyte*, and may contain NaOH, H_2, and unreacted NaCl (27). ECA has been used for many years and was popularized mainly in Russia and Japan (28, 29). ECA is also used in other countries in Europe and

South America. The main applications of ECA are in medicine, food industry, and waste water treatment, and more recently in dentistry because of its disinfectant, antiseptic, and antimicrobial properties. ECA produces a hypochlorous acid solution that is biocompatible, antimicrobial, and possesses a detergent effect. The antimicrobial properties are characteristic of the high oxidation potential of the anolyte solution produced, while the strong detergent effect is due to the high reduction potential of the catholyte solution (28–31).

A simple schematic of the process is shown in Figure 12.1.

In medicine, because of proven antimicrobial properties, ECA has been used in several countries during surgical procedures to disinfect endoscopy units, to prevent potential postoperative infection, and has also been used for the treatment of infectious skin, peritonitis, and to improve wound healing (32–35). The actual composition of the anolyte and catholyte will vary according to many factors, including the electrode material, electrode surface area, rate of electrolyte flow, amplitude of the electric current, and salt composition. The anolyte and catholyte have strong but opposite characteristics:

Anolyte

- Low pH, usually ranging from 2 to 8
- High oxidizing potential, usually in the range of +400 to +1200 mV
- Strong antibacterial, antifungal, and viral characteristics
- There are three types: acidic (anolyte), neutral, or alkaline (anolyte neutral cathodic) depending on the pH

Catholyte

- pH usually ranging from 7 to 12

- High reducing potential, usually in the range of −800 to −1200 mV
- Strong cleaning (detergent) effect

The anolyte solution is used extensively in the health field following the antimicrobial, antiviral, and antifungal properties (36, 37).

Other terms are also used to describe the same basic product. For example, OPW stands for oxidative potential water and SOW stands for superoxidized water. In the same manner, other researchers and equipment manufacturers use many different terms for what is essentially an ECA solution. Clearly, what is important is the physical and chemical characteristics of ECA solutions, rather than the name. In this chapter, we use the term *ECA*.

A popular ECA system in the USA, Sterilox® (PuriCore, Malvern, PA) has a pH between 5.0 and 6.5 with a oxidation potential of greater than

Table 12.2   Summary of Studies Evaluating ECA for Canal Cleanliness and Antimicrobial Action

Study	Type of solution	Aim	Effectiveness
Hata *et al.* (44)	Acidic anolyte solution	Canal cleanliness/smear layer	Effective
Marais (30)	Catholyte followed by anolyte	Canal cleanliness/smear layer	Effective and superior than NaOCl
Solovyeva and Dummer (45)	Anolyte solution pH 7.7	Canal cleanliness/smear layer	Effective at the apical third
Serper *et al.* (46)	Not specified	Canal cleanliness/smear layer	Not effective
Marais and Williams (47)	Anolyte solution (pH 7 and 9)	Antimicrobial effect	Lack of antimicrobial activity when compared to 3.5% NaOCl
Gulabilava *et al.* (48)	Neutral and acidic anolyte, catholyte, and catholyte/neutral anolyte with and without ultrasonic activation	Antimicrobial effect	Not as effective as 3% NaOCl
Heydrich *et al.* (49)	Several combinations	Canal cleanliness/smear layer	Not effective
Davis *et al.* (50)	Dermacyn (superoxidized water)	Antimicrobial effect	No antimicrobial activity against *E. faecalis*
Rossi-Fedele *et al.* (51)	Anolyte solution	Antimicrobial effect	No antimicrobial activity against *E. faecalis* when compared to 4.0% NaOCl
Garcia *et al.* (52)	Anolyte pH 6	Canal cleanliness/smear layer	Similar effect as 6% NaOCl following rinse with 17% EDTA

Summary of studies evaluating ECA for canal cleanliness and antimicrobial action (by author).

+950 mV. Sterilox has been demonstrated to be an effective antimicrobial and antifungal solution within 24 h of its production (36). In the food industry and medicine, there is enough *in-vitro* evidence of the antimicrobial and antiviral activities of ECA solutions against *Clostridium difficile* spores, *Helicobacter pylori*, vancomycin resistant *Enterococcus* species, *C. albicans*, and several *Mycobacterium* species (36), *P. aeruginosa* (38), *S. aureus* (39), and *Salmonella enteritidis* (40).

In dentistry, ECA is used for biofilm removal in dental unit water lines (41) and it became popular in endodontics following low cytotoxicity (42) and corrosion of instruments caused by irrigation solutions such as sodium hypochlorite (43). In endodontics, two main areas evaluate ECA: canal cleanliness and antimicrobial action (Table 12.2).

The removal of smear layer prior to obturation was advocated several years ago and is commonly achieved by the use of irrigants and chelating agents (53). With the introduction of ECA in endodontics, a few studies examined the capability of these solutions on smear layer removal. However, because of several discrepancies in the methodology the results are contradictory. Hata *et al.* (44) demonstrated the removal of smear layer following irrigation with OPW and advocated it as a potential irrigant solution in endodontics. In a later study, Hata and his group (54) showed oxidative water following instrumentation with 5% NaOCl to have a similar results when compared to NaOCl and 15% ethylenediaminetetraaceticacid (EDTA) on both debris and smear layer removal. Solovyeva and Dummer (45) showed that the combination of anolyte and catholyte solutions resulted in more opened dentinal tubules on the apical third of the canal system. They also noticed that a thinner smear layer with a more even surface was produced following the irrigation with ECA solutions. When a tooth model contaminated with *E. faecalis* biofilm was used, it was noted that ECA solution was as effective as 6% NaOCl in the presence of a chelating agent (52). However, Heydrich *et al.* (48) examined the use of different combinations of ECA solutions on canal cleanliness and determined they had no effect on the cleanliness of the canal system when smear layer and opened dentinal tubules were examined under SEM. Serper *et al.* (46) also demonstrated the inability of OPW on removing the smear layer.

The antimicrobial effect of ECA was investigated by Rossi-Fedele *et al.* (51) comparing Sterilox's Aquatine Alpha Electrolyte® with NaOCl using a bovine root canal model, and the conclusion reached was that NaOCl eliminated *E. faecalis* better. These findings were in agreement with the research by other investigators who concluded that ECA solutions were not as effective in eliminating bacteria from the root canal system (47).

We examined the antimicrobial effect of Sterilox and Qmix against *E. faecalis* biofilm using quantitative real time polymerase chain reaction (PCR) in the mesial buccal roots and isthmus of mandibular first molars. Both solutions had a reduction of more than 90% pre- and postirrigation; however, the difference between each solution was not statistically significant.

Currently, we cannot ignore the fact that Regenerative Endodontics is a viable and important alternative to our field. In a recent study, it was demonstrated that irrigation with Sterilox better preserved the survival and attachment of dental

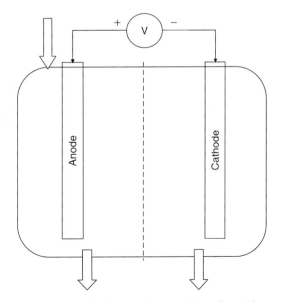

Figure 12.1 Simple schematic showing electrochemical process in an electrolyzed water generator.

pulp stem cells to the dentinal wall as compared to other solutions (55).

There is no strong evidence in favor of the use of ozone and ECA solutions in dentistry and more studies are needed in this field. Owing to a new era in which Regenerative Endodontics plays a major role in the specialty, antimicrobial solutions with reduced cytotoxicity are important for a successful outcome.

References

1. Carmichael, N.G., Winder, C., Borges, S.H., Backhouse, B.L. & Lewis, P.D. (1982) Minireview: the health implications of water treatment with ozone. *Life Sciences*, **30** (2), 117–129, PubMed PMID: 7033710.

2. Bocci, V.A. (2006) Scientific and medical aspects of ozone therapy. State of the art. *Archives of Medical Research*, **37** (4), 425–435, PubMed PMID: 16624639.

3. Bocci, V., Zanardi, I. & Travagli, V. (2011) Oxygen/ozone as a medical gas mixture. A critical evaluation of the various methods clarifies positive and negative aspects. *Medical Gas Research*, **1** (1), 6, PubMed PMID: 22146387; Pubmed Central PMCID: 3231820.

4. Sagai, M. & Bocci, V. (2011) mechanisms of action involved in ozone therapy: is healing induced via a mild oxidative stress? *Medical Gas Research.*, **1**, 29, PubMed PMID: 22185664. Pubmed Central PMCID: 3298518.

5. Seidler, V., Linetskiy, I., Hubalkova, H., Stankova, H., Smucler, R. & Mazanek, J. (2008) Ozone and its usage in general medicine and dentistry. A review article. *Prague Medical Report*, **109** (1), 5–13, PubMed PMID: 19097384.

6. Zhang, Y.Q., Wu, Q.P., Zhang, J.M. & Yang, X.H. (2011) Effects of ozone on membrane permeability and ultrastructure in Pseudomonas aeruginosa. *Journal of Applied Microbiology*, **111** (4), 1006–1015, PubMed PMID: 21790913.

7. Gulmen, S., Kurtoglu, T., Meteoglu, I., Kaya, S. & Okutan, H. (2013) Ozone therapy as an adjunct to vancomycin enhances bacterial elimination in methicillin resistant Staphylococcus aureus mediastinitis. *The Journal of Surgical Research*, **185** (1), 64–69, PubMed PMID: 23809152.

8. Azarpazhooh, A. & Limeback, H. (2008) The application of ozone in dentistry: a systematic review of literature. *Journal of Dentistry*, **36** (2), 104–116, PubMed PMID: 18166260.

9. Saini, R. (2011) Ozone therapy in dentistry: a strategic review. *Journal of Natural Science, Biology, and Medicine.*, **2** (2), 151–153, PubMed PMID: 22346227. Pubmed Central PMCID: 3276005.

10. Baysan, A., Whiley, R.A. & Lynch, E. (2000) Antimicrobial effect of a novel ozone- generating device on micro-organisms associated with primary root carious lesions in vitro. *Caries Research*, **34** (6), 498–501, PubMed PMID: 11093025.

11. Holmes, J. (2003) Clinical reversal of root caries using ozone, double-blind, randomised, controlled 18-month trial. *Gerodontology*, **20** (2), 106–114, PubMed PMID: 14697022.

12. Huth, K.C., Paschos, E., Brand, K. & Hickel, R. (2005) Effect of ozone on non-cavitated fissure carious lesions in permanent molars. A controlled prospective clinical study. *American Journal of Dentistry*, **18** (4), 223–228, PubMed PMID: 16296426.

13. Polydorou, O., Pelz, K. & Hahn, P. (2006) Antibacterial effect of an ozone device and its comparison with two dentin-bonding systems. *European Journal of Oral Sciences*, **114** (4), 349–353, PubMed PMID: 16911107.

14. Muller, P., Guggenheim, B. & Schmidlin, P.R. (2007) Efficacy of gasiform ozone and photodynamic therapy on a multispecies oral biofilm in vitro. *European Journal of Oral Sciences*, **115** (1), 77–80, PubMed PMID: 17305720.

15. Cadenaro, M., Delise, C., Antoniollo, F., Navarra, O.C., Di Lenarda, R. & Breschi, L. (2009) Enamel and dentin bond strength following gaseous ozone application. *The Journal of Adhesive Dentistry*, **11** (4), 287–292, PubMed PMID: 19701509.

16. Schmidlin, P.R., Zimmermann, J. & Bindl, A. (2005) Effect of ozone on enamel and dentin bond strength. *The Journal of Adhesive Dentistry*, **7** (1), 29–32, PubMed PMID: 15892361.

17. Garcia, E.J., Serrano, A.P., Urruchi, W.I. *et al.* (2012) Influence of ozone gas and ozonated water application to dentin and bonded interfaces on resin–dentin bond strength. *The Journal of Adhesive Dentistry*, **14** (4), 363–370, PubMed PMID: 22282748.

18. Azarpazhooh, A., Limeback, H., Lawrence, H.P. & Fillery, E.D. (2009) Evaluating the effect of an ozone delivery system on the reversal of dentin hypersensitivity: a randomized, double-blinded clinical trial. *Journal of Endodontics*, **35** (1), 1–9, PubMed PMID: 19084115.

19. Elgalaid, T. (2010) Ozone treatment had no effect on tooth hypersensitivity. *Evidence-Based Dentistry*, **11** (3), 70, PubMed PMID: 20938468.

20. Nagayoshi, M., Fukuizumi, T., Kitamura, C., Yano, J., Terashita, M. & Nishihara, T. (2004) Efficacy of ozone on survival and permeability of oral microorganisms. *Oral Microbiology and Immunology*, **19** (4), 240–246, PubMed PMID: 15209994.

21. Virtej, A., MacKenzie, C.R., Raab, W.H., Pfeffer, K. & Barthel, C.R. (2007) Determination of the performance of various root canal disinfection methods after in situ carriage. *Journal of Endodontics*, **33** (8), 926–929, PubMed PMID: 17878076.

22. Hems, R.S., Gulabivala, K., Ng, Y.L., Ready, D. & Spratt, D.A. (2005) An in vitro evaluation of the ability of ozone to kill a strain of Enterococcus faecalis. *International Endodontic Journal*, **38** (**1**), 22–29, PubMed PMID: 15606819.

23. Estrela, C., Estrela, C.R.A., Decurcio, D.A., Hollanda, A.C.B. & Silva, J.A. (2007) Antimicrobial efficacy of ozonated water, gaseous ozone, sodium hypochlorite and chlorhexidine in infected human root canals. *International Endodontic Journal*, **40** (**2**), 85–93, PubMed PMID: WOS:000243404100001. English.

24. Cardoso, M.G., de Oliveira, L.D., Koga-Ito, C.Y. & Jorge, A.O. (2008) Effectiveness of ozonated water on Candida albicans, Enterococcus faecalis, and endotoxins in root canals. *Oral Surgery, Oral Medicine, Oral Pathology, Oral Radiology, and Endodontics*, **105** (**3**), e85–e91, PubMed PMID: 18280954.

25. Case, P.D., Bird, P.S., Kahler, W.A., George, R. & Walsh, L.J. (2012) Treatment of root canal biofilms of Enterococcus faecalis with ozone gas and passive ultrasound activation. *Journal of Endodontics*, **38** (**4**), 523–526, PubMed PMID: 22414842.

26. Lynch, E. (2008) Evidence-based efficacy of ozone for root canal irrigation. *Journal of Esthetic and Restorative Dentistry: Official Publication of the American Academy of Esthetic Dentistry*, **20** (**5**), 287–293, PubMed PMID: 18837750.

27. Hsu, S.Y. (2005) Effects of flow rate, temperature and salt concentration on chemical and physical properties of electrolyzed oxidizing water. *Journal of Food Engineering*, **66** (**2**), 171–176, PubMed PMID: WOS:000224283200004. English.

28. Bakhir, V.M. (1997) Electrochemical activation: theory and practice. *Proceedings of the First International Symposium on Electrochemical Activation*, pp. 38–45. Moscow.

29. Leonov, B.I. (1997) Electrochemical activation of water and aqueous solutions: past, present and future. *Proceedings of the First International Symposium on Electrochemical Activation*, pp. 11–27. Moscow.

30. Marais, J.T. (2000) Cleaning efficacy of a new root canal irrigation solution: a preliminary evaluation. *International Endodontic Journal*, **33** (**4**), 320–325, PubMed PMID: 11307206.

31. Shimizu, Y. & Hurusawa, T. (1992) Antiviral, antibacterial, and antifungal actions of electrolyzed oxidizing water through electrolysis. *Dental Journal*, **37**, 1055–1062.

32. Selkon, J.B. (2001) Sterilox disinfection of endoscopes. *The Journal of Hospital Infection*, **48** (**2**), 154–155, PubMed PMID: 11428885.

33. Inoue, Y., Endo, S., Kondo, K., Ito, H., Omori, H. & Saito, K. (1997) Trial of electrolyzed strong acid aqueous solution lavage in the treatment of peritonitis and intraperitoneal abscess. *Artificial Organs*, **21** (**1**), 28–31, PubMed PMID: 9012903.

34. Ohno, H., Higashidate, M. & Yokosuka, T. (2000) Mediastinal irrigation with superoxidized water after open-heart surgery: the safety and pitfalls of cardiovascular surgical application. *Surgery Today*, **30** (**11**), 1055–1056, PubMed PMID: 11110409.

35. Piaggesi, A., Goretti, C., Mazzurco, S. *et al.* (2010) A randomized controlled trial to examine the efficacy and safety of a new super-oxidized solution for the management of wide postsurgical lesions of the diabetic foot. *The International Journal of Lower Extremity Wounds*, **9** (**1**), 10–15, PubMed PMID: 20207618.

36. Shetty, N., Srinivasan, S., Holton, J. & Ridgway, G.L. (1999) Evaluation of microbicidal activity of a new disinfectant: Sterilox 2500 against Clostridium difficile spores, Helicobacter pylori, vancomycin resistant Enterococcus species, Candida albicans and several Mycobacterium species. *The Journal of Hospital Infection*, **41** (**2**), 101–105, PubMed PMID: 10063471.

37. Robinson, G.M., Lee, S.W., Greenman, J., Salisbury, V.C. & Reynolds, D.M. (2010) Evaluation of the efficacy of electrochemically activated solutions against nosocomial pathogens and bacterial endospores. *Letters in Applied Microbiology*, **50** (**3**), 289–294, PubMed PMID: 20070511.

38. Kiura, H., Sano, K., Morimatsu, S. *et al.* (2002) Bactericidal activity of electrolyzed acid water from solution containing sodium chloride at low concentration, in comparison with that at high concentration. *Journal of Microbiological Methods*, **49** (**3**), 285–293, PubMed PMID: 11869793.

39. Park, H., Hung, Y.C. & Kim, C. (2002) Effectiveness of electrolyzed water as a sanitizer for treating different surfaces. *Journal of Food Protection*, **65** (**8**), 1276–1280, PubMed PMID: 12182480.

40. Venkitanarayanan, K.S., Ezeike, G.O., Hung, Y.C. & Doyle, M.P. (1999) Efficacy of electrolyzed oxidizing water for inactivating Escherichia coli O157:H7, Salmonella enteritidis, and Listeria monocytogenes. *Applied and Environmental Microbiology*, **65** (**9**), 4276–4279, PubMed PMID: 10473453; Pubmed Central PMCID: 99778.

41. Walker, J.T., Bradshaw, D.J., Fulford, M.R. & Marsh, P.D. (2003) Microbiological evaluation of a range of disinfectant products to control mixed-species biofilm contamination in a laboratory model of a dental unit water system. *Applied and Environmental Microbiology*, **69** (**6**), 3327–3332, PubMed PMID: 12788733; Pubmed Central PMCID: 161510.

42. Gatot, A., Arbelle, J., Leiberman, A. & Yanai-Inbar, I. (1991) Effects of sodium hypochlorite on soft tissues after its inadvertent injection beyond the root apex. *Journal of Endodontics*, **17** (**11**), 573–574, PubMed PMID: 1812208.

43. Berutti, E., Angelini, E., Rigolone, M., Migliaretti, G. & Pasqualini, D. (2006) Influence of sodium

hypochlorite on fracture properties and corrosion of ProTaper Rotary instruments. *International Endodontic Journal*, **39** (**9**), 693–699, PubMed PMID: 16916358.

44. Hata, G., Uemura, M., Weine, F.S. & Toda, T. (1996) Removal of smear layer in the root canal using oxidative potential water. *Journal of Endodontics*, **22** (**12**), 643–645, PubMed PMID: 9220747.

45. Solovyeva, A.M. & Dummer, P.M. (2000) Cleaning effectiveness of root canal irrigation with electrochemically activated anolyte and catholyte solutions: a pilot study. *International Endodontic Journal*, **33** (**6**), 494–504, PubMed PMID: 11307252.

46. Serper, A., Calt, S., Dogan, A.L., Guc, D., Ozcelik, B. & Kuraner, T. (2001) Comparison of the cytotoxic effects and smear layer removing capacity of oxidative potential water, NaOCl and EDTA. *Journal of Oral Science*, **43** (**4**), 233–238, PubMed PMID: 11848188.

47. Marais, J.T. & Williams, W.P. (2001) Antimicrobial effectiveness of electro-chemically activated water as an endodontic irrigation solution. *International Endodontic Journal*, **34** (**3**), 237–243, PubMed PMID: 12193270.

48. Seal, GJ, Ng YL, Spratt D, Bhatti M, Gulabivala K. (2002) An in vitro comparison of the bactericidal efficacy of lethal photosensitization or sodium hypochlorite irrigation on Streptococcus intermedius biofilms in root canals. *Int Endod J.*, **35** (**3**), 268–274.

49. Heydrich, R., Varella, C., Vertucci, F. & Pileggi, R. (2008) A quantitative SEM analysis of canal cleanliness utilizing different irrigating solutions. *Journal of Endodontics*, **34**, 343.

50. Davis, J.M., Maki, J., Bahcall, J.K. (2007) An in vitro comparison of the antimicrobial effects of various endodontic medicaments on Enterococcus faecalis. *J Endod*, **33** (**5**), 567–569.

51. Rossi-Fedele, G., Figueiredo, J.A., Steier, L., Canullo, L., Steier, G. & Roberts, A.P. (2010) Evaluation of the antimicrobial effect of super-oxidized water (Sterilox(R)) and sodium hypochlorite against Enterococcus faecalis in a bovine root canal model. *Journal of Applied Oral Science: Revista FOB*, **18**(**5**), 498–502, PubMed PMID: 21085808.

52. Garcia, F., Murray, P.E., Garcia-Godoy, F. & Namerow, K.N. (2010) Effect of aquatine endodontic cleanser on smear layer removal in the root canals of ex vivo human teeth. *Journal of Applied Oral Science: Revista FOB*, **18** (**4**), 403–408, PubMed PMID: 20835577.

53. Haapasalo, M., Shen, Y., Qian, W. & Gao, Y. (2010) Irrigation in endodontics. *Dental Clinics of North America*, **54** (**2**), 291–312, PubMed PMID: 20433979.

54. Hata, G., Hayami, S., Weine, F.S. & Toda, T. (2001) Effectiveness of oxidative potential water as a root canal irrigant. *International Endodontic Journal*, **34** (**4**), 308–317, PubMed PMID: 11482143.

55. Ring, K.C., Murray, P.E., Namerow, K.N., Kuttler, S. & Garcia-Godoy, F. (2008) The comparison of the effect of endodontic irrigation on cell adherence to root canal dentin. *Journal of Endodontics*, **34** (**12**), 1474–1479, PubMed PMID: 19026877.

13 Intracanal Medication in Root Canal Disinfection

Lea Assed Bezerra da Silva, Raquel Assed Bezerra da Silva, and Paulo Nelson-Filho

Department of Pediatric Dentistry, School of Dentistry of Ribeirão Preto. University of Sao Paulo, Riberao Preto, Brazil

Nestor Cohenca

Department of Endodontics and Pediatric Dentistry, University of Washington, Seattle, WA, USA

Introduction

Considering that apical periodontitis is a disease caused primarily by microorganisms and/or their by-products infecting the root canal system (1), the key for the success of endodontic treatment and apical repair is infection control (2–4). It is known that microorganisms aggregated in well-established biofilms are more resistant to killing (5) and that residual endodontic infection can cause the persistence of apical periodontitis (4). In a clinical study, Sjogren *et al.* verified that postendodontic treatment success rate was significantly lower in teeth with apical periodontitis compared with teeth without the disease (6). Therefore, the primary goal of the endodontic treatment in teeth with chronic apical periodontitis and a long-term infectious process

should be eliminating the microbial infection from the root canal system (2, 7–10). In addition, root canal treatment should be done as early as possible because apical periodontitis causes tissue destruction, involving loss of periodontal ligament fiber attachment, concomitantly with cementum and bone resorption (Figure 13.1a,b), which might culminate in tooth loss (11).

It has been discussed whether the biomechanical preparation alone can eradicate endodontic infection in teeth with apical periodontitis. In these cases, microorganisms are disseminated throughout the root canal system, namely main canal, lateral, accessory and secondary canals, dentinal tubules (Figure 13.2), cemental lacunae (Figure 13.3), apical delta ramifications (Figure 13.4a,b), apical foramen, apical erosions,

Disinfection of Root Canal Systems: The Treatment of Apical Periodontitis, First Edition. Edited by Nestor Cohenca.
© 2014 John Wiley & Sons, Inc. Published 2014 by John Wiley & Sons, Inc.

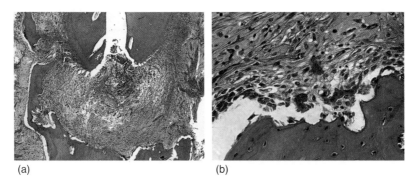

Figure 13.1　Apical periodontitis: tissue destruction, loss of periodontal ligament fiber attachment, cementum, and bone resorption (a, b). Hematoxilin and eosin.

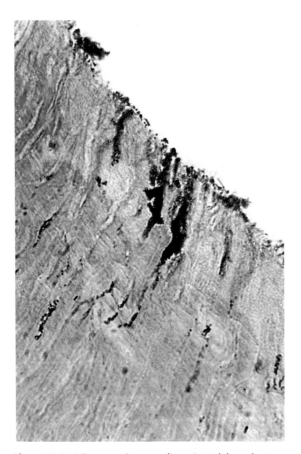

Figure 13.2　Microorganisms are disseminated throughout the dentinal tubules in teeth with apical periodontitis. Brown and Brenn staining.

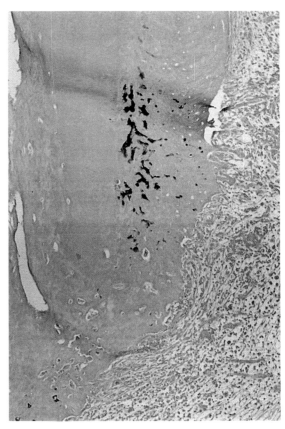

Figure 13.3　Microorganisms found in cemental lacunae in teeth with apical periodontitis. Brown and Brenn staining.

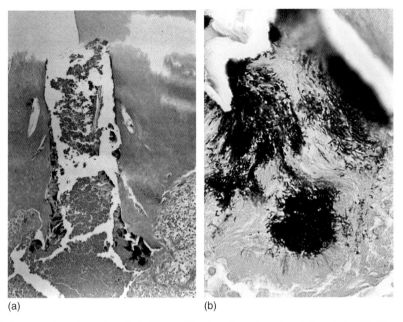

(a)   (b)

Figure 13.4   (a, b) Microorganisms found in apical delta ramifications in teeth with apical periodontitis. Brown and Brenn staining.

and are even organized as biofilms on the external surfaces of the apical root third (Figure 13.5a,b)(12, 13), which are areas inaccessible to the biomechanical preparation and to the body defense system (14–18).

Historically, different substances and medications have been used as intracanal medication between endodontic treatment sessions to assist in the control of microbial infection, including calcium hydroxide-based pastes, polyantibiotic pastes, formalin tricresol, camphorated paramonochlorophenol, and chlorhexidine alone or in combination with other substances.

At the same time, studies using microbial culture and biomolecular techniques in permanent teeth have established that the infection in teeth with pulp necrosis and apical periodontitis is of polymicrobial nature, with predominance of anaerobic microorganisms (19–21), mainly Gram-positive. bacteria (20). These characteristics have also been demonstrated in primary teeth (22, 23).

In addition to generating toxic products and by-products to the tissues, Gram-positive bacteria present as a major component of its cell wall endotoxin, also known as *LPS* following its lipopolysaccharide nature (24, 25), that acts as

one of the most important virulence factors of these microorganisms (26–29). Bacterial endotoxin is released after the death or multiplication of microorganisms and causes a series of biological events that activate immunocompetent cells. In sequence, this activation leads to the release of several proinflammatory cytokines and mediators that are responsible for establishing an inflammatory response (24, 30–33), osteoclastogenesis and cemental and bone resorption (34–36), thus contributing to the genesis (Figure 13.6), development, and persistence of apical periodontitis (25, 37). A positive association has also been observed between the amount of bacterial endotoxin in the root canals and the presence of clinical symptoms, such as pain, tenderness to percussion and palpation, edema, and purulent exudate (38).

Bacterial endotoxin has long been recognized as a potential stimulator of several host's cells via receptors, such as lipopolysaccharide-binding protein (LBP), CD14 receptor (39), and toll-like receptors (TLRs) (39, 40), causing the expression of proinflammatory cytokines and amplification of the host's response. The bacterial endotoxin acts on macrophages and other cell types (24) by stimulating the expression of the tumor necrosis

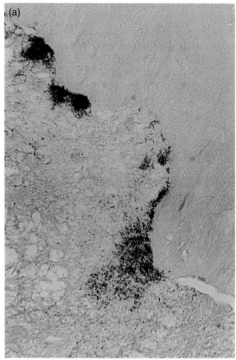

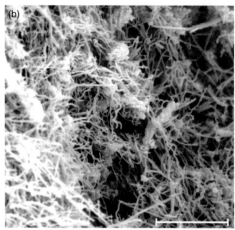

Figure 13.5 Microorganisms organized as biofilms on the external surfaces of the apical root third. Brown and Brenn staining (a) and scanning electronic microscopy (b).

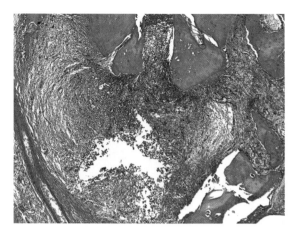

Figure 13.6 Apical inflammatory response and osteoclastogenesis, resulting in apical periodontitis development. Hematoxilin and eosin.

metabolism, and complement system (44, 45), and acts as a pyrogen agent inducing fever (46), being involved in inflammatory response events, such as the increase of vascular permeability, neutrophil and macrophage chemotaxis, and release of lysozymes and lymphokines (44). It has been suggested that the LPS-mediated sensitization of nociceptors is one of the mechanisms responsible for the pain associated with endodontic and apical infections (47).

In addition to causing inflammatory reaction, bacterial endotoxin adheres to mineralized tissues, stimulating bone resorption (37), synthesis, and release of osteoclast-activating cytokines (36, 48), and osteoclastogenesis (36). Thus, in teeth with apical periodontitis, the use of an intracanal medication between sessions is indicated to assist in the elimination of endodontic infection and inactivate bacterial endotoxin. Several materials with antimicrobial activity have been evaluated to inactivate the bacterial endotoxin, other bacterial cell wall components with and without effective results, including calcium hydroxide (33, 36, 37, 49, 50), polymyxin B (51), formocresol (52), chlorhexidine (53) Er:YAG laser (54), ultrasound (55), ozonized water (56), and sodium hypochlorite at different concentrations (53, 57, 58).

The chances of having bacterial endotoxin and viable microorganisms in the canal at the filling stage are greater in single-session endodontic treatments. Theoretically, most of the residual bacteria would be killed because of the contact of the filling

factor (TNF) (41), interleukin-1, interleukin-6 (30), and interleukin-8 (30, 42). In addition, bacterial endotoxin acts as a potential inductor of nitric oxide production (13).

Bacterial endotoxin also activates the Hageman factor (coagulation factor XII) (43), arachidonic acid material or would remain entombed inside the dentinal tubules and die from starvation following scarcity of nutrients. Also, considering the complex canal anatomy and the small number and low pathogenicity of the residual bacteria, it is assumed that those who survived would not reach the apical tissues. However, it should be considered that fillings do not provide hermetic apical and cervical seals. In addition, residual microorganisms could reach the periapex through the interface between the filling material and the canal walls, and through the dentinal tubules, apical cementum, and apical delta canals. Microorganisms may also persist after single-session endodontic treatment in aggregates adhered to cementum surface (apical biofilm). For these reasons, a significant correlation has been demonstrated between endodontic failures and microorganisms surviving after root canal filling.

Traditionally, the root canal treatment of teeth with necrotic pulp and apical periodontitis has been done in multiple sessions with the use of an interappointment intracanal medication being accepted as a safe and effective therapy (59). The philosophy of completing the root canal treatment of these teeth in one visit has been proposed only to shorten treatment duration and is based on achieving similar outcome rates in clinical and radiographic evaluations after single-session treatments (60–65). However, this is still a controversial topic within the endodontic literature (65) mainly considering the relatively short follow-up periods of some studies (63, 64). In addition, some of those who adopt single-session endodontic treatments consider partial apical repair in asymptomatic teeth as success, which increases their treatment success rates.

It is incontestable that the persistence of apical periodontitis or even partial posttreatment radiographic repair indicates the existence of residual infection in the root canal system or on the external apical root surfaces. This condition may impede the occurrence of complete repair, resulting in the maintenance of a chronic apical inflammatory infiltrate and formation of areas of cemental and bone resorption (Figure 13.7).

It is known that *clinical silence* may remain for several months or years. This condition together with radiographic apical repair, often partial, refers

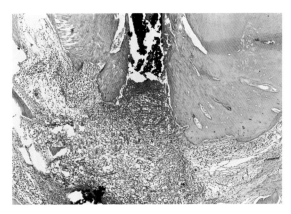

Figure 13.7 Persistence of apical periodontitis following root canal treatment indicating the existence of residual infection in the root canal system or on the external apical root surfaces. Hematoxilin and eosin.

to an *evolutive phase* of the healing process without recovery of the lamina dura, and therefore it does not represent an ideal histological repair. In a histopathological analysis, apical lesions with partial radiographic resolution present accentuated tissue disorganization and persistence of inflammatory response events.

Following the discussion above, we can conclude that the intracanal medication of choice should be an antiseptic medication without adverse effects to the apical tissues and the capacity to stimulate the occurrence of repair.

Intracanal medication—definition

Intracanal medication can be defined as a medication or substance used after biomechanical preparation of root canals between treatment sessions to

— eliminate the endodontic infection and the microbial proliferation in the root canal system and neutralize the bacterial endotoxin in teeth with pulp necrosis and apical periodontitis;
— reduce the intensity of apical and apical inflammatory responses;
— act as a physical and chemical barrier, preventing canal reinfection and minimizing coronal leakage through the temporary restoration; and
— increase the pH of the region.

Basic requisites for an interappointment intracanal medication

A substance or medication to be used as an interappointment intracanal medication should (66)

— have a broad spectrum of antimicrobial activity;
— eliminate residual microorganisms in the canals after instrumentation and neutralize bacterial endotoxin;
— present physicochemical properties that permit its diffusion through the root canal system and sufficient action time to reach the microorganisms at different canal sites;
— reduce apical tissue inflammation;
— act as a barrier against coronal leakage through the temporary restorative material;
— assist in the control of persistent exudation; and
— have tissue compatibility to favor the repair without causing additional irritation to the apical tissues.

Materials used as interappointment intracanal medication

Calcium hydroxide

Contemporary endodontics seeks substances that combine antibacterial and anti-inflammatory properties and capacity to induce mineralized tissue formation in such a way that the interrelation of these properties results in a medication with a beneficial effect to the repair of the apical tissues.

Calcium hydroxide is an odorless white powder with molecular weight of 74.08 and low solubility in water (~1.2 g/l at 25 °C, decreasing with the increase of temperature) (67). Its coefficient of dissociation of 0.17 permits a slow and controlled release of calcium and hydroxyl ions (68). The low solubility is a favorable characteristic because a long period is necessary before the solubilization of the material in direct contact with the tissue fluids. Calcium hydroxide has an alkaline pH (~12.5–12.8) and is chemically classified as a strong base (69). Its main properties—antimicrobial activity and capacity of inducing mineralized tissue deposition (70)— is a result of its ionic dissociation.

Calcium hydroxide has been traditionally considered as the intracanal medication of choice (2, 68, 71) because of its simultaneous multiplicity of actions that include antimicrobial activity (14, 72–75), even against *Enterococcus faecalis* (76, 77); indirect antimicrobial action by environmental carbon dioxide absorption (78) and consequent stimulation of apical and apical repair; assistance in the control of apical exudation (74, 79) following its hygroscopic propriety; capacity to dissolve necrotic material (80); reduction of the amount of matrix metalloproteinases (81); release of inflammatory mediators (74) and the inactivation of the lipoteichoic acid from *E. faecalis* (50); anti-inflammatory activity (82); participation in mineralized tissue formation (16, 83, 84), with alkaline phosphatase activation and collagen synthesis (85); increase of extracellular calcium levels, inducing differentiation of periodontal ligament cementoblasts and cementogenesis (86); and, most importantly, tissue compatibility (16, 87–89) (Figure 13.8a–c).

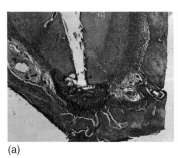
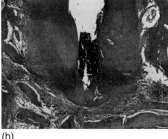
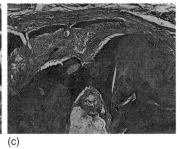

(a)   (b)   (c)

Figure 13.8   Mineralized tissue formation (cementogenesis) as a result of calcium hydroxide root canal dressing and filling (a, b, c). This response indicates tissue compatibility. Hematoxilin and eosin and Mallory Trichrome.

Calcium hydroxide also has the capacity to penetrate into the dentinal tubules (90), increasing the pH on the root periphery. This property contributes to the regression of resorption processes because the alkalinization of regions with acidic pH creates unfavorable conditions to the action of osteoclasts. In addition, calcium hydroxide has been widely used in dentistry to stimulate mineralization because of its dissociation into hydroxyl and calcium ions. The hydroxyl ions are responsible for maintaining an alkaline pH while the calcium ions have a direct effect on extracellular matrix mineralization (91). Furthermore, the increase of intracellular calcium levels activates the calcium/calmodulin-dependent pathways, which regulates osteoblast differentiation via phosphorylated extracellular signal-regulated kinases (ERK-1/ERK-2) and c-fos protein expression (92).

An important aspect to be considered is that, to date, calcium hydroxide is the only intracanal medication that presents effective results on bacterial endotoxin inactivation (35, 36, 41, 49, 58, 93–95), without causing damage to tissue repair (33).

On the basis of all these considerations and in agreement with health promotion principles, calcium hydroxide should be the medication of choice when the use of an interappointment intracanal medication is required.

Vehicle

Calcium hydroxide does not have good physical properties presenting low flow, viscosity, and adherence to canal walls, in addition to being radiolucent. Therefore, to be used in the form of paste under clinical conditions, calcium hydroxide must be combined with an aqueous, viscous, or oily vehicle, for example, distilled water, saline, anesthetic solution, methylcellulose, cresatin, polyethylene glycol (PEG), propylene glycol, and olive oil. On the other hand, the potential interferences of the different vehicles on the action of calcium hydroxide must be carefully examined because the type of vehicle determines the velocity of ionic dissociation and the capacity of paste solubilization (96), which might alter its antimicrobial activity (97), tissue compatibility (87), and the mineralized tissue-inductive capacity (98).

Aqueous vehicles permit a rapid ionic dissociation. Nevertheless, viscous vehicles like PEG 400 or propyleneglycol allow for a slow but sustained release of hydroxyl ions, maintaining an alkaline environment for a longer period (98). At the same time, it has been suggested that such pH elevation resulting from the release of hydroxyl ions could start or favor the mineralization process (90).

The use of a commercial calcium hydroxide paste in aqueous vehicle supplemented with blood salts, Calasept® (Speiko, Darmstadt, Germany), in the endodontic treatment of immature teeth with vital pulp resulted in the formation of mineralized tissue barriers at the apical level and the absence of inflammatory and normal periodontal ligament thickness (98).

A commercial calcium hydroxide paste using PEG 400 as vehicle (Calen®; S. S. White; Artigos Dentários Ltda., Rio de Janeiro, RJ, Brazil) has been shown to maintain calcium hydroxide for a longer time in the region of interest, prolonging its action, decreasing its solubilization in the fluids, and increasing its capacity of penetrating the tubular root dentin (98). Calen presents pH around 12.4 (87), high antimicrobial activity and tissue compatibility (16, 87). Theoretically, the low PEG 400 dispersion results in slower dissolution rates of the paste with consequent lower release of calcium ions compared with the use of distilled water as a vehicle. This is relevant, considering the changes of intracanal medication during the treatment and the need of maintaining an alkaline pH and calcium and hydroxyl ion release.

The mild tissue aggression caused by Calen could be explained by the fact that the hydroxyl ions released from this paste do not remain free for a long time because they react with the hydrogen ions released from PEG 400 ionization in water (neutralization reaction). In the commercial calcium hydroxide paste with distilled water (Calasept), on the other hand, the hydroxyl ions released from calcium hydroxide dissociation are not neutralized because there are no free hydrogen ions in the solution. However, even though Calasept causes an initially more severe tissue aggression than Calen, both pastes have been shown to offer a similar tissue repair in the later periods of evaluation (87, 98).

Aqueous and viscous vehicles should be preferred to calcium hydroxide-based intracanal medications. Oily vehicles are not indicated because they impede ion dissociation from the paste (99).

Endodontic treatment of teeth with apical periodontitis

Single session × multiple sessions
While some clinical and radiographic studies have found no difference between the single- and two-session endodontic treatments using a calcium hydroxide-based intracanal medication (60, 62, 63, 65, 100–108), or that the single-session treatment can be more effective (64), other clinical, radiographic and histopathological studies have found higher success when an intracanal medication was placed between sessions (16, 86, 109–117). A fact that is worth mentioning is that in most studies that found no difference between single- and two-session treatments, the intracanal medication was left in the canal for only 7 days, a period that is considered insufficient (118), as is discussed later in this chapter.

As emphasized before, another relevant aspect to be discussed is that after completion of an endodontic treatment, we should be aware that the absence of postoperative pain or "clinical silence" *per se* does not necessarily indicate treatment success. For both primary and permanent teeth with pulp necrosis and chronic apical periodontitis, no endodontic treatment can be considered as successful based only on the findings of clinical and radiographic examinations. The results of tomographic (clinical trials) and histopathological (research studies) analyses must be computed as well, as several authors have found higher success rates of root canal treatment performed with the use of a calcium hydroxide-based intracanal medication between sessions compared with one-visit treatment (16, 86, 112, 115, 117). Endodontic techniques that reach success at all these levels should be the ones of choice for use in clinical practice.

Intracanal medication: how to perform?
In order to obtain a deeper penetration of the paste into the dentinal tubules, the instrumented root canals should be filled with EDTA for 3 min under agitation with a K-file to remove the smear layer (119). Next, the canals should be copiously irrigated, dried with paper points, and filled with a calcium hydroxide-based paste in aqueous or viscous vehicle with slight apical overflow to reach the apical biofilm.

Duration of calcium hydroxide therapy
A minimal period of 14-21 days is necessary for calcium hydroxide to diffuse through the regions that may harbor microorganisms responsible for endodontic failure (e.g., dentinal tubules, apical cementum, and accessory/collateral canals) (112), increasing the pH of the external apical root surface and killing microorganisms and eliminating bacterial endotoxin from these regions (112, 118, 120, 121).

Although the usual duration of an interappointment intracanal medication is 7 days, this time is not sufficient to eliminate residual microorganisms from the root canal system. The interappointment intracanal medication should be maintained for, at least, 14 days (112), which is the time necessary for a greater release of calcium and hydroxyl ions (118) and for these ions to penetrate deeply into the entire dentin thickness, reaching the external apical root cementum.

From a histopathological standpoint, the best results of apical and apical repair are obtained after 15 and 30 days of calcium hydroxide therapy, while the worst results are observed when an intracanal medication is not used or is left for only 7 days. For this reason, the calcium hydroxide paste should be used as an interappointment intracanal medication in teeth with pulp necrosis and apical periodontitis for no less than 14 days.

From a mechanical and clinical perspective, new evidence has demonstrated that removal of calcium hydroxide by additional instrumentation in a second appointment may lead to canal transportation with higher incidence in curved canals (122), and residual medication might remain in the root canal system (123). Furthermore, calcium hydroxide has recently been associated with reduced fracture resistance of the dental hard tissues when applied for more than 30 days (124, 125). The intracanal placement of calcium hydroxide weakened the microtensile fracture strength of teeth with an average of 0.157 MPa *per* day (126). The authors also reported a statistically significant difference between 7 days (45.7 MPa) and 28 days (35.6 MPa) and also between 7 and 84 days (31.8 MPa).

Periapical radiograph × computed tomography

Apical radiolucency is the main suggestive sign of apical periodontitis. Conventional and digital Apical radiographs are the main auxiliary resources for diagnosing and following up apical periodontitis resolution after root canal treatment. It is generally accepted that posttreatment follow-up of apical periodontitis for confirmation of complete healing requires at least 4 years of radiographic examination (127–129). Nevertheless, radiographic findings are frequently divergent from clinical or microscopic features in teeth with apical periodontitis. These outcomes indicate that, in many situations, apical periodontitis may persist for several years after root canal filling, even in the absence of clinical and radiographic signs and symptoms (111).

These divergences result from the fact that the radiographs produce two-dimensional images of a three-dimensional structure, which impedes the detection of apical lesions confined to the cancellous bone, especially in areas with thicker cortical bone (130–132). In addition, apical radiographs provide images of teeth in the sagittal plane (mesiodistal direction), and images in the coronal plane cannot be obtained. This fact is a limitation for evaluating the buccolingual extension of the apical lesion and determining cortical bone tissue resorption level (133–135).

Computed tomography (CT) has been widely used in medicine since 1970 and it was gradually introduced to dentistry, more specifically to endodontics, in 1989 (136). However, the use of this computed-assisted imaging technology has become widespread in endodontics only in the past few years thanks to the development of a high-resolution tomography called *cone beam computed tomography* (CBCT) (137–141). The importance of CT has been demonstrated in previous studies in which apical radiolucencies identified by CT were not detected by apical radiography (142–144). Computed tomography may also produce data about pre- and postendodontic treatment bone mineral density (145).

In a previous study, comparison of the size of experimentally induced apical periodontitis obtained with apical radiography and CBCT scans showed that the tomographic evaluation detected lesions with larger mesiodistal extension while radiographic evaluation underestimated the size of lesions (146) (Figure 13.9a,b). In addition, the sensitivity and accuracy of CBCT for detection of apical periodontitis has been shown to be superior to that of conventional apical radiography (147, 148), considering microscopic evaluation as the gold standard (149). The divergence between CT and conventional apical radiography could be because of the superimposition of three-dimensional structures in the two-dimensional radiographic image, which can mask the real size of the lesion. Conversely, CBCT can provide a sequence of serial slices that allow for determining the real dimension of apical periodontitis, using a thin slice

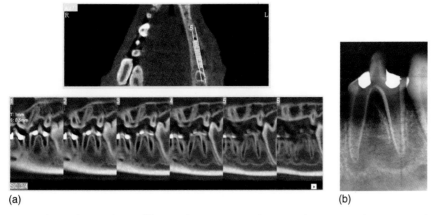

(a)   (b)

Figure 13.9 Large apical periodontitis detected by cone beam computed tomograph (CBCT) evaluation (a). Apical radiograph of the same tooth showing the underestimated mesiodistal extension of the lesions (b).

containing only the cancellous bone region (135, 139, 142, 150, 151).

The superiority of CBCT in the detection and evaluation of apical periodontitis size has been demonstrated when apical lesions with mean mesiodistal diameter of 2.8 mm, not detected by conventional apical radiography, could be detected by tomographic evaluation (142). Another study showed that during the development of apical periodontitis, the radiographic examination did not detect radiolucent areas 14 days after root canal contamination, while CT detected apical radiolucency in 33% of the specimens. These results were similar to those obtained 21 days after contamination, when conventional apical radiography and CT detected apical lesions in 47% and 83% of the specimens, respectively (143). In teeth subjected to endodontic retreatment, superiority of CT over conventional apical radiography for detection of apical lesions has been attributed to the lower possibility of false-negative results (152).

According to Paula-Silva *et al.* (149), teeth with apical disease subjected to single-visit endodontic treatment evaluated by CBCT, apical radiography, and histological analysis (gold standard) showed discontinuity of the lamina dura and radiolucent areas suggestive of apical periodontitis. The fact that the lesions in these teeth were larger compared with those of the other groups evaluated in the study allowed all diagnostic methods to have a similar performance in lesion detection, which also occurred in the teeth with experimentally induced apical periodontitis not subjected to root canal treatment. On the other hand, in the teeth with apical periodontitis subjected to endodontic treatment using a calcium hydroxide intracanal medication, discontinuity of the lamina dura and presence of radiolucent areas suggestive of apical periodontitis were detected in 71.4% of the specimens by apical radiography, while CBCT allowed this detection in 100% of specimens, similar to the microscopic evaluation. These divergent tomographic and radiographic results could be because of the fact that the lesions in this group had a smaller mesiodistal extension with larger amount of surrounding bone tissue increasing the superimposition of sound bone structure (Figure 13.10a,b).

A previous study showed a positive correlation between microscopic and microtomographic measurements of apical lesion size, as well as between the area and volume of the lesions measured by microtomography (135). On the other hand, conventional apical radiography has shown low reliability to detect the presence of apical lesions and the reduction of lesion size, which could be attributed to the fact that the buccolingual expansion of the lesion in the cancellous bone cannot be visualized in a sagittal plane (153–157). In these situations, the increase in the lesion size can be revealed only by volumetric measurements, as provided by CT (130, 158).

In experimental studies, unfavorable outcomes have been found more frequently in teeth subjected to a single-session endodontic treatment compared with those in which a calcium hydroxide intracanal

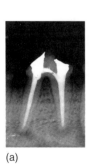 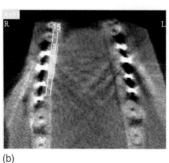

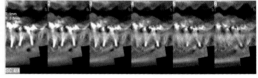

(a)   (b)

Figure 13.10   Persistent apical periodontitis detection following root canal treatment is divergent in cone beam computed tomograph (CBCT) and radiographic evaluations. Superimposition of sound bone structure indicated smaller mesiodistal extension in the radiograph (a) compared with the CBCT scan (b).

medication was used between two or more treatment sessions (16, 111, 112, 115, 117). On the other hand, clinical and radiographic studies in humans for the posttreatment follow-up of root canals have found no difference in the outcome of endodontic treatment completed in one or two-session procedures (60, 101, 102, 110, 159, 160), possibly because of the limitations of clinical research design, especially regarding the sample size and the methods used for apical lesion detection.

There are divergences in the literature over the time required to confirm radiographic success or failure after endodontic treatment. Currently, the European Society of Endodontics recommends a clinical-radiographic follow-up of 1 year after root canal filling, with annual evaluation during a period of 4 years in order to determine treatment success or failure (161). The American Association of Endodontists recommends a minimum of 4–5 years for root canal treatment follow-up (162). Considering that apical lesions confined to the cancellous bone might pass undetected radiographically during or after the follow-up period (130–132, 153–156, 163), the use of CT might establish new follow-up periods to determine the tomographic success of root canal treatment. The fact that CT is useful for determining the actual lesion size and its spatial relationship with the different anatomic sites indicates that this imaging method should be considered a valid option for the follow-up of apical lesion repair after root canal treatment (164). Other advantages of CT over conventional apical radiography include measurement of bone tissue thickness at different planes, precise location of the mandibular canal and its relation to the tooth apexes, differentiation of lingual from buccal root canals by coronal tooth slicing, and detection of vertical root fractures in endodontically and nonendodontically treated teeth (135, 139, 142, 150, 165–169).

Combination of calcium hydroxide with chlorhexidine

Chlorhexidine is a cationic bisbiguanide. Structurally, its molecule consists of two symmetrical chlorophenol rings (4-chlorophenyl) and two bisbiguanide groups united by a central hexamethylene chain that provides its hydrophilic and hydrophobic properties (170). It presents a broad spectrum of action (171) against gram-positive, gram-negative bacteria, aerobes, anaerobes, yeasts, fungi, and viruses (10, 172–176), and binds to the mineralized tissues, with prolonged release at specific therapeutic levels (71, 177, 178). The antimicrobial activity of chlorhexidine is the result of its ionic interaction with the negatively charged bacterial cell surfaces, causing cell wall damage, enzymatic inhibition, and irreversible loss of cytoplasmic content (176). An important property of chlorhexidine is its substantivity (179–182), which permits a sustained residual effect without causing microbial resistance (177, 182).

The use of calcium hydroxide in combination with chlorhexidine has been investigated as an intracanal medication (17, 23, 77, 82, 83, 115, 182–186). Although chlorhexidine alone is not capable to inactivate the bacterial endotoxin (53, 58, 95, 187) and dissolve necrotic tissues (188), such a combination could produce a synergic antimicrobial effect (7, 77, 171, 183) and increase the antimicrobial action of the medication against resistant microorganisms (7, 71, 172, 189–192). Even at low concentrations, the efficacy of chlorhexidine against the most prevalent microorganisms in endodontic infections has been demonstrated (193). The potential additional benefits of this combination for the root canal treatment of teeth with chronic apical periodontitis has raised scientific interest and has been investigated *in-vitro*, *ex-vivo*, and *in-vivo* (23, 115, 171, 183, 190, 194).

On the other hand, it has been demonstrated that the addition of chlorhexidine does not increase the antimicrobial capacity of calcium hydroxide pastes (195), although the antimicrobial activity of calcium hydroxide is not affected. Ercan *et al.* compared the *in-vitro* antimicrobial activity of calcium hydroxide p.a. in combination as well as alone with 2% chlorhexidine against E. *faecalis* and concluded that chlorhexidine alone was significantly more effective than when combined with calcium hydroxide (184).

In this regard, a reasonable question to be posed could be why the antimicrobial activity of calcium hydroxide is maintained and the antimicrobial activity of chlorhexidine is reduced when these materials are combined in a single medication. A possible answer could be related to the fact that the antimicrobial properties of calcium hydroxide are directly related to its pH (196, 197), that is, its capacity to release hydroxyl ions. According to Haenni *et al.*, the pH of the paste is not altered with the addition of chlorhexidine because calcium hydroxide is a highly alkaline substance (195). The combination of materials does not cause alterations on ion release, maintaining the alkaline pH and, consequently, calcium hydroxide's antimicrobial activity. On the other hand, the combination with calcium hydroxide (pH ~12.5) inhibits the antimicrobial activity of chlorhexidine probably because this bisbiguanide is deprotonated at pH 10 or higher, which results in the reduction of solubility and alterations on the interaction with the microbial surfaces because of changes on molecule charge (198). According to Gomes *et al.*, the antimicrobial action of chlorhexidine is reduced when it is combined with calcium hydroxide possibly because of chlorhexidine precipitation at high pH conditions (199). Further physicochemical and antimicrobial studies are required to elucidate the mechanism involved in the potential loss of chlorhexidine efficacy when combined with calcium hydroxide.

An important and conflicting aspect refers to the toxicity of chlorhexidine used alone as an intracanal medication. Although some authors have claimed that chlorhexidine presents low toxicity (170, 200) and beneficial effects (201–203), not affecting collagen synthesis or surgical wound repair, other authors have reported that chlorhexidine presents toxic effects to various cell types, according to its concentration (82, 83, 204–206). Delay of granulation tissue formation (207), induction of microcirculatory alterations (208), and delay of tissue repair (209–211) have also been associated with the use of chlorhexidine. Some studies have demonstrated that subcutaneous injection of chlorhexidine at different concentrations induced inflammatory tissue reactions (200, 212).

There have also been reports that the use of chlorhexidine intracanal medication could affect protein synthesis (213, 214) and cell proliferation (215) at different levels; cause endoplasmic reticulum (ER) stress as a consequence of protein accumulation in the ER cisterns; induce apoptotic or necrotic cell death via ER stress; and increase cellular stress-related protein expression (216).

It should be emphasized that these effects are dose-dependent (211). In a previous study, the addition of 0.4% chlorhexidine to a commercial calcium hydroxide paste (Calen paste) did not result in immunostimulatory effects, with no increase of nitric oxide (NO) production and consequently no cytotoxicity (82). Nevertheless, in another study, the same calcium hydroxide paste added with 0.4% chlorhexidine did not increase the osteogenic potential (83).

Regarding tissue compatibility, the use of a calcium hydroxide and 1% chlorhexidine paste as intracanal medication resulted in a significant reduction in the mean size of the radiographic image and improvement in the histopathological healing of apical radiolucent images in comparison with single-session endodontic treatment of dog's teeth. However, although the use of this paste provided remarkably better results compared with the completion of root canal treatment in a single session, some adverse effects associated with the chlorhexidine concentration (1%) in the paste were observed (115).

The results of studies obtained so far indicate that the incorporation of chlorhexidine to calcium hydroxide-based intracanal medications does not offer any additional beneficial effects and is therefore unnecessary.

Triple antibiotic paste

Antibiotics have been used as intracanal medication in root canal treatment since the 1950s (217). However, local application of antibiotics in endodontics has been restricted because of the polymicrobial nature of apical alterations and the risks of adverse effects, such as hypersensitivity, toxicity, development of microbial resistance, and favorable conditions for fungal growth (218–220). In spite of this, the interest for using a combination of antibiotics as an intracanal medication has reemerged with the introduction of a paste containing three antibiotics. It has appeared as an alternative conservative treatment option, especially in young permanent teeth with immature roots, for root canal disinfection (221, 222), and revascularization of necrotic pulps (223–227).

The triple antibiotic regimen was first tested *in-vitro* by Sato *et al.* (228) followed by Hoshino *et al.* (229). The so-called triple antibiotic paste is prepared by mixing 20 mg of ciprofloxacin, minocycline, and metronidazole antibiotics with sterile distilled water and is used as an intracanal medication usually for 2 weeks (221).

Despite the recognized antimicrobial activity of this paste (3, 230), it should be emphasized that the use of antibiotic-based intracanal medications may result in clinical and biological side effects, including crown darkening (225, 231, 232) (Figure 13.11), development of microbial resistance (233) and allergic reactions (234–236). In addition, minocycline, one of the active components of the triple antibiotic paste, has been associated with angiogenesis inhibition (237, 238).

It should also be considered that the use of the triple antibiotic paste is based fundamentally on the reports of clinical cases in immature teeth with pulp necrosis (224, 226, 227) and mature teeth with pulp necrosis and extensive apical periodontitis in which conventional intracanal medication had failed (239–241).

As emphasized by Mohammadi (220) in a literature review article, indication of any medication should be preceded by evaluation of whether the expected benefits outweigh the risks involved (242). Despite the claimed clinical and radiographic success and possible undesirable side effects, few histopathological studies have evaluated tissue compatibility of the triple antibiotic paste (243, 244).

Yoshiba *et al.* (243) evaluated pulp tissue response to the combination of tricalcium phosphate and triple antibiotic paste in cavities prepared in monkey's teeth (whether they were left exposed or not) to the oral cavity for 24 h. After 4 weeks, a well-defined inflammatory infiltrate was observed without evidence of mineralized tissue deposition in all teeth, regardless of the exposure to microbial contamination. This indicates that the paste promoted an effective disinfection of the pulp tissue, without destroying the healthy tissue. However, mineralized tissue formation was delayed by the mixture of antibiotics, compared with the use of a calcium hydroxide paste.

Silva *et al.* (244) evaluated *in-vivo* the apical and apical repair in immature dog's teeth with experimentally induced apical periodontitis after root canal instrumentation and intracanal medication with the triple antibiotic paste compared with the use of EndoVac. The authors found a significantly more intense inflammatory cell infiltrate and a less advanced repair process when the paste was used (Figure 13.12a,b).

A recent study tested the hypothesis that intracanal medications at high concentrations would be toxic to the human stem cells of the apical papilla (245). The authors concluded that the antibiotics at high concentrations present in the triple antibiotic paste had a detrimental effect on cell survival and that calcium hydroxide at all tested concentrations was conducive with the survival and proliferation of the human stem cells of the apical papilla. These results reinforce the importance of using intracanal medications at concentrations that produce a bactericidal effect without harming the dental papilla stem cells in order to permit regenerative endodontic procedures. It seems reasonable to assume that as root canal disinfection can be achieved with the use of biological medications that do not cause side effects, the use of the triple antibiotic paste is undesirable and unnecessary.

Tricresol formalin/formocresol

Tricresol formalin is a formaldehyde and cresol-based compound that, because of its chemical bond with proteins, has a bactericidal action but is also a highly irritating substance to live tissues. This medication acts both by direct contact and at distance, reaching the apical tissues and causing adverse reactions. Formaldehyde recognizably causes strong harmful effects in contact with the cells (246).

Although formaldehyde-based materials had been largely used in dentistry, the International Agency for Research on Cancer (IARC), a branch of

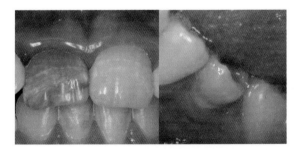

Figure 13.11 Crown discoloration as the result of a revascularization procedure performed with triantibiotic intracanal medication.

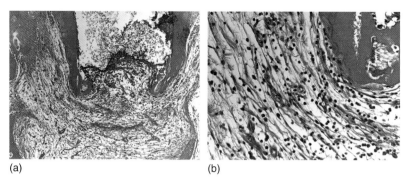

(a)   (b)

Figure 13.12   Intense inflammatory cell infiltrate in apical periodontitis of immature teeth after intracanal medication with the triple antibiotic paste (a, b). Hematoxilin and eosin.

the World Health Organization, issued an official statement in June 2004 classifying formaldehyde as definitely carcinogenic to humans, contraindicating its use in contact with live tissues, supported by research-based evidence evaluated by 26 researchers from 10 countries (247). In June 2011, the National Toxicology Program—Report on Carcinogens stated that "formaldehyde is known to be a human carcinogen based on sufficient evidence of carcinogenicity from studies in humans and supporting data on mechanisms of carcinogenesis." These data suggest that the use of tricresol formalin and formocresol should be discontinued, as proposed by Lewis (248).

In addition, the clinical use of formocresol for pulpotomy in children causes chromosomal breaks (isochromatid gaps, chromatid breaks, isochromatid breaks, total aberrations, and other chromosomal alterations). In view of these results, and considering that genotoxicity is cumulative with age and that pulpotomies are usually performed in very young patients aged 5–10 years, these children might be more vulnerable to future health hazards, and thus caution is advised for the use of formocresol in pediatric dentistry (249). Therefore, although formocresol and its derivatives have been used as intracanal medications for a long time, they should no longer be indicated because of their systemic distribution and their potential adverse effects such as allergies and carcinogenesis (2).

Root canal disinfection—future perspectives

New techniques have been proposed to promote a synergic effect to the use of sodium hypochlorite during biomechanical canal preparation in permanent and primary teeth, among which Antimicrobial Photodynamic Therapy (APDT) and Drug Delivery Systems stand out.

Antimicrobial photodynamic therapy (APDT)

aPDT, also known as *Light-Activated Disinfection (LAD)*, Antimicrobial Photodynamic Chemotherapy and Photoactivated Disinfection, involves the irradiation of a nontoxic light-sensitive compound (known as *photosensitizer*) with a light of specific wavelength matched to the peak absorption of the photosensitizer, which is applied on the target tissue. Absorption of light by the photosensitizer results in conversion of existing oxygen into reactive oxygen species, such as singlet oxygen, which are highly reactive and act at different sites of the bacteria, such as nucleic acids, plasma membrane proteins, and cell wall, causing irreversible damage that leads to their death (250–252). This photodynamic inactivation mechanism results in a broad spectrum of antimicrobial action and low risk of microbial resistance development (253).

The most frequently used light sources are laser and light-emitting diode (LED) (254–258), while the most common photosensitizing drugs used in aPDT are toluidine blue (256), methylene blue (253, 259), phenothiazine chloride (257), erythrosine or tetraiodide fluorescein (260, 261), malachite green or aniline green (262, 263), and rose Bengal (261, 264).

There is not yet any standardization in the literature with respect to the type of light source or to the type and concentration of photosensitizing drugs, as few studies have investigated their effects on the wide range of microorganisms. A recent study (262) evaluating oxygen singlet production and *Streptococcus mutans* viability after exposure to six photosensitizing drugs and two light sources found varied levels of antimicrobial action, with better photodynamic inactivation of the microorganism with toluidine blue and malachite green.

Vilela *et al.* (263) have demonstrated that malachite green, toluidine blue, and methylene blue photosensitizers can have different actions on the photodynamic inactivation of *Staphylococcus aureus and Escherichia coli*, depending on drug concentration during therapy. In addition, aPDT efficacy could be affected by the presence of tissue inhibitors (265). Shrestha and Kishen (253) investigated the antimicrobial action of aPDT using methylene blue and rose Bengal photosensitizers on culture medium containing *E. faecalis* and in the presence of various tissue inhibitors such as dentin, dentin matrix, pulp tissue rests, and bacterial endotoxin. These authors observed that although aPDT was more effective using methylene blue photosensitizer than rose Bengal, the photodynamic inactivation in both protocols was reduced in the presence of tissue inhibitors.

Photosensitizing drugs should also present high selectivity to eliminate microorganisms without causing deleterious effect to the viability of host's cells (256, 266). Goulart *et al.* (264) demonstrated that aPDT using rose Bengal photosensitizer caused a substantial decrease of *Aggregatibacter actinomycetemcomitans* viability in planktonic and biofilm cultures, without affecting the viability of gingival fibroblasts. On the other hand, while this photosensitizer was efficient to eliminate *S. aureus*, it also caused morphological alterations and reduced the viability of neutrophils. These side effects were not observed when methylene blue and toluidine blue photosensitizers were used (259).

The aPDT has been used for the photokilling of bacteria in several areas of Dentistry as an adjuvant in the treatment of *Candida albicans* infections (267), oral carcinomas (268), caries lesions (269, 270), periodontal disease (271, 272), and peri-implantitis (273). In endodontics, aPDT has been widely tested *in-vitro* and *in-vivo* for root canal disinfection as an adjuvant to the standard endodontic treatment, with promising and encouraging preliminary results (253–258, 274, 275). In a recent study in dog's teeth (257), it was observed that although the expected apical closure by mineralized tissue deposition was not achieved, the absence of inflammatory cells, moderate neoangiogenesis, and fibrogenesis in the periapex of teeth subjected to aPDT suggests that this can be a promising supplemental therapy to cleaning and shaping procedures in teeth with pulp necrosis and apical periodontitis subjected to single-session endodontic treatment.

There is also no consensus on the type of light source to be used for activating the photosensitizing drug, and different devices are used, including light-curing units. Recent studies have evaluated a system developed for photodynamic applications, consisting of a red LED system to be used with a specific photosensitizer, and found adjunctive effects of aPDT in periodontal treatment (276) and lack of cytotoxicity to human periodontal ligament fibroblasts (277).

As shown above, although recent studies have demonstrated the efficacy of aPDT as an adjuvant to the standard root canal treatment, further studies are required to establish parameters such as type, intensity, and wavelength of the light source, type and concentration of the photosensitizer, and application time, in order to obtain an effective antimicrobial activity without damage to the host's cells and tissues.

Drug delivery systems

Drug delivery systems (DDS) have been used widely to increase the pharmacological effect of different drugs, reducing their side effects as, in most forms of administrations, only a small amount of the administered dose actually reaches the infected target site, while the majority of the drug distributes throughout the rest of the body according to its physicochemical properties (278). For this reason, nanoparticles, solid polymer, and colloidal particles with diameters ranging from 1 to 1000 nm have been evaluated as drug carriers in root canal disinfection procedures. Natural or synthetic polymers can be used for the fabrication of nanoparticles and can be denominated nanospheres or nanocapsules, depending on the preparation process (278). Nanoparticles can be introduced into the dentinal tubules during root canal treatment by ultrasound activation (253, 279).

Biodegradable polymer nanoparticles present advantages over conventional materials, such as broad spectrum of antimicrobial activity, tissue compatibility, and long-term stability (253, 280, 281).

Currently, chitosan nanoparticles stand out among the most employed nanoparticles. Chitosan is a natural water-soluble polymer, coming from the deacetylation of chitin, which is obtained mainly from the exoskeleton of crabs, shrimps, and lobsters, but is also found in some fungi and yeasts. This polysaccharide combines ideal properties of a drug carrier, namely tissue compatibility, biodegradability, bioadhesion, no toxicity to the human body, and low cost. Because of these properties, chitosan has been widely explored for pharmacological applications (278, 282), namely parenteral administration of antifungal drugs and vaccines, administration of insulin, and is also applicable for mucosal routes of administration, that is, oral, nasal, and ocular mucosa, which are noninvasive routes (278). Its mechanism of action consists of an electrostatic interaction with the bacterial wall, which increases membrane permeability and results in the release of cellular components, which culminate in the death of bacteria (253, 283).

It is well accepted in dentistry that nanoparticles are effective drug carriers against the most prevalent microorganisms in endodontic infections, such as E. faecalis (281, 284, 285). In addition to increasing the antimicrobial activity, chitosan nanoparticles do not alter the physical properties of the materials, which they are incorporated to, like zinc oxide and eugenol and mineral trioxide aggregate (284, 286).

In this regard, Lee et al. (287) evaluated the use of chitosan nanoparticles to assist in the sustained release of chlorhexidine in the root canal system, thereby demonstrating that this is a promising combination of materials for more effective root canal disinfection. Ballal et al. (288) evaluated calcium ion release and pH alteration after calcium hydroxide was incorporated into chitosan nanoparticles in extracted human teeth 30 days after root canal filling. From the obtained results, those authors concluded that the chitosan nanoparticles used as calcium hydroxide carriers were able to provide a slow release of calcium ions for a prolonged period of time and maintain an adequate pH. As chitosan has various other biological properties, it could be a promising vehicle for calcium hydroxide-based materials for the sustained release of calcium ions in the root canal system.

The use of nanoparticles that composed of poly (D,L-lactic-co-glycolic acid) (PLGA) copolymers has also been evaluated for root canal disinfection during endodontic treatment. This carrier is quite a promising bioabsorbable polymer because it undergoes hydrolytic degradation, generating products that are absorbed by the body, such as lactic and glycolic acids. PLGA nanoparticles have low toxicity, low allergenic potential, and excellent tissue compatibility (289–295). In the same way as chitosan nanoparticles, the efficacy of PLGA nanoparticles as carriers of materials to reach the entire root canal system has been demonstrated (285, 287, 295). However, like aPDT, their antimicrobial activity may be influenced in different ways by the presence of tissue inhibitors, such as dentin, pulp tissue, dentin matrix, and bovine serum albumin (BSA) remnants (253).

References

1. Sundqvist, G. (1992) Associations between microbial species in dental root canal infections. *Oral Microbiology and Immunology*, 7 (5), 257–262.
2. Kawashima, N., Wadachi, R., Suda, H., Yeng, T. & Parashos, P. (2009) Root canal medicaments. *International Dental Journal*, 59 (1), 5–11.
3. Cohenca, N., Heilborn, C., Johnson, J.D., Flores, D.S., Ito, I.Y. & da Silva, L.A. (2010) Apical negative pressure irrigation versus conventional irrigation plus triantibiotic intracanal dressing on root canal disinfection in dog teeth. *Oral Surgery, Oral Medicine, Oral Pathology, Oral Radiology, and Endodontics*, 109 (1), e42–e46.
4. Vieira, A.R., Siqueira, J.F. Jr., Ricucci, D. & Lopes, W.S. (2012) Dentinal tubule infection as the cause of recurrent disease and late endodontic treatment

failure: a case report. *Journal of Endodontics*, **38** (**2**), 250–254.

5. Wang, Z., Shen, Y. & Haapasalo, M. (2012) Effectiveness of endodontic disinfecting solutions against young and old *Enterococcus faecalis* biofilms in dentin canals. *Journal of Endodontics*, **38** (**10**), 1376–1379.

6. Sjogren, U., Hagglund, B., Sundqvist, G. & Wing, K. (1990) Factors affecting the long-term results of endodontic treatment. *Journal of Endodontics*, **16** (**10**), 498–504.

7. Evans, M.D., Baumgartner, J.C., Khemaleelakul, S.U. & Xia, T. (2003) Efficacy of calcium hydroxide: chlorhexidine paste as an intracanal medication in bovine dentin. *Journal of Endodontics*, **29** (**5**), 338–339.

8. Wuerch, R.M., Apicella, M.J., Mines, P., Yancich, P.J. & Pashley, D.H. (2004) Effect of 2% chlorhexidine gel as an intracanal medication on the apical seal of the root-canal system. *Journal of Endodontics*, **30** (**11**), 788–791.

9. Kanisavaran, Z.M. (2008) Chlorhexidine gluconate in endodontics: an update review. *International Dental Journal*, **58** (**5**), 247–257.

10. Mohammadi, Z. & Abbott, P.V. (2009) Antimicrobial substantivity of root canal irrigants and medicaments: a review. *Australian Endodontic Journal*, **35** (**3**), 131–139.

11. Marton, I.J. & Kiss, C. (2000) Protective and destructive immune reactions in apical periodontitis. *Oral Microbiology and Immunology*, **15** (**3**), 139–150.

12. Leonardo, M.R., Rossi, M.A., Silva, L.A., Ito, I.Y. & Bonifácio, K.C. (2002) EM evaluation of bacterial biofilm and microorganisms on the apical external root surface of human teeth. *Journal of Endodontics*, **28** (**12**), 815–881.

13. Rocha, C.T., Rossi, M.A., Leonardo, M.R., Rocha, L.B., Nelson-Filho, P. & Silva, L.A. (2008) Biofilm on the apical region of roots in primary teeth with vital and necrotic pulps with or without radiographically evident apical pathosis. *International Endodontic Journal*, **41** (**8**), 664–669.

14. Shuping, G.B., Orstavik, D., Sigurdsson, A. & Trope, M. (2000) Reduction of intracanal bacteria using nickel-titanium rotary instrumentation and various medications. *Journal of Endodontics*, **26** (**12**), 751–755.

15. Faria, G., Nelson-Filho, P., Freitas, A.C., Assed, S. & Ito, I.Y. (2005) Antibacterial effect of root canal preparation and calcium hydroxide paste (Calen) intracanal dressing in primary teeth with apical periodontitis. *Journal of Applied Oral Science*, **13** (**4**), 351–355.

16. Leonardo, M.R., Hernandez, M.E., Silva, L.A. & Tanomaru-Filho, M. (2006) Effect of a calcium hydroxide-based root canal dressing on periapical repair in dogs: a histological study. *Oral Surgery, Oral Medicine, Oral Pathology, Oral Radiology, and Endodontics*, **102** (**5**), 680–685.

17. Soares, J.A., Leonardo, M.R., da Silva, L.A., Tanomaru-Filho, M. & Ito, I.Y. (2006) Histomicrobiologic aspects of the root canal system and periapical lesions in dogs' teeth after rotary instrumentation and intracanal dressing with Ca(OH)2 pastes. *Journal of Applied Oral Science*, **14** (**5**), 355–364.

18. Lee, Y., Han, S.H., Hong, S.H., Lee, J.K., Ji, H. & Kum, K.Y. (2008) Antimicrobial efficacy of a polymeric chlorhexidine release device using in vitro model of *Enterococcus faecalis* dentinal tubule infection. *Journal of Endodontics*, **34** (**7**), 855–858.

19. Sundqvist, G. (1992) Ecology of the root canal flora. *Journal of Endodontics*, **18** (**9**), 427–430.

20. Assed, S., Ito, I.Y., Leonardo, M.R., Silva, L.A. & Lopatin, D.E. (1996) Anaerobic microorganisms in root canals of human teeth with chronic apical periodontitis detected by indirect immunofluorescence. *Endodontics & Dental Traumatology*, **12** (**2**), 66–69.

21. Rôças, I.N., Alves, F.R., Santos, A.L., Rosado, A.S. & Siqueira, J.F. Jr. (2010) Apical root canal microbiota as determined by reverse-capture checkerboard analysis of cryogenically ground root samples from teeth with apical periodontitis. *Journal of Endodontics*, **36** (**10**), 1617–1621.

22. Ruviere, D.B., Leonardo, M.R., da Silva, L.A., Ito, I.Y. & Nelson-Filho, P. (2007) Assessment of the microbiota in root canals of human primary teeth by checkerboard DNA-DNA hybridization. *Journal of Dentistry for Children*, **74** (**2**), 118–123.

23. Ito, I.Y., Junior, F.M., Paula-Silva, F.W., Da Silva, L.A., Leonardo, M.R. & Nelson-Filho, P. (2011) Microbial culture and checkerboard DNA-DNA hybridization assessment of bacteria in root canals of primary teeth pre- and post-endodontic therapy with a calcium hydroxide/chlorhexidine paste. *International journal of paediatric dentistry*, **21** (**5**), 353–360.

24. Rietschel, E.T. & Brade, H. (1992) Bacterial endotoxins. *Scientific American*, **267** (**2**), 54–61.

25. Leonardo, M.R., Silva, R.A., Assed, S. & Nelson-Filho, P. (2004) Importance of bacterial endotoxin (LPS) in endodontics. *Journal of Applied Oral Science*, **12** (**2**), 93–98.

26. Pitts, D.L., Williams, B.L. & Morton, T.H. Jr. (1982) Investigation of the role of endotoxin in periapical inflammation. *Journal of Endodontics*, **8** (**1**), 10–18.

27. Schein, B. & Schilder, H. (1975) Endotoxin content in endodontically involved teeth. *Journal of Endodontics*, **1 (1)**, 19–21.

28. Hong, C.Y., Lin, S.K., Kok, S.H. *et al.* (2004) The role of lipopolysaccharide in infectious bone resorption of periapical lesion. *Journal of Oral Pathology & Medicine*, **33 (3)**, 162–169.

29. Mohammadi, Z. (2011) Endotoxin in endodontic infections: a review. *Journal of the California Dental Association*, **39 (3)**, 152–155., 158–161

30. Matsushita, K., Tajima, T., Tomita, K., Takada, H., Nagaoka, S. & Torii, M. (1999) Inflammatory cytokine production and specific antibody responses to lipopolysaccharide from endodontopathic black-pigmented bacteria in patients with multilesional periapical periodontitis. *Journal of Endodontics*, **25 (12)**, 795–799.

31. Martinho, F.C. & Gomes, B.P. (2008) Quantification of endotoxins and cultivable bacteria in root canal infection before and after chemomechanical preparation with 2.5% sodium hypochlorite. *Journal of Endodontics*, **34 (3)**, 268–272.

32. Sosroseno, W., Bird, P.S. & Seymour, G.J. (2009) Nitric oxide production by a human osteoblast cell line stimulated with Aggregatibacter actinomycetemcomitans lipopolysaccharide. *Oral Microbiology and Immunology*, **24 (1)**, 50–55.

33. Silva, L., Nelson-Filho, P., Leonardo, M.R., Rossi, M.A. & Pansani, C.A. (2002) Effect of calcium hydroxide on bacterial endotoxin in vivo. *Journal of Endodontics*, **28 (2)**, 94–98.

34. Stashenko, P. (1990) Role of immune cytokines in the pathogenesis of periapical lesions. *Endodontics & Dental Traumatology*, **6 (3)**, 89–96.

35. Nelson-Filho, P., Leonardo, M.R., Silva, L.A. & Assed, S. (2002) Radiographic evaluation of the effect of endotoxin (LPS) plus calcium hydroxide on apical and periapical tissues of dogs. *Journal of Endodontics*, **28 (10)**, 694–696.

36. Jiang, J., Zuo, J., Chen, S.H. & Holliday, L.S. (2003) Calcium hydroxide reduces lipopolysaccharide-stimulated osteoclast formation. *Oral Surgery, Oral Medicine, Oral Pathology, Oral Radiology and Endodontics*, **95 (3)**, 348–354.

37. da Silva, L.A., da Silva, R.A., Branco, L.G., Navarro, V.P. & Nelson-Filho, P. (2008) Quantitative radiographic evaluation of periapical bone resorption in dog's teeth contaminated or not with calcium hydroxide. *Brazilian Dental Journal*, **19 (4)**, 296–300.

38. Jacinto, R.C., Gomes, B.P., Shah, H.N., Ferraz, C.C., Zaia, A.A. & Souza-Filho, F.J. (2005) Quantification of endotoxins in necrotic root canals from symptomatic and asymptomatic teeth. *Journal of Medical Microbiology*, **54 (Pt 8)**, 777–783.

39. Ren, L., Leung, W.K., Darveau, R.P. & Jin, L. (2005) The expression profile of lipopolysaccharide-binding protein, membrane-bound CD14, and toll-like receptors 2 and 4 in chronic periodontitis. *Journal of Periodontology*, **76 (11)**, 1950–1959.

40. da Silva, R.A., Ferreira, P.D., De Rossi, A., Nelson-Filho, P. & Silva, L.A. (2012) Toll-like receptor 2 knockout mice showed increased periapical lesion size and osteoclast number. *Journal of Endodontics*, **38 (6)**, 803–813.

41. Barthel, C.R., Levin, L.G., Reisner, H.M. & Trope, M. (1997) TNF-alpha release in monocytes after exposure to calcium hydroxide treated Escherichia coli LPS. *International Endodontic Journal*, **30 (3)**, 155–159.

42. He, W., Qu, T., Yu, Q. *et al.* (2012) LPS induces IL-8 expression through TLR4, MyD88, NF-kappaB and MAPK pathways in human dental pulp stem cells. *International endodontic journal*, **46 (2)**, 128–136.

43. Morrison, D.C. & Cochrane, C.G. (1974) Direct evidence for Hageman factor (factor XII) activation by bacterial lipopolysaccharides (endotoxins). *The Journal of Experimental Medicine*, **140 (3)**, 797–811.

44. Morrison, D.C. & Kline, L.F. (1977) Activation of the classical and properdin pathways of complement by bacterial lipopolysaccharides (LPS). *Journal of Immunology*, **118 (1)**, 362–368.

45. Horiba, N., Maekawa, Y., Yamauchi, Y., Ito, M., Matsumoto, T. & Nakamura, H. (1992) Complement activation by lipopolysaccharides purified from gram-negative bacteria isolated from infected root canals. *Oral Surgery, Oral Medicine, and Oral Pathology*, **74 (5)**, 648–651.

46. Navarro, V.P., Rocha, M.J. & Branco, L.G. (2007) Reduced central c-fos expression and febrile response to repeated LPS injection into periodontal tissue of rats. *Brain Research*, **1152**, 57–63.

47. Ferraz, C.C., Henry, M.A., Hargreaves, K.M. & Diogenes, A. (2011) Lipopolysaccharide from Porphyromonas gingivalis sensitizes capsaicin-sensitive nociceptors. *Journal of Endodontics*, **37 (1)**, 45–48.

48. Katagiri, T. & Takahashi, N. (2002) Regulatory mechanisms of osteoblast and osteoclast differentiation. *Oral Diseases*, **8 (3)**, 147–159.

49. Safavi, K.E. & Nichols, F.C. (1994) Alteration of biological properties of bacterial lipopolysaccharide by calcium hydroxide treatment. *Journal of Endodontics*, **20 (3)**, 127–129.

50. Baik, J.E., Jang, K.S., Kang, S.S. *et al.* (2011) Calcium hydroxide inactivates lipoteichoic acid from Enterococcus faecalis through deacylation of the lipid moiety. *Journal of Endodontics*, **37 (2)**, 191–196.

51. Oliveira, L.D., Leao, M.V., Carvalho, C.A. *et al.* (2005) In vitro effects of calcium hydroxide and polymyxin B on endotoxins in root canals. *Journal of Dentistry*, **33** (**2**), 107–114.

52. Sant'anna, A.T., Spolidorio, L.C. & Ramalho, L.T. (2008) Histological analysis of the association between formocresol and endotoxin in the subcutaneous tissue of mice. *Brazilian Dental Journal*, **19** (**1**), 40–45.

53. Silva, L.A., Leonardo, M.R., Assed, S. & Tanomaru, F.M. (2004) Histological study of the effect of some irrigating solutions on bacterial endotoxin in dogs. *Brazilian Dental Journal*, **15** (**2**), 109–114.

54. Rocha, R.A., Silva, R.A., Assed, S., Medeiros, A.I., Faccioli, L.H., Pécora, J.D. & Nelson-Filho, P. (2009) Nitric oxide detection in cell culture exposed to LPS after Er:YAG laser irradiation. *International Endodontic Journal*, **42** (**11**), 992–996.

55. Liu, G.X., Wang, Q. & Su, L.W. (2009) Endotoxin deactivation in artificial glass root canals with ultrasonic treatment. *Hua xi kou qiang yi xue za zhi*, **27** (**3**), 280–282.

56. Noguchi, F., Kitamura, C., Nagayoshi, M., Chen, K.K., Terashita, M. & Nishihara, T. (2009) Ozonated water improves lipopolysaccharide-induced responses of an odontoblast-like cell line. *Journal of Endodontics*, **35** (**5**), 668–672.

57. Buttler, T.K. & Crawford, J.J. (1982) The detoxifying effect of varying concentrations of sodium hypochlorite on endotoxins. *Journal of Endodontics*, **8** (**2**), 59–66.

58. de Oliveira, L.D., Jorge, A.O., Carvalho, C.A., Koga-Ito, C.Y. & Valera MC. (2007) In vitro effects of endodontic irrigants on endotoxins in root canals. *Oral Surgery, Oral Medicine, Oral Pathology, Oral Radiology and Endodontics*, **104** (**1**), 135–142.

59. Sathorn, C., Parashos, P. & Messer, H. (2009) Australian endodontists' perceptions of single and multiple visit root canal treatment. *International Endodontic Journal*, **42** (**9**), 811–818.

60. Figini, L., Lodi, G., Gorni, F. & Gagliani, M. (2008) Single versus multiple visits for endodontic treatment of permanent teeth: a Cochrane systematic review. *Journal of Endodontics*, **34** (**9**), 1041–1047.

61. Kvist, T., Molander, A., Dahlen, G. & Reit, C. (2004) Microbiological evaluation of one- and two-visit endodontic treatment of teeth with apical periodontitis: a randomized, clinical trial. *Journal of Endodontics*, **30** (**8**), 572–576.

62. Molander, A., Warfvinge, J., Reit, C. & Kvist, T. (2007) Clinical and radiographic evaluation of one- and two-visit endodontic treatment of asymptomatic necrotic teeth with apical periodontitis: a randomized clinical trial. *Journal of Endodontics*, **33** (**10**), 1145–1148.

63. Penesis, V.A., Fitzgerald, P.I., Fayad, M.I., Wenckus, C.S., BeGole, E.A. & Johnson, B.R. (2008) Outcome of one-visit and two-visit endodontic treatment of necrotic teeth with apical periodontitis: a randomized controlled trial with one-year evaluation. *Journal of Endodontics*, **34** (**3**), 251–257.

64. Waltimo, T., Trope, M., Haapasalo, M. & Orstavik, D. (2005) Clinical efficacy of treatment procedures in endodontic infection control and one year follow-up of periapical healing. *Journal of Endodontics*, **31** (**12**), 863–866.

65. Su, Y., Wang, C. & Ye, L. (2011) Healing rate and post-obturation pain of single- versus multiple-visit endodontic treatment for infected root canals: a systematic review. *Journal of Endodontics*, **37** (**2**), 125–132.

66. Chong, B.S. & Pitt Ford, T.R. (1992) The role of intracanal medication in root canal treatment. *International Endodontic Journal*, **25** (**2**), 97–106.

67. Farhad, A. & Mohammadi, Z. (2005) Calcium hydroxide: a review. *International Dental Journal*, **55** (**5**), 293–301.

68. Mohammadi, Z., Shalavi, S. & Yazdizadeh, M. (2012) Antimicrobial activity of calcium hydroxide in endodontics: a review. *Chonnam Medical Journal*, **48** (**3**), 133–140.

69. Hermann, B. (1920) Calcium hydroxid als Mittelzurn, Behandeln und Fullen von Wurzelkanalen Wurzburg.

70. Mohammadi, Z. & Dummer, P.M. (2011) Properties and applications of calcium hydroxide in endodontics and dental traumatology. *International Endodontic Journal*, **44** (**8**), 697–730.

71. Almyroudi, A., Mackenzie, D., McHugh, S. & Saunders, W.P. (2002) The effectiveness of various disinfectants used as endodontic intracanal medications: an in vitro study. *Journal of Endodontics*, **28** (**3**), 163–167.

72. Bystrom, A., Claesson, R. & Sundqvist, G. (1985) The antibacterial effect of camphorated paramonochlorophenol, camphorated phenol and calcium hydroxide in the treatment of infected root canals. *Endodontics & Dental Traumatology*, **1** (**5**), 170–175.

73. Georgopoulou, M., Kontakiotis, E. & Nakou, M. (1993) In vitro evaluation of the effectiveness of calcium hydroxide and paramonochlorophenol on anaerobic bacteria from the root canal. *Endodontics & Dental Traumatology*, **9** (**6**), 249–253.

74. Tavares, W.L., de Brito, L.C., Henriques, L.C. *et al.* (2012) Effects of calcium hydroxide on cytokine expression in endodontic infections. *Journal of Endodontics*, **38** (**10**), 1368–1371.

75. Paiva, S.S., Siqueira, J.F. Jr., Rocas, I.N. *et al.* (2013) Clinical antimicrobial efficacy of NiTi rotary instrumentation with NaOCl irrigation, final rinse with chlorhexidine and interappointment medication: a molecular study. *International Endodontic Journal*, **46** (3), 225–233.

76. Javidi, M., Zarei, M. & Afkhami, F. (2011) Antibacterial effect of calcium hydroxide on intraluminal and intratubular *Enterococcus faecalis*. *Iranian Endodontic Journal*, **6** (3), 103–106.

77. Lima, R.K., Guerreiro-Tanomaru, J.M., Faria-Junior, N.B. & Tanomaru-Filho, M. (2012) Effectiveness of calcium hydroxide-based intracanal medicaments against *Enterococcus faecalis*. *International Endodontic Journal*, **45** (4), 311–316.

78. Kontakiotis, E., Nakou, M. & Georgopoulou, M. (1995) In vitro study of the indirect action of calcium hydroxide on the anaerobic flora of the root canal. *International Endodontic Journal*, **28** (6), 285–289.

79. Heithersay, G.S. (1970) Periapical repair following conservative endodontic therapy. *Australian Dental Journal*, **15** (6), 511–518.

80. Hasselgren, G., Olsson, B. & Cvek, M. (1988) Effects of calcium hydroxide and sodium hypochlorite on the dissolution of necrotic porcine muscle tissue. *Journal of Endodontics*, **14** (3), 125–127.

81. Paula-Silva, F.W., da Silva, L.A. & Kapila, Y.L. (2010) Matrix metalloproteinase expression in teeth with apical periodontitis is differentially modulated by the modality of root canal treatment. *Journal of Endodontics*, **36** (2), 231–237.

82. da Silva, R.A., Leonardo, M.R., da Silva, L.A., Faccioli, L.H. & de Medeiros, A.I. (2008) Effect of a calcium hydroxide-based paste associated to chlorhexidine on RAW 264.7 macrophage cell line culture. *Oral Surgery, Oral Medicine, Oral Pathology, Oral Radiology, and Endodontics*, **106** (5), e44–e51.

83. da Silva, R.A., Leonardo, M.R., da Silva, L.A., de Castro, L.M., Rosa, A.L. & de Oliveira, P.T. (2008) Effects of the association between a calcium hydroxide paste and 0.4% chlorhexidine on the development of the osteogenic phenotype in vitro. *Journal of Endodontics*, **34** (12), 1485–1489.

84. Almushayt, A., Narayanan, K., Zaki, A.E. & George, A. (2006) Dentin matrix protein 1 induces cytodifferentiation of dental pulp stem cells into odontoblasts. *Gene Therapy*, **13** (7), 611–620.

85. Schroder, U. (1985) Effects of calcium hydroxide-containing pulp-capping agents on pulp cell migration, proliferation, and differentiation. *Journal of Dental Research*, (**64** Spec No), 541–548.

86. Paula-Silva, F.W., Ghosh, A., Arzate, H., Kapila, S., da Silva, L.A. & Kapila, Y.L. (2010) Calcium hydroxide promotes cementogenesis and induces cementoblastic differentiation of mesenchymal periodontal ligament cells in a CEMP1- and ERK-dependent manner. *Calcified Tissue International*, **87** (2), 144–157.

87. Nelson-Filho, P., Silva, L.A., Leonardo, M.R., Utrilla, L.S. & Figueiredo, F. (1999) Connective tissue responses to calcium hydroxide-based root canal medicaments. *International Endodontic Journal*, **32** (4), 303–311.

88. Lu, Y., Liu, T., Li, X., Li, H. & Pi, G. (2006) Histologic evaluation of direct pulp capping with a self-etching adhesive and calcium hydroxide in beagles. *Oral Surgery, Oral Medicine, Oral Pathology, Oral Radiology, and Endodontics*, **102** (4), e78–e84.

89. Queiroz, A.M., Assed, S., Consolaro, A. *et al.* (2011) Subcutaneous connective tissue response to primary root canal filling materials. *Brazilian Dental Journal*, **22** (3), 203–211.

90. Tronstad, L., Andreasen, J.O., Hasselgren, G., Kristerson, L. & Riis, I. (1981) pH changes in dental tissues after root canal filling with calcium hydroxide. *Journal of Endodontics*, **7** (1), 17–21.

91. Fava, L.R. & Saunders, W.P. (1999) Calcium hydroxide pastes: classification and clinical indications. *International Endodontic Journal*, **32** (4), 257–282.

92. Zayzafoon, M., Fulzele, K. & McDonald, J.M. (2005) Calmodulin and calmodulin-dependent kinase IIalpha regulate osteoblast differentiation by controlling c-fos expression. *The Journal of Biological Chemistry*, **280** (8), 7049–7059.

93. Safavi, K.E. & Nichols, F.C. (1993) Effect of calcium hydroxide on bacterial lipopolysaccharide. *Journal of Endodontics*, **19** (2), 76–78.

94. Maekawa, L.E., Valera, M.C., Oliveira, L.D., Carvalho, C.A., Koga-Ito, C.Y. & Jorge, A.O. (2011) In vitro evaluation of the action of irrigating solutions associated with intracanal medications on Escherichia coli and its endotoxin in root canals. *Journal of Applied Oral Science : Revista FOB*, **19** (2), 106–112.

95. Buck, R.A., Cai, J., Eleazer, P.D., Staat, R.H. & Hurst, H.E. (2001) Detoxification of endotoxin by endodontic irrigants and calcium hydroxide. *Journal of Endodontics*, **27** (5), 325–327.

96. Camargo, C.H., Bernardineli, N., Valera, M.C. *et al.* (2006) Vehicle influence on calcium hydroxide pastes diffusion in human and bovine teeth. *Dental Traumatology: Official Publication of International Association for Dental Traumatology*, **22** (6), 302–306.

97. Pacios, M.G., Silva, C., Lopez, M.E. & Cecilia, M. (2012) Antibacterial action of calcium hydroxide vehicles and calcium hydroxide pastes. *Journal of Investigative and Clinical Dentistry*, **3** (**4**), 264–270.

98. Leonardo, M.R., da Silva, L.A., Leonardo Rde, T., Utrilla, L.S. & Assed, S. (1993) Histological evaluation of therapy using a calcium hydroxide dressing for teeth with incompletely formed apices and periapical lesions. *Journal of Endodontics*, **19** (**7**), 348–352.

99. Blanscet, M.L., Tordik, P.A. & Goodell, G.G. (2008) An agar diffusion comparison of the antimicrobial effect of calcium hydroxide at five different concentrations with three different vehicles. *Journal of Endodontics*, **34** (**10**), 1246–1248.

100. Pekruhn, R.B. (1981) Single-visit endodontic therapy: a preliminary clinical study. *Journal of the American Dental Association*, **103** (**6**), 875–877.

101. Naito, T. (2008) Single or multiple visits for endodontic treatment? *Evidence-Based Dentistry*, **9** (**1**), 24.

102. Sathorn, C., Parashos, P. & Messer, H.H. (2005) Effectiveness of single- versus multiple-visit endodontic treatment of teeth with apical periodontitis: a systematic review and meta-analysis. *International Endodontic Journal*, **38** (**6**), 347–355.

103. Paredes-Vieyra, J. & Enriquez, F.J. (2012) Success rate of single- versus two-visit root canal treatment of teeth with apical periodontitis: a randomized controlled trial. *Journal of Endodontics*, **38** (**9**), 1164–1169.

104. Sathorn, C., Parashos, P. & Messer, H. (2008) The prevalence of postoperative pain and flare-up in single- and multiple-visit endodontic treatment: a systematic review. *International Endodontic Journal*, **41** (**2**), 91–99.

105. Balto, K. (2009) Single- or multiple-visit endodontics: which technique results in fewest postoperative problems? *Evidence-Based Dentistry*, **10** (**1**), 16.

106. El Mubarak, A.H., Abu-bakr, N.H. & Ibrahim, Y.E. (2010) Postoperative pain in multiple-visit and single-visit root canal treatment. *Journal of Endodontics*, **36** (**1**), 36–39.

107. Prashanth, M.B., Tavane, P.N., Abraham, S. & Chacko, L. (2011) Comparative evaluation of pain, tenderness and swelling followed by radiographic evaluation of periapical changes at various intervals of time following single and multiple visit endodontic therapy: an in vivo study. *The Journal of Contemporary Dental Practice*, **12** (**3**), 187–191.

108. Singh, S. & Garg, A. (2012) Incidence of post-operative pain after single visit and multiple visit root canal treatment: a randomized controlled trial. *Journal of Conservative Dentistry : JCD*, **15** (**4**), 323–327.

109. Sjogren, U., Figdor, D., Persson, S. & Sundqvist, G. (1997) Influence of infection at the time of root filling on the outcome of endodontic treatment of teeth with apical periodontitis. *International Endodontic Journal*, **30** (**5**), 297–306.

110. Trope, M., Delano, E.O. & Orstavik, D. (1999) Endodontic treatment of teeth with apical periodontitis: single vs. multivisit treatment. *Journal of Endodontics*, **25** (**5**), 345–350.

111. Katebzadeh, N., Sigurdsson, A. & Trope, M. (2000) Radiographic evaluation of periapical healing after obturation of infected root canals: an in vivo study. *International Endodontic Journal*, **33** (**1**), 60–66.

112. Holland, R., Otoboni Filho, J.A., de Souza, V., Nery, M.J., Bernabe, P.F. & Dezan, E. Jr. (2003) A comparison of one versus two appointment endodontic therapy in dogs' teeth with apical periodontitis. *Journal of Endodontics*, **29** (**2**), 121–124.

113. Oginni, A.O. & Udoye, C.I. (2004) Endodontic flare-ups: comparison of incidence between single and multiple visit procedures in patients attending a Nigerian teaching hospital. *BMC Oral Health*, **4** (**1**), 4.

114. Yoldas, O., Topuz, A., Isci, A.S. & Oztunc, H. (2004) Postoperative pain after endodontic retreatment: single- versus two-visit treatment. *Oral Surgery, Oral Medicine, Oral Pathology, Oral Radiology, and Endodontics*, **98** (**4**), 483–487.

115. De Rossi, A., Silva, L.A., Leonardo, M.R., Rocha, L.B. & Rossi, M.A. (2005) Effect of rotary or manual instrumentation, with or without a calcium hydroxide/1% chlorhexidine intracanal dressing, on the healing of experimentally induced chronic periapical lesions. *Oral Surgery, Oral Medicine, Oral Pathology, Oral Radiology, and Endodontics*, **99** (**5**), 628–636.

116. Hargreaves, K.M. (2006) Single-visit more effective than multiple-visit root canal treatment? *Evidence-Based Dentistry*, **7** (**1**), 13–14.

117. Silveira, A.M., Lopes, H.P., Siqueira, J.F. Jr., Macedo, S.B. & Consolaro, A. (2007) Periradicular repair after two-visit endodontic treatment using two different intracanal medications compared to single-visit endodontic treatment. *Brazilian Dental Journal*, **18** (**4**), 299–304.

118. Nerwich, A., Figdor, D. & Messer, H.H. (1993) pH changes in root dentin over a 4-week period following root canal dressing with calcium hydroxide. *Journal of Endodontics*, **19** (**6**), 302–306.

119. da Silva, L.A., Sanguino, A.C., Rocha, C.T., Leonardo, M.R. & Silva, R.A. (2008) Scanning electron microscopic preliminary study of the efficacy of SmearClear and EDTA for smear layer removal after root canal instrumentation in

permanent teeth. *Journal of Endodontics*, **34** (**12**), 1541–1544.

120. Anthony, D.R., Gordon, T.M. & del Rio, C.E. (1982) The effect of three vehicles on the pH of calcium hydroxide. *Oral Surgery, Oral Medicine, and Oral Pathology*, **54** (**5**), 560–565.

121. Simon, S.T., Bhat, K.S. & Francis, R. (1995) Effect of four vehicles on the pH of calcium hydroxide and the release of calcium ion. *Oral Surgery, Oral Medicine, Oral Pathology, Oral Radiology, and Endodontics*, **80** (**4**), 459–464.

122. Goldberg, F., Alfie, D. & Roitman, M. (2004) Evaluation of the incidence of transportation after placement and removal of calcium hydroxide. *Journal of Endodontics*, **30** (**9**), 646–648.

123. Wiseman, A., Cox, T.C., Paranjpe, A., Flake, N.M., Cohenca, N. & Johnson, J.D. (2011) Efficacy of sonic and ultrasonic activation for removal of calcium hydroxide from mesial canals of mandibular molars: a microtomographic study. *Journal of Endodontics*, **37** (**2**), 235–238.

124. Andreasen, J.O., Farik, B. & Munksgaard, E.C. (2002) Long-term calcium hydroxide as a root canal dressing may increase risk of root fracture. *Dental Traumatology : Official Publication of International Association for Dental Traumatology*, **18** (**3**), 134–137.

125. Doyon, G.E., Dumsha, T. & von Fraunhofer, J.A. (2005) Fracture resistance of human root dentin exposed to intracanal calcium hydroxide. *Journal of Endodontics*, **31** (**12**), 895–897.

126. Rosenberg, B., Murray, P.E. & Namerow, K. (2007) The effect of calcium hydroxide root filling on dentin fracture strength. *Dental Traumatology: Official Publication of International Association for Dental Traumatology*, **23** (**1**), 26–29.

127. Orstavik, D., Kerekes, K. & Eriksen, H.M. (1987) Clinical performance of three endodontic sealers. *Endodontics & Dental Traumatology*, **3** (**4**), 178–186.

128. Ørstavik, D. & Pitt-Ford, T.R. (1998) Apical periodontitis: microbial infection and host responses. In: Ørstavik, D. & Pitt-Ford, T.R. (eds), *Essential Endodontology*. Blackwell Science, Oxford, pp. 1–8.

129. Endodontology ESo (2006) Quality guidelines for endodontic treatment: consensus report of the European Society of Endodontology. *International Endodontic Journal*, **39** (**12**), 921–930.

130. Huumonen, S. & Ørstavik, D. (2002) Radiological aspects of apical periodontitis. *Endod Topics*, **1**, 3–25.

131. Ricucci, D. & Bergenholtz, G. (2003) Bacterial status in root-filled teeth exposed to the oral environment by loss of restoration and fracture or caries--a histo-bacteriological study of treated cases. *International Endodontic Journal*, **36** (**11**), 787–802.

132. Wu, M.K., Dummer, P.M. & Wesselink, P.R. (2006) Consequences of and strategies to deal with residual post-treatment root canal infection. *International Endodontic Journal*, **39** (**5**), 343–356.

133. Schwarz, M.S., Rothman, S.L., Rhodes, M.L. & Chafetz, N. (1987) Computed tomography: Part II. Preoperative assessment of the maxilla for endosseous implant surgery. *The International Journal of Oral & Maxillofacial Implants*, **2** (**3**), 143–148.

134. Schwarz, M.S., Rothman, S.L., Rhodes, M.L. & Chafetz, N. (1987) Computed tomography: Part I. Preoperative assessment of the mandible for endosseous implant surgery. *The International Journal of Oral & Maxillofacial Implants*, **2** (**3**), 137–141.

135. von Stechow, D., Balto, K., Stashenko, P. & Muller, R. (2003) Three-dimensional quantitation of periradicular bone destruction by micro-computed tomography. *Journal of Endodontics*, **29** (**4**), 252–256.

136. Trope, M., Pettigrew, J., Petras, J., Barnett, F. & Tronstad, L. (1989) Differentiation of radicular cyst and granulomas using computerized tomography. *Endodontics & Dental Traumatology*, **5** (**2**), 69–72.

137. Cohenca, N., Simon, J.H., Mathur, A. & Malfaz, J.M. (2007) Clinical indications for digital imaging in dento-alveolar trauma. Part 2: root resorption. *Dental Traumatology: Official Publication of International Association for Dental Traumatology*, **23** (**2**), 105–113.

138. Cohenca, N., Simon, J.H., Roges, R., Morag, Y. & Malfaz, J.M. (2007) Clinical indications for digital imaging in dento-alveolar trauma. Part 1: traumatic injuries. *Dental Traumatology: Official Publication of International Association for Dental Traumatology*, **23** (**2**), 95–104.

139. Cotton, T.P., Geisler, T.M., Holden, D.T., Schwartz, S.A. & Schindler, W.G. (2007) Endodontic applications of cone-beam volumetric tomography. *Journal of Endodontics*, **33** (**9**), 1121–1132.

140. Patel, S., Dawood, A., Ford, T.P. & Whaites, E. (2007) The potential applications of cone beam computed tomography in the management of endodontic problems. *International Endodontic Journal*, **40** (**10**), 818–830.

141. Patel, S. & Horner, K. (2009) The use of cone beam computed tomography in endodontics. *International Endodontic Journal*, **42** (**9**), 755–756.

142. Lofthag-Hansen, S., Huumonen, S., Grondahl, K. & Grondahl, H.G. (2007) Limited cone-beam CT and intraoral radiography for the diagnosis of periapical pathology. *Oral Surgery, Oral Medicine, Oral Pathology, Oral Radiology, and Endodontics*, **103** (**1**), 114–119.

143. Jorge, E.G., Tanomaru-Filho, M., Goncalves, M. & Tanomaru, J.M. (2008) Detection of periapical lesion development by conventional radiography or computed tomography. *Oral Surgery, Oral Medicine, Oral Pathology, Oral Radiology, and Endodontics*, **106** (**1**), e56–e61.

144. Vandenberghe, B., Jacobs, R. & Yang, J. (2008) Detection of periodontal bone loss using digital intraoral and cone beam computed tomography images: an in vitro assessment of bony and/or infrabony defects. *Dento Maxillo Facial Radiology*, **37** (**5**), 252–260.

145. Kaya, S., Yavuz, I., Uysal, I. & Akkus, Z. (2012) Measuring bone density in healing periapical lesions by using cone beam computed tomography: a clinical investigation. *Journal of Endodontics*, **38** (**1**), 28–31.

146. de Paula-Silva, F.W., Wu, M.K., Leonardo, M.R., da Silva, L.A. & Wesselink, P.R. (2009) Accuracy of periapical radiography and cone-beam computed tomography scans in diagnosing apical periodontitis using histopathological findings as a gold standard. *Journal of Endodontics*, **35** (**7**), 1009–1012.

147. Abella, F., Patel, S., Duran-Sindreu, F., Mercade, M., Bueno, R. & Roig, M. (2012) Evaluating the periapical status of teeth with irreversible pulpitis by using cone-beam computed tomography scanning and periapical radiographs. *Journal of Endodontics*, **38** (**12**), 1588–1591.

148. Ma, L., Zhan, F.L., Qiu, L.H. & Xue, M. (2012) The application of cone-beam computed tomography in diagnosing the lesions of apical periodontitis of posterior teeth. *Shanghai kou qiang yi xue*, **21** (**4**), 442–446.

149. de Paula-Silva, F.W., Santamaria, M. Jr., Leonardo, M.R., Consolaro, A. & da Silva, L.A. (2009) Cone-beam computerized tomographic, radiographic, and histologic evaluation of periapical repair in dogs' post-endodontic treatment. *Oral Surgery, Oral Medicine, Oral Pathology, Oral Radiology, and Endodontics*, **108** (**5**), 796–805.

150. Simon, J.H., Enciso, R., Malfaz, J.M., Roges, R., Bailey-Perry, M. & Patel, A. (2006) Differential diagnosis of large periapical lesions using cone-beam computed tomography measurements and biopsy. *Journal of Endodontics*, **32** (**9**), 833–837.

151. Stavropoulos, A. & Wenzel, A. (2007) Accuracy of cone beam dental CT, intraoral digital and conventional film radiography for the detection of periapical lesions. An ex vivo study in pig jaws. *Clinical Oral Investigations*, **11** (**1**), 101–106.

152. Huumonen, S., Kvist, T., Grondahl, K. & Molander, A. (2006) Diagnostic value of computed tomography in re-treatment of root fillings in maxillary molars. *International Endodontic Journal*, **39** (**10**), 827–833.

153. Bender, I.B. & Seltzer, S. (2003) Roentgenographic and direct observation of experimental lesions in bone: II. 1961. *Journal of Endodontics*, **29** (**11**), 707–712.; discussion 701

154. Bender, I.B. & Seltzer, S. (2003) Roentgenographic and direct observation of experimental lesions in bone: I. 1961. *Journal of Endodontics*, **29** (**11**), 702–706.; discussion 701

155. Bender, I.B. (1982) Factors influencing the radiographic appearance of bony lesions. *Journal of Endodontics*, **8** (**4**), 161–170.

156. van der Stelt, P.F. (1985) Experimentally produced bone lesions. *Oral Surgery, Oral Medicine, and Oral Pathology*, **59** (**3**), 306–312.

157. Green, T.L., Walton, R.E., Taylor, J.K. & Merrell, P. (1997) Radiographic and histologic periapical findings of root canal treated teeth in cadaver. *Oral Surgery, Oral Medicine, Oral Pathology, Oral Radiology, and Endodontics*, **83** (**6**), 707–711.

158. Gielkens, P.F., Schortinghuis, J., de Jong, J.R. et al. (2008) A comparison of micro-CT, microradiography and histomorphometry in bone research. *Archives of Oral Biology*, **53** (**6**), 558–566.

159. Weiger, R., Rosendahl, R. & Lost, C. (2000) Influence of calcium hydroxide intracanal dressings on the prognosis of teeth with endodontically induced periapical lesions. *International Endodontic Journal*, **33** (**3**), 219–226.

160. Peters, L.B. & Wesselink, P.R. (2002) Periapical healing of endodontically treated teeth in one and two visits obturated in the presence or absence of detectable microorganisms. *International Endodontic Journal*, **35** (**8**), 660–667.

161. European Society of Endodontology (2006) Quality guidelines for endodontic treatment: consensus report of the European Society of Endodontology. *International Endodontic Journal*, **39** (**12**), 921–930.

162. Ng, Y.L., Mann, V., Rahbaran, S., Lewsey, J. & Gulabivala, K. (2007) Outcome of primary root canal treatment: systematic review of the literature - part 1. Effects of study characteristics on probability of success. *International Endodontic Journal*, **40** (**12**), 921–939.

163. Stabholz, A., Friedman, S. & Tamse, A. (1994) Endodontic failures and re-treatment. In: Cohen, S. & Burns, R.C. (eds), *Pathways of the pulp*. Mosby, St Louis, pp. 692–723.

164. Cotti, E., Vargiu, P., Dettori, C. & Mallarini, G. (1999) Computerized tomography in the management and follow-up of extensive periapical lesion. *Endodontics & Dental Traumatology*, **15** (**4**), 186–189.

165. Tachibana, H. & Matsumoto, K. (1990) Applicability of X-ray computerized tomography in endodontics. *Endodontics & Dental Traumatology*, **6** (**1**), 16–20.

166. Kassebaum, D.K., Reader, C.M., Kleier, D.J. & Averbach, R.E. (1991) Localization of anatomic structures before endodontic surgery with tomograms. Report of a case. *Oral Surgery, Oral Medicine, and Oral Pathology*, **72** (**5**), 610–613.

167. Velvart, P., Hecker, H. & Tillinger, G. (2001) Detection of the apical lesion and the mandibular canal in conventional radiography and computed tomography. *Oral Surgery, Oral Medicine, Oral Pathology, Oral Radiology, and Endodontics*, **92** (**6**), 682–688.

168. Nair, M.K. & Nair, U.P. (2007) Digital and advanced imaging in endodontics: a review. *Journal of Endodontics*, **33** (**1**), 1–6.

169. Hassan, B., Metska, M.E., Ozok, A.R., van der Stelt, P. & Wesselink, P.R. (2009) Detection of vertical root fractures in endodontically treated teeth by a cone beam computed tomography scan. *Journal of Endodontics*, **35** (**5**), 719–722.

170. Greenstein, G., Berman, C. & Jaffin, R. (1986) Chlorhexidine. An adjunct to periodontal therapy. *Journal of Periodontology*, **57** (**6**), 370–377.

171. Mohammadi, Z. & Shalavi, S. (2012) Is chlorhexidine an ideal vehicle for calcium hydroxide? A microbiologic review. *Iranian Endodontic journal*, **7** (**3**), 115–122.

172. Heling, I., Steinberg, D., Kenig, S., Gavrilovich, I., Sela, M.N. & Friedman, M. (1992) Efficacy of a sustained-release device containing chlorhexidine and Ca(OH)2 in preventing secondary infection of dentinal tubules. *International Endodontic Journal*, **25** (**1**), 20–24.

173. Heling, I., Sommer, M., Steinberg, D., Friedman, M. & Sela, M.N. (1992) Microbiological evaluation of the efficacy of chlorhexidine in a sustained-release device for dentine sterilization. *International Endodontic Journal*, **25** (**1**), 15–19.

174. Vahdaty, A., Pitt Ford, T.R. & Wilson, R.F. (1993) Efficacy of chlorhexidine in disinfecting dentinal tubules in vitro. *Endodontics & Dental Traumatology*, **9** (**6**), 243–248.

175. Jeansonne, M.J. & White, R.R. (1994) A comparison of 2.0% chlorhexidine gluconate and 5.25% sodium hypochlorite as antimicrobial endodontic irrigants. *Journal of Endodontics*, **20** (**6**), 276–278.

176. Shen, Y., Stojicic, S. & Haapasalo, M. (2011) Antimicrobial efficacy of chlorhexidine against bacteria in biofilms at different stages of development. *Journal of Endodontics*, **37** (**5**), 657–661.

177. Komorowski, R., Grad, H., Wu, X.Y. & Friedman, S. (2000) Antimicrobial substantivity of chlorhexidine-treated bovine root dentin. *Journal of Endodontics*, **26** (**6**), 315–317.

178. Hidalgo, E. & Dominguez, C. (2001) Mechanisms underlying chlorhexidine-induced cytotoxicity. *Toxicology In Vitro: An International Journal Published in Association with BIBRA*, **15** (**4-5**), 271–276.

179. Jenkins, S., Addy, M. & Wade, W. (1988) The mechanism of action of chlorhexidine. A study of plaque growth on enamel inserts in vivo. *Journal of Clinical Periodontology*, **15** (**7**), 415–424.

180. Leonardo, M.R., Tanomaru-Filho, M., Silva, L.A., Nelson-Filho, P., Bonifacio, K.C. & Ito, I.Y. (1999) In vivo antimicrobial activity of 2% chlorhexidine used as a root canal irrigating solution. *Journal of Endodontics*, **25** (**3**), 167–171.

181. Lenet, B.J., Komorowski, R., Wu, X.Y. *et al.* (2000) Antimicrobial substantivity of bovine root dentin exposed to different chlorhexidine delivery vehicles. *Journal of Endodontics*, **26** (**11**), 652–655.

182. Rosenthal, S., Spangberg, L. & Safavi, K. (2004) Chlorhexidine substantivity in root canal dentin. *Oral Surgery, Oral Medicine, Oral Pathology, Oral Radiology, and Endodontics*, **98** (**4**), 488–492.

183. Zerella, J.A., Fouad, A.F. & Spangberg, L.S. (2005) Effectiveness of a calcium hydroxide and chlorhexidine digluconate mixture as disinfectant during retreatment of failed endodontic cases. *Oral Surgery, Oral Medicine, Oral Pathology, Oral Radiology, and Endodontics*, **100** (**6**), 756–761.

184. Ercan, E., Dalli, M. & Dulgergil, C.T. (2006) In vitro assessment of the effectiveness of chlorhexidine gel and calcium hydroxide paste with chlorhexidine against *Enterococcus faecalis* and Candida albicans. *Oral Surgery, Oral Medicine, Oral Pathology, Oral Radiology, and Endodontics*, **102** (**2**), e27–e31.

185. Oncag, O., Cogulu, D. & Uzel, A. (2006) Efficacy of various intracanal medicaments against *Enterococcus faecalis* in primary teeth: an in vivo study. *The Journal of Clinical Pediatric Dentistry*, **30** (**3**), 233–237.

186. Manzur, A., Gonzalez, A.M., Pozos, A., Silva-Herzog, D. & Friedman, S. (2007) Bacterial quantification in teeth with apical periodontitis related to instrumentation and different intracanal medications: a randomized clinical trial. *Journal of Endodontics*, **33** (**2**), 114–118.

187. Aibel, K. & Stevens, R. (1999) Effect of chlorhexidine on IL-6 induction by LPS. *Journal of Endodontics*, **25**, 282.

188. Zehnder, M., Grawehr, M., Hasselgren, G. & Waltimo, T. (2003) Tissue-dissolution capacity and dentin-disinfecting potential of calcium hydroxide mixed with irrigating solutions. *Oral Surgery, Oral Medicine, Oral Pathology, Oral Radiology, and Endodontics*, **96** (**5**), 608–613.

189. Waltimo, T.M., Siren, E.K., Orstavik, D. & Haapasalo, M.P. (1999) Susceptibility of oral Candida species to calcium hydroxide in vitro. *International Endodontic Journal*, **32** (**2**), 94–98.

190. Basrani, B., Ghanem, A. & Tjaderhane, L. (2004) Physical and chemical properties of chlorhexidine and calcium hydroxide-containing medications. *Journal of Endodontics*, **30** (**6**), 413–417.

191. Basrani, B., Santos, J.M., Tjaderhane, L. *et al.* (2002) Substantive antimicrobial activity in chlorhexidine-treated human root dentin. *Oral Surgery, Oral Medicine, Oral Pathology, Oral Radiology, and Endodontics*, **94** (**2**), 240–245.

192. Podbielski, A., Spahr, A. & Haller, B. (2003) Additive antimicrobial activity of calcium hydroxide and chlorhexidine on common endodontic bacterial pathogens. *Journal of Endodontics*, **29** (**5**), 340–345.

193. do Amorim, C.V., Aun, C.E. & Mayer, M.P. (2004) Susceptibility of some oral microorganisms to chlorhexidine and paramonochlorophenol. *Brazilian Oral Research*, **18** (**3**), 242–246.

194. Soares, J.A., Leonardo, M.R., Tanomaru-Filho, M., Silva, L.A. & Ito, I.Y. (2007) Residual antibacterial activity of chlorhexidine digluconate and camphorated p-monochlorophenol in calcium hydroxide-based root canal dressings. *Brazilian Dental Journal*, **18** (**1**), 8–15.

195. Haenni, S., Schmidlin, P.R., Mueller, B., Sener, B. & Zehnder, M. (2003) Chemical and antimicrobial properties of calcium hydroxide mixed with irrigating solutions. *International Endodontic Journal*, **36** (**2**), 100–105.

196. Bystrom, A. & Sundqvist, G. (1985) The antibacterial action of sodium hypochlorite and EDTA in 60 cases of endodontic therapy. *International Endodontic Journal*, **18** (**1**), 35–40.

197. Evans, M., Davies, J.K., Sundqvist, G. & Figdor, D. (2002) Mechanisms involved in the resistance of *Enterococcus faecalis* to calcium hydroxide. *International Endodontic Journal*, **35** (**3**), 221–228.

198. Jones, D.S., Brown, A.F., Woolfson, A.D., Dennis, A.C., Matchett, L.J. & Bell, S.E. (2000) Examination of the physical state of chlorhexidine within viscoelastic, bioadhesive semisolids using raman spectroscopy. *Journal of Pharmaceutical Sciences*, **89** (**5**), 563–571.

199. Gomes, B.P., Vianna, M.E., Sena, N.T., Zaia, A.A., Ferraz, C.C. & de Souza-Filho, F.J. (2006) In vitro evaluation of the antimicrobial activity of calcium hydroxide combined with chlorhexidine gel used as intracanal medicament. *Oral Surgery, Oral Medicine, Oral Pathology, Oral Radiology, and Endodontics*, **102** (**4**), 544–550.

200. Yesilsoy, C., Whitaker, E., Cleveland, D., Phillips, E. & Trope, M. (1995) Antimicrobial and toxic effects of established and potential root canal irrigants. *Journal of Endodontics*, **21** (**10**), 513–515.

201. Hirst, R.C., Egelberg, J., Hornbuckle, G.C., Oliver, R.C. & Rathbun, W.E. (1973) Microscopic evaluation of topically applied chlorhexidine gluconate on gingival wound healing in dogs. *Journal - Southern California Dental Association*, **41** (**4**), 311–317.

202. Brennan, S.S., Foster, M.E. & Leaper, D.J. (1986) Antiseptic toxicity in wounds healing by secondary intention. *The Journal of Hospital Infection*, **8** (**3**), 263–267.

203. Heitz, F., Heitz-Mayfield, L.J. & Lang, N.P. (2004) Effects of post-surgical cleansing protocols on early plaque control in periodontal and/or periimplant wound healing. *Journal of Clinical Periodontology*, **31** (**11**), 1012–1018.

204. Knuuttila, M. & Soderling, E. (1981) Effect of chlorhexidine on the release of lysosomal enzymes from cultured macrophages. *Acta Odontologica Scandinavica*, **39** (**5**), 285–289.

205. Mariotti, A.J. & Rumpf, D.A. (1999) Chlorhexidine-induced changes to human gingival fibroblast collagen and non-collagen protein production. *Journal of Periodontology*, **70** (**12**), 1443–1448.

206. Patel, P., Ide, M., Coward, P. & Di Silvio, L. (2006) The effect of a commercially available chlorhexidine mouthwash product on human osteoblast cells. *The European Journal of Prosthodontics and Restorative Dentistry*, **14** (**2**), 67–72.

207. Paunio, K.U., Knuttila, M. & Mielitynen, H. (1978) The effect of chlorhexidine gluconate on the formation of experimental granulation tissue. *Journal of Periodontology*, **49** (**2**), 92–95.

208. Luostarinen, V., Soderling, E., Knuuttila, M. & Paunio, K. (1977) Effect of chlorhexidine on the hamster cheek pouch. Microcirculation and penetration studies. *Journal of Periodontology*, **48** (**7**), 421–424.

209. Bassetti, C. & Kallenberger, A. (1980) Influence of chlorhexidine rinsing on the healing of oral mucosa and osseous lesions. *Journal of Clinical Periodontology*, **7** (**6**), 443–456.

210. Saatman, R.A., Carlton, W.W., Hubben, K., Streett, C.S., Tuckosh, J.R. & DeBaecke, P.J. (1986) A wound healing study of chlorhexidine digluconate in guinea pigs. *Fundamental and Applied Toxicology: Official Journal of the Society of Toxicology*, **6** (**1**), 1–6.

211. Silva, R.A., Assed, S., Nelson-Filho, P., Silva, L.A. & Consolaro, A. (2009) Subcutaneous tissue response of isogenic mice to calcium hydroxide-based pastes with chlorhexidine. *Brazilian Dental Journal*, **20** (**2**), 99–106.

212. Oncag, O., Hosgor, M., Hilmioglu, S., Zekioglu, O., Eronat, C. & Burhanoglu, D. (2003) Comparison of antibacterial and toxic effects of various root canal irrigants. *International Endodontic Journal*, **36** (**6**), 423–432.

213. Goldschmidt, P., Cogen, R. & Taubman, S. (1977) Cytopathologic effects of chlorhexidine on human cells. *Journal of Periodontology*, **48** (**4**), 212–215.

214. Pucher, J.J. & Daniel, J.C. (1992) The effects of chlorhexidine digluconate on human fibroblasts in vitro. *Journal of Periodontology*, **63** (**6**), 526–532.

215. Lucarotti, M.E., White, H., Deas, J., Silver, I.A. & Leaper, D.J. (1990) Antiseptic toxicity to breast carcinoma in tissue culture: an adjuvant to conservation therapy? *Annals of the Royal College of Surgeons of England*, **72** (**6**), 388–392.

216. Faria, G., Celes, M.R., De Rossi, A., Silva, L.A., Silva, J.S. & Rossi, M.A. (2007) Evaluation of chlorhexidine toxicity injected in the paw of mice and added to cultured l929 fibroblasts. *Journal of Endodontics*, **33** (**6**), 715–722.

217. Grossman, L.I. (1951) Polyantibiotic treatment of pulpless teeth. *Journal of the American Dental Association*, **43** (**3**), 265–278.

218. Marrie, T.J., Haldane, E.V., Swantee, C.A. & Kerr, E.A. (1981) Susceptibility of anaerobic bacteria to nine antimicrobial agents and demonstration of decreased susceptibility of Clostridium perfringens to penicillin. *Antimicrobial Agents and Chemotherapy*, **19** (**1**), 51–55.

219. Longman, L.P., Preston, A.J., Martin, M.V. & Wilson, N.H. (2000) Endodontics in the adult patient: the role of antibiotics. *Journal of Dentistry*, **28** (**8**), 539–548.

220. Mohammadi, Z. (2009) Antibiotics as intracanal medicaments: a review. *Journal of the California Dental Association*, **37** (**2**), 98–108.

221. Windley, W. 3rd, Teixeira, F., Levin, L., Sigurdsson, A. & Trope, M. (2005) Disinfection of immature teeth with a triple antibiotic paste. *Journal of Endodontics*, **31** (**6**), 439–443.

222. Akgun, O.M., Altun, C. & Guven, G. (2009) Use of triple antibiotic paste as a disinfectant for a traumatized immature tooth with a periapical lesion: a case report. *Oral Surgery, Oral Medicine, Oral Pathology, Oral Radiology, and Endodontics*, **108** (**2**), e62–e65.

223. Iwaya, S.I., Ikawa, M. & Kubota, M. (2001) Revascularization of an immature permanent tooth with apical periodontitis and sinus tract. *Dental Traumatology : Official Publication of International Association for Dental Traumatology*, **17** (**4**), 185–187.

224. Banchs, F. & Trope, M. (2004) Revascularization of immature permanent teeth with apical periodontitis: new treatment protocol? *Journal of Endodontics*, **30** (**4**), 196–200.

225. Reynolds, K., Johnson, J.D. & Cohenca, N. (2009) Pulp revascularization of necrotic bilateral bicuspids using a modified novel technique to eliminate potential coronal discolouration: a case report. *International Endodontic Journal*, **42** (**1**), 84–92.

226. Ding, R.Y., Cheung, G.S., Chen, J., Yin, X.Z., Wang, Q.Q. & Zhang, C.F. (2009) Pulp revascularization of immature teeth with apical periodontitis: a clinical study. *Journal of Endodontics*, **35** (**5**), 745–749.

227. Nosrat, A., Seifi, A. & Asgary, S. (2011) Regenerative endodontic treatment (revascularization) for necrotic immature permanent molars: a review and report of two cases with a new biomaterial. *Journal of Endodontics*, **37** (**4**), 562–567.

228. Sato, I., Ando-Kurihara, N., Kota, K., Iwaku, M. & Hoshino, E. (1996) Sterilization of infected root-canal dentine by topical application of a mixture of ciprofloxacin, metronidazole and minocycline in situ. *International Endodontic Journal*, **29** (**2**), 118–124.

229. Hoshino, E., Kurihara-Ando, N., Sato, I. *et al.* (1996) In-vitro antibacterial susceptibility of bacteria taken from infected root dentine to a mixture of ciprofloxacin, metronidazole and minocycline. *International Endodontic Journal*, **29** (**2**), 125–130.

230. Velasco-Loera, N., De Alba-Vazquez, Y., Garrocho-Rangel, A., Gonzalez-Amaro, A.M., Flores-Reyes, H. & Pozos-Guillen, A.J. (2012) Comparison of the antibacterial effect of modified 3-mix paste versus Ultrapex over anaerobic microorganisms from infected root canals of primary teeth: an in vitro study. *The Journal of Clinical Pediatric Dentistry*, **36** (**3**), 239–244.

231. McKenna, B.E., Lamey, P.J., Kennedy, J.G. & Bateson, J. (1999) Minocycline-induced staining of the adult permanent dentition: a review of the literature and report of a case. *Dental Update*, **26** (**4**), 160–162.

232. Kim, J.H., Kim, Y., Shin, S.J., Park, J.W. & Jung, I.Y. (2010) Tooth discoloration of immature permanent incisor associated with triple antibiotic therapy: a case report. *Journal of Endodontics*, **36** (**6**), 1086–1091.

233. Greenstein, G. & Polson, A. (1998) The role of local drug delivery in the management of periodontal diseases: a comprehensive review. *Journal of Periodontology*, **69** (**5**), 507–520.

234. de Paz, S., Perez, A., Gomez, M., Trampal, A. & Dominguez, L.A. (1999) Severe hypersensitivity reaction to minocycline. *Journal of Investigational Allergology & Clinical Immunology : Official Organ of the International Association of Asthmology*, **9** (**6**), 403–404.

235. Hausermann, P., Scherer, K., Weber, M. & Bircher, A.J. (2005) Ciprofloxacin-induced acute generalized exanthematous pustulosis mimicking bullous drug eruption confirmed by a positive patch test. *Dermatology*, **211** (**3**), 277–280.

236. Madsen, J.T., Thormann, J., Kerre, S., Andersen, K.E. & Goossens, A. (2007) Allergic contact dermatitis to topical metronidazole - 3 cases. *Contact Dermatitis*, **56** (**6**), 364–366.

237. Tamargo, R.J., Bok, R.A. & Brem, H. (1991) Angio-genesis inhibition by minocycline. *Cancer Research*, **51** (**2**), 672–675.

238. Gilbertson-Beadling, S., Powers, E.A., Stamp-Cole, M. *et al.* (1995) The tetracycline analogs minocycline and doxycycline inhibit angiogenesis in vitro by a non-metalloproteinase-dependent mechanism. *Cancer Chemotherapy and Pharmacology*, **36** (**5**), 418–424.

239. Er, K., Kustarci, A., Ozan, U. & Tasdemir, T. (2007) Nonsurgical endodontic treatment of dens invaginatus in a mandibular premolar with large periradicular lesion: a case report. *Journal of Endodontics*, **33** (**3**), 322–324.

240. Kusgoz, A., Yildirim, T., Er, K. & Arslan, I. (2009) Retreatment of a resected tooth associated with a large periradicular lesion by using a triple antibiotic paste and mineral trioxide aggregate: a case report with a thirty-month follow-up. *Journal of Endodontics*, **35** (**11**), 1603–1606.

241. Taneja, S., Kumari, M. & Parkash, H. (2010) Nonsurgical healing of large periradicular lesions using a triple antibiotic paste: a case series. *Contemporary Clinical Dentistry*, **1** (**1**), 31–35.

242. Dabbagh, B., Alvaro, E., Vu, D.D., Rizkallah, J. & Schwartz, S. (2012) Clinical complications in the revascularization of immature necrotic permanent teeth. *Pediatric Dentistry*, **34** (**5**), 414–417.

243. Yoshiba, K., Yoshiba, N. & Iwaku, M. (1995) Effects of antibacterial capping agents on dental pulps of monkeys mechanically exposed to oral microflora. *Journal of Endodontics*, **21** (**1**), 16–20.

244. da Silva, L.A., Nelson-Filho, P., da Silva, R.A. *et al.* (2010) Revascularization and periapical repair after endodontic treatment using apical negative pressure irrigation versus conventional irrigation plus triantibiotic intracanal dressing in dogs' teeth with apical periodontitis. *Oral Surgery, Oral Medicine, Oral Pathology, Oral Radiology, and Endodontics*, **109** (**5**), 779–787.

245. Ruparel, N.B., Teixeira, F.B., Ferraz, C.C. & Diogenes, A. (2012) Direct effect of intracanal medicaments on survival of stem cells of the apical papilla. *Journal of Endodontics*, **38** (**10**), 1372–1375.

246. Kobayashi, M., Tsutsui, T.W., Kobayashi, T. *et al.* (2013) Sensitivity of human dental pulp cells to eighteen chemical agents used for endodontic treatments in dentistry. *Odontology / the Society of the Nippon Dental University*, **101** (**1**), 43–51.

247. International Agency for Research on Cancer (2004) World Health Organization, Press Release No. 153. IARC Classifies Formalhadeyde as carcinogenic to humans [cited 2004 June 15]. http://www.iarc.fr/en/media-centre/pr/2004/pr153.html [accessed on 10 February 2014]

248. Lewis, B. (2010) The obsolescence of formocresol. *Journal of the California Dental Association*, **38** (**2**), 102–107.

249. Lucas Leite, A.C., Rosenblatt, A., da Silva, C.M., da Silva, C.M. & Santos, N. (2012) Genotoxic effect of formocresol pulp therapy of deciduous teeth. *Mutation Research*, **747** (**1**), 93–97.

250. Hamblin, M.R. & Hasan, T. (2004) Photodynamic therapy: a new antimicrobial approach to infectious disease? *Photochemical & Photobiological Sciences : Official Journal of the European Photochemistry Association and the European Society for Photobiology*, **3** (**5**), 436–450.

251. George, S. & Kishen, A. (2008) Influence of photosensitizer solvent on the mechanisms of photoactivated killing of *Enterococcus faecalis*. *Photochemistry and Photobiology*, **84** (**3**), 734–740.

252. Mortman, R.E. (2011) Technologic advances in endodontics. *Dental clinics of North America*, **55** (**3**), 461–480.vii-viii

253. Shrestha, A. & Kishen, A. (2012) The effect of tissue inhibitors on the antibacterial activity of chitosan nanoparticles and photodynamic therapy. *Journal of Endodontics*, **38** (**9**), 1275–1278.

254. Nunes, M.R., Mello, I., Franco, G.C. *et al.* (2011) Effectiveness of photodynamic therapy against *Enterococcus faecalis*, with and without the use of an intracanal optical fiber: an in vitro study. *Photomedicine and Laser Surgery*, **29** (**12**), 803–808.

255. Poggio, C., Arciola, C.R., Dagna, A. *et al.* (2011) Photoactivated disinfection (PAD) in endodontics: an in vitro microbiological evaluation. *The International Journal of Artificial Organs*, **34** (**9**), 889–897.

256. Rios, A., He, J., Glickman, G.N., Spears, R., Schneiderman, E.D. & Honeyman, A.L. (2011) Evaluation of photodynamic therapy using a light-emitting diode lamp against *Enterococcus faecalis* in extracted human teeth. *Journal of Endodontics*, **37** (**6**), 856–859.

257. Silva, L.A., Novaes, A.B. Jr., de Oliveira, R.R., Nelson-Filho, P., Santamaria, M. Jr. & Silva, R.A. (2012) Antimicrobial photodynamic therapy for the treatment of teeth with apical periodontitis: a histopathological evaluation. *Journal of Endodontics*, **38** (**3**), 360–366.

258. Yao, N., Zhang, C. & Chu, C. (2012) Effectiveness of photoactivated disinfection (PAD) to kill *Enterococcus faecalis* in planktonic solution and in an infected tooth model. *Photomedicine and Laser Surgery*, **30** (**12**), 699–704.

259. Tanaka, M., Kinoshita, M., Yoshihara, Y. *et al.* (2012) Optimal photosensitizers for photodynamic therapy of infections should kill bacteria but spare neutrophils. *Photochemistry and Photobiology*, **88** (**1**), 227–232.

260. Rossoni, R.D., Junqueira, J.C., Santos, E.L., Costa, A.C. & Jorge, A.O. (2010) Comparison of the efficacy of Rose Bengal and erythrosin in photodynamic therapy against Enterobacteriaceae. *Lasers in Medical Science*, **25** (**4**), 581–586.

261. Ishiyama, K., Nakamura, K., Ikai, H. *et al.* (2012) Bactericidal action of photogenerated singlet oxygen from photosensitizers used in plaque disclosing agents. *PloS One*, **7** (**5**), e37871.

262. Rolim, J.P., de-Melo, M.A., Guedes, S.F. *et al.* (2012) The antimicrobial activity of photodynamic therapy against *Streptococcus mutans* using different photosensitizers. *Journal of Photochemistry and Photobiology. B, Biology*, **106**, 40–46.

263. Vilela, S.F., Junqueira, J.C., Barbosa, J.O., Majewski, M., Munin, E. & Jorge, A.O. (2012) Photodynamic inactivation of *Staphylococcus aureus* and *Escherichia coli* biofilms by malachite green and phenothiazine dyes: an in vitro study. *Archives of Oral Biology*, **57** (**6**), 704–710.

264. Goulart Rde, C., Bolean, M., Paulino Tde, P. *et al.* (2010) Photodynamic therapy in planktonic and biofilm cultures of *Aggregatibacter actinomycetemcomitans*. *Photomedicine and Laser Surgery*, **28** (**Suppl 1**), S53–S60.

265. Soukos, N.S., Chen, P.S., Morris, J.T. *et al.* (2006) Photodynamic therapy for endodontic disinfection. *Journal of Endodontics*, **32** (**10**), 979–984.

266. Lee, M.T., Bird, P.S. & Walsh, L.J. (2004) Photo-activated disinfection of the root canal: a new role for lasers in endodontics. *Australian Endodontic Journal*, **30** (**3**), 93–98.

267. Mima, E.G., Vergani, C.E., Machado, A.L. *et al.* (2012) Comparison of Photodynamic Therapy versus conventional antifungal therapy for the treatment of denture stomatitis: a randomized clinical trial. *Clinical Microbiology and Infection*, **18** (**10**), E380–E388.

268. Ahn, M.Y., Kwon, S.M., Kim, Y.C., Ahn, S.G. & Yoon, J.H. (2012) Pheophorbide a-mediated photodynamic therapy induces apoptotic cell death in murine oral squamous cell carcinoma in vitro and in vivo. *Oncology Reports*, **27** (**6**), 1772–1778.

269. Guglielmi Cde, A., Simionato, M.R., Ramalho, K.M., Imparato, J.C., Pinheiro, S.L. & Luz, M.A. (2011) Clinical use of photodynamic antimicrobial chemotherapy for the treatment of deep carious lesions. *Journal of Biomedical Optics*, **16** (**8**), 088003.

270. Nagata, J.Y., Hioka, N., Kimura, E. *et al.* (2012) Antibacterial photodynamic therapy for dental caries: evaluation of the photosensitizers used and light source properties. *Photodiagnosis and Photodynamic Therapy*, **9** (**2**), 122–131.

271. Al-Zahrani, M.S. & Austah, O.N. (2011) Photodynamic therapy as an adjunctive to scaling and root planing in treatment of chronic periodontitis in smokers. *Saudi Medical Journal*, **32** (**11**), 1183–1188.

272. Garcia, V.G., Gualberto Junior, E.C., Fernandes, L.A. *et al.* (2012) Adjunctive antimicrobial photodynamic treatment of experimentally induced periodontitis in ovariectomized rats. *Journal of Periodontology*, **84** (**4**), 556–565.

273. Salmeron, S., Rezende, M.L., Consolaro, A. *et al.* (2012) Laser therapy as an effective method for implant surface decontamination: a histomorphometric study in rats. *Journal of Periodontology*, **84** (**5**), 641–649.

274. Upadya, M., Shrestha, A. & Kishen, A. (2011) Role of efflux pump inhibitors on the antibiofilm efficacy of calcium hydroxide, chitosan nanoparticles, and light-activated disinfection. *Journal of Endodontics*, **37** (**10**), 1422–1426.

275. Gursoy, H., Ozcakir-Tomruk, C., Tanalp, J. & Yilmaz, S. (2012) Photodynamic therapy in dentistry: a literature review. *Clinical Oral Investigations*, **17** (**4**), 1113–1125.

276. Mongardini, C., Di Tanna, G.L. & Pilloni, A. (2012) Light-activated disinfection using a light-emitting diode lamp in the red spectrum: clinical and microbiological short-term findings on periodontitis patients in maintenance. A randomized controlled split-mouth clinical trial. *Lasers in Medical Science*, **2** (**1**), 1–8.

277. Gambarini, G., Plotino, G., Grande, N.M. *et al.* (2011) In vitro evaluation of the cytotoxicity of FotoSan light-activated disinfection on human fibroblasts. *Medical Science Monitor*, **17** (**3**), MT21–MT25.

278. Tiyaboonchai, W. (2003) Chitosan nanoparticles: a promising system for drug delivery. *Naresuan University Journal*, **11** (**Sep**), 51–66.

279. Shrestha, A., Fong, S.W., Khoo, B.C. & Kishen, A. (2009) Delivery of antibacterial nanoparticles into dentinal tubules using high-intensity focused ultrasound. *Journal of Endodontics*, **35** (**7**), 1028–1033.

280. Shrestha, A. & Kishen, A. (2012) Polycationic chitosan-conjugated photosensitizer for antibacterial photodynamic therapy. *Photochemistry and Photobiology*, **88** (**3**), 577–583.

281. Shrestha, A., Shi, Z., Neoh, K.G. & Kishen, A. (2010) Nanoparticulates for antibiofilm treatment and effect of aging on its antibacterial activity. *Journal of Endodontics*, **36** (**6**), 1030–1035.

282. Illum, L. (1998) Chitosan and its use as a pharmaceutical excipient. *Pharmaceutical Research*, **15** (**9**), 1326–1331.

283. Rabea, E.I., Badawy, M.E., Stevens, C.V., Smagghe, G. & Steurbaut, W. (2003) Chitosan as antimicrobial agent: applications and mode of action. *Biomacromolecules*, **4** (**6**), 1457–1465.

284. Kishen, A., Shi, Z., Shrestha, A. & Neoh, K.G. (2008) An investigation on the antibacterial and antibiofilm efficacy of cationic nanoparticulates for root canal disinfection. *Journal of Endodontics*, **34** (**12**), 1515–1520.

285. Pagonis, T.C., Chen, J., Fontana, C.R. *et al.* (2010) Nanoparticle-based endodontic antimicrobial photodynamic therapy. *Journal of Endodontics*, **36** (**2**), 322–328.

286. Budiraharjo, R., Neoh, K.G., Kang, E.T. & Kishen, A. (2010) Bioactivity of novel carboxymethyl chitosan scaffold incorporating MTA in a tooth model. *International Endodontic Journal*, **43** (**10**), 930–939.

287. Lee, D.Y., Spangberg, L.S., Bok, Y.B., Lee, C.Y. & Kum, K.Y. (2005) The sustaining effect of three polymers on the release of chlorhexidine from a controlled release drug device for root canal disinfection. *Oral Surgery, Oral Medicine, Oral Pathology, Oral Radiology, and Endodontics*, **100** (**1**), 105–111.

288. Ballal, N.V., Shavi, G.V., Kumar, R., Kundabala, M. & Bhat, K.S. (2010) In vitro sustained release of calcium ions and pH maintenance from different vehicles containing calcium hydroxide. *Journal of Endodontics*, **36** (**5**), 862–866.

289. Johansen, P., Men, Y., Merkle, H.P. & Gander, B. (2000) Revisiting PLA/PLGA microspheres: an analysis of their potential in parenteral vaccination. *European Journal of Pharmaceutics and Biopharmaceutics*, **50** (**1**), 129–146.

290. Prior, S., Gamazo, C., Irache, J.M., Merkle, H.P. & Gander, B. (2000) Gentamicin encapsulation in PLA/PLGA microspheres in view of treating Brucella infections. *International Journal of Pharmaceutics*, **196** (**1**), 115–125.

291. Blanco-Prieto, M., Lecaroz, C., Renedo, M., Kunkova, J. & Gamazo, C. (2002) In vitro evaluation of gentamicin released from microparticles. *International Journal of Pharmaceutics*, **242** (**1-2**), 203–206.

292. Mandal, T.K., Bostanian, L.A., Graves, R.A. & Chapman, S.R. (2002) Poly(D,L-lactide-co-glycolide) encapsulated poly(vinyl alcohol) hydrogel as a drug delivery system. *Pharmaceutical Research*, **19** (**11**), 1713–1719.

293. Graves, R.A., Pamujula, S., Moiseyev, R., Freeman, T., Bostanian, L.A. & Mandal, T.K. (2004) Effect of different ratios of high and low molecular weight PLGA blend on the characteristics of pentamidine microcapsules. *International Journal of Pharmaceutics*, **270** (**1-2**), 251–262.

294. Schnieders, J., Gbureck, U., Thull, R. & Kissel, T. (2006) Controlled release of gentamicin from calcium phosphate-poly(lactic acid-co-glycolic acid) composite bone cement. *Biomaterials*, **27** (**23**), 4239–4249.

295. Sousa, F.F., Luzardo-Alvarez, A., Perez-Estevez, A., Seoane-Prado, R. & Blanco-Mendez, J. (2010) Development of a novel AMX-loaded PLGA/zein microsphere for root canal disinfection. *Biomedical Materials*, **5** (**5**), 055008.

14 Emerging Technologies in Root Canal Disinfection

Anil Kishen and Annie Shrestha

Discipline of Endodontics, University of Toronto, Toronto, ON, Canada

Nestor Cohenca

Department of Endodontics and Pediatric Dentistry, University of Washington, Seattle, WA, USA

Introduction

Inactivating biofilm bacteria and their by-product in the root canal systems is one of the main goals in root canal disinfection. In this context, bacteria existing as a biofilm pose a major challenge as they confer them greater immunity against antimicrobials and disinfectants (Figures 14.1 and 14.2). Disruption of the biofilm polymeric structure and killing of the resident microbes would provide a comprehensive approach in improving root canal system disinfection. Different antimicrobials and/or treatment strategies either single or in combination could be applied to eliminate biofilms (Figure 14.3). It includes the application of antimicrobials that (i) produces slow destruction of the biofilm structure, (ii) destroys persister cell or quorum sensing signals in a biofilm, (iii) diffuses into the biofilm structure producing biofilm bacterial killing, (iv) is used in combination with other strategies that enhance its diffusion into the biofilm structure, and (v) destroys both the biofilm matrix and resident bacteria in a biofilm structure (1).

Recently, antibiofilm strategies are also directed toward preventing biofilm formation. Toward this purpose, biomaterial surfaces are modified with chemicals or surface preparations to hinder bacterial adherence and subsequently biofilm formation (3, 4). Considering the nature of challenges offered by the root canal environment and microbes, ideal disinfection strategies should eliminate the biofilm structure and destroy the resident bacteria completely even from the uninstrumented portions and anatomical complexities of the root canal system. During this process, it is crucial that the therapeutic method does not cause any physical, mechanical,

Disinfection of Root Canal Systems: The Treatment of Apical Periodontitis, First Edition. Edited by Nestor Cohenca.
© 2014 John Wiley & Sons, Inc. Published 2014 by John Wiley & Sons, Inc.

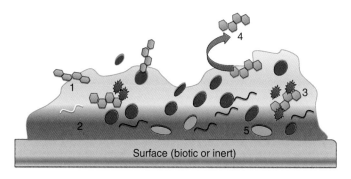

Biofilms resist antimicrobials due to
1. Decreased penetration: presence of extracellular polysaccharide
2. Decreased efficacy: altered environment (low O_2)
3. Trapped and destroyed by the enzymes
4. Expression of genes: efflux pumps
5. Inactive: Persister cells
       Actively growing biofilm bacteria on the surface
       Biofilm persister bacteria
       Antimicrobials
       Antimicrobial neutralizing enzyme

Figure 14.1   Schematic diagram showing different methods by which bacteria in a biofilm gain resistance against antimicrobials.

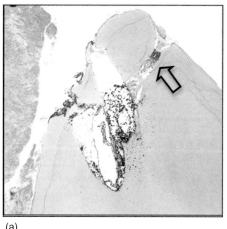

(a)

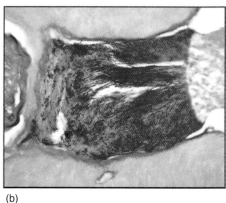

(b)

Figure 14.2   Histopathologic evaluation of a root-end section from a retreatment case with symptoms of persistent infection. (a) The overview of the mesiobuccal root tip. Three ramifications are present. Soft tissue does not appear in close contact with the root tip. This is an artifact caused by partial detachment during surgical procedure (Taylor's modified Brown and Brenn, original magnification ×25). (b) Ramification on the right side in (arrow). Its lumen is filled with a large biofilm arranged against inflammatory cells (Taylor's modified Brown and Brenn, original magnification×400). (Ricucci *et al.* (2). Reproduced with permission of Elsevier.)

and/or chemical changes to the root dentin. Moreover, inadvertent seepage of antimicrobials into the apical region should not cause cytotoxic effects in the apical tissues. Different emerging disinfection methods that are developed and tested in endodontics are discussed in this chapter.

Antibacterial nanoparticles

Nanoparticles are particles with at least three of its external dimensions in the nanoscale. Typically nanoscale size ranges from 1 to 100 nm.

The quantum size effect of nanoparticles provides them unique physicochemical properties

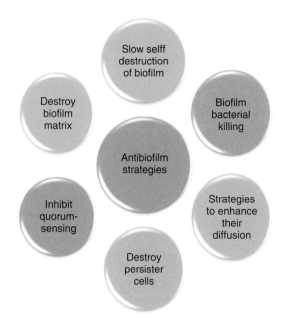

Figure 14.3   Schematic diagram showing different antibiofim strategies.

that are different from their bulk or powder counterparts. One of the key features of antibacterial nanoparticles is the broad spectrum of antimicrobial activity and far lower propensity to induce microbial resistance than antibiotics. The antibacterial activity of nanoparticles also depends on the material (i.e., organic/polymeric or inorganic/metallic), size/surface area, and charge density (5). The electrostatic interaction between positively charged nanoparticles and negatively charged bacterial cells and the accumulation of large number of nanoparticles on the bacterial cell membrane has been associated with the loss of membrane permeability and rapid loss of membrane function.

Heavy metal ions are known to have different effects on bacterial cell functions (6–8). Copper ions induced oxidative stresses (9) and affected the redox cycling, resulting in cell membrane and DNA damages. Zinc ions, above the essential threshold level, inhibited bacterial enzymes including dehydrogenase, which in turn impeded the metabolic activity (10). Silver ions inactivated proteins and inhibited the ability of DNA to replicate (11). Metallic nanoparticles synthesized from powders of silver (Ag), copper oxide (CuO), and zinc oxide

(ZnO) are currently used for their antimicrobial activity (12).

The initial interaction of microorganism with a tissue or biomaterial surface is adherence and is recognized to be an important step in the establishment of biofilm-mediated infections (13–15). Bacterial adherence experiments have highlighted that endodontic irrigants reduced the posttreatment adherence of *Enterococcus faecalis* to root dentin. Nevertheless, chemicals that alter the physicochemical properties of dentin may influence the nature of bacterial adherence and adhesion force to dentin. Final irrigation with ethylenediaminetetraaceticacid (EDTA) following sodium hypochlorite (5.2%) produced minimum reduction (33%) in the bacterial adherence to root dentin. EDTA (17%, pH 7.3) after 5 min application produced 20–30 µm zone of demineralization in dentin (16, 17). The exposed collagen fibers in this demineralized dentin served as an excellent substrate for the binding of *E. faecalis*. Thus care should be practiced to flush the root canal with sodium hypochlorite as the final irrigant to minimize the propensity of bacterial adherence (18, 19).

The quantum size effect of nanoparticles permits them to exhibit superior interaction with bacteria and dentin substrate. When cationic nanoparticles in an aqueous suspension are allowed to settle onto dentin surface, they adhered to the dentin surface by electrostatic interaction. Although this interaction between nanoparticles and dentin is weak and easily disrupted, they can impede bacterial recolonization and biofilm formation (18). Different studies pertaining to the use of nanoparticles for root canal disinfection has been summarized in Table 14.1 (3, 20–26). Among the polymeric nanoparticles, chitosan has been researched extensively owing to its excellent antimicrobial and antifungal activities. Chitosan is a natural nontoxic polymer derived by the deacetylation of chitin. Though the exact mechanisms of antibacterial action of chitosan and its derivatives are still not vivid, the electrostatic interaction between the positively charged chitosan nanoparticles and negatively charged bacterial cell membrane is believed to alter bacterial cell permeability and loss of function (27). A recent study examined the antimicrobial properties of ZnO and resin based root canal sealers loaded with chitosan and ZnO nanoparticles (3). This study highlighted that the

Table 14.1   Summary of relevant studies carried out using antimicrobial nanoparticles in endodontics.

No	Author/date	Objectives and materials	Methodology	Conclusion
1	Waltimo et al. (2007)	To test the hypothesis that nanometric bioactive glass 45S5 releases more alkaline species, and consequently has a better antimicrobial effect, than the currently available micron-sized 45S5 bioactive glass	Ionic dissolution profiles were monitored in simulated body fluid. Antimicrobial efficacy was assessed against clinical isolates of E. faecalis (planktonic form)	Micron to nanosize treatment materials afforded a 10-fold increase in silica release and solution pH Substantially increased killing efficacy
2	Kishen et al. (2008)	(1) To investigate the physical and antibacterial properties of different nanoparticulates and nanoparticulates-mixed zinc oxide-eugenol-based endodontic sealer (2) To examine the ability of different nanoparticulates-treated dentin to prevent adherence of E. faecalis	E. faecalis in planktonic Zinc oxide nanoparticulates, chitosan (CS) nanoparticulates, a mixture of zinc oxide and CS nanoparticulates, and zinc oxide nanoparticulates with multilayered coating of CS were tested	Significant reduction in the adherence of Enterococcus faecalis to nanoparticulates-treated dentin CS-highest antibacterial Combination-highest leaching property
3	Waltimo et al. (2009)	To assess the continuous release of alkaline species and antibacterial effect of Bioactive glass-Nano/Micron combination	Antimicrobial effectiveness was tested in extracted human premolars mono-infected with 3 weeks old E. faecalis biofilm	Nano BAG did not show any antibacterial efficacy
4	Mortazavi et al. (2010)	To evaluate the antibacterial effect of bioactive glass nanopowders (58S, 63S, and 72S) of different size and compositions	The antibacterial activity was studied using Escherichia coli, Pseudomonas aeruginosa, Salmonella typhi, and Staphylococcus aureus. Cytotoxicity of the samples was evaluated using mouse fibroblast L929 cell line	Antibacterial activity decreased with decrease in size and showed no cytotoxicity
5	Pagonis et al. (2010)	To study the in-vitro effects of poly(lactic-co-glycolic acid) (PLGA) nanoparticles loaded with the photosensitizer methylene blue (MB) and light against Enterococcus faecalis (ATCC 29212)	3 days old E. faecalis biofilm in root canals E. faecalis species were sensitized in planktonic phase and in experimentally infected root canals of human extracted teeth with MB-loaded nanoparticles	Significant reduction of biofilm Colony forming units (CFU) levels were significantly lower than controls and MB-loaded nanoparticles without light PLGA nanoparticles encapsulated with photoactive drugs may be a promising adjunct in antimicrobial endodontic treatment

Table 14.1   *(Continued)*

No	Author/date	Objectives and materials	Methodology	Conclusion
6	Chogle *et al.* (2011)	To evaluate two nanoparticle-enhanced polymer root-end filling materials (NERP1 and NERP2) on the initial apical seal as compared to a polymer-based commercial compomer C18 organoclay	Dual-chamber leakage apparatus and inoculated coronally with *Enterococcus faecalis* Turbidity of the apical broth was assessed daily for 4 weeks as a sign of initial leakage	The addition of C18-nanoparticles to a monomer matrix significantly reduced apical microleakage in an *in-vitro* environment
7	Shrestha (Kishen*) *et al.* (2010)	To test (1) the efficacy of chitosan (CS-np) and zinc oxide (ZnO-np) in disinfecting and disrupting biofilm bacteria and (2) the long-term efficacy of these nanoparticulates following aging	*E. faecalis* in planktonic and biofilms	• Total elimination of planktonic • Significant reduction of biofilms • Retained antibacterial property after aging
8	Shrestha and Kishen (2012)	CS in the presence of tissue inhibitors	*E. faecalis* in planktonic	Pulp and bovine serum albumin (BSA) significantly inhibited the antibacterial effect

addition of antibacterial nanoparticles in root canal sealers would improve the direct (based on direct antibacterial assay) and diffusible antibacterial effects (based on a membrane-restricted antibacterial assay) in root canal sealers. Studies also showed that the application of chitosan nanoparticles reduced the adherence of *E. faecalis* to root dentin.

Root dentin treated with chlorhexidine and subsequently with nanoparticulate showed the maximum reduction (97%) in bacterial adherence (3). Antibacterial substantivity have been highlighted after using 2% chlorhexidine gel (28); however, chlorhexidine did not entirely remove bacteria from the dentinal tubules of teeth that were infected with *E. faecalis* (29). Addition of nanoparticles into the root canal sealers showed improved antibacterial property and did not affect the flow characteristics of the root canal sealer. Also, ZnO nanoparticles were able to diffuse out from the sealer and exert antibacterial activity, which is definitely advantageous in a posttreated root canal environment (3). These polymeric and

metallic nanoparticles were also able to eliminate bacterial biofilm and withstand the effect of aging for 90 days (conditioning with tissue fluids) on their antibacterial properties. The planktonic *E. faecalis* were totally eliminated in contrast to the biofilm bacteria. Longer duration of interaction and higher concentration of nanoparticles were required to reduce the biofilm bacteria in significant numbers (Figure 14.4) (22).

Microparticles and nanoparticles of bioactive glass received considerable interest in root canal disinfection following its antibacterial properties. The bioactive glass consists of SiO_2, Na_2O, CaO_2, and P_2O_5 at different concentrations. The antibacterial mechanism of bioactive glass has been attributed to a combination of several factors such as (i) high pH, (ii) increase in osmotic effects, and (iii) Ca/P precipitation (30). The feasibility of using bioactive glass for root canal disinfection has been tested *in-vitro* (31–33). However, bioactive glass showed shortcomings such as significantly less antibacterial effect when compared with calcium hydroxide (32) and ineffective in preventing

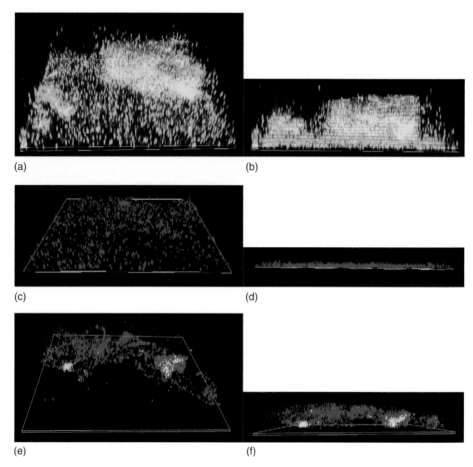

(a)   (b)

(c)   (d)

(e)   (f)

Figure 14.4   The three-dimensional confocal laser scanning microscopy (CLSM) reconstruction of *Enterococcus faecalis* (ATCC 29212) biofilm (a, b) and after treatment with antibacterial ZnO-np (c, d) and CS-np (e, f). The number of live bacterial cells was reduced significantly, and the three-dimensional structure was also disrupted. (b, d, and f show the sagittal sections of the biofilm structure) (original magnification, 60×). (Shrestha *et al.* (22). Reproduced with permission of Elsevier.)

recontamination of instrumented root canals (31). 45S5 bioactive glass suspensions/slurries for root canal disinfection should combine the ability to induce high pH with the capacity to continuously release alkaline species (21).

The bioactive glass nanometric slurry with a 12-fold higher specific surface area than the micrometric counterpart was expected to possess better antibacterial properties. Nevertheless, the microparticles of bioactive glass produced considerably higher alkalinity and antimicrobial efficacy and this did not support the previous report by the same group that showed higher antibacterial efficacy with the shift from micron- to nanosized

treatment materials (20). In another related application, bioactive glass was used to promote mineral deposition within the root canal, which could ultimately replace the use of endodontic sealers. Toward this end, a combination of polyisoprene or polycaprolactone and nanometric bioactive glass 45S5 was employed. Incorporation of bioactive glass fillers into polyisoprene and polycaprolactone rendered the resulting composite material bioactive and permitted improved mineralization (34). These initial observations need further research to apply the composite of polyisoprene, polycaprolactone, and bioactive glass as a "single" root canal filling material.

The studies so far showed that most tested nanoparticles possess high antibacterial properties when compared to their powder counterpart. Though they have the ability to diffuse antimicrobial components deep into the dentin tissue, additional research is needed to study their ability to inactivate bacterial biofilms in the anatomical complexities and uninstrumented portion of the root canal system. Their interaction with host tissues/immune cells also requires further investigations. Nevertheless, the successful application of nanoparticles in endodontic disinfection will depend on both the effectiveness of antimicrobial nanoparticles and the delivery method used within the root canal system.

Antimicrobial photodynamic therapy

Photodynamic therapy applies a photosensitizer, that is, a light sensitive chemical at extremely low and nontoxic concentration, which, when activated with a specific wavelength of light, produces activated oxygen radicals that cause toxic effects on the bacterial cells.

Antimicrobial Photodynamic Therapy (APDT) involves two specific steps for achieving disinfection. Step-1 is the photosensitization of the infected tissue with photosensitizer to allow uptake into the bacterial cells and Step-2 is the irradiation of the photosensitized tissue to result in the destruction of bacteria and infected tissue. The light should be at a specific wavelength, which corresponds to the absorption wavelength of the photosensitizer used. The photosensitizer in the triplet state is extremely reactive, which reacts further by one or both of the following pathways to destroy the cell. (1) *Type I reaction*: the photosensitizer triplet state can react with a target, other than oxygen by hydrogen or electron transfer resulting in radical ions that can react with oxygen, yielding cytotoxic species such as hydrogen peroxide, superoxide anion, hydroxyl, and lipid derived radicals. (2) *Type II reaction*: the photosensitizer triplet state can transfer the excitation energy to ground state molecular oxygen to produce excited state singlet oxygen ($^1O_2$) (35) (Figure 14.5).

Singlet oxygen is a strong oxidizing agent and thus highly reactive, with a lifetime of less than $0.04\,\mu s$ in a biological environment and a radius of action of less than $0.02\,\mu m$ (36). The reactions of singlet oxygen with the cellular targets lead to cell death. The two basic mechanisms that have been proposed to account for this lethal damage to the bacterial cell are DNA damage and cytoplasmic membrane damage. APDT on gram-positive and gram-negative bacteria have reported breaks in both single and double-stranded DNA and the disappearance of the plasmid supercoiled fraction (37, 38). Previous studies have shown that the photo-oxidative effect caused by phenothiazinium photosensitizer in bacteria could lead to damage of multiple targets in bacterial cells such as DNA (37), membrane integrity (39), protease activity, and lipopolysaccharide (LPS) (40). George and Kishen (41) reported functional impairment of cell wall, extensive damage to chromosomal DNA, and degradation of membrane proteins following methylene blue mediated APDT of *E. faecalis*. These findings support the hypothesis that APDT can be a feasible alternative to antibiotics as the mode of action is markedly different from that of most antibiotics.

In endodontic literature, Meire *et al.* (42) and George and Kishen (43, 44) used APDT to enhance the root canal disinfection. They showed that biofilms of *E. faecalis* could be effectively killed by APDT with photosensitizer such as methylene blue and toluidine blue O (TBO) along with red light. Soukos *et al.* (45) conducted APDT experiments on a range of endodontic pathogens (methylene blue as photosensitizer) and reported complete elimination of all bacteria except *E. faecalis* (53%). In yet another study, significant antibacterial effect on suspensions of *Streptococcus intermedius*, *Peptostreptococcus micros*, *Prevotella intermedia*, and *Fusobacterium nucleatum* were reported by Williams *et al.* (46) following APDT with TBO and red light. Some of the tissue specific challenging factors in the application of APDT for endodontic disinfection are the penetration of the activating light energy into the infected tissue, penetration of optimum photosensitizer concentration into the infected tissue, limited availability of environmental oxygen in the infected tissue, the ability of excess photosensitizer to induce discoloration of dentin, and reduction or neutralization of antimicrobial activities following the presence of tissue and serum within the root canals.

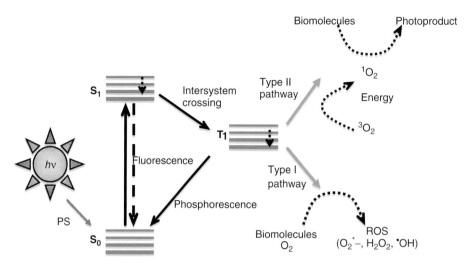

Figure 14.5   Schematic diagram of possible mechanism of photodynamic therapy where the excited photosensitizer (PS) after light irradiation could follow different pathways to return to its stable ground state. The PS on photoactivation absorbs a photon and goes to the excited singlet state (S_1). The S_1 can come back to the ground state by releasing fluorescence or relax back to excited-triplet PS state (T_1). The long-lived T1 state can phosphoresce and come back to S_0. Or else T_1 can interact with molecular oxygen following two specific pathways Type I and Type II mechanism, resulting in the generation of reactive oxygen species or singlet oxygen, respectively. The singlet oxygen generated in Type II mechanism then interacts with biomolecules to produce the resultant PDT effect (photoproduct).

In an approach to improve the antimicrobial efficacy of APDT in root canal system (tissue specific approach), George and Kishen dissolved methylene blue in different formulations: water, 70% glycerol, 70% polyethylene glycol, and a mixture of glycerol:ethanol:water (MIX) in a ratio of 30:20:50, and analyzed for the photophysical, photochemical, and photobiological characteristics (43). They showed that aggregation of methylene blue molecules was significantly higher in water when compared to other formulations. Other than this, the MIX based methylene blue formulation had effective penetration into dentinal tubules, enhanced singlet oxygen generation, which in turn improved bactericidal action. A significantly higher impairment of bacterial cell wall and extensive damage to chromosomal DNA was observed when methylene blue in a MIX based formulation was used, when compared to water (41). The same group also showed that the incorporation of an oxidizer and oxygen carrier with photosensitizer formulation in the form of an emulsion would produce significant photo-oxidation capabilities, which in turn facilitated comprehensive disruption of matured endodontic biofilm structure (44).

The selectivity of APDT toward microbial cells elimination over host cells, at the suggested photosensitization periods and light fluence, presents itself as a preferable choice among antibacterial alternatives. Soukos et al. compared the effect of APDT using a combination of TBO and red light against *Streptococcus sanguis* and human gingival keratinocytes and fibroblasts. They reported no reduction in the human cell viability whereas the bacteria were effectively killed (47). Soncin et al. reported the selective killing of *Staphylococcus aureus* over human fibroblasts and keratinocytes (four to sixfold) when subjected to APDT using cationic pthalocyanine and relatively low light fluencies (48). George and Kishen (49) demonstrated a 97.7% killing of E. faecalis compared to a 30% human fibroblast dysfunction following methylene blue mediated APDT. All these *in-vitro* studies suggested the targeted killing efficacy of APDT.

Conjugating photosensitizer to various agents or chemical moieties can result in improved photosensitizers for APDT. These modified photosensitizers are expected to bind to the outer membrane of bacteria and on activation generated reactive oxygen species, which then diffused into cells, resulting in cell death (50, 51). Therefore, photogenerated oxidative species is confined to the cell wall and its vicinity, which is a highly susceptible domain for photodynamic action. Soukos and coworkers formed a hypothesis that by covalently conjugating a suitable photosensitizer to a *poly-l-lysine* chain, a bacteria-targeted photosensitizer delivery vehicle could be constructed that would efficiently inactivate both gram-positive and gram-negative species (51). This was demonstrated by preparing a conjugate of chlorin (e6) and a *poly-l-lysine* chain (20 lysine residues), which after 1 min incubation and illumination with red light, killed greater than 99% of the gram-positive *Actinomyces viscosus* and gram-negative *Porphyromonas gingivalis* (51). Photosensitizer conjugated with positively charged chitosan has also been shown to be highly effective in removing biofilms of gram-positive and gram-negative bacteria (52). Shrestha *et al.* (53) showed that the rose-bengal conjugated chitosan presented a synergistic effect of the antimicrobial polymer chitosan and singlet oxygen generated following photoactivation.

Tissue remnants and serum products compromised the antimicrobial efficacy of not only the common endodontic irrigants (54), but also the APDT efficacy (23). Most studies concerning the APDT of microbial pathogens use deionized water or phosphate buffered saline to dissolve the photosensitizer. In some studies, photosensitizer was dissolved in brain heart infusion broth wherein reduced bactericidal effect with the tested photosensitizer was reported. This reduction in antibacterial effect was attributed to the presence of serum proteins in the broth (45, 55). Constituents of the infected root canal such as tissue remnants (pulp), serum, and dentin matrix have also been shown to significantly reduce the APDT effect *in-vitro* (23). This is either because of the cross-linking action or the compromised half-life of singlet oxygen in the presence of proteins. Light sources used for APDT can be coherent (lasers) or noncoherent (lamps). The choice of light source is dictated by the location, required light dose, and the choice of photosensitizer. Laser provides monochromatic, coherent, and collimated light, offering a wide range of output power. Laser light can be easily coupled into a fiber optic cable, which can serve as a delivery system (probe) while irradiating complex anatomy such as a root canal.

Nd:YAG, KTP, HeNe, GaAlAs and diode lasers, light emitting diodes (LEDs), and xenon-arc lamps have been employed for APDT. The superiority of one type of light source over the other has not been clearly demonstrated and hence the use of lasers or lamps depends on the specific application (56).

Different *in-vivo* studies that examined the efficacy of APDT in root canal disinfection has been summarized in Table 14.2 (57–60). These studies concluded that a combination of chemomechanical preparation and APDT would bring about maximum reduction in microbial loads. Currently research is directed toward potential antibiofilm efficacy of APDT by combining the advantages of photodynamic effect with bioactive microparticles (52, 53, 61) and nanoparticles (26). Further research is mandatory to improve the antibiofilm efficacy of APDT in the presence of tissue inhibitors, to optimize light delivery within the root canal, to optimize new photosensitizers, and/or to formulate applications within the root canal. A standardized protocol for photosensitization and light activation is paramount for endodontic disinfection.

Lasers assisted root canal disinfection

A laser is a device that emits electromagnetic radiation through a process of light amplification based on stimulated emission of photons. The light emitted from a laser device has all the photons in a coherent state (usually with the same frequency and phase) and produces lethal effect on bacteria.

Different types of lasers may produce different effects on the same tissue, and the same laser may have varying effects on different tissues. The nature of laser–tissue interaction is influenced by (i) the properties of laser such as wavelength, energy density, and pulse duration. (ii) The optical characteristics of the tissue such as reflection, absorption, transmission, and scattering. Generally, the laser effects on a tissue will depend on its interaction with the tissue and the depth of penetration. Nevertheless, the parameters to be controlled during operation are (i) applied power (power density), (ii) total energy applied over a given area of tissue (energy density), (iii) rate and duration of laser irradiation (pulse repetition), and

Table 14.2   Summary of relevant *in-vivo* studies carried out using antimicrobial photodynamic therapy.

No	Author/date	Objective and materials	Methodology	Conclusion
1	Bonsor *et al.* (2006)	Aimed to evaluate the antimicrobial efficacy of root canal disinfection by combining conventional endodontic treatment with PDT Clinical study on 32 root canals from 14 patients	Irrigation with 20% citric acid and 2.25% sodium hypochlorite PDT with TBO and diode laser (12.7 mg/l, 100 mW, 120 s) Samples collected by filing	Cleaning and shaping resulted in complete bacterial killing in 86.7% of samples Combination of cleaning and shaping + PDT resulted in complete bacterial killing in 96.7% of samples
2	Bonsor *et al.* (2006)	Aimed to compare the effect of a combination of 20% citric acid and PDT with the use of 20% citric acid and 2.25% sodium hypochlorite on bacterial load in prepared root canals 64 patients were used	Procedure similar to previous study	Combination of 20% citric acid and PDT resulted in complete bacterial killing in 91% of samples 20% citric acid and 2.25% sodium hypochlorite resulted in complete bacterial killing in 82% of samples
3	Garcez *et al.* (2008)	Aimed to analyze the antimicrobial effect of PDT in association with endodontic treatment 20 patients were selected First session of cleaning and shaping + PDT At the end of first session, the root canal was filled with $Ca(OH)_{(2)}$, and after 1 week, a second session of PDT was performed	Irrigation with 2.5% sodium hypochlorite, 3% hydrogen peroxide, and 17% EDTA PDT with polyethylenimine (PEI) chlorin (e6 [ce6]) conjugate (2 min, 9.6 J, 240 s) Paper point sampling	First session produced 98.5% bacterial reduction (1.83 log reduction) Second session produced 99.9% bacterial reduction (1.14 log reduction) Second session PDT was observed to be more effective than first session
4	Garcez *et al.* (2010)	Studied antimicrobial effect of PDT combined with endodontic treatment in patients with necrotic pulp infected with microflora resistant to a previous antibiotic therapy 30 teeth from 21 patients with apical lesions that had been treated with conventional endodontic treatment and antibiotic therapy were selected	PDT used polyethylenimine chlorin(e6) as a photosensitizer and a diode laser (40 mW, 4 min, 9.6 J)	Endodontic therapy alone produced a significant reduction in the number of microbial species (only three teeth were free of bacteria) The combination of endodontic therapy with PDT eliminated all drug-resistant species and all teeth were bacteria-free

(iv) mode of energy delivery (continuous/pulsed energy; direct/indirect tissue contact) (62).

Currently, lasers are employed in root canal disinfection mainly to enhance the degree of microbial elimination subsequent to the cleaning and shaping procedure. Laser assisted root canal disinfection requires the root canals to be prepared (shaped) as the parameters of the laser used for disinfection does not produce marked ablative effects on dentin tissue (62, 63). Infrared lasers such as CO_2, Nd:YAG, diode, and Erbium lasers have been applied for endodontic disinfection. The bactericidal effect of lasers depends on the wavelength characteristics and laser energy used, and in most case, their thermal effects are counted on. The laser induced thermal effect will produce alteration in the bacterial cell wall, leading to changes in osmotic gradients, swelling, and cell death. The gram-negative bacteria showed a higher resistance against laser irradiation than gram-positive bacteria. This higher resistance of gram-negative bacteria was attributed to their cell wall characteristics (62).

The delivery of laser energy throughout the root canal system and absorption of laser energy by dentin tissue are important issues to consider in laser assisted root canal disinfection (64). This will influence the degree of structural alteration in dentin and elimination of bacterial biofilm from root canal system. In a study, to increase the effect of disinfection in the infected root canals, black Indian ink or 38% silver ammonium solution was placed in the root canal before irradiating with pulsed Nd:YAG laser (1064 nm). They reported disinfection rates of 80–90% with Nd:YAG laser within the primary root canal (65). Schoop *et al.* (64) showed that the Nd:YAG laser presented a bacterial reduction of 85% at 1 mm depth within the dentin when compared to diode laser (810 nm), which produced 63% bacterial reduction at a depth of 750 μm into the dentin. Bergmans *et al.* tried to define the role of the laser as a disinfecting tool by using Nd:YAG laser irradiation on certain endodontic pathogens *in-vitro*. They concluded that Nd:YAG laser irradiation is not an alternative but a possible supplement to existing protocols for root canal disinfection (66). The bactericidal effect of Erbium laser in root canal model was observed to be inferior to that of Nd:YAG laser. The thermal energy produced by the Erbium laser is absorbed mostly by the surface structure because of their high affinity to water molecules, thus exerting higher bactericidal effect on the surface of the root canal wall (67). Contradictory finding supporting the superior antibacterial effect of Er:YAG laser in combination with hypochlorite as compared to Nd:YAG laser has been shown in a study (68).

Despite all these studies, it was suggested that endodontic pathogens grow, as biofilms are difficult targets to eradicate even on direct laser exposure. In addition to this, there are several limitations that may be associated with the intracanal use of high-power lasers that cannot be overlooked. The emission of laser energy from the tip of the optical fiber or laser guide is directed along the root canal and not necessarily laterally to the root canal walls. Thus it is almost impossible to obtain uniform coverage of the canal surface using a laser (69, 70). The safety of such a procedure is another limitation, as potential thermal damage to the apical tissues is possible. Direct emission of laser irradiation from the tip of the optical fiber in the vicinity of the apical foramen may result in the transmission of irradiation beyond the apical foramen, which may adversely affect the supporting apical tissues. This effect can be hazardous in teeth with close proximity to the mental foramen or to the mandibular nerve (70). A modified beam delivery system has been tested for Er:YAG laser. This system consists of a hollow tube allowing lateral emission of the radiation (side firing), rather than direct emission through a single opening at its terminal end (70). This new endodontic side firing spiral tip was designed to fit the shape and volume of root canals prepared by nickel–titanium rotary instrumentation. It emits the Er:YAG laser irradiation laterally to the walls of the root canal through a spiral slit located all along the tip. The tip is sealed at its far end, preventing the transmission of irradiation to and through the apical foramen of the tooth (71). This tip improvement is aimed at improving the ability of laser to penetrate and destroy the microbes in the lateral walls of the root canal and dentinal tubules.

The antibiofilm effect of Er:YAG laser on *in-vitro* monospecies biofilm of *Actinomyces naeslundii*, *E. faecalis*, *Lactobacillus casei*, *Propionibacterium acnes*, *F. nucleatum*, *P. gingivalis*, and *Prevotella nigrescens* grown on hydroxyapatite disks for 21 days (aerobically for 7 days and anaerobically for 14 days) was investigated (72). It was reported that

Er:YAG irradiation produced significant reduction in the numbers of viable cells in most of the biofilms tested. Nevertheless, complete elimination of biofilm structure/bacteria was not possible. Er:YAG laser irradiation at all tested energy densities could not disinfect *L. casei* biofilm cells. It was mentioned that the *L. casei* decalcified the high availability (HA) disks at a depth of about 200 μm and invaded the porous decalcified layer. It was speculated that the laser could not reach the base of the decalcified layer inhabited by *L. casei* cells (72). It is important to realize the surface degradation and microbial penetration, deep within the anatomical complexities and dentinal tubules in an endodontically infected tooth. The antibiofilm actions of the Er:YAG laser are influenced by the water content, components of extracellular matrix, cell density, and absorption properties. The temperature increase during irradiation ranged from 7.3 °C at 20 mJ to 40.2 °C at 80 mJ. In another study, Yavari examined the ability of high-power settings of Er, Cr:YSGG laser irradiation (2 and 3 W output powers for 16 s) to eradicate *in-vitro* monospecies biofilm of *E. faecalis* (48 h). It was concluded that though 2- and 3-W of Er, Cr:YSGG laser showed antibacterial properties on *E. faecalis* in root canal models, their effect was less remarkable than that of NaOCl solution (73). Similar comparison of two different lasers Er:YAG and Nd:YAG with NaOCl was tested on a relatively young *E. faecalis* biofilms. Meire *et al.* (74) confirmed that even though Er:YAG laser treatment (100 mJ pulses) showed strong reductions of biofilm bacteria, NaOCl proved to be the most effective in biofilm elimination (74).

The changes in the ultrastructure of radicular dentin as a concomitant/adverse effect to root canal disinfection have been reported. The use of near- and midinfrared lasers produced characteristic thermal effects on dentin when used in a dry root canal. Human dentin presents low absorption coefficients in the near-infrared range. Nonetheless, Nd:YAG laser irradiation is still able to melt the dentin surface (75). Moriyama *et al.* showed that morphological changes in dentin are induced by Nd:YAG laser irradiation following laser induced thermal processes. In this case, the smear layer is only partially removed and the dentinal tubules are primarily closed because of the melting of inorganic dentin material, and cracks are formed. Longer pulses produce more evident effects of deeper resolidified structures because of the larger volume of melted material. Thus increasing the number of pulses may result in a more regular surface. Nonetheless, high number of thermal cycles may lead to cracks (76).

During photothermal interaction, the tissue molecules absorb photons, resulting in the generation of heat, which is dissipated into the tissue. As the tissue needs some time to propagate the heat, longer pulses will result in higher temperatures in deeper regions of the tissue, whereas for shorter pulses using the same average energy, higher temperatures are observed at the surface (77). The thermal damage in tissue is a temperature/time-dependent process. The resultant confinement of thermal stress would depend on the laser pulse duration and the tissue absorption coefficient (μ_a). The use of longer pulses will lead to longer interaction times, resulting in more evident thermal effects (78). Presence of water/irrigation solutions limits the thermal interaction of laser beam on dentinal wall. The irradiation of root dentin with diode laser (2.5 W, 15 Hz) and Nd:YAG laser (1.5 W, 100 mJ, 15 Hz) after irrigation with the irrigating solution produce better dentin morphology (79, 80). It was also shown that the presence of water in root canal space prevented undesirable effects on dentin during the application of Erbium laser (81). Table 14.3 summarizes relevant clinical studies that examined the antimicrobial efficacy of high-power laser in endodontics (82, 83). There is no strong evidence currently available to support the application of high-power laser in endodontic disinfection.

Understanding liquid irrigant laser interaction is a new area of research interest. This concept forms the basis for *laser-activated irrigation* and *photon-initiated photoacoustic streaming* in root canal disinfection (84–86). The mechanism of interaction of Er, Cr:YSGG laser with liquid irrigant in the root canal is attributed to efficient absorption of the midinfrared wavelength light by water. The aspects of *laser-activated irrigation* and *photon-initiated photoacoustic streaming* are covered elsewhere in this book.

Ozone

Ozone (O_3) is an energized, unstable gaseous form of oxygen that dissociates readily back into oxygen

Table 14.3 Summary of relevant *in-vivo* studies carried out using laser assisted disinfection.

No	Author/date	Objective and materials	Methodology	Conclusion
1	Koba *et al.* (1999)	Evaluated the postoperative symptoms and healing after root canal treatment with pulsed Nd:YAG laser

44 teeth from 38 patients

Radiological evaluation used to assess the reduction of apical lesions at 3 and 6 months | Nd:YAG (1 W, 15 pps for 1 s)

5% NaOCl and 3% H_2O_2 used to disinfect (control) | No significant differences were found between the groups regarding apical healing |
| 2 | Dostálová *et al.* (2002) | Studied the ability of Er:YAG laser radiation with a movable waveguide to disinfect root canals

Root canal of 44 premolars and molars were treated using a step-back technique; 10 teeth were then treated with calcium hydroxide; 22 teeth were irradiated with the waveguide | 5.25% NaOCl used to disinfect (control)

Er:YAG (100 mJ, 30 pulses, repetition rate 4 Hz)

Before and after treatment, the colony-forming units were counted to determine 21 different microorganisms | Conventional treatment was effective in 60% of the root canal

Application of calcium hydroxide was effective in 80% of the root canal

Er:YAG laser irradiation via movable waveguide was effective in 100% of the root canal |
| 3 | Leonardo *et al.* (2005) | Evaluated the antimicrobial effect of Er:YAG laser applied after the cleaning and shaping of root canals of dog's teeth with apical periodontitis

40 root canals of dogs' premolar teeth with apical lesions were used | Group I-cleaning and shaping only

Group II-cleaning and shaping and Er:YAG laser application (63-mJ output/15 Hz).

After coronal sealing, the root canals were left empty for 7 days before microbiological analysis | Er:YAG laser applied after cleaning and shaping did not reduce microorganisms in the root canal system |

(O_2), liberating a reactive form of oxygen, the singlet oxygen (O_1), which is capable of oxidizing the cells.

Ozone is an unstable, allotrope of oxygen that is formed naturally in the ozone layer from atmospheric oxygen by electric discharge or exposure to ultraviolet radiation. Ozone presents a broad range of antibacterial efficacy without developing drug resistance (87, 88). Ozone gas is currently used clinically for endodontic treatment. But, the results of studies on its efficacy against endodontic pathogens have been inconsistent. This inconsistency is attributed to the lack of information about the optimum duration of application and concentration to be used within the root canal (89–91). In order to achieve a concentration, which is relatively nontoxic toward apical and oral mucosal tissues, the ozone gas concentration currently used in endodontics is $4\,g/m^3$. This concentration has been shown to be slightly less cytotoxic than NaOCl (2.5%). Aqueous ozone (up to $20\,\mu g/ml$) showed essentially no toxicity to oral cells *in-vitro* (92–94).

Ozone demonstrated substantial antibacterial effect *in-vitro* when tested against *E. faecalis*. Hems *et al.* (91) tested ozone against *E. faecalis*, in both planktonic and biofilm cultures (48 h old biofilm grown on cellulose nitrate membrane filter). Different interaction time ranging from 30 to 240 s was applied in both cultures. It was concluded that ozone had an antibacterial effect on planktonic *E. faecalis* cells and those suspended in fluid, but little effect when embedded in a biofilm structure. Its antibacterial efficacy was not comparable with that of sodium hypochlorite under the conditions tested in this study (91, 92). Another study assessed the antimicrobial efficacy of aqueous (1.25–20 μg/ml) and gaseous ozone (1–53 g/m³) as an alternative antiseptic against endodontic pathogens in suspension and a biofilm model (95). *E. faecalis*, *Candida albicans*, *P. micros*, and *Pseudomonas aeruginosa* were grown in planktonic culture or in monospecies biofilms in root canals for 3 weeks. The antibacterial efficacy of ozone in the gaseous and aqueous forms depended on the concentration, strain, and time of interaction against the tested microorganisms in suspension and the biofilm test model.

Pseudomonas fluorescens as planktonic and biofilms were tested in another study. Planktonic form was completely eliminated by low concentrations of ozone (0.1 ± 0.3 ppm) within 15 or 30 min contact time. The disinfectant action of ozone on biofilm models was less effective with only a decrease of two orders of magnitude, and increased contact time was not helpful (96). Kuştarci *et al.* evaluated the antimicrobial activity of potassium-titanyl-phosphate (KTP) laser and gaseous ozone in experimentally infected root canals. It was found that both KTP laser and gaseous ozone have a significant antibacterial effect on infected root canals, with the gaseous ozone being more effective than the KTP laser. However, 2.5% NaOCl was superior in its antimicrobial abilities compared with KTP laser and gaseous ozone (97). Table 14.4 enlists relevant antimicrobial studies carried out using ozone. A recent study has claimed that ozone dissolved in oil can be used as an intracanal medicament (98). Studies on the effect of surface tension on the flow characteristics of ozonized oil, chemical stability of ozonized oil, and their interaction with root dentin and obturating material is justified before ozone can be applied in endodontics (99).

Table 14.4 Summary of relevant antimicrobial studies carried out using ozone.

No	Author/date	Objective/methodology	Conclusion
1	Estrela *et al.* (2007)	To determine the antimicrobial efficacy of ozonated water, gaseous ozone, 2.5% sodium hypochlorite, and 2% chlorhexidine in human root canals infected by *E. faecalis* for 60 days	The irrigation of infected human root canals with ozonated water, 2.5% NaOCl, 2% chlorhexidine, and the application of gaseous ozone for 20 min were not sufficient to inactivate *E. faecalis*
2	Hems *et al.* (2005)	To evaluate the potential of ozone as an antibacterial agent using *E. faecalis*. The antibacterial efficacy of ozone was tested against both broth and biofilm cultures. Ozone was sparged for 30, 60, 120, and 240 s	NaOCl was found to be superior to ozonated water in killing *E. faecalis* in broth culture and in biofilms
3	Nagayoshi *et al.* (2004)	To evaluate the effect of ozonated water against *E. faecalis* and *S. mutans* infected dentin of bovine incisors	Ozonated water application might be useful for root canal irrigation
4	Kuştarci *et al.* (2009)	To evaluate the antimicrobial activity of potassium-titanyl-phosphate (KTP) laser and gaseous ozone in experimentally infected root canals (*E. faecalis* for 24 h)	2.5% NaOCl was superior in its antimicrobial abilities compared with KTP laser and gaseous ozone

The reduced effectiveness of ozone against sessile bacteria when compared to planktonic bacteria is because of the characteristics of biofilm (96). The polymeric layer may form a physical/chemical barrier preventing deeper penetration of the dissolved ozone into the biofilm structure (100). In addition, blockage of water channels in biofilm by the oxidation products of ozone may impede further penetration of ozone to the inner layers of biofilm structure (101). In a systematic review by Azarpazhooh and Limeback, ozone has been highlighted for its biocompatibility with human oral epithelial cells, gingival fibroblast, and periodontal cells, though conflicting evidence of antimicrobial efficacy of ozone in root canal disinfection cannot not be overlooked (102).

Conclusion

Current understanding emphasizes the fact that endodontic disease is a biofilm-mediated infection, and the elimination of bacterial biofilm from the root canal system remains to be the primary challenge in the management of endodontic disease. In the haste to introduce newer and advanced antibacterial strategies, it is important not to neglect potential constraining factors associated with their application in root canal disinfection. The key to the successful application of newer antibacterial strategies in root canal disinfection is to address all the challenges prevailing in root canal system in entirety rather than focusing only on the antibacterial aspect.

References

1. Prince, A.S. (2002) Biofilms, antimicrobial resistance, and airway infection. *The New England Journal of Medicine*, **347**, 1110–1111.
2. Ricucci, D., Siqueira, J.F., Bate, A.L. & Pitt Ford, T.R. (2009) Histologic investigation of root canal-treated teeth with apical periodontitis: a retrospective study from twenty-four patients. *Journal of Endodontics*, **35**, 493–502.
3. Kishen, A., Shi, Z., Shrestha, A. & Neoh, K.G. (2008) An investigation on the antibacterial and antibiofilm efficacy of cationic nanoparticulates for root canal disinfection. *Journal of Endodontics*, **34**, 1515–1520.
4. An, Y.H., Stuart, G.W., McDowell, S.J., McDaniel, S.E., Kang, Q. & Friedman, R.J. (1996) Prevention of bacterial adherence to implant surfaces with a crosslinked albumin coating in vitro. *Journal of Orthopaedic Research*, **14**, 846–849.
5. Sawai, J., Shoji, S., Igarashi, H. *et al.* (1998) Hydrogen peroxide as an antibacterial factor in zinc oxide powder slurry. *Journal of Fermentation and Bioengineering*, **86**, 521–522.
6. Stohs, S.J. & Bagchi, D. (1995) Oxidative mechanisms in the toxicity of metal-ions. *Free Radical Biology and Medicine*, **18**, 321–336.
7. Yoon, K.Y., Byeon, J.H., Park, J.H. & Hwang, J. (2007) Susceptibility constants of Escherichia coli and Bacillus subtilis to silver and copper nanoparticles. *Science of the Total Environment*, **373**, 572–575.
8. Reddy, K.M., Feris, K., Bell, J., Wingett, D.G., Hanley, C. & Punnoose, A. (2007) Selective toxicity of zinc oxide nanoparticles to prokaryotic and eukaryotic systems. *Applied Physics Letters*, **90**, 213902-1–213902-3.
9. Cioffi, N., Ditaranto, N., Torsi, L. *et al.* (2005) Analytical characterization of bioactive fluoropolymer ultra-thin coatings modified by copper nanoparticles. *Analytical and Bioanalytical Chemistry*, **381**, 607–616.
10. Beard, S.J., Hughes, M.N. & Poole, R.K. (1995) Inhibition of the cytochrome Bd-terminated NADH oxidase system in Escherichia-Coli K-12 by divalent metal-cations. *FEMS Microbiology Letters*, **131**, 205–210.
11. Feng, Q.L., Wu, J., Chen, G.Q., Cui, F.Z., Kim, T.N. & Kim, J.O. (2000) A mechanistic study of the antibacterial effect of silver ions on Escherichia coli and Staphylococcus aureus. *Journal of Biomedical Materials Research*, **52**, 662–668.
12. Kim, J.S., Kuk, E., Yu, K.N. *et al.* (2007) Antimicrobial effects of silver nanoparticles. *Nanomedicine: Nanotechnology, Biology and Medicine*, **3**, 95–101.
13. Jefferson, K.K. (2004) What drives bacteria to produce a biofilm? *FEMS Microbiology Letters*, **236**, 163–173.
14. Busscher, H.J. & van der Mei, H.C. (1997) Physico-chemical interactions in initial microbial adhesion and relevance for biofilm formation. *Advances in Dental Research*, **11**, 24–32.
15. An, Y.H. & Friedman, R.J. (1998) Concise review of mechanisms of bacterial adhesion to biomaterial surfaces. *Journal of Biomedical Materials Research*, **43**, 338–348.
16. Marshall, G.W., Balooch, M., Kinney, J.H. & Marshall, S.J. (1995) Atomic-force microscopy of conditioning agents on dentin. *Journal of Biomedical Materials Research*, **29**, 1381–1387.
17. Habelitz, S., Balooch, M., Marshall, S.J., Balooch, G. & Marshall, G.W. Jr. (2002) In situ atomic force microscopy of partially demineralized human

dentin collagen fibrils. *Journal of Structural Biology*, **138**, 227–236.

18. Kishen, A., Sum, C.P., Mathew, S. & Lim, C.T. (2008) Influence of irrigation regimens on the adherence of Enterococcus faecalis to root canal dentin. *Journal of Endodontics*, **34**, 850–854.

19. Basrani, B.R., Manek, S., Sodhi, R.N.S., Fillery, E. & Manzur, A. (2007) Interaction between sodium hypochlorite and chlorhexidine gluconate. *Journal of Endodontics*, **33**, 966–969.

20. Waltimo, T., Brunner, T.J., Vollenweider, M., Stark, W.J. & Zehnder, M. (2007) Antimicrobial effect of nanometric bioactive glass 45S5. *Journal of Dental Research*, **86**, 754–757.

21. Waltimo, T., Mohn, D., Paque, F. *et al.* (2009) Fine-tuning of bioactive glass for root canal disinfection. *Journal of Dental Research*, **88**, 235–238.

22. Shrestha, A., Shi, Z., Neoh, K.G. & Kishen, A. (2010) Nanoparticulates for antibiofilm treatment and effect of aging on its antibacterial activity. *Journal of Endodontics*, **36**, 1030–1035.

23. Shrestha, A. & Kishen, A. (2012) The effect of tissue inhibitors on the antibacterial activity of chitosan nanoparticles and photodynamic therapy. *Journal of Endodontics*, **38**, 1275–1278.

24. Mortazavi, V., Nahrkhalaji, M.M., Fathi, M.H., Mousavi, S.B. & Esfahani, B.N. (2010) Antibacterial effects of sol–gel-derived bioactive glass nanoparticle on aerobic bacteria. *Journal of Biomedical Materials Research. Part A*, **94**, 160–168.

25. Chogle, S.M., Duhaime, C.F., Mickel, A.K. *et al.* (2011) Preliminary evaluation of a novel polymer nanocomposite as a root-end filling material. *International Endodontic Journal*, **44**, 1055–1060.

26. Pagonis, T.C., Chen, J., Fontana, C.R. *et al.* (2010) Nanoparticle-based endodontic antimicrobial photodynamic therapy. *Journal of Endodontics*, **36**, 322–328.

27. Rabea, E.I., Badawy, M.E., Stevens, C.V., Smagghe, G. & Steurbaut, W. (2003) Chitosan as antimicrobial agent: applications and mode of action. *Biomacromolecules*, **4**, 1457–1465.

28. Wang, C.S., Arnold, R.R., Trope, M. & Teixeira, F.B. (2007) Clinical efficiency of 2% chlorhexidine gel in reducing intracanal bacteria. *Journal of Endodontics*, **33**, 1283–1289.

29. Buck, R.A., Eleazer, P.D., Staat, R.H. & Scheetz, J.P. (2001) Effectiveness of three endodontic irrigants at various tubular depths in human dentin. *Journal of Endodontics*, **27**, 206–208.

30. Stoor, P., Soderling, E. & Salonen, J.I. (1998) Antibacterial effects of a bioactive glass paste on oral microorganisms. *Acta Odontologica Scandinavica*, **56**, 161–165.

31. Gubler, M., Brunner, T.J., Zehnder, M., Waltimo, T., Sener, B. & Stark, W.J. (2008) Do bioactive glasses convey a disinfecting mechanism beyond a mere increase in pH? *International Endodontic Journal*, **41**, 670–678.

32. Zehnder, M., Luder, H.U., Schatzle, M., Kerosuo, E. & Waltimo, T. (2006) A comparative study on the disinfection potentials of bioactive glass S53P4 and calcium hydroxide in contra-lateral human premolars ex vivo. *International Endodontic Journal*, **39**, 952–958.

33. Zehnder, M., Soderling, E., Salonen, J. & Waltimo, T. (2004) Preliminary evaluation of bioactive glass S53P4 as an endodontic medication in vitro. *Journal of Endodontics*, **30**, 220–224.

34. Mohn, D., Bruhin, C., Luechinger, N.A., Stark, W.J., Imfeld, T. & Zehnder, M. (2010) Composites made of flame-sprayed bioactive glass 45S5 and polymers: bioactivity and immediate sealing properties. *International Endodontic Journal*, **43**, 1037–1046.

35. Dai, T., Huang, Y.Y. & Hamblin, M.R. (2009) Photodynamic therapy for localized infections—state of the art. *Photodiagnosis and Photodynamic Therapy*, **6**, 170–188.

36. Moan, J. & Berg, K. (1991) The photodegradation of porphyrins in cells can be used to estimate the lifetime of singlet oxygen. *Photochemistry and Photobiology*, **53**, 549–553.

37. Menezes, S., Capella, M.A.M. & Caldas, L.R. (1990) Photodynamic-action of methylene-blue – repair and mutation in Escherichia-Coli. *Journal of Photochemistry and Photobiology B*, **5**, 505–517.

38. Bertoloni, G., Lauro, F.M., Cortella, G. & Merchat, M. (2000) Photosensitizing activity of hematoporphyrin on Staphylococcus aureus cells. *Biochimica et Biophysica Acta - General Subjects*, **1475**, 169–174.

39. Wakayama, Y., Takagi, M. & Yano, K. (1980) Photosensitized inactivation of E. coli cells in toluidine blue-light system. *Photochemistry and Photobiology*, **32**, 601–605.

40. Komerik, N., Wilson, M. & Poole, S. (2000) The effect of photodynamic action on two virulence factors of gram-negative bacteria. *Photochemistry and Photobiology*, **72**, 676–680.

41. George, S. & Kishen, A. (2008) Influence of photosensitizer solvent on the mechanisms of photoactivated killing of Enterococcus faecalis. *Photochemistry and Photobiology*, **84**, 734–740.

42. Meire, M.A., De Prijck, K., Coenye, T., Nelis, H.J. & De Moor, R.J.G. (2009) Effectiveness of different laser systems to kill Enterococcus faecalis in aqueous suspension and in an infected tooth model. *International Endodontic Journal*, **42**, 351–359.

43. George, S. & Kishen, A. (2007) Photophysical, photochemical, and photobiological characterization of methylene blue formulations for light-activated root canal disinfection. *Journal of Biomedical Optics*, **12**, 034029.

44. George, S. & Kishen, A. (2008) Augmenting the antibiofilm efficacy of advanced noninvasive light activated disinfection with emulsified oxidizer and oxygen carrier. *Journal of Endodontics*, **34**, 1119–1123.

45. Soukos, N.S., Chen, P.S., Morris, J.T. *et al.* (2006) Photodynamic therapy for endodontic disinfection. *Journal of Endodontics*, **32**, 979–984.

46. Williams, J.A., Pearson, G.J. & Colles, M.J. (2006) Antibacterial action of photoactivated disinfection {PAD} used on endodontic bacteria in planktonic suspension and in artificial and human root canals. *Journal of Dentistry*, **34**, 363–371.

47. Soukos, N.S., Wilson, M., Burns, T. & Speight, P.M. (1996) Photodynamic effects of toluidine blue on human oral keratinocytes and fibroblasts and Streptococcus sanguis evaluated in vitro. *Lasers in Surgery and Medicine*, **18**, 253–259.

48. Soncin, M., Fabris, C., Busetti, A. *et al.* (2002) Approaches to selectivity in the Zn(II)-phthalocyanine-photosensitized inactivation of wild-type and antibiotic-resistant Staphylococcus aureus. *Photochemical and Photobiological Sciences*, **1**, 815–819.

49. George, S. & Kishen, A. (2007) Advanced noninvasive light-activated disinfection: assessment of cytotoxicity on fibroblast versus antimicrobial activity against Enterococcus faecalis. *Journal of Endodontics*, **33**, 599–602.

50. Gross, S., Brandis, A., Chen, L. *et al.* (1997) Protein-A-mediated targeting of Bacteriochlorophyll-IgG to Staphylococcus aureus: a model for enhanced site-specific photocytotoxicity. *Photochemistry and Photobiology*, **66**, 872–878.

51. Soukos, N.S., Hamblin, M.R. & Hasan, T. (1997) The effect of charge on cellular uptake and phototoxicity of polylysine chlorin(e6) conjugates. *Photochemistry and Photobiology*, **65**, 723–729.

52. Shrestha, A. & Kishen, A. (2011) Polycationic chitosan conjugated photosensitizer for antibacterial photodynamic therapy (dagger). *Photochemistry and Photobiology*, **83 (3)**, 577–583.

53. Shrestha, A., Hamblin, M.R. & Kishen, A. (2012) Characterization of a conjugate between Rose Bengal and chitosan for targeted antibiofilm and tissue stabilization effects as a potential treatment of infected dentin. *Antimicrobial Agents and Chemotherapy*, **56**, 4876–4884.

54. Portenier, I., Haapasalo, H., Orstavik, D., Yamauchi, M. & Haapasalo, M. (2002) Inactivation of the antibacterial activity of iodine potassium iodide and chlorhexidine digluconate against Enterococcus faecalis by dentin, dentin matrix, type-I collagen, and heat-killed microbial whole cells. *Journal of Endodontics*, **28**, 634–637.

55. Foschi, F., Fontana, C.R., Ruggiero, K. *et al.* (2007) Photodynamic inactivation of Enterococcus faecalis in dental root canals in vitro. *Lasers in Surgery and Medicine*, **39**, 782–787.

56. Prasad, P.N. (2003) *Introduction to Biophotonics*. John Wiley & Sons, Hoboken, NJ.

57. Bonsor, S.J., Nichol, R., Reid, T.M. & Pearson, G.J. (2006) Microbiological evaluation of photo-activated disinfection in endodontics (an in vivo study). *British Dental Journal*, **200**, 337–341, discussion 329.

58. Bonsor, S.J., Nichol, R., Reid, T.M.S. & Pearson, G.J. (2006) An alternative regimen for root canal disinfection. *British Dental Journal*, **201**, 101–105.

59. Garcez, A.S., Nunez, S.C., Hamblin, M.R. & Ribeiro, M.S. (2008) Antimicrobial effects of photodynamic therapy on patients with necrotic pulps and periapical lesion. *Journal of Endodontics*, **34**, 138–142.

60. Garcez, A.S., Nunez, S.C., Hamblim, M.R., Suzuki, H. & Ribeiro, M.S. (2010) Photodynamic therapy associated with conventional endodontic treatment in patients with antibiotic-resistant microflora: a preliminary report. *Journal of Endodontics*, **36**, 1463–1466.

61. Wainwright, M. & Giddens, R.M. (2003) Phenothiazinium photosensitisers: choices in synthesis and application. *Dyes and Pigments*, **57**, 245–257.

62. Miserendino, L.J. & Pick, R.M. (1995) *Lasers in Dentistry*. Quintessence Publishing, Hanover Park, IL.

63. Moshonov, J., Orstavik, D., Yamauchi, S., Pettiette, M. & Trope, M. (1995) Nd:YAG laser irradiation in root canal disinfection. *Endodontics and Dental Traumatology*, **11**, 220–224.

64. Schoop, U., Kluger, W., Moritz, A., Nedjelik, N., Georgopoulos, A. & Sperr, W. (2004) Bactericidal effect of different laser systems in the deep layers of dentin. *Lasers in Surgery and Medicine*, **35**, 111–116.

65. Rooney, J., Midda, M. & Leeming, J. (1994) A laboratory investigation of the bactericidal effect of a NdYAG laser. *British Dental Journal*, **176**, 61–64.

66. Bergmans, L., Moisiadis, P., Teughels, W., Van Meerbeek, B., Quirynen, M. & Lambrechts, P. (2006) Bactericidal effect of Nd:YAG laser irradiation on some endodontic pathogens ex vivo. *International Endodontic Journal*, **39**, 547–557.

67. Wang, Q.Q., Zhang, C.F. & Yin, X.Z. (2007) Evaluation of the bactericidal effect of Er,Cr:YSGG, and Nd:YAG lasers in experimentally infected root canals. *Journal of Endodontics*, **33**, 830–832.

68. Cheng, X., Guan, S., Lu, H. *et al.* (2012) Evaluation of the bactericidal effect of Nd:YAG, Er:YAG, Er,Cr:YSGG laser radiation, and antimicrobial photodynamic therapy (APDT) in experimentally infected root canals. *Lasers in Surgery and Medicine,* **44**, 824–831.

69. Goodis, H.E., Pashley, D. & Stabholz, A. (2002) Pulpal effects of thermal and mechanical irritant. In: Seltzer & Benderís (eds), *Dental Pulp.* Quintessence Publishing, Hanover Park, IL, pp. 371–410.

70. Stabholz, A., Zeltser, R., Sela, M. *et al.* (2003) The use of lasers in dentistry: principles of operation and clinical applications. *Compendium of Continuing Education in Dentistry,* **24**, 935–948.

71. George, R. & Walsh, L.J. (2011) Performance assessment of novel side firing safe tips for endodontic applications. *Journal of Biomedical Optics,* **16**, 048004.

72. Noiri, Y., Katsumoto, T., Azakami, H. & Ebisu, S. (2008) Effects of Er:YAG laser irradiation on biofilm-forming bacteria associated with endodontic pathogens in vitro. *Journal of Endodontics,* **34**, 826–829.

73. Yavari, H.R., Rahimi, S., Shahi, S. *et al.* (2010) Effect of Er, Cr: YSGG laser irradiation on Enterococcus faecalis in infected root canals. *Photomedicine and Laser Surgery,* **28 (Suppl. 1)**, S91–S96.

74. Meire, M.A., Coenye, T., Nelis, H.J. & De Moor, R.J. (2012) Evaluation of Nd:YAG and Er:YAG irradiation, antibacterial photodynamic therapy and sodium hypochlorite treatment on Enterococcus faecalis biofilms. *International Endodontic Journal,* **45**, 482–491.

75. Fried, D., Glena, R.E., Featherstone, J.D. & Seka, W. (1995) Nature of light scattering in dental enamel and dentin at visible and near-infrared wavelengths. *Applied Optics,* **34**, 1278–1285.

76. Moriyama, E.H., Zangaro, R.A., Villaverde, A.B. *et al.* (2004) Dentin evaluation after Nd:YAG laser irradiation using short and long pulses. *Journal of Clinical Laser Medicine & Surgery,* **22**, 43–50.

77. Armon, E. & Laufer, G. (1995) Analysis to determine the beam parameters which yield the most extensive cut with the least secondary damage. *Journal of Biomechanical Engineering,* **107**, 286–290.

78. van Leeuwen, T.G., Jansen, E.D., Motamedi, M., Borst, C. & Welch, A.J. (1995) Pulsed laser ablation of soft tissue. In: Welch, A.J. & van Gemert, M.J.C. (eds), *Optical–Thermal Response of Laser-Irradiated Tissue.* Plenum Press, New York.

79. Marchesan, M.A., Brugnera, A., Souza-Gabriel, A.E., Correa-Silva, S.R. & Sousa-Neto, M.D. (2008) Ultrastructural analysis of root canal dentine irradiated with 980-nm diode laser energy at different parameters. *Photomedicine and Laser Surgery,* **26**, 235–240.

80. Gurbuz, T., Ozdemir, Y., Kara, N., Zehir, C. & Kurudirek, M. (2008) Evaluation of root canal dentin after Nd:YAG laser irradiation and treatment with five different irrigation solutions: a preliminary study. *Journal of Endodontics,* **34**, 318–321.

81. Yamazaki, R., Goya, C., Yu, D.G., Kimura, Y. & Matsumoto, K. (2001) Effects of erbium, chromium:YSGG laser irradiation on root canal walls: a scanning electron microscopic and thermographic study. *Journal of Endodontics,* **27**, 9–12.

82. Dostalova, T., Jelinkova, H., Housova, D. *et al.* (2002) Endodontic treatment with application of Er:YAG laser waveguide radiation disinfection. *Journal of Clinical Laser Medicine and Surgery,* **20**, 135–139.

83. Leonardo, M.R., Guillen-Carias, M.G., Pecora, J.D., Ito, I.Y. & Silva, L.A.B. (2005) Er:YAG laser: antimicrobial effects in the root canals of dogs' teeth with pulp necrosis and chronic periapical lesions. *Photomedicine and Laser Surgery,* **23**, 295–299.

84. Kimura, Y., Tanabe, M., Imai, H., Amano, Y., Masuda, Y. & Yamada, Y. (2011) Histological examination of experimentally infected root canals after preparation by Er:YAG laser irradiation. *Lasers in Medical Science,* **26**, 749–754.

85. Blanken, J., De Moor, R.J., Meire, M. & Verdaasdonk, R. (2009) Laser induced explosive vapor and cavitation resulting in effective irrigation of the root canal. Part 1: a visualization study. *Lasers in Surgery and Medicine,* **41**, 514–519.

86. De Moor, R.J., Blanken, J., Meire, M. & Verdaasdonk, R. (2009) Laser induced explosive vapor and cavitation resulting in effective irrigation of the root canal. Part 2: evaluation of the efficacy. *Lasers in Surgery and Medicine,* **41**, 520–523.

87. Restaino, L., Frampton, E.W., Hemphill, J.B. & Palnikar, P. (1995) Efficacy of ozonated water against various food-related microorganisms. *Applied and Environmental Microbiology,* **61**, 3471–3475.

88. Paraskeva, P. & Graham, N.J.D. (2002) Ozonation of municipal wastewater effluents. *Water Environment Research,* **74**, 569–581.

89. Nagayoshi, M., Kitamura, C., Fukuizumi, T., Nishihara, T. & Terashita, M. (2004) Antimicrobial effect of ozonated water on bacteria invading dentinal tubules. *Journal of Endodontics,* **30**, 778–781.

90. Arita, M., Nagayoshi, M., Fukuizumi, T. *et al.* (2005) Microbicidal efficacy of ozonated water against Candida albicans adhering to acrylic denture plates. *Oral Microbiology and Immunology,* **20**, 206–210.

91. Hems, R.S., Gulabivala, K., Ng, Y.L., Ready, D. & Spratt, D.A. (2005) An in vitro evaluation of the

ability of ozone to kill a strain of Enterococcus faecalis. *International Endodontic Journal*, **38**, 22–29.

92. Estrela, C., Estrela, C.R.A., Decurcio, D.A., Hollanda, A.C.B. & Silva, J.A. (2007) Antimicrobial efficacy of ozonated water, gaseous ozone, sodium hypochlorite and chlorhexidine in infected human root canals. *International Endodontic Journal*, **40**, 85–93.

93. Ebensberger, U., Pohl, Y. & Filippi, A. (2002) PCNA-expression of cementoblasts and fibroblasts on the root surface after extraoral rinsing for decontamination. *Dental Traumatology*, **18**, 262–266.

94. Noguchi, F., Kitamura, C., Nagayoshi, M., Chen, K.K., Terashita, M. & Nishihara, T. (2009) Ozonated water improves lipopolysaccharide-induced responses of an odontoblast-like cell line. *Journal of Endodontics*, **35**, 668–672.

95. Huth, K.C., Jakob, F.M., Saugel, B. *et al.* (2006) Effect of ozone on oral cells compared with established antimicrobials. *European Journal of Oral Sciences*, **114**, 435–440.

96. Viera, M.R., Guiamet, P.S., de Mele, M.F.L. & Videla, H.A. (1999) Use of dissolved ozone for controlling planktonic and sessile bacteria in industrial cooling systems. *International Biodeterioration & Biodegradation*, **44**, 201–207.

97. Kustarci, A., Sumer, Z., Altunbas, D. & Kosum, S. (2009) Bactericidal effect of KTP laser irradiation against Enterococcus faecalis compared with gaseous ozone: an ex vivo study. *Oral Surgery, Oral Medicine, Oral Pathology, Oral Radiology, and Endodontics*, **107**, e73–e79.

98. Silveira, A.M., Lopes, H.P., Siqueira, J.F. Jr., Macedo, S.B. & Consolaro, A. (2007) Periradicular repair after two-visit endodontic treatment using two different intracanal medications compared to single-visit endodontic treatment. *Brazilian Dental Journal*, **18**, 299–304.

99. Guinesi, A.S., Andolfatto, C., Bonetti Filho, I., Cardoso, A.A., Passaretti Filho, J. & Farac, R.V. (2011) Ozonized oils: a qualitative and quantitative analysis. *Brazilian Dental Journal*, **22**, 37–40.

100. Stoodley, P., Debeer, D. & Lewandowski, Z. (1994) Liquid flow in biofilm systems. *Applied and Environmental Microbiology*, **60**, 2711–2716.

101. Lawrence, J.R., Wolfaardt, G.M. & Korber, D.R. (1994) Determination of diffusion coefficients in biofilms by confocal laser microscopy. *Applied and Environmental Microbiology*, **60**, 1166–1173.

102. Azarpazhooh, A. & Limeback, H. (2008) The application of ozone in dentistry: a systematic review of literature. *Journal of Dentistry*, **36**, 104–116.

Part 3

Apical Response and Surgery

15

Healing of Apical Lesions: How Do They Heal, Why Does the Healing Take So Long, and Why Do Some Lesions Fail to Heal?

Zvi Metzger and Anda Kfir

Department of Endodontology, Tel Aviv University, Tel Aviv, Israel

Introduction

Apical lesions are radiolucent lesions that appear in the bone surrounding portals of exit from infected root canal systems. Because most lesions of this type occur in the apical area, and for the convenience of the reader, the term *apical lesion* is used in this chapter. Many but not all apical lesions will heal in response to adequate debridement, disinfection, and obturation of the root canal. Such healing may be a prolonged process, and some lesions will fail to heal. To understand why the healing process is often prolonged and why some lesions fail to heal, the nature of these lesions and the processes leading to their development must be understood. Because the healing of apical lesions occurs via the regrowth of bone into the area, an understanding of the osteogenic signals that lead to and control the apposition of new bone is also important.

Some apical lesions fail to respond to intracanal endodontic treatment. However, many of them will heal after subsequent apical surgery has been applied. The reasons for such failures are discussed in an attempt to understand why apical surgery does lead to healing in many cases that originally failed to heal. This discussion is extended beyond the simple concept of a retrograde approach to the root canal system, to include the eradication of extraradicular infection and the removal of cystic formations and other factors, the elimination of which may represent additional factors contributing to the success of apical surgical intervention.

What is the apical lesion?

A protective host response with a price tag

Apical lesions represent a protective activity of the host response that is successful most of the time. Nevertheless, this protection has a price tag, which is destruction of the surrounding apical bone. Bone destruction is one of the primary indicative signs of an apical lesion. The gradual disappearance of the bone defect that was caused by this destructive response is commonly used as a major clinical sign and tool to monitor the healing of these lesions (1–6).

Disinfection of Root Canal Systems: The Treatment of Apical Periodontitis, First Edition. Edited by Nestor Cohenca.
© 2014 John Wiley & Sons, Inc. Published 2014 by John Wiley & Sons, Inc.

The protective response

The apical lesion represents a successful attempt of the host to prevent highly pathogenic bacteria present in the infected root canal from spreading into the adjacent bone and to other more remote places in the body (Figure 15.1). Some bacterial species that are often found in the apical part of the infected root canals, such as *Porphyromonas gingivalis*, *Fusobacterium nucleatum*, and *Prevotella nigrescens*, are extremely pathogenic (7, 8). Some strains of *P. gingivalis* can kill a mouse into which they are injected within 24 h (8), while other strains may cause severe spreading abscesses at the site of injection (7, 8). Furthermore, cooperation between strains of *F. nucleatum* and *P. gingivalis* in the form of coaggregation (9) may make these strains 1000 times more pathogenic than each one alone (10). Osteomyelitis of the maxilla or the mandible is extremely rare. The protective mechanisms in the apical lesion are highly effective and contain the hazardous bacteria within the lesion in most cases. Occasional failures may occur, resulting in the development of an acute abscess.

The host response to bacteria is mediated by several processes: (i) the effective recruitment of polymorphonuclear granulocyte neutrophils (PMNs) to the site of bacterial penetration; (ii) effective opsonization with both specific immunoglobulin G (IgG) (11) and the complement component C3b; and (iii) effective phagocytosis of the bacteria, followed by intracellular killing by oxidative mechanisms. The host response in the apical lesion may be viewed as a complex mechanism for the recruitment of PMNs to the site at which the bacteria emerge from the root canal and for assisting the PMNs in effective phagocytosis of these bacteria (Figure 15.1) (12–14).

Prolonged exposure of the host to bacteria residing in the infected root canal is likely to result in the production of specific immunoglobulins against these bacteria. IgG specific to root canal bacteria have been found in human apical lesions (15–17). Although these specific IgGs may come from the systemic sensitization of the host, local production of such IgGs by plasma cells present in human apical lesions has also been reported by Baumgartner and Falkler (18) (Figure 15.1). Thus, bacteria emerging from the root canal are likely to encounter specific IgGs that attach to their surfaces. Such

attachment will in turn activate the complement system, resulting in the generation of three signals: (i) the C3b elements of the complement system will attach to the surface of the bacteria and, together with the already attached IgG, will serve as effective opsonization mediators that permit subsequent phagocytosis by PMNs; (ii) the C3a and C5a complement components will cause the degranulation of local mast cells, which will release vasoactive amines; these released agents will cause the increased permeability of blood vessels in the area, in turn resulting in an increased supply of complement and specific IgG in the area; and (iii) C5a molecules will serve as a chemotactic signal for

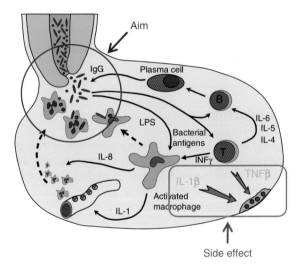

Figure 15.1   Host response in apical granuloma. The aim of the host response is to kill bacteria emerging from the infected root canal. To serve this aim, specific IgGs are required. These IgGs may be produced locally by activation of B-lymphocytes, which then become plasma cells secreting the IgG. This process requires prior local activation of antigen-specific T-lymphocytes. Activated lymphocytes produce an array of cytokines, some of which are required for B-lymphocyte activation and maturation to plasma cells. Gamma-interferon is another T-lymphocyte-derived cytokine that activates local macrophages and causes them to produce IL-1, which in turn induces the expression of attachment molecules on local endothelial cells. This causes PMNs to attach to the local endothelium, making them available for recruitment by chemotaxis to the site where bacteria emerge. Two of the cytokines produced by locally activated lymphocytes and macrophages, TNFβ and IL-1β, are the primary signals that induce local osteoclastic bone resorption. Such bone resorption may be viewed as a destructive side effect of the local activity of the host response.

PMNs, directing them from the vicinity of the local blood vessels to the site of bacterial penetration.

PMNs normally circulate in the bloodstream and must be "told" where to exit the blood vessels so they can reach the invading bacteria. Interleukin-1 (IL-1), which is produced by activated macrophages in the apical lesion (19–21), serves as such a signal (Figure 15.1). When capillary endothelial cells are exposed to IL-1, they express attachment molecules such as ICAM-1 (inter cellular adhesion molecule-1) on their surfaces (22–25). PMNs in the blood bind to these attachment molecules and thus become concentrated and "marginated" in the area in which they are required. Guided by the concentration gradient of C5a molecules, the PMNs migrate into the tissue and move in the direction of the bacteria in a process known as *directed chemotactic movement*. It is important to note that PMNs are not resident cells of the apical tissue. Every PMN observed in a histological section of the tissue has been "captured" during the process of such chemotactic migration (13).

Once PMNs reach the bacteria, specific receptors for C3b and for the Fc portion of IgG allow the PMN to attach to opsonized bacteria that carry this dual signal on their surfaces. The PMN then internalize the bacteria through a process of phagocytosis, followed by the oxidative killing of the bacteria within the PMN.

Macrophage activation is essential for the local production of IL-1. Such activation is mediated by the cytokine gamma-interferon (γ-INF), which is produced by activated T-lymphocytes within the lesion (26–31) (Figure 15.1). The activation of T-lymphocytes is antigen-specific. Bacteria emerging from the root canal are phagocytized by antigen-presenting cells in the lesion, which process their specific antigens and present them to antigen-specific T-lymphocytes. This antigen presentation signal, together with IL-1, which is also produced by the antigen-presenting cells, causes the T-lymphocytes to become activated and produce many cytokines, one of which is γ INF, which is essential in turn for the activation of the macrophages. Other cytokines produced by the activated T-Lymphocytes such as IL-4, IL-5, and IL-6 are essential for the proliferation of antigen-specific B-lymphocytes and their maturation to plasma cells that will produce the antigen-specific IgG (Figure 15.1).

Thus, the apical lesion may be viewed as a complex mechanism that is designed to facilitate and support a single primary target: the phagocytosis and killing of bacteria by PMNs (13).

Development of apical lesions

The body's response to the bacteria emerging from the apical foramen is initiated in the adjacent periodontal ligament in the form of apical periodontitis. This response, which is aimed at containing and killing the bacteria, also causes local damage to the host in the form of bone resorption (Figure 15.1). Among the cytokines that are produced by the cells of the apical inflammatory response, IL-1β and tumor necrosis factor β (TNF β) have the capacity to activate local osteoclastic bone resorption. The first (IL-1β) is produced mainly by activated macrophages, while the second (TNF β) is a product of activated T-lymphocytes.

IL-1β and TNF β are the primary causes of the local apical bone resorption (32). When lining cells of the bone are exposed to these cytokines, they express on their surfaces a signaling molecule, the receptor activator of nuclear factor kappa β-ligand (RANKL) (33–38). This ligand engages the RANK receptor, which is present on the surface of the neighboring preosteoclasts and osteoclasts, thus causing the maturation of preosteoclasts into mature osteoclasts and the activation of existing osteoclasts, which express ruffled borders and begin the bone resorbing actively (39–44).

The resulting local bone resorption is first radiographically expressed as a widening of the apical periodontal space; this space gradually increases, eventually resulting in a radiolucent lesion in the apical bone, that is, an apical lesion.

Apical bone resorption may thus be considered a side effect of the protective host response (Figure 15.1). The activation of an effective host response that is aimed at eliminating harmful bacteria results in the local production of cytokines that cause resorption of the surrounding bone (12, 13).

Granuloma versus abscess

Lesions of apical periodontitis usually contain inflammatory tissue in which lymphocytes, macrophages, and the resident cells of

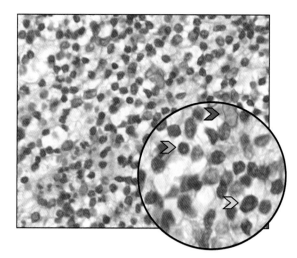

Figure 15.2   Apical granuloma. Histological section of an apical granuloma. Green arrow: Lymphocyte. Yellow arrow: Macrophage. Blue arrow: Fibroblast.

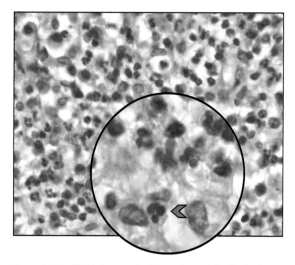

Figure 15.3   PMNs in an apical granuloma. Histological section of an apical granuloma. Blue arrow: PMN.

the periodontium, fibroblasts, are the dominant cells (Figure 15.2) (12, 45–49). Inflammatory lesions with such constituents are termed *granulomas*. Varying numbers of PMNs (Figure 15.3) may be found in granulomatous lesions, mainly adjacent to the apical foramen. It should be kept in mind that while lymphocytes, macrophages, and fibroblasts are long-lived cells, PMNs are not.

Any PMN observed in a lesion of apical periodontitis is recruited from the bloodstream and is

in the process of migrating to the site of bacterial penetration, guided by chemotactic signals that consist of C5a components of the complement system. Every such PMN will die a preprogrammed death within 24–48 h of leaving the bloodstream (50).

When PMNs die, the proteolytic enzymes contained within them are released. These enzymes attack and damage or destroy the collagen and hyaluronic acid components of the connective tissue matrix (51). As long as the number of PMNs reaching the apical site per day is limited, the damage to the tissue is effectively repaired by local macrophages. The macrophages phagocytize the damaged tissue components and the remains of dead bacteria released from the PMN, thus performing a "cleanup" function. The macrophages also signal the fibroblasts to form new collagen and hyaluronic acid, resulting in the repair of the damage caused by the enzymes released from the dead PMNs. Conversely, if excessive numbers of PMNs reach the site, massive proteolysis of tissue components may occur, which is beyond the "cleanup" and repair capacity of the macrophages in the area. Under such conditions, local liquefaction of the tissue occurs and pus forms (13).

The appearance of an abscess within a granuloma may be viewed as the result of a disturbance of the equilibrium between the damage caused by the released PMN enzymes and the cleanup and repair capacity of the macrophages (12, 13). Because the number of macrophages in the lesion is more or less stable, any event that results in massive recruitment of PMNs is likely to induce an abscess within the granuloma. Such an event may be transient in nature, such as accidental pushing of bacteria into the apical lesion by an endodontic file. In such a case, the abscess will eventually subside, and with time, the macrophages will remove the damaged tissue and induce repair by fibroblasts. In other cases, there may be a persistent and continuous influx of large numbers of PMNs. This can occur when bacteria that have phagocytosis-evading mechanisms (7, 52–55) or bacteria that collaborate with other bacteria to form aggregates or biofilms (10, 56–59) are present in the root canal (see below). In such cases, the continuous influx of PMNs will result in continuous and persistent formation of pus and in the development of a chronic abscess with a permanently draining sinus tract.

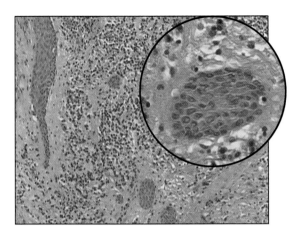

Figure 15.4 Epithelial proliferation in an apical granuloma. Strands of epithelium in an apical granuloma. Some strands were cut longitudinally; others were cut diagonally, giving the impression of isolated isles.

Apical granulomas often contain epithelial elements originating from the rests of Malassez (60) (Figure 15.4). This epithelium may proliferate in response to root canal infection (20, 21, 61–65) or overinstrumentation and filling beyond the apex of the tooth (66). Such proliferation may eventually lead to development into cystic formations (see below).

The lumen of such cystic formations may or may not be infected, and they may be either bay (pseudo) cysts or true cysts (62, 67) (see below).

How does an apical lesion heal?

Basic concepts of osteogenesis

Bone formation in the apical area, as well as elsewhere in the body, is dependent on the activity of osteoblasts, the bone-forming cells. Osteoblasts originate as mesenchymal stem cells in the bone marrow (Figure 15.5). Under the influence of bone morphogenic proteins (BMPs), these stem cells are induced to differentiate and give rise to spindle-shaped osteoprogenitor cells. Growth factors such as transforming growth factor β (TGFβ), fibroblast-derived growth factor (FGF), BMPs, platelet-derived growth factor (PDGF), and colony-stimulating factor (CSF) can induce and/or increase the proliferation of and are chemotactic to osteoprogenitor cells (68). Osteoprogenitor cells

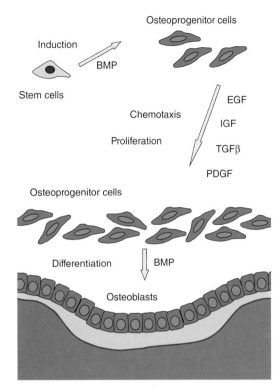

Figure 15.5 Apposition of new bone. Osteoprogenitor cells are required for the formation of new osteoblasts and new bone. Osteoprogenitor cells originate as bone marrow mesenchymal stem cells that are induced by BMPs to become osteoprogenitor cells. Certain growth factors, including epidermal growth factor (EGF), insulin-like growth factor (IGF), TGFβ, and PDGF, are chemotactic to the osteoprogenitor cells and cause them to proliferate. Consequently, spindle-shaped osteoprogenitor cells accumulate next to the future site of bone apposition. BMPs cause the final differentiation of the osteoprogenitor cells into cuboidal, metabolically active osteoblasts that line the bone surface and produce osteoid (shown in pink) that will later mineralize and turn into bone (shown in purple).

may accumulate at a future site of bone formation by local proliferation, by the chemotactic attraction of osteoprogenitor cells from adjacent sites, or both processes (68) (Figure 15.5).

BMPs induce the final differentiation of the osteoprogenitor cells into cuboidal, metabolically active osteoblasts that line the bone surface and begin the process of bone apposition (68). The osteoblasts secrete collagen and BMPs as well as several growth factors and form the osteoid that will eventually mineralize and form bone. When osteoid apposition is completed, the osteoblasts differentiate into flat lining cells that cover the new bone.

Sources of osteogenic factors in the apical lesion

The tissues of the apical lesion and the surrounding bone are rich sources of the cells and signals required for the generation of active osteoblasts. Osteoprogenitor cells are found in the bone marrow, from which they can be attracted by chemotactic signals (68). Osteoprogenitor cells were also demonstrated to be present within the apical granulomas (69). Macrophages, which are abundant in apical granulomas, are a rich source of signals such as TGFβ, FGF, PDGF, and CSF, which are required for the recruitment and proliferation of osteoprogenitor cells. Platelets in blood clots formed after apical surgery are a particularly rich source of PDGF. BMPs, which are required for the final maturation of osteoblasts, are released locally from the resorbing bone matrix and are produced by neighboring osteoblasts (68). Thus, the apical granuloma and its surrounding bone are rich sources of components that together represent substantial osteogenic potential.

The remodeling process

Bone apposition is not a continuous process. The initially formed bone will eventually be resorbed and replaced by new bone formations in cycles of a process known as *bone remodeling*. Evidence for such resorption–apposition cycles can later be seen in the bone in the form of apposition lines (Figure 15.6a). Thus, one may envision the process of bone healing in the apical lesion as involving repeated cycles of apposition and remodeling. Such process is schematically illustrated in Figure 15.6b,c.

Healing of the apical lesion

The persistence of an apical lesion and its size are likely to be an expression of the local balance between the osteoclastic activity within the lesion and the osteogenic potential that surrounds it (Figure 15.7). The bacteria emerging from the

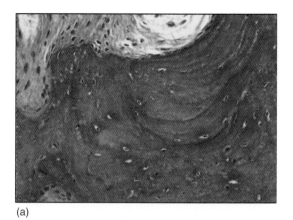
(a)

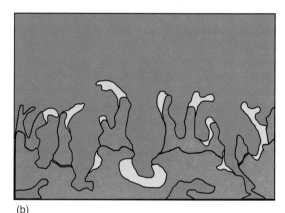
(b)

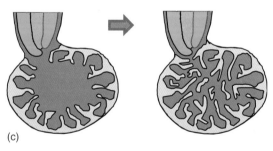
(c)

Figure 15.6 Bone remodeling. The process of bone formation occurs in cycles of formation and resorption that determine the final bone structure. (a) Reversal lines in bone representing cycles of resorption and apposition within the bone. (Reproduced with permission of Prof. Miron Weinreb, Tel Aviv University.) (b) Schematic presentation of the formation of bone trabeculae. Pink: Recently formed bone. Purple: Older calcified bone, with resting lines representing older bone resorption and apposition cycles. (Adopted from Aanan *et al.* (70). Reproduced with permission of Lippincott Williams & Wilkins.) (c) Schematic representation of bone formation in an apical lesion.

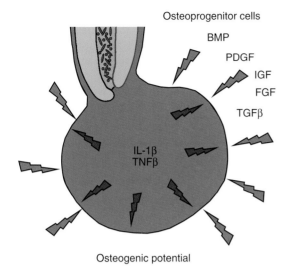

Osteoprogenitor cells

BMP

PDGF

IGF

FGF

TGFβ

IL-1β
TNFβ

Osteogenic potential

Figure 15.7 Osteoclastic versus osteogenic potential in an apical granuloma. The cytokines TNFβ and IL-1β, which are produced by activated T-lymphocytes and activated macrophages in the lesion, serve as the primary main signals that induce osteoclastic bone resorption in an apical granuloma. The surrounding bone is a rich source of osteoprogenitor cells that, together with locally produced EGF, IGF, TGFβ, PDGF, and BMPs, provide osteoblastic potential. Once bacteria are eliminated from the root canal, gradual yet slow reduction of the local production of TNFβ and IL-1β occurs, and the osteogenic potential begins to dominate, causing healing of the lesion by new bone apposition.

infected root canal provide a stimulus for activation of T-lymphocytes and macrophages thus maintaining the osteoclastic signals in the lesion. When these bacteria have been eliminated by root canal treatment and the canal has been properly sealed, this stimulus ceases to exist, and with time, the response to the bacteria subsides. The osteoclastic activity, initiated by IL-1β and TNFβ, will then diminish, and the surrounding osteogenic potential will take over (Figure 15.7). The gradual apposition of new bone, followed by its remodeling and further cycles of apposition, will eventually result in the healing of the bone defect that was initially caused by the response to the bacteria, and the apical lesion will heal (Figure 15.6c).

How long does it take the lesion to heal?

Several large-scale follow-up studies indicate that 74–85% of apical lesions heal within 48 months (1, 2, 4–6).

Ørstavik's study (1) found that 85% of such lesions healed within 48 months. Of the lesions that eventually healed, only 50% were healed or in a process of healing at 6 months after treatment, namely 42.5% of the total number of lesions that were studied (50% of 85%). At 12 months, 88% of the lesions that eventually healed were healed or in the process of healing, namely 75% of the total number of lesions (88% of 85%) (1).

Thus, healing of an apical lesion is a rather prolonged process. If a cavity of similar size is surgically formed in the bone, healing occurs much more rapidly (71).

Why does healing often take so long?

Macrophage activation

Activated macrophages and activated lymphocytes are the primary sources of IL-1β and TNFβ cytokines, which represent the main osteoclast-stimulating activity in the apical lesion (32) (Figure 15.1). Animal studies have shown that macrophage activation that is induced, for example, by the subcutaneous injection of streptococcal cell walls may persist for a very long period of time (72).

A potential explanation for the extended time required for apical lesions to heal may be the persistence of an activated state of macrophages and lymphocytes within the lesion. Such an activated state may outlive its biological purpose as a pivotal element of the host's defensive response in the area of the lesion (12, 13). As long as such activation persists and these cytokines are produced, the osteoclastic potential of the lesion persists, keeping the vast surrounding osteogenic potential at bay. When the osteoclastic activity subsides, the lesion finally heals (12, 13).

Potential pharmacological intervention sites

A better understanding of the processes that are involved in the production and effects of the bone-resorbing cytokines may in the future permit pharmacological intervention in the balance between osteoclastic and osteogenic activities in the apical lesion and make it possible to favorably affect the kinetics of the healing process. Several potential targets for such pharmacological intervention are the local production and release of cytokines that induce osteoclastic activity (27, 73–76), the receptors for these cytokines on local target cells (77) and the bone-resorbing activity of the osteoclasts themselves (12, 13).

The effect of apical debridement

Another approach to enhancing the kinetics of the healing of apical lesions is the mechanical removal of the granuloma. A study by Kvist and Reit (71) compared the healing of apical lesions after retreatment and after apical surgery. The apical surgery used in that study did not include retrograde filling. Although healing after 48 months was similar in the two groups, healing after 12 months was substantially greater in the group in which the apical lesions were surgically removed (71).

A more recent study applied a microinvasive method to remove the bulk of the tissues from apical lesions with no open-flap surgery (78, 79) (see below). When the apical tissue was removed and allowed to be replaced by a blood clot that, in turn, developed into fresh, "uncommitted" granulation tissue, the healing kinetics were substantially enhanced (see below).

Taken together, these two studies support the idea that residual activated cells of the apical tissue remaining in the bony crypt of the lesion after the elimination of the bacteria from the root canal are the likely cause of the extremely long time that bony defects of this type sometimes require to heal (13).

Why do some lesions fail to heal?

Residual infection within the root canal system

Residual infection in the root canal system is commonly perceived as the reason for the failure of apical lesions to heal. It is indeed the most common reason, but it is not the only one, as discussed below.

The root canal system often includes components that are inaccessible to intracanal debridement and disinfection. Lateral canals, delta-like ramifications of the canal, and fin-like recesses of the main canal are among such inaccessible components. The ramifications of the canal are more common in the apical part of the canal; cutting off the tip of the root during apical surgery is expected to eliminate this part of the root canal system, along with the infection that it contains (80).

Radiographic image versus the 3D reality of the root canal

The challenge of oval canals

An apical lesion that fails to heal in spite of adequate root canal treatment is often perceived as an enigma; in the radiograph, good quality root filling of the desired length, adequate enlargement of the canal, and well-condensed filling are observed. Nevertheless, the apical lesion fails to heal and, in some cases, is even symptomatic.

One of the common reasons for such presentation is an oval canal that is treated as if it were a canal with a round cross-section. Oval canals are rather common; 25% of roots contain an oval canal (81). In certain teeth, the presence of an oval canal is the rule, and such a canal is present in up to 90% of all cases (81). The oval cross-section of the canal is not seen on a regular apical radiograph, because the flatness of the canal is in the bucco-lingual direction, which is parallel to the X-ray beam. Consequently, oval canals may be incorrectly identified by the operator as simple round canals and treated as such (82). When a minimal access cavity is prepared and rotary files are used for canal preparation, it is easy to finish a case that will look satisfactory in the apical radiograph but nevertheless contains uninstrumented buccal and/or lingual recesses in which infected debris remains (Figure 15.8a,b) (82). Such debris-containing recesses also represent a weak link in the obturation of the canal because no root filling system will be able to adequately fill a recess in which debris remains (83–85).

Isthmuses between two canals in the same root provide another example of often-inaccessible areas of the root canal that may contain infected debris (Figure 15.8c,d). Recent studies indicate that the use of rotary files further complicates this problem by actively packing such isthmuses with

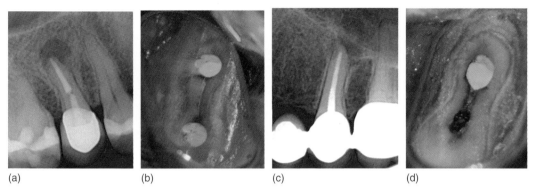

(a)   (b)   (c)   (d)

Figure 15.8   Inadequate preparation and obturation of root canal systems. (a) The radiograph shows an apparently good root canal filling. Nevertheless, the case was failing. (Metzger *et al.* (82), Figure 20a. Reproduced with permission of Quintessence.) (b) Apical surgery revealed an uninstrumented isthmus that was likely to contain infected material. (Metzger *et al.* (82), Figure 20b. Reproduced with permission of Quintessence.) (c) The radiograph shows an apparently good root canal filling. Nevertheless, the case was failing. (Metzger *et al.* (82), Figure 20c. Reproduced with permission of Quintessence.) (d) Apical surgery revealed that the case, which was treated as if it had a single, round canal, had a long oval flat canal, the buccal side of which was not instrumented and contained infected material that caused the case to fail. (Metzger *et al.* (82), Figure 20a. Reproduced with permission of Quintessence.)

dentin chips (86–88) that cannot be completely removed from the isthmus even using passive ultrasonic irrigation (87).

Inadequate cleaning and obturation of the root canal is often discovered during apical surgery (Figure 15.8). Sealing the canal by retrograde filling may isolate the residual infection from the apical tissues and allow the lesion to heal (80, 89).

Cystic apical lesion

Cystic formations within the apical lesion may also prevent healing (90, 91). Radiographs alone do not permit differentiation between cystic and noncystic lesions (92–94). Recently, it has been shown that methods such as ultrasound real-time imaging (95), ultrasound (96), and cone-beam computed tomography scanning (97) may make it possible to distinguish between apical granulomas and apical cysts.

Apical granulomas often contain proliferating epithelium originating from the epithelial rests of Malassez (60, 66, 98) (Figure 15.4). The epithelial rests of Malassez are stable cells and possess the potential to undergo cell division if appropriate extracellular mitogenic signals are present to stimulate their entry into the cell cycle (99).

Two types of cysts may develop in the lesion: a bay (pocket) cyst, the lumen of which is continuous with the space of the infected root canal, and a true cyst that is completely enclosed by lining epithelium and may or may not be attached to the root apex by a cord of epithelium (62, 97).

Only serial histological sectioning of lesions removed *in toto* can correctly differentiate between the two types of cysts, resulting in a discrepancy in the reported incidence of apical cysts, which varies from 6% to 55% (62). Nair *et al.* (62) histologically examined 256 apical lesions and found that 9% of them contained apical true cysts while 6% of them contained apical pocket cysts.

In apical pocket cysts, the irritants are in the canal and can usually be eliminated by nonsurgical endodontic procedures. Epithelial cell proliferation in the apical tissues may then subside by the elimination of inflammatory mediators, proinflammatory cytokines, and growth factors. Epithelial cell apoptosis may also be induced by positive extracellular signals such as Fas-L, TNF, or by the removal of survival factors (100). However, in apical true cysts, in addition to intracanal irritants that triggered its formation, other irritants such as cholesterol (Figure 15.9) or possibly unidentified antigens (90, 101, 102) may be present within the cyst. These agents cannot be removed and are not affected by root canal treatment and will continuously sustain the inflammatory stimulation of the cystic epithelium.

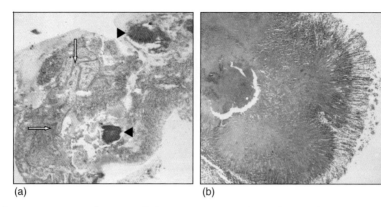

(a)   (b)

Figure 15.9 Apical actinomycosis. A refractory endodontic case. (a) Apical granuloma with cystic formation (thin arrows) and aggregates ("granules") of *Actinomyces* organisms. (b) Magnification of an aggregate of *Actinomyces* organisms resembling "rays" on its surface. Bacteria in such aggregates are protected from the host response. Continued recruitment of large amounts of PMNs to the area caused persistent pus formation and a sinus tract that persisted after root canal treatment and was the reason for the surgical removal of this sample. (Hirshberg *et al.* (103). Reproduced with permission of Mosby, Inc.)

Cystic lesions that fail to respond to conventional endodontic treatment may also be the cause of a nonhealing apical lesion. Because irritants in apical true cysts cannot be eliminated by nonsurgical endodontic procedures, an apical true cyst must be treated surgically (62, 67, 90, 104).

Extraradicular infection: aggregates

An extraradicular infection that does not respond to conventional endodontic treatment has been associated with certain types of bacteria such as *Actinomyces israelli* and *Rothia* spp. (105, 106). In such cases, bacterial cohesive colonies that have become established extraradicularly in the form of "granules" have been found in the apical tissue (Figure 15.10). The cohesive colony protects the bacteria within it from phagocytosis by PMNs and allows these bacteria to survive in the tissue in spite of the continuous attack by PMNs. Consequently, they are able to perpetuate the inflammation even after meticulous root canal treatment (105–109, 103) (Figure 15.10).

The coaggregation of different bacterial strains has also been studied as a potential way by which bacteria may avoid phagocytosis. Animal studies involving the coinoculation of *F. nucleatum* strains and *P. gingivalis* strains showed that when injected in combination, the bacteria could survive in the host tissues, while neither of the strains survived when injected individually (10, 58, 59, 110, 111),

Bacterial granules were present in the puss of the resulting lesions (110).

When coaggregating strains of *F. nucleatum* and *P. gingivalis* were coinoculated into a subcutaneous chamber, in another study (10), the minimal infective dose (MID_{100}) could be reduced by 1000-fold compared to inoculating each bacterium separately (10).

It is likely that the aggregation or coaggregation of bacteria serves as a phagocytosis-evading mechanism that allows bacteria to survive in the apical lesion independent of the infection in the root canal, thus preventing the healing of the lesions. Such bacteria may survive despite the continuous massive recruitment of PMNs into the area, resulting in persistent pus formation that is clinically expressed as a persistent sinus tract. Surgical removal of the apical tissue is likely to remove such bacterial aggregates and allow healing of the lesion.

Extraradicular infection: biofilm

In some cases that failed to respond to conventional root canal treatment, bacterial biofilms were found to be attached to the outer surface of the root within the apical lesion (57, 106, 112) (Figure 15.11). Such biofilms were initially reported by Tronstad *et al.* (106) and by Siqueira and Lopes (112). Noguchi *et al.* (57) studied the bacterial content of such biofilms on the outer surfaces of 14 root tips that were removed during the apical surgery

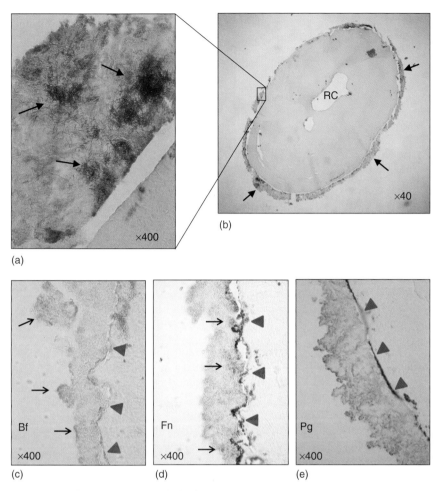

Figure 15.10 Extraradicular infection in the form of a biofilm. (a) Gram-negative rods and filamentous microorganisms located in an extraradicular biofilm on the outer surface of a root that was surgically removed in a case of refractory apical lesion. (b) Section of an apical part of the root. RC: root canal. The arrows indicate a 30–40 μm thick bacterial biofilm on the outer surface of the root. The square indicates the area which is magnified in "a". (c) Frozen section with immunohistochemical staining for *T. forsythensis* (Tf), revealing that this bacterium was located mainly in the surface layers of the extraradicular biofilm. (d) Frozen section with immunohistochemical staining for *F. nucleatum* (Fn), revealing that this bacterium was located mainly in the inner layers of the extraradicular biofilm. (e) Frozen section with immunohistochemical staining for *P. gingivalis* (Pg), revealing that this bacterium was evenly distributed in the extraradicular biofilm. Brown triangles in "c", "d", and "e" indicate the surface of the radicular dentin. (Courtesy of Prof. Yuichiro Noiri, Osaka University, Osaka, Japan.)

performed in these refractory cases. They found organized biofilms that were 30–40 μm thick and contained *F. nucleatum* (14 of 14 samples), *P. gingivalis* (12 of 14 samples), and *Tannellera forsythensis* (8 of 14 samples), as well as other bacteria. In these biofilms, *P. gingivalis* was immunohistochemically detected in all parts of the extraradicular biofilms, while *F. nucleatum* was located mainly in the middle layer, and *T. forsythensis* was located mainly in the outer layer of the biofilm (Figure 15.11c).

Such extraradicular biofilms may also represent an effective mechanism by which bacteria may evade phagocytosis, which in turn may allow their persistent survival in the presence of a continuous flow of PMNs. Such a frustrated attempt of the host response to eradicate these bacteria is often expressed as continuous pus draining from a sinus tract.

Extraradicular biofilms most likely originate from infection in the root canal; however, once

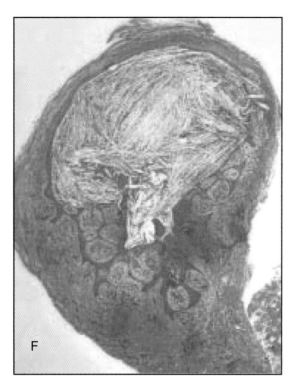

F

Figure 15.11 (a–c) Cholesterol crystals. Apical cyst filled with cholesterol crystals that appear as "clefts" in the histological section. ((a–c) Lin *et al.* (126). Reproduced with permission of Lippincott, Williams, and Wilkins.)

formed, they are not likely to respond to conventional root canal treatment. Surgical intervention during which the root tip is removed is likely to eliminate such extraradicular biofilms and allow healing.

Extraradicular foreign materials

Extraradicular foreign materials have been reported as another cause of the persistence of apical lesions (113, 114). Such foreign materials may include materials used in root canal treatment, such as minute contaminated particles of gutta-percha (115, 116), cellulose particles originating from paper points and cotton wool that were extruded into the apical tissues (113, 117), especially when associated with trauma to the apical tissue (118), and endodontic sealants and calcium salts derived from apically extruded $Ca(OH)_2$ (114). Another possible source of foreign material is food that is pushed into

a root canal that is left open during treatment, as in a case in which leguminous seeds (pulses) were found in an apical granuloma that did not respond to treatment (119, 120). The presence of such foreign materials that are extruded during root canal treatment may keep the macrophages in the apical lesion in a perpetually activated state, thus preventing the healing of the lesion.

Of particular interest are infected dentin particles and debris originating from the walls of a necrotic and infected root canal. Such particles may be extruded into the apical lesion through overinstrumentation during root canal treatment. In this situation, microorganisms within the dentinal tubules of the dentin particles may be protected from the host defense mechanisms and can survive within the apical lesion, thus maintaining apical inflammation, as reported by Yusuf (121).

Such apical extrusion of debris should be considered not only in the context of potential flare-ups and postoperative symptoms but also as a potential contributing factor to the prevention of healing of apical lesions (121, 122). The extent of apical extrusion of debris by different file systems has recently been studied and compared and it seems that the recently introduced reciprocating files have a greater tendency to extrude debris apically than traditional rotary multifile systems (122).

Apical surgery will remove the tissue of the apical lesion, along with any foreign material contained within it, thus allowing the healing of the lesion.

Apical debridement with no open surgery

The importance of the abovementioned factors in preventing the healing of apical lesions or in delaying such healing was recently demonstrated in a study in which apical debridement was performed during primary endodontic treatment with no open-flap surgery and no removal of the root tip (79).

Surgically treated apical lesions show enhanced healing kinetics compared with lesions that are treated nonsurgically (71). This enhancement is commonly attributed to the removal of the root tip and to the sealing of the root canal by the retrograde filling. Nevertheless, surgical removal of the apical, chronically inflamed tissue may also be an important factor. Such procedure may remove any extraradicular factors that cause the osteoclastic potential to persist while allowing a fresh blood clot to form, thereby converting a chronic inflammatory lesion into new "noncommitted" granulation tissue in which healing is likely to proceed much more rapidly (12, 13).

The Apexum procedure and what it demonstrates

The Apexum procedure was designed as a complementary treatment for teeth with infected root canals and apical lesions (78, 79). Debridement and disinfection of the root canal was first accomplished, as in any endodontic treatment, using conventional cleaning and shaping procedures. Then, a device made of nickel–titanium wire (Apexum NiTi Ablator, Apexum Ltd., Or-Yehuda, Israel) (Figure 15.12a, left) was inserted through the apical foramen and into the apical lesion (79) (Figure 15.12b). The soft tissue content of the lesion was then minced by rotating the Apexum NiTi Ablator device at 300 rpm for 30 s. This was followed by the use of a second device (Apexum PGA Ablator) (Figure 15.12a, right) made of a polyglycolic acid fiber, which was rotated in the lesion at 3000 rpm for 30 s, thus turning the soft tissue of the lesion into a thin suspension (79). The resulting suspension was washed out with sterile saline solution, while the backflow passively drained through the root canal. The root canal was then filled using gutta-percha and AH-26, with lateral compaction (79) (Figure 15.12c).

This debridement process removed the bulk of the apical tissue and allowed a fresh blood clot to form. All of this was accomplished with no opening of the flap and no resection of the root tip.

Follow-up radiography showed that after 6 months, 95% of the lesions had healed or were in advanced stages of healing, while only 39% of the lesions were at such stages in a control group (79) (Figure 15.13). This result represents a major improvement in both the kinetics of healing and in the healing rate of apical lesions compared with those of the control group within the study and with the previously reported healing rates and healing kinetics (1) (Figure 15.13).

The observed enhancement of the healing process (Figure 15.12c,d) likely resulted from the removal of one or more of the following factors by this minimally invasive procedure: (i) the bulk of tissue containing activated macrophages and lymphocytes; (ii) epithelial cystic formations; (iii) extraradicular infection in the form of coaggregates

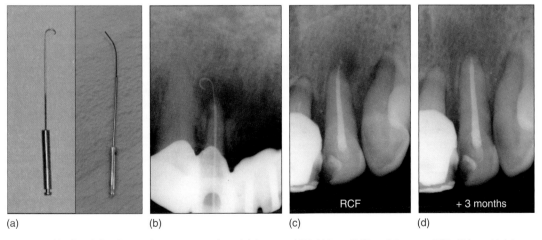

(a)   (b)   (c)   (d)

Figure 15.12   Healing following an Apexum procedure. (a) Apexum NiTi Ablator (left) and Apexum PGA Ablator (right). (b) Apexum NiTi Ablator inserted into an apical lesion. (c, d) The Apexum procedure was applied after the completion of conventional cleaning and shaping. The procedure removed the major bulk of the apical tissue by homogenizing it and washing it out through the root canal. (c) Root canal filling after completion of the procedure. (d) Advanced healing of the lesion after 3 months. ((a–d) Metzger et al. (79). Reproduced with permission of Lippincott, Williams & Wilkins)

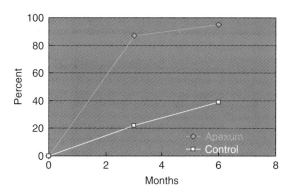

Figure 15.13　Healing after apical debridement by the Apexum procedure. Healing of lesions in the control group, which received conventional root canal treatment alone, reached 39% at 6 months, a value that is consistent with the results of published large-scale surveys (1). In the Apexum-treated group, the percent of lesions showing complete or advanced healing was 87% and 95% at 3 and 6 months, respectively. The difference in the healing rate can be attributed to the (i) removal of activated lymphocytes and macrophages and (ii) removal of other factors that may interfere with the healing of the lesion, such as extraradicular infection, epithelial and cystic formations, and foreign materials extruded apically while cleaning and shaping the root canal. (Metzger et al. (79). Reproduced with permission of Lippincott, Williams & Wilkins.)

in the tissue or biofilm on the outer root surface; and (iv) any foreign material that may have been extruded apically.

No removal of the root tip was involved, and curetting of all tissue from the surface of the bony crypt was not attempted. Nevertheless, a substantial change in the healing kinetics was observed. Thus, the removal of the apical tissue and allowing a fresh blood clot to organize into a new "uncommitted" granulation tissue may alone enhance apical healing. This finding, in turn, provides support for the concept expressed above that factors within the lesion other than and in addition to actual residual infection within the root canal system may play a role in slowing down (12, 13) or preventing the healing of apical lesions (123, 124).

Conclusions

The healing rate of apical lesions in response to conventional endodontic treatment is at best approximately 80%, and such healing shows rather

slow kinetics and may take many months to occur. In cases that fail to heal, apical surgery may be called for; it has a high success rate and often results also in faster healing kinetics.

Apical surgery usually consists of three separate processes: (i) removal of the soft tissue of the apical lesion; (ii) removal of the root tip that is present within the lesion; and (iii) retrograde root canal treatment and filling. The last process is usually the focus of attention of the operator; the first two processes are often looked on as a means of reaching the goal of sealing the root canal system with a retrograde filling.

Studies in which debridement alone was performed with no retrograde filling resulted in apical healing with faster kinetics and higher healing rates than expected with conventional root canal treatment (79), providing support for the idea that the removal of factors other than the persistent infection in the root canal may also play an important role in the high success rate achieved using apical surgery (80, 89, 125).

References

1. Ørstavik, D. (1996) Time-course and risk analyses of the development and healing of chronic apical periodontitis in man. *International Endodontic Journal*, **29**, 150–155.
2. Hoskinson, S.E., Ng, Y.-L., Hoskinson, A.E., Moles, D.R. & Gulabivala, K. (2002) A retrospective comparison of outcome or root canal treatment using two different protocols. *Oral Surgery, Oral Medicine, Oral Pathology, Oral Radiology, and Endodontics*, **93**, 705–715.
3. Friedman, S. (2002) Prognosis of initial endodontic therapy. *Endodontic Topics*, **2**, 59–88.
4. Ørstavik, D., Qvist, V. & Stoltze, K. (2004) A multivariate analysis of the outcome of endodontic treatment. *European Journal of Oral Sciences*, **112**, 224–230.
5. de Chevigny, C., Dao, T.T., Basrani, B. *et al.* (2008) Treatment outcome in endodontics: the Toronto study- phase 4: initial treatment. *Journal of Endodontics*, **34**, 258–263.
6. Siqueira, J.F. Jr., Rôças, I.N., Riche, F.N.S.J. & Provenzano, J.C. (2008) Clinical outcome of the endodontic treatment of teeth with apical periodontitis using an antimicrobial protocol. *Oral Surgery, Oral Medicine, Oral Pathology, Oral Radiology, and Endodontics*, **106**, 757–762.

7. Sundqvist, G., Figdor, D., Hanstrom, L., Sorlin, S. & Sandstrom, G. (1991) Phagocytosis and virulence of different strains of *Porphyromonas gingivalis*. *Scandinavian Journal of Dental Research*, **99**, 117–129.

8. Genco, C.A., Cutler, C.W., Kapczynski, D., Maloney, K. & Arnold, R.R. (1991) A novel mouse model to study the virulence of and host response to *Porphyromonas (Bacteroides) gingivalis*. *Infection and Immunity*, **59**, 1255–1263.

9. Kolenbrander, P.E. & Andersen, R.N. (1989) Inhibition of coaggregation between *Fusobacterium nucleatum* and *Porphyromonas (Bacteroides) gingivalis* by lactose and related sugars. *Infection and Immunity*, **57**, 3204–3209.

10. Metzger, Z., Lin, Y., DiMeo, F., Ambrose, W., Trope, M. & Arnold, R.R. (2009) Synergistic pathogenicity of *Porphyromonas gingivalis* and *Fusobacterium nucleatum* in the mouse subcutaneous chamber model. *Journal of Endodontics*, **35**, 86–94.

11. Cutler, C.W., Kalmar, J.R. & Arnold, R.R. (1991) Phagocytosis of virulent *Porphyromonas gingivalis* by human polymorphonuclear leukocytes requires specific immunoglobulin G. *Infection and Immunity*, **59**, 2097–2104.

12. Metzger, Z. (2000) Macrophages in periapical lesions. *Endodontics and Dental Traumatology*, **16**, 1–8.

13. Metzger, Z. & Abramovitz, I. (2009) Periapical lesions of endodontic origin. In: Ingle, J.I., Bakland, L.K. & Baumgartner, J.C. (eds), *Ingle's Endodontics*, 6 edn. BC Decker, Hamilton, ON, Canada, pp. 494–519.

14. Metzger, Z., Abramovitz, I. & Bergenholtz, G. (2009) Apical periodontitis. In: Bergenholtz, G., Horsted-Bindslev, P. & Reit, C. (eds), *Textbook of Endodontology*, 2 edn. Wiley-Blackwell Munksgaard, Chichester, UK, pp. 113–127.

15. Baumgartner, J.C. & Falkler, W.A. Jr. (1991) Detection of immunoglobulins from explant cultures of periapical lesions. *Journal of Endodontics*, **17**, 105–110.

16. Baumgartner, J.C. & Falkler, W.A. Jr. (1991) Reactivity of IgG from explant cultures of periapical lesions with implicated microorganisms. *Journal of Endodontics*, **17**, 207–212.

17. Kettering, J.D., Torabinejad, M. & Jones, S.L. (1991) Specificity of antibodies present in human periapical lesions. *Journal of Endodontics*, **17**, 213–216.

18. Baumgartner, J.C. & Falkler, W.A. Jr. (1991) Biosynthesis of IgG in periapical lesion explant cultures. *Journal of Endodontics*, **17**, 143–146.

19. Artese, L., Piattelli, A., Quaranta, M., Colasante, A. & Musani, P. (1991) Immunoreactivity for interleukin 1-beta and tumor necrosis factor-alpha and ultrastructural features of monocytes/macrophages in periapical granulomas. *Journal of Endodontics*, **17**, 483–487.

20. Tani-Ishii, N., Wang, C.Y. & Stashenko, P. (1995) Immunolocalization of bone-resorptive cytokines in rat pulp and periapical lesions following surgical pulp exposure. *Oral Microbiology and Immunology*, **10**, 213–219.

21. Hamachi, T., Anan, H., Akamine, A., Fujise, O. & Maeda, K. (1995) Detection of interleukin-1 beta mRNA in rat periapical lesions. *Journal of Endodontics*, **21**, 118–121.

22. Lane, T.A., Lamkin, G.E. & Wancewicz, E.V. (1990) Protein kinase C inhibitors block the enhanced expression of intercellular adhesion molecule-1 on endothelial cells activated by interleukin-1, lipopolysaccharide and tumor necrosis factor. *Biochemical and Biophysical Research Communications*, **172**, 1273–1281.

23. Luscinskas, F.W., Cybulsky, M.I., Kiely, J.M., Peckins, C.S., Davis, V.M. & Gimbrone, M.A. Jr. (1991) Cytokine-activated human endothelial monolayers support enhanced neutrophil transmigration via a mechanism involving both endothelial-leukocyte adhesion molecule-1 and intercellular adhesion molecule-1. *Journal of Immunology*, **146**, 1617–1625.

24. Issekutz, A.C., Rowter, D. & Springer, T.A. (1999) Role of ICAM-1 and ICAM-2 and alternate CD11/CD18 ligands in neutrophil transendothelial migration. *Journal of Leukocyte Biology*, **65**, 117–126.

25. Kabashima, H., Nagata, K., Maeda, K. & Iijima, T. (2002) Involvement of substance P, mast cells, TNF-alpha and ICAM-1 in the infiltration of inflammatory cells in human periapical granulomas. *Journal of Oral Pathology & Medicine*, **31**, 175–180.

26. Dinarello, C.A. (1988) Interleukin-1. *Annals of the New York Academy of Sciences*, **546**, 122–132.

27. Politis, A.D., Sivo, J., Driggers, P.H., Ozato, K. & Vogel, S.N. (1992) Modulation of interferon consensus sequence binding protein mRNA in murine peritoneal macrophages. Induction by IFN-gamma and down-regulation by IFN-alpha, dexamethasone, and protein kinase inhibitors. *Journal of Immunology*, **148**, 801–887.

28. Alshwaimi, E., Purcell, P., Kawai, T. *et al.* (2009) Regulatory T cells in mouse periapical lesions. *Journal of Endodontics*, **35**, 1229–1233.

29. Colić, M., Gazivoda, D., Vucevic, D., Vasilijic, S., Rudolf, R. & Lukic, A. (2009) Proinflammatory and immunoregulatory mechanisms in periapical lesions. *Molecular Immunology*, **47**, 101–113.

30. Colić, M., Gazivoda, D., Vucević, D. *et al.* (2009) Regulatory T-cells in periapical lesions. *Journal of Dental Research*, **88**, 997–1002.

31. Fukada, S.Y., Silva, T.A., Garlet, G.P., Rosa, A.L., da Silva, J.S. & Cunha, F.Q. (2009) Factors involved in the T helper type 1 and type 2 cell commitment and osteoclast regulation in inflammatory apical diseases. *Oral Microbiology and Immunology*, **24**, 25–31.

32. Wang, C.Y. & Stashenko, P. (1993) Characterization of bone-resorbing activity in human periapical lesions. *Journal of Endodontics*, **19**, 107–111.

33. Lacey, D.L., Timms, E., Tan, H.L., Kelley, M.J., Dunstan, C.R. & Burgess, T. (1998) Osteoprotegerin ligand is a cytokine that regulates osteoclast differentiation and activation. *Cell*, **93**, 165–176.

34. Suda, T., Takahashi, N., Udagawa, N., Jimi, E., Gillespie, M.T. & Martin, T.J. (1999) Modulation of osteoclast differentiation and function by the new members of the tumor necrosis factor receptor and ligand families. *Endocrine Reviews*, **20**, 345–357.

35. Hofbauer, L.C., Khosla, S., Dunstan, C.R., Lacey, D.L., Boyle, W.J. & Riggs, B.L. (2000) The roles of osteoprotegerin and osteoprotegerin ligand in the paracrine regulation of bone resorption. *Journal of Bone and Mineral Research*, **15**, 2–12.

36. Teitelbaum, S.L. (2000) Bone resorption by osteoclasts. *Science*, **289**, 1504–1508.

37. Hofbauer, L.C. & Heufelder, A.E. (2001) Role of receptor activator of nuclear factor-kappa B ligand and osteoprotegerin in bone cell biology. *Journal of Molecular Medicine*, **79**, 243–253.

38. Hofbauer, L.C., Kuhne, C.A. & Viereck, V. (2004) The OPG/RANKL/RANK system in metabolic bone diseases. *Journal of Musculoskeletal and Neuronal Interactions*, **4**, 268–275.

39. Zhang, X. & Peng, B. (2005) Immunolocalization of receptor activator of NF kappa B ligand in rat periapical lesions. *Journal of Endodontics*, **31**, 574–577.

40. Sabeti, M., Simon, J., Kermani, V. & Rostein, I. (2005) Detection of receptor activator of NF-κ β ligand in apical periodontitis. *Journal of Endodontics*, **31**, 17–18.

41. Vernal, R., Dezerega, A., Dutzan, N., Chaparro, A., Leon, R. & Chandia, S. (2006) RANKL in human periapical granuloma: possible involvement in periapical bone destruction. *Oral Diseases*, **12**, 283–289.

42. Kawashima, N., Suzuki, N., Yang, G. *et al.* (2007) Kinetics of RANKL, RANK and OPG expressions in experimentally induced rat periapical lesions. *Oral Surgery, Oral Medicine, Oral Pathology, Oral Radiology, and Endodontics*, **103**, 707–711.

43. Menezes, R., Garlet, T.P., Letra, A. *et al.* (2008) Differential patterns of receptor activator of nuclear factor kappa B ligand/osteoprotegerin expression in human periapical granulomas: possible association with progressive or stable nature of the lesions. *Journal of Endodontics*, **34**, 932–938.

44. Graves, D.T., Oates, T. & Garlet, G.P. (2011) Review of osteoimmunology and the host response in endodontic and periodontal lesions. *Journal of Oral Microbiology*, **3**, 5304. doi:10.3402/jom.v3i0.5304

45. Kopp, W. & Schwarting, R. (1989) Differentiation of T lymphocyte subpopulations, macrophages, and HLA-DR-restricted cells of apical granulation tissue. *Journal of Endodontics*, **15**, 72–75.

46. Piattelli, A., Artese, L., Rosini, S., Quaranta, M. & Musiani, P. (1991) Immune cells in periapical granuloma: morphological and immunohistochemical characterization. *Journal of Endodontics*, **17**, 26–29.

47. Matsuo, T., Ebisu, S., Shimabukuro, Y., Ohtake, T. & Okada, H. (1992) Quantitative analysis of immunocompetent cells in human periapical lesions: correlations with clinical findings of the involved teeth. *Journal of Endodontics*, **18**, 497–500.

48. Marton, I.J. & Kiss, C. (1993) Characterization of inflammatory cell infiltrate in dental periapical lesions. *International Endodontic Journal*, **26**, 131–136.

49. Kawashima, N., Okiji, T., Kosaka, T. & Suda, H. (1996) Kinetics of macrophages and lymphoid cells during the development of experimentally induced periapical lesions in rat molars: a quantitative immunohistochemical study. *Journal of Endodontics*, **22**, 311–316.

50. Savill, J.S., Wyllie, A.H., Henson, J.E. *et al.* (1989) Macrophage phagocytosis of aging neutrophils in inflammation. Programmed cell death in the neutrophil leads to its recognition by macrophages. *Journal of Clinical Investigation*, **3**, 865–875.

51. Cochrane, C.G. (1968) Immunologic tissue injury mediated by neutrophilic leukocytes. *Advances in Immunology*, **9**, 97–165.

52. Sundqvist, G.K., Carlsson, J., Herrmann, B.F., Hofling, J.F. & Vaatainen, A. (1984) Degradation in vivo of the C3 protein of guinea-pig complement by a pathogenic strain of *Bacteroides gingivalis*. *Scandinavian Journal of Dental Research*, **92**, 14–24.

53. Sundqvist, G., Carlsson, J., Herrmann, B. & Tarnvik, A. (1985) Degradation of human immunoglobulins G and M and complement factors C3 and C5 by black-pigmented *Bacteroides*. *Journal of Medical Microbiology*, **19**, 85–94.

54. Cutler, C.W., Arnold, R.R. & Schenkein, H.A. (1993) Inhibition of C3 and IgG proteolysis enhances phagocytosis of *Porphyromonas gingivalis*. *Journal of Immunology*, **151**, 7016–7029.

55. Jansen, H.J., van-der Hoeven, J., van-den Kieboom, C., Goertz, J.H., Camp, P.J. & Bakkeren, J.A. (1994) Degradation of immunoglobulin G by periodontal bacteria. *Oral Microbiology and Immunology*, **9**, 345–351.

56. Weiss, E.I., Shaniztki, B., Dotan, M., Ganeshkumar, N., Kolenbrander, P.E. & Metzger, Z. (2000) Attachment of *Fusobacterium nucleatum* PK1594 to mammalian cells and its coaggregation with periopathogenic bacteria are mediated by the same galactose-binding adhesion. *Oral Microbiology and Immunology*, **15**, 371–377.

57. Noguchi, N., Noiri, Y., Narimatsu, M. & Ebisu, S. (2005) Identification and localization of extraradicular biofilm-forming bacteria associated with refractory endodontic pathogens. *Applied and Environmental Microbiology*, **71**, 8738–8743.

58. Khemaleelakul, S., Baumgartner, J.C. & Pruksakom, S. (2006) Autoaggregation and coaggregation of bacteria associated with acute endodontic infections. *Journal of Endodontics*, **32**, 312–318.

59. Metzger, Z., Blasbalg, Y., Dotan, M. & Weiss, E.I. (2009) Characterization of coaggregation of *Fusobacterium nucleatum* PK1594 with six *Porphyromonas gingivalis* strains. *Journal of Endodontics*, **35**, 50–54.

60. Ten Cate, A.R. (1972) The epithelial cell rests of Malassez and the genesis of the dental cyst. *Oral Surgery, Oral Medicine, Oral Pathology, Oral Radiology, and Endodontics*, **34**, 956–964.

61. Bergenholtz, G., Lekholm, U., Liljenberg, B. & Lindhe, J. (1983) Morphometric analysis of chronic inflammatory periapical lesions in root filled teeth. *Oral Surgery, Oral Medicine, and Oral Pathology*, **55**, 295–301.

62. Nair, P.N., Pajarola, G. & Schroeder, H.E. (1996) Types and incidence of human periapical lesions obtained with extracted teeth. *Oral Surgery, Oral Medicine, Oral Pathology, Oral Radiology, and Endodontics*, **81**, 93–102.

63. Torabinejad, M. & Bakland, L. (1980) Prostaglandins: their possible role in the pathogenesis of pulpal and periapical disease. Part 2. *Journal of Endodontics*, **6**, 769–776.

64. Matsumoto, A., Anan, H. & Maeda, K. (1998) An immunohistochemical study of the behavior of cells expressing interleukin-1 and interleukin-1within experimentally induced periapical lesions in rats. *Journal of Endodontics*, **24**, 811–816.

65. Honma, M., Hayakawa, Y., Kosugi, H. & Koizumi, F. (1998) Localization of mRNA for inflammatory cytokines in radicular cyst tissue by in situ hybridization, and induction of inflammatory cytokines by human gingival fibroblasts in response to radicular cyst contents. *Journal of Oral Pathology and Medicine*, **27**, 399–404.

66. Seltzer, S., Bender, I.B., Smith, J., Freedman, I. & Nazimov, H. (1967) Endodontic failures – an analysis based on clinical, roentgenographic and histologic findings. Parts I and II. *Oral Surgery, Oral Medicine, and Oral Pathology*, **23**, 500–530.

67. Simon, J.H.S. (1980) Incidence of periapical cysts in relation to the root canal. *Journal of Endodontics*, **6**, 845–848.

68. Liberman, R., Daluiski, A. & Einhorn, T.A. (2002) The role of growth factors in the repair of bone. Biology and clinical applications. *Journal of Bone and Joint Surgery*, **84**, 1032–1044.

69. Maeda, H., Wada, N., Nakamuta, H. & Akamine, A. (2004) Human periapical granulation tissue contains osteogenic cells. *Cell and Tissue Research*, **315**, 203–208.

70. Lin, L.M., Ricucci, D. & Rosenberg, P.A. (2009) Nonsurgical root canal therapy of large cyst-like inflammatory apical lesions and inflammatory apical cysts. *Journal of Endodontics*, **35**, 607–615.

71. Kvist, T. & Reit, C. (1999) Results of endodontic retreatment: a randomized clinical study comparing surgical and nonsurgical procedures. *Journal of Endodontics*, **25**, 814–817.

72. Ginsburg, I. (1972) Mechanisms of cell and tissue injury induced by group A Streptococci: relation to poststreptococcal sequelae. *Journal of Infectious Diseases*, **126**, 294–340.

73. Schultz, R.M., Chirigos, M.A., Stoychkov, J.N. & Pavilidis, R.J. (1979) Factors affecting macrophage cytotoxic activity with particular emphasis on corticosteroids and acute stress. *Journal of the Reticuloendothelial Society*, **26**, 83–91.

74. Shapira, L., Barak, V., Soskolne, W.A., Halabi, A. & Stabholz, A. (1998) Effects of tetracyclines on the pathologic activity of endotoxin: in vitro and in vivo studies. *Advances in Dental Research*, **12**, 119–122.

75. Metzger, Z., Klein, H., Klein, A. & Tagger, M. (2002) Periapical lesion development in rats inhibited by dexamethasone. *Journal of Endodontics*, **28**, 643–645.

76. Metzger, Z., Belkin, D., Kariv, N., Dotan, M. & Kfir, A. (2008) Low-dose doxycycline inhibits development of periapical lesions in rats. *International Endodontic Journal*, **41**, 303–309.

77. Stashenko, P., Teles, R. & D'Souza, R. (1998) Periapical inflammatory responses and their modulation. *Critical Reviews in Oral Biology and Medicine*, **9**, 498–521.

78. Metzger, Z., Huber, R., Tobis, I. & Better, H. (2009) Enhancement of healing kinetics of periapical lesions in dogs by the Apexum procedure. *Journal of Endodontics*, **35**, 40–45.

79. Metzger, Z., Huber, R., Tobis, I. & Better, H. (2009) Healing kinetics of periapical lesions enhanced by the Apexum procedure: a clinical trial. *Journal of Endodontics*, **35**, 153–159.

80. Kim, S. & Kratchman, S. (2006) Modern endodontic surgery concepts and practice: a review. *Journal of Endodontics*, **32**, 601–623.

81. Wu, M.-K., R'oris, A., Barkis, D. & Wesselink, P.R. (2000) Prevalence and extent of long oval canals in the apical third. *Oral Surgery, Oral Medicine, Oral Pathology, Oral Radiology, and Endodontics*, **89**, 739–743.

82. Metzger, Z., Kfir, A., Abramovitz, I., Weissman, A. & Solomonov, M. (2013) *The Self-Adjusting File System*. ENDO, London, in press.

83. De-Deus, G., Gurgel-Filho, E.D., Magalhães, K.M. & Coutinho-Filho, T. (2006) A laboratory analysis of gutta-percha filled area obtained using thermafil, system B and lateral condensation. *International Endodontic Journal*, **39**, 378–383.

84. De-Deus, G., Reis, C., Beznos, D., Gruetzmacher-de-Abranches, A.M., Coutinho-Filho, T. & Pacionrik, S. (2008) Limited ability of three commonly used thermoplasticised gutta-percha techniques in filling oval-shaped canals. *Journal of Endodontics*, **34**, 1401–1405.

85. De-Deus, G., Barino, B., Marins, J., Magalhães, K., Thuanne, E. & Kfir, A. (2012) Self-Adjusting File cleaning-shaping-irrigation system optimizes the filling of oval-shaped canals with thermoplasticized gutta-percha. *Journal of Endodontics*, **38**, 846–849.

86. Paqué, F., Laib, A., Gautschi, H. & Zehnder, M. (2009) Hard-tissue debris accumulation analysis by high-resolution computed tomography scans. *Journal of Endodontics*, **35**, 1044–1047.

87. Paqué, F., Boessler, C. & Zehnder, M. (2011) Accumulated hard tissue debris levels in mesial roots of mandibular molars after sequential irrigation steps. *International Endodontic Journal*, **44**, 148–153.

88. Paqué, F., Al-Jadaa, A. & Kfir, A. (2012) Hard tissue debris accumulation caused by conventional rotary versus Self-Adjusting File instrumentation in mesial root canal systems of mandibular molars. *International Endodontic Journal*, **45**, 413–418.

89. Rubinstein, R.A. & Kim, S. (1999) Short-term observation of the results of endodontic surgery with the use of a surgical operation microscope and super-EBA as root-end filling material. *Journal of Endodontics*, **25**, 43–48.

90. Nair, P.N.R., Sjögren, U., Schumacher, E. & Sundqvist, G. (1993) Radicular cyst affecting a root-filled human tooth: a long-term post-treatment follow-up. *International Endodontic Journal*, **26**, 225–233.

91. Nair, P.N.R. (2003) Non-microbial etiology: periapical cysts sustain post-treatment apical periodontitis. *Endodontic Topics*, **6**, 114–134.

92. Bhaskar, S.N. (1966) Periapical lesion-types, incidence and clinical features. *Oral Surgery, Oral Medicine, and Oral Pathology*, **21**, 657–671.

93. Lalonde, E.R. (1970) A new rationale for the management of periapical granulomas and cysts, an evaluation of histopathological and radiographic findings. *Journal of the American Dental Association*, **80**, 1056–1059.

94. Mortensen, H., Winter, J.E. & Birn, H. (1970) Periapical granulomas and cysts. *Scandinavian Journal of Dental Research*, **78**, 241–250.

95. Cotti, E., Campisi, G., Ambu, R. & Dettori, C. (2003) Ultrasound real-time imaging in the differential diagnosis of periapical lesions. *International Endodontic Journal*, **36**, 556–563.

96. Gundappa, M., Ng, S.Y. & Whaites, E.J. (2006) Comparison of ultrasound, digital and conventional radiography in differentiating periapical lesions. *Dento Maxillo Facial Radiology*, **35**, 326–333.

97. Simon, J.H.S., Enciso, R., Malfaz, J.M., Roges, R., Bailey-Perry, M. & Patel, A. (2006) Differential diagnosis of large periapical lesions using cone-beam computed tomography measurements and biopsy. *Journal of Endodontics*, **32**, 833–837.

98. Harris, M. & Toller, P. (1975) The pathogenesis of dental cysts. *British Medical Bulletin*, **31**, 159–163.

99. D'Sousa, R. (2002) Development of the pulpodentin complex. In: Hargreaves, K.M. & Goodies, H.E. (eds), *Dental Pulp*. Quintessence Publishing Co, Inc., Chicago, IL.

100. Matsushime, H., Roussel, M.F., Ashmun, R.A. & Sherr, C.J. (1991) Colony-stimulating factor 1 regulates novel cyclins during the G1 phase of the cell cycle. *Cell*, **65**, 701–713.

101. Shear, M. (1985) Cysts of the jaw: recent advances. *Journal of Oral Pathology*, **14**, 43–59.

102. Trott, J.R., Chebib, F. & Galindo, Y. (1973) Factors related to cholesterol formation in cysts and granulomas. *Journal of Canadian Dental Association*, **38**, 76–78.

103. Hirshberg, A., Tsesis, I., Metzger, Z. & Kaplan, I. (2003) Periapical actinomycosis associated with radicular cysts – a clinicopathological study. *Oral Surgery, Oral Medicine, Oral Pathology, Oral Radiology, and Endodontics*, **95**, 600–620.

104. Nair, P.N.R., Sjögren, U. & Sundqvist, G. (1998) Cholesterol crystals as an etiological factor in non-resolving chronic inflammation: an experimental study in guinea pigs. *European Journal of Oral Sciences*, **106**, 644–650.

105. Sjogren, U., Happonen, R.P., Kahnberg, K.E. & Sundqvist, G. (1988) Survival of Arachnia propionica in periapical tissue. *International Endodontic Journal*, **21**, 277–282.

106. Tronstad, L., Barnett, F. & Cervone, F. (1990) Periapical bacterial plaque in teeth refractory to endodontic treatment. *Endodontics and Dental Traumatology*, **6**, 3–77.

107. Happonen, R.P., Soderling, E., Viander, M., Linko, K.L. & Pelliniemi, L.J. (1985) Immunocytochemical demonstration of *Actinomyces* species and *Arachnia propionica* in periapical infections. *Journal of Oral Pathology*, **14**, 405–413.

108. Happonen, R.P. (1986) Periapical actinomycosis: a follow-up study of 16 surgically treated cases. *Endodontics and Dental Traumatology*, **2**, 205–209.

109. Figdor, D., Sjögren, U., Sorlin, S., Sundqvist, G. & Nair, P.N.R. (1992) Pathogenicity of *Actinomyces israelii* and *Arachnia propionica*: experimental infection in guinea pigs and phagocytosis and intracellular killing by human polymorphonuclear leukocytes *in vitro*. *Oral Microbiology and Immunology*, **7**, 129–136.

110. Baumgartner, J.C., Falkler, W.J. & Beckerman, T. (1992) Experimentally induced infection by oral anaerobic microorganisms in a mouse model. *Oral Microbiology and Immunology*, **7**, 253–256.

111. Feuille, F., Ebersole, J.L., Kesavalu, L., Stepfen, M.J. & Holt, S.C. (1996) Mixed infection with *Porphyromonas gingivalis* and *Fusobacterium nucleatum* in a murine lesion model: potential synergistic effects on virulence. *Infection and Immunity*, **64**, 2094–2100.

112. Siqueira, J.F. Jr. & Lopes, H.P. (2001) Bacteria on the apical root surfaces of untreated teeth with periradicular lesions: a scanning electron microscopy study. *International Endodontic Journal*, **34**, 216–220.

113. Koppang, H.S., Koppang, R., Solheim, T., Aarnes, H. & Stolen, S.Ø. (1989) Cellulose fibers from endodontic paper points as an etiologic factor in postendodontic periapical granulomas and cysts. *Journal of Endodontics*, **15**, 369–372.

114. Koppang, H.S., Koppang, R. & Stolen, S.Ø. (1992) Identification of common foreign material in postendodontic granulomas and cysts. *Journal of the Dental Association of South Africa*, **47**, 210–216.

115. Kerekes, K. & Tronstad, L. (1979) Long-term results of endodontic treatment performed with standardized technique. *Journal of Endodontics*, **5**, 83–90.

116. Sjögren, U., Hägglund, B., Sundqvist, G. & Wing, K. (1990) Factors affecting the long-term results of endodontic treatment. *Journal of Endodontics*, **16**, 498–504.

117. Sedglev, C.M. & Messer, H. (1993) Long-term retention of a paper-point in the periapical tissues: a case report. *Endodontics and Dental Traumatology*, **9**, 120–123.

118. Saxen, L. & Myallarniemi, H. (1968) Foreign material postoperative adhesions. *New England Journal of Medicine*, **279**, 200–202.

119. King, O.H. Giant cell hyaline angiopathy: pulse granuloma by another name? *Presented at the 32nd Annual Meeting of the American Academy of Oral Pathologists*. Fort Lauderdale.

120. Simon, J.H.S., Chimenti, Z. & Mintz, G. (1982) Clinical significance of the pulse granuloma. *Journal of Endodontics*, **8**, 116–119.

121. Yusuf, H. (1982) The significance of the presence of foreign material periapically as a cause of failure of root treatment. *Oral Surgery, Oral Medicine, and Oral Pathology*, **54**, 566–574.

122. Bürklein, S. & Schäfer, E. (2012) Apically extruded debris with reciprocating single-file and full-sequence rotary instrumentation systems. *Journal of Endodontics*, **38**, 850–852.

123. Siqueira, J.F. Jr. (2001) Aetiology of root canal treatment failure: why well-treated teeth can fail. *International Endodontic Journal*, **34**, 1–10.

124. Nair, P.N.R. (2004) Pathogenesis of apical periodontitis and the causes of endodontic failures. *Critical Reviews in Oral Biology & Medicine*, **15**, 348–381.

125. Rubinstein, R.A. & Kim, S. (2002) Long-term follow-up of cases considered healed one year after apical microsurgery. *Journal of Endodontics*, **28**, 378–383.

126. Anan, H., Matsumoto, A., Hamachi, T., Yoshimine, Y. & Maeda, K. (1996) Effects of a combination of an antibacterial agent (Ofloxacin) and a collagenase inhibitor (FN-439) on healing of rat periapical lesions. *Journal of Endodontics*, **22**, 668–673.

16 Surgical Endodontics: The Complimentary Approach

Richard Rubinstein and Alireza Aminlari

Department of Cariology, University of Michigan, Ann Arbor, MI, USA;
Private Practice, Farmington Hills, MI, USA

Introduction

Treatment of apical periodontitis aims at eliminating the microbial contamination infection from the root canal system and preventing reinfection by sealing the root canal space. However, even when the most careful clinical procedures are followed, a proportion of lesions may persist because of the anatomical complexity of the root canal system, which are inaccessible to mechanical and chemical debridement (1), as well as microorganisms capable of surviving and proliferating in apical tissues, thus enabling a persistent infection interfering with posttreatment healing of the lesion (2–5). Ricucci and Siqueira demonstrated that when pulp necrosis reached the apical third, all lateral canals and apical ramifications contained either partially or completely necrotic tissue (6). Chemomechanical preparation partially removed necrotic tissue from the entrance of the lateral canals and apical ramifications, whereas the adjacent tissue remained

inflamed, sometimes infected, and associated with apical disease.

The debate whether chronic apical lesions are infected is still a subject of controversy. Kronfeld stated bacteria were always found within the root canal while apical tissue is not an area in which bacteria live but are destroyed (7). In contrast, Stewart, in 1947, proposed that bacteria were present in apical lesions (8). Few years later, Hedman demonstrated that 68% of 82 apical lesions contained bacteria (9). Tronstad *et al.* demonstrated that bacteria can survive in apical lesions and proved endodontic infections (4, 10). Advanced molecular biology and polymerase chain reaction (PCR) permitted identification of more species of microbes capable of inhabiting apical lesions and providing strong evidence that extraradicular infection might be the cause of many failed endodontic treatment (11). In 2000, Sunde *et al.* examined whether bacteria were present in apical lesions of asymptomatic teeth before sampling or were transferred there

Disinfection of Root Canal Systems: The Treatment of Apical Periodontitis, First Edition. Edited by Nestor Cohenca.
© 2014 John Wiley & Sons, Inc. Published 2014 by John Wiley & Sons, Inc.

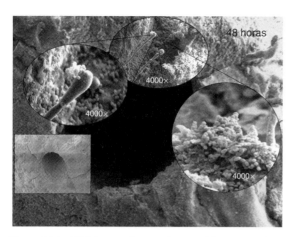

Figure 16.1 High power showing the apical foramen and cementum covered by a biofilm. Another area of the external surface of the apical surface covered by a biofilm. Note interaction and synergy between *Enterococcus faecalis* and *Candida*. (Image courtesy of Dr. Ana Maria Gonzalez.)

during sampling (3). The predominant cultivable bacteria were anaerobic and clearly different from the bacteria present at the neighboring sites and appeared to have been there before sampling. Siqueira and Ricucci found actinomycosis and arachnea in apical lesions (5, 12). Although no stainable bacteria were observed in the apparently well-treated main canal, apical ramifications were clogged with dense bacterial biofilms that were contiguous to extraradicular actinomycotic aggregates (5). Current literature supports the fact that extraradicular biofilms are related to refractory apical periodontitis, mostly by aggregation of numerous filamentous or spirochete-shaped bacterial cells (13, 14) (Figure 16.1). Clinically this implies that even if the tooth is extracted (ultimate root canal), apical periodontitis might persevere and develop a residual cyst (Figure 16.2). Thus the etiology is outside the root canal system and surgical intervention (along with orthograde treatment) is necessary to achieve apical healing.

Although the pathogenesis of apical periodontitis has been well described (15–17), it must be emphasized that the composition of lesions of apical periodontitis at any time depends on the balance between the microbial factors and the host defenses. Consequently, a great deal of morphological heterogeneity is common for chronic apical periodontitis.

Extraradicular endodontic plaque

In 1987, Tronstad *et al.* (10) demonstrated the presence of extraradicular endodontic plaque on the external surface of necrotic teeth. In a clinical and histopathologic study, Ricucci and Siqueira observed the presence of extraradicular biofilms in 6% of the cases (18). This has been substantiated with the visualization of biofilms under Scanning Electron Microscopy (SEM) (Figure 16.3).

Bacteria and apical actinomycosis

Actinomycosis is a chronic, granulomatous, infectious disease in man and animals caused by the genera *Actinomyces and Propionibacterium* (which normally colonize the mouth, colon, and vagina). Invasion of the microorganism is usually a result of the disruption of the mucosal barrier after trauma or dental manipulation (1). The endodontic infections of *actinomyces* are a sequel to caries and are caused by *Actinomyces israelii* and *Propionibacterium propionicum*, commensals of the oral cavity. Because of the ability of the actinomycotic organisms to establish in apical tissues, they can perpetuate the inflammation, even after orthograde root canal therapy. Among the most commonly isolated are *A. israelii and P. propionicum*, which are associated with refractory lesion (19). The properties that enable these bacteria to establish in the apical tissues are not fully understood, but appear to involve their ability to build cohesive colonies that enable them to escape the host defense system. There are only limited data on the frequency of apical actinomycosis among apical lesions or on the correlation between apical and cervicofacial actinomycosis (19).

Virus

Within the past decade, researchers have reported the presence of certain viruses in inflamed apical tissues and suggested as a possible etiological pathogenic factor related to apical periodontitis. Both Cytomegalovirus and Epstein–Barr viruses are present in almost all humans in latent form from previous primary infections (1). Sabeti *et al.* (20) investigated the occurrence of herpes viruses

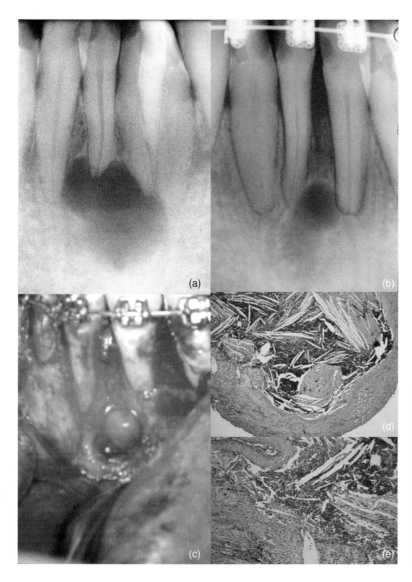

Figure 16.2 (a) Clinical radiograph of a lower lateral incisor with an apical lesion. The tooth was extracted for orthodontic reasons. The apical area was not curetted. (b) Postextraction radiograph with orthodontic treatment in progress. (c) Surgical removal of the persistent lesion. (d) Biopsy showing an epithelial lining cholesterol clefts and chronic inflammation consistent with the diagnosis of a residual cyst. (e) Higher power of the lesion showing epithelium, cholesterol clefts, and inflammation in the connective tissue.

in apical granulomas. cDNA identification of genes transcribed late during the infectious cycle of herpes viruses was used to indicate an active herpes virus infection. The authors proposed that herpes viruses may cause apical pathosis as a direct result of virus infection and replication or as a result of virally induced damage to the host defense (21). In addition, a strong association of human Cytomegalovirus and Epstein–Barr virus with the acute exacerbation of apical lesions has been reported (20, 22). Apical lesions harboring dual Cytomegalovirus and Epstein–Barr virus infection

tended to exhibit elevated occurrence of anaerobic bacteria, be symptomatic, and show large-size radiographic bone destruction. Cytomegalovirus and Epstein–Barr virus, in cooperation with specific bacterial species, have also been associated with various types of advanced marginal odontitis and several nonoral infectious diseases (22). Slots *et al.* have postulated that virus may initiate lesions by attacking and inactivating dendritic cells, thus processing and presenting the antigen by the dendritic cells to the B and T cells (21). This weakens the immune and inflammatory response

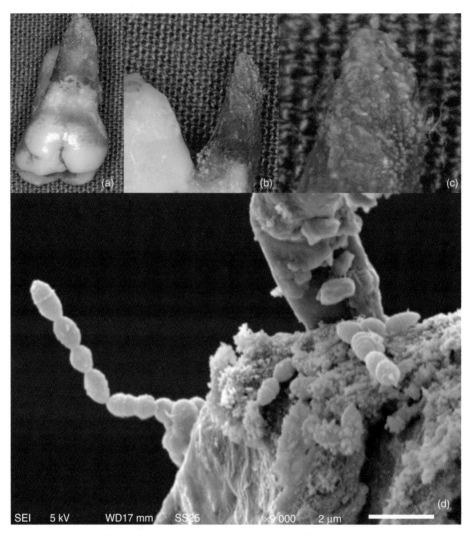

Figure 16.3   (a–c) Extracted maxillary molar demonstrating the presence of biofilm covering the external surface of the palatal root. (d) Scanning electron micrograph of the extraradicular biofilm at high power (×9000) showing the diversity of bacteria.

allowing bacteria to follow the viruses into the PA lesion.

Fungi

Fungi have also isolated in apical lesions but in far rear instances. They are thought to be the secondary contaminants following bacteria through the apical foramen. Among fungi, *Candida* is the most frequently found, although other fungi have been

cultivated. It has been detected in therapy-resistant apical lesions (23) (Figure 16.4).

Cholesterol

As a result of the inflammatory process with bacterial and cellular destruction, cholesterol is a usual component of apical lesions. Nair has stated that the body cannot destroy cholesterol and thus is a reason for the nonhealing of nonsurgical root

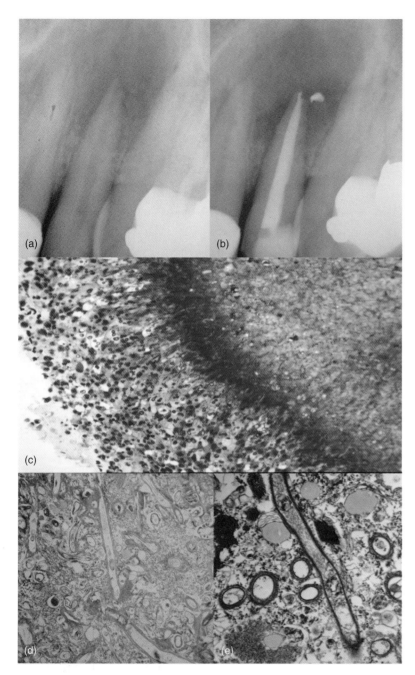

Figure 16.4 (a) Preoperative radiograph of a maxillary lateral incisor with an apical radiolucency. (b) Three-month recall demonstrating an increase in the size of the lesion. (c) One micron section prior to electron microscopy and stained with methylene blue. The inflammatory cells are attacking the antigen. (d) Low power electron micrograph showing fungal hyphae. (e) Higher power showing the presence of the fungus.

canal treatment (24). It can span from only several cholesterol clefts to the predominant component of the lesion. Thoma and Goldman classified these lesions as cholesteatoma where cholesterol is the dominating feature of the lesion (25). These lesions do not appear to heal with orthograde treatment and must be surgically removed for healing to occur (Figure 16.5).

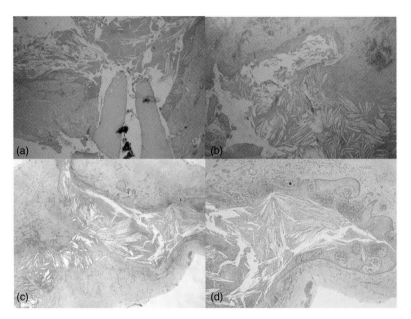

Figure 16.5 (a) Biopsy of a large lesion with the previously treated root tip. Note the cyst's lumen filled with cholesterol clefts. (b) Another part of the same lesion showing an epithelial lining and cholesterol clefts. (c) Epithelium and cholesterol clefts consistent with a cystic cholesteatoma. (d) Higher power of the same lesion.

Foreign bodies

Theoretically, anything that is in the mouth is capable of penetrating into the canal system and if small enough into the apical area. Numerous reports of foreign bodies and materials that penetrate the apical foramen along with bacteria show a foreign body giant cell reaction. Along with the usual acute and chronic inflammatory response, the macrophages coalesce to form giant cells in an attempt to degrade the foreign material. These lesions must be curetted in order to effect healing (Figure 16.6).

Anatomical complexities

Walter Hess (26), a Swiss dentist, first published his landmark anatomical studies in the early 1920s. When his work was first published many clinicians felt that the anatomical complexities he reported were artifacts created by injecting vulcanite rubber under too much pressure (Figures 16.7 and 16.8). However, more progressive thinkers of that time believed the results had merit and sought more effective ways to clean, shape, and obturate root canal systems. More recently, Takahashi and Kishi (27), using a dye infusion process, also studied

anatomical complexities. These models clearly show the majesty and grace of the human dental pulp (Figures 16.9–16.12). Weller *et al.* (28) studied the incidence and location of the isthmus in the mesial buccal root of the maxillary first molar and found a partial or complete isthmus 100% of the time at the 4 mm level of resection. West (29) looked at the relationship between failed endodontics and unfilled or underfilled portals of exit (POE's). Using a centrifuged dye, he identified that 100% of the failed specimens studied had at least one underfilled or unfilled POE. As 93% of the canal ramifications occur in the apical 3 mm (27), it is logical that the clinicians attempt to treat the root canal system to the full extent of the anatomy. Failure to address these anatomical concerns will leave the etiology of failure unattended and reinfection, even after the removal of a apical lesion, may occur. Clearly, root canal systems are more complex than previously thought. Significant pulpal anatomy such as accessory canals and isthmuses has to be considered when performing both conventional endodontic treatment and apical surgery. The acceptance of the significance of these anatomic complexities and the need to disinfect them may in fact have been the genesis of modern apical surgery, which could further be appreciated with the introduction of magnification and microsurgical armamentarium.

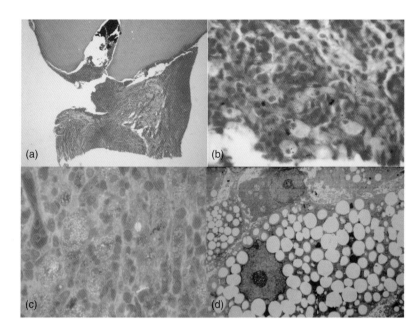

Figure 16.6   (a) Histologic section of an extracted tooth with attached lesion. Note foreign material in the canal. The bottom part of the lesion was used for the transmission electron microscope. (b) High power of the lesion showing macrophages and foreign material. (c) One micron section stained with methylene blue showing the macrophages full of foreign material. (d) A macrophage full to bursting with lipid. Note the absence of organelles and impingement on the nucleus.

Apical microsurgery

In order to understand the objectives of apical microsurgery, one can divide the procedure into multiple stages or sections. Among these are flap design, flap reflection, flap retraction, osteotomy, apical curettage, biopsy, hemostasis, apical resection, resected apex evaluation, apical preparation, apical preparation evaluation, drying the apical preparation, selecting retrofilling materials, mixing retrofilling materials, placing retrofilling materials, condensing retrofilling materials, carving retrofilling materials, finishing retrofilling materials, and flap closure.

After anesthesia is obtained, and prior to incising the surgical flap, the oral cavity should be rinsed with a disinfectant solution such as chlorhexidine. A 0.12% chlorhexidine rinse has been shown to significantly reduce the bacterial count in the oral cavity in advance of operative procedures (30).

Microscalpels (Figure 16.13) (SybronEndo, Orange, CA) are used in the design of the flap to delicately incise the interdental papillae when full-thickness flaps are required. Microscalpels cause less trauma than conventional scalpels resulting in less scarring and more favorable cosmetic outcomes. Vertical incisions are made 1.5–2 times longer than in conventional apical surgery to assure that the flap can easily be reflected out of the light path of the microscope.

Historically, flaps have been reflected with a Molt 2–4 curette or variation of the Molt 2–4. This instrument is double ended and the cross-sectional diameters of the working ends are 3.5 and 7 mm. Under low-range magnification it can readily be seen that even the smallest end of this instrument is too large to place beneath the interdental papilla without causing significant tearing and trauma to the delicate tissues. Rubinstein Mini-Molts (Figure 16.14) (JEDMED, St. Louis, MO) are available in two configurations whose working ends are 2 and 3.5 and 2 and 7 mm. The smaller ends of these instruments provide for atraumatic elevation of the interdental papilla making flap reflection more predictable and gentle to the tissues. The recently introduced PR-1 and PR-2 (Figure 16.15) (G. Hartzell & Son, Concord, CA) have similar geometries and also accomplish the goals of atraumatic flap reflection.

Once the flap has been reflected, instruments such as the Minnesota retractor have been used to retract the flap away from the surgical field while assuring visual access. Maintaining pressure on this instrument for even a short period of time often causes restriction of blood flow to the fingers of the operator and using it can be quite uncomfortable.

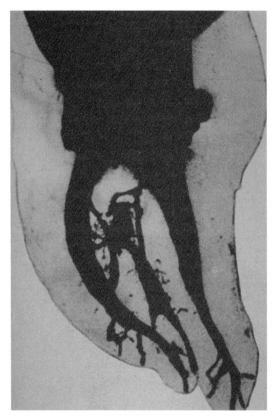

Figure 16.7   Hess model of a mandibular molar showing anatomical complexities throughout the root canal system.

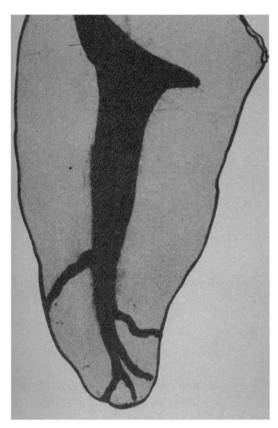

Figure 16.8   Hess model of a mandibular bicuspid showing anatomical complexities in the apical terminus.

A series of six retractors (JEDMED, St. Louis, MO) (Figure 16.16) and a new universal positioning retractor offering a variety of serrated contact surfaces that are flat, notched, and recessed allow the operator several options for secure placement in areas of anatomical concern. Among these are placements over nasal spine, canine eminence, and mental nerve. These retractors decrease the chance of slippage, which can cause trauma to the flap and delicate gingival mucosa. The blades of the retractors are designed to retract both the flap and the lip and are bent at 110° to keep the retractor and operator's hand out of the light path of the microscope. The handles are ergonomically designed to decrease cramping and fatigue and can be held in a variety of grips.

Because we can see better with the surgical operating microscope (SOM), bone removal can be more conservative. Handpieces such as the Impact

Air 45™ (SybronEndo, Orange, CA) introduced by oral surgeons to facilitate sectioning mandibular third molars, are also suggested for apical surgery to gain better access to the apices of maxillary and mandibular molars. When using the handpiece, the water spray is aimed directly into the surgical field but the air stream is ejected out through the back of the handpiece, thus eliminating much of the splatter that occurs with conventional high-speed handpieces. Because there is no pressurized air or water, the chances of producing pyemia and emphysema are significantly reduced.

Burs such as Lindemann bone cutters (Brasseler USA, Savannah. GA) are extremely efficient and are recommended for hard tissue removal. They are 9 mm in length and have only four flutes, which result in less clogging. With the use of an SOM, the Impact Air 45 and high-speed surgical burs can be placed even in areas of anatomical jeopardy

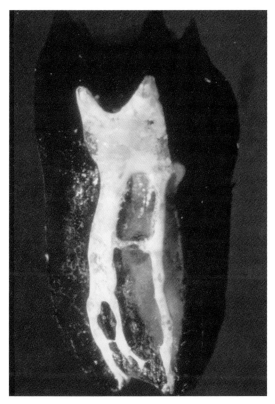

Figure 16.9 Takahashi model of the mesial view of the mesial root of a mandibular molar. Note the mid-root isthmus and the apical bifidity of the buccal canal. Also note the multiple apical termini.

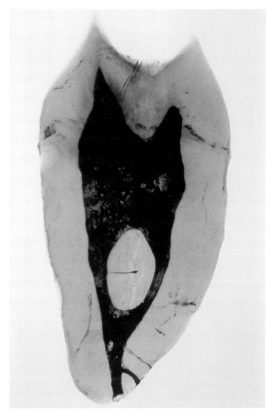

Figure 16.10 Takahashi model of a mandibular second bicuspid. Note how the single canal bifurcates, rejoins, and then splits once more at the canal terminus.

with a high degree of confidence and accuracy (Figure 16.17). The size of the osteotomy should be as small as practical so that healing will not be impaired, yet large enough to allow for complete debridement of the bony crypt and access for root-end procedures that will follow.

With the SOM, apical curettage is facilitated because bony margins can be scrutinized for completeness of tissue removal. A Columbia 13–14 curette is recommended in small crypts because it is curved and can reach to the lingual aspect of a root. After the Columbia 13–14 is used, the Jacquette 34/35 scaler is recommended to remove the remainder of granulomatous tissue. Because of its sharp edge, the Jacquette 34/35 is an excellent instrument for removing granulomatous tissue from the junction of the cemental root surface and the bony crypt. The more tissue that can be

removed results in less work for the body to do relative to wound healing. In addition, any foreign material present in the bony crypt should be removed as it could cause persistent irritation and may prevent complete healing of the tissues (31). After the bony crypt has been physically debrided, it should be rinsed thoroughly with sterile saline.

There is general agreement that the main cause of failure in conventional endodontic treatment is the clinician's inability to adequately shape, disinfect, and obturate the entire root canal system (32). As previously stated (27–29), the majority of this untreated anatomy is located in the apical 3 mm and for this reason a 3 mm resection is recommended. With the introduction of ultrasonics for creating root-end preparations, a second reason for a 3 mm resection has emerged. Layton *et al.*

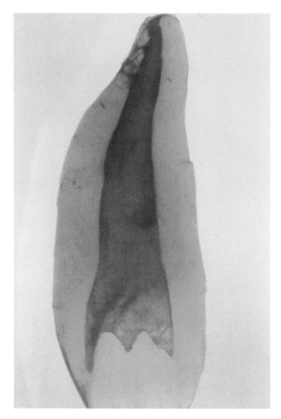

Figure 16.11   Takahashi model of a maxillary central incisor. Note the multiple portals of exit in the apical third of the root.

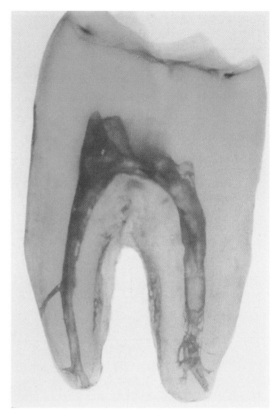

Figure 16.12   Takahashi model of a mandibular molar. Note the anatomical complexities present in both roots.

(33), Beling *et al.* (34), Min *et al.* (35), Morgan and Marshall (36) and Rainwater *et al.* (37) have studied the incidence of craze line, cracks, and fractures in the root and cemental surfaces after ultrasonic root-end preparations. While all of these studies showed a statistically significant increase, none has shown any clinical significance as a result of their findings. In as much as the greatest cross-sectional diameter of a root in the apical 6 mm is typically at the 3 mm level, it is suggested that this be the location of the resection in order to create an adequate buffer or cushion to absorb the potential deleterious effects of ultrasonic energy.

Traditionally, a long bevel was created in order to provide access for a microhead handpiece. With the introduction of apical ultrasonics, little to no bevel is needed. This results in fewer cut dentinal tubules and less chance of leakage. The Impact Air 45 handpiece and 1701 tapered fissure bur have

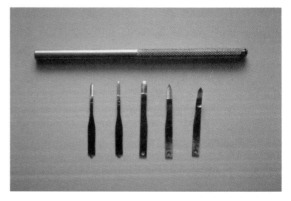

Figure 16.13   A variety of microscalpels sized 1–5 used for precise incision.

been the instruments of choice to resect the root. However, because of the size of the head of the handpiece, visual access is often impaired,

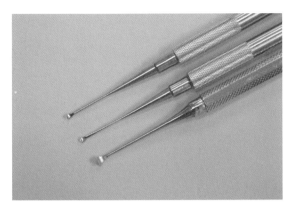

Figure 16.14   A comparison of the small ends of two mini-Molts and a standard Molt 2–4 curette.

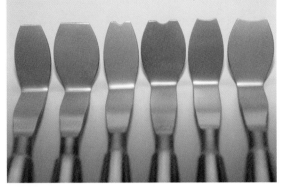

Figure 16.16   Blade and contact surfaces of the Rubinstein retractors 1–6.

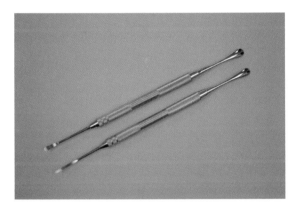

Figure 16.15   PR-1 and PR-2 periosteal elevators.

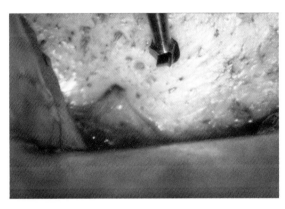

Figure 16.17   Impact Air 45™ and surgical length bur in close proximity to the mental nerve 8×.

especially in the posterior regions of the mouth. Recent advancements in electric motor design and straight handpieces afford the clinician opportunities for direct visualization of the root-end while performing root resection and the creation of axial bevels that approximate zero degrees. One such unit is the Aseptico 7000 motor and NSK 2:1 nose-cone handpiece (Figures 16.18 and 16.19). The unit drives the handpiece at 80,000 rpm's and is more than sufficient to atraumatically cut cortical bone and root. A variety of burs are available in 44.5 and 65 mm lengths allowing access into difficult to reach areas. A saline solution spray is directed over the bur and cools the bone and root surfaces. Saline has the advantage over distilled water and city water in that it is physiologic and sterile. The Aseptico 7000 motor and NSK

nose-cone handpiece can also be used to prepare the osteotomy.

After the root-end resection has been completed, the beveled surface of the root can be examined under mid-range magnification. Using a small CX-1 micro explorer (SybronEndo, Orange, CA), small micro fractures, isthmuses, and POEs can readily be seen (Figures 16.20 and 16.21).

Since the introduction of apical ultrasonic technology in the early 1990s by Carr (38), apical preparations have been made with ultrasonic tips. These tips are driven by a variety of commercially available ultrasonic units, which are self-tuning regardless of the changes in tip or load, for maximum stability during operation. A piezoelectric crystal made of quartz or ceramic located in the handpiece is vibrated at 28,000–40,000 cycles per

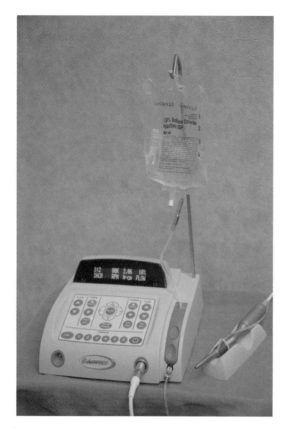

Figure 16.18 Aseptico 7000 motor and NSK 2 : 1 nose-cone handpiece.

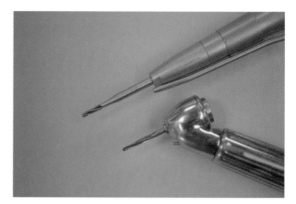

Figure 16.19 A comparison of Impact Air 45™ and NSK 2 : 1 nose-cone handpiece and surgical length burs.

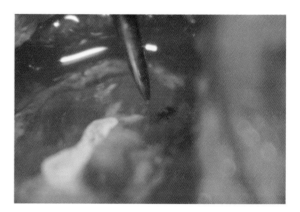

Figure 16.20 CX-1 explorer locating an untreated POE on the beveled surface of a previously retrofilled root at 20×.

second and the energy is transferred to the ultrasonic tip in a single plane. Dentin is then abraded microscopically and gutta-percha is thermoplasticized. Continuous irrigation along the tip cools the cutting surface while maximizing debridement and cleaning.

From their initial introduction, a variety of tips and tip configurations have been introduced to accommodate virtually any access situation. Most ultrasonic tips are .25 mm in diameter and approximately 3 mm in length. When used, they are placed in the long axis of the root so that the walls of the preparation will be parallel and encompass about 3 mm of the apical morphology. As the piezoelectric crystal in the handpiece is activated, the energy is transferred to the ultrasonic tip, which then moves forward and backward in a single plane and dentin is "brush cut" away in gentle strokes. The combination of the SOM and ultrasonic tips

make previously challenging cases routine. By combining magnification and ultrasonic technology, apical preparation can be visualized and executed with a high level of confidence that was previously unattainable.

Brent *et al.* (39) studied the incidence of intradentin and canal cracks in apical preparations made with stainless steel and diamond-coated ultrasonic tips. They found that diamond-coated tips do not result in significant root-end cracking and can remove cracks caused by prior instruments. For this reason diamond-coated tips are suggested as the last ultrasonic tip to be used in root-end preparation. Furthermore, clinical use of diamond tips has shown that they are more efficient at removing gutta-percha when compared to stainless steel

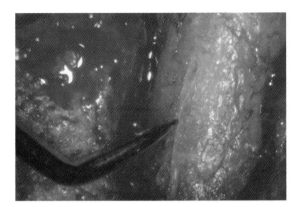

Figure 16.21   CX-1 explorer locating a crack on the facial surface of a root at 20×.

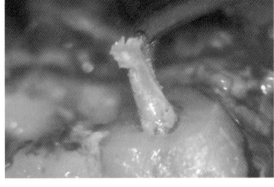

Figure 16.23   Thermoplasticized gutta-percha "walking" out of the preparation at 16×.

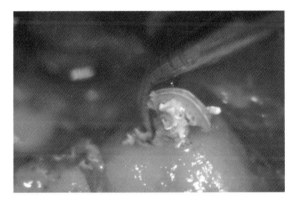

Figure 16.22   Thermoplasticized gutta-percha spinning around a stainless steel tip at 16x.

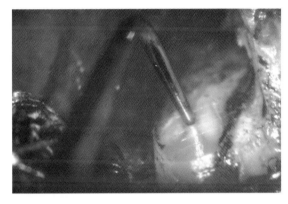

Figure 16.24   Off axis angulation with ultrasonic tip at 16×.

tips. The irregular surface of the diamond coating appears to grab and hold the gutta-percha facilitating removal. When using smooth-surfaced ultrasonic tips, the gutta-percha just spins on the smooth surface making removal difficult (Figures 16.22 and 16.23).

When using ultrasonic tips, the clinician should use gentle brush strokes with the smallest tip possible to conserve root dentin. This procedure should be observed while using mid-range magnification of the SOM. Pressure on the tip should be gentle. If resistance is met, it is assumed that the tip is lingual verted. The operator should then back off to low-range magnification and ensure that the tip is aligned in the long axis of the root. If this step is not taken and a lingual verted path is continued, a perforation of the root might occur (Figure 16.24).

There have been no clear guidelines on how to make the apical preparation until Gilheany *et al.* (40) studied the angle of the bevel and the depth of the preparation from the facial wall necessary to affect an adequate apical seal. They reported a 1 mm preparation was necessary with a 0° bevel, a 2.1 mm preparation was necessary with a 30° bevel, and a 2.5 mm preparation was necessary with a 45° bevel. They further recommended a 3.5 mm deep preparation when measured radiographically to account for errors in vertical angulation. This study raised the question as to whether preparation of an isthmus, which is so common (27–29), should be treated differently from the preparation of the main canals. Clearly, to satisfy the criteria set forth by Gilheany *et al.*, the clinician needs to create a 3 mm circumferential preparation in the long axis of the root, which includes all the anatomical ramifications of the pulp space including the isthmus. The inability to adequately clean and disinfect the isthmus with orthograde techniques was shown by Ricucci and Siqueira (18). This makes the surgical treatment of the isthmus even more critical and detailed attention must be used to thoroughly treat this space. This presents a conundrum for the clinician perfuming orthograde treatment or retreatment, as we are seldom able to instrument and irrigate these isthmuses and ramifications. Siqueira (41) proposed that all retreatment cases be regarded as infected and that the microorganisms reside mainly in the isthmuses, fins, dentin debris, apical deltas, and root filling voids. These microorganisms are in the form of a biofilm as described by Nair (42). Nair suggested that biofilms could not be eradicated by the host's defense system or chemotherapy, but rather by mechanical dislocation and disruption of the biofilm. The only way to achieve this is to surgically remove the portion of the root containing the isthmus and to ultrasonically clean this space. According to Teixeira (43), most isthmuses are found 3–5 mm from the apex. Research by Mannocci (44), Degerness (45), and others are in agreement with this finding. Therefore, a minimum of 3 mm of apical root structure should be removed to eliminate the apical delta. Additional debris and biofilm contained in the isthmus and fins are addressed by retropreping a minimum of 3 mm coronally to further decrease the number of microorganisms remaining in the root. Currently, we are not able to assess whether the ultrasonic action of retro-tips adds to the mechanical removal of biofilm created by the microabrasion of dentinal walls. Assuming that the mechanism of this action is the same as orthograde ultrasonic irrigation (46) one can assume most of the bacteria will be removed from the isthmus.

There are clinical situations where a post has been placed without orthograde treatment. The untreated canal space is usually filled with pulpal remnants and bacterial contamination. Endo Success Apical Surgery Tips address this problem (Figure 16.25). The tip lengths are 3, 6, and 9 mm. When used in progressive sequence, up to 9 mm of canal space can be cleaned and debrided. Longer pluggers are available to condense retrofilling materials to length.

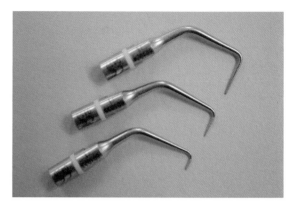

Figure 16.25   Endo success apical surgery tips.

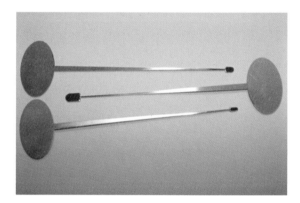

Figure 16.26   Zinni ENT micromirrors.

Another development in apical microsurgery has been the introduction of the surgical micromirror. Among the early pioneers of micromirrors was Dr. Carlo Zinni, an otorhinolaryngologist from Parma Italy (Carlo Zinni (C.Z.) Personal interview with the author. 1997). Being an early user of the microscope, Zinni recognized the need to indirectly view the pharynx and larynx for proper diagnosis. Zinni crafted the first polished stainless steel mirrors from which the early endodontic micromirrors were developed (Figure 16.26).

Micromirrors come in a variety of shapes and sizes and have diameters ranging from 1 to 5 mm. There have been many surfaces used on micromirrors. Among them have been polished stainless steel, polished tungsten carbide, and diamond-like coating. Recently introduced micromirrors utilize a rhodium coating. Rhodium is extremely hard

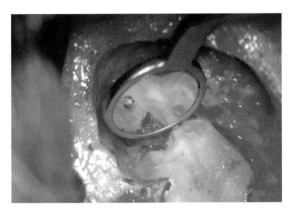

Figure 16.27   Rhodium micromirror view of the beveled surface of the root at 13×.

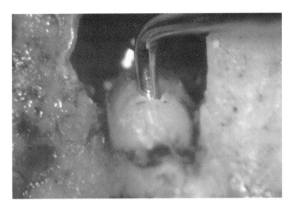

Figure 16.29   Condensing thermoplasticized gutta-percha away from the facial wall and compressing it coronally at 16×.

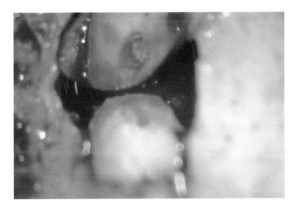

Figure 16.28   Micromirror view of gutta-percha and debris on the facial wall of the apical preparation at 16×.

and durable and is unsurpassed in reflectivity, clarity, and brightness. They are front surface, scratch resistant, and autoclavable (JEDMED, St. Louis. MO) (Figure 16.27). Using the SOM, it is now possible to look up into the apical preparation to check for completeness of tissue removal. Before using micromirrors, it was impossible to assess the thoroughness of apical preparation. Failure to completely remove old root canal filling material and debris from the facial wall of the apical preparation (Figure 16.28) may lead to facial wall leakage and eventual failure if not cleaned before the placement of an apical seal. Clearly, it is necessary to circumferentially remove all debris from the apical preparation to satisfy the criteria set forth by Gilheany *et al.* (40) and Ricucci and Siqueira (18).

Debris can be removed from the facial wall by capturing the maximum cushion of thermoplasticized gutta-percha with a small plugger (Figure 16.29) and condensing it coronally. A variety of small pluggers ranging in diameters from 0.25 mm to 0.75 mm are available for this purpose. Facial wall debris can further be addressed by the removal with a back action ultrasonic tip. Virtually all modern day ultrasonic tips have some degree of back action in their design. This angle can vary between 70° and 80°.

Once the apical preparation has been examined, it should be rinsed and dried. Traditionally, apical preparations were dried with paper points before placing retrofilling materials. This allowed for thorough adaptation of retrofilling materials against the walls of the cavity preparation and decreased the chances of creating material voids. Microcontrol of air and water is now accomplished by using a small blunt irrigating needle (Ultradent Products, Inc., South Jordan, UT) mounted in a Stropko Irrigator (SybronEndo, Orange, CA). The irrigator fits over a triflow syringe and allows for the directional microcontrol of air and water (Figure 16.30). Air pressure can be regulated down to 4 psi. Now the beveled root surface and the apical preparation can be completely rinsed and dried before inspection with microsurgical mirrors. Anatomical complexities, isthmuses, and tissue remnants are more easily seen when the cut surfaces are thoroughly rinsed and then desiccated (Figure 16.31).

Prior to selecting and placing retrofilling materials, it is essential to have established good

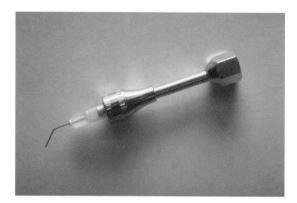

Figure 16.30 Stropko irrigator with an attached blunt irrigating needle.

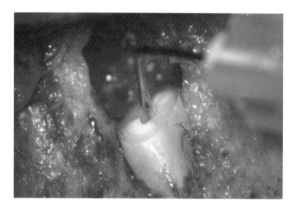

Figure 16.31 Blue Micro Tip™ drying the apical preparation at 13×. Note the chalky dry beveled surface.

hemostasis. Hemostasis begins on reviewing the patient's health questionnaire. In addition to the many anticoagulants that patients are prescribed, herbal supplements and a variety of vitamins can complicate hemostasis. It is critical to evaluate the various pharmaceutical cocktails that patients may be consuming. Consultation with the patient's physician may be necessary. Anesthesia must be profound with adequate vasoconstrictor. In most cases intraoperative hemostasis is not necessary. Should this not be the case, a variety of materials are available to choose from. Such a list could include ferric sulfate, aluminum chloride, collagen, hemostatic gauze, racemic epinephrine, and electro cautery. When selecting hemostatic agents, one should consider their effect on hard and soft tissues and whether their use could compromise healing.

After the apical preparation is rinsed and dried, retrofilling materials such as SuperEBA™ (Harry J. Bosworth Co, Skokie, Il) and ProRoot™ MTA (Dentsply Tulsa Dental, Tulsa, OK) are then placed into the apical preparation. The question as to which material has a higher success rate was studied by Song *et al.* (47) and reported as a prospective randomized controlled study. They reported that there was no significant difference in the clinical outcomes of endodontic microsurgery when SuperEBA and MTA were used as root-end filling materials. The surgical technique may then have a greater bearing on the result than the root-end filling material.

The clinician should select instruments and carriers that allow for direct observation of placement so he can see how the materials perform as they are placed into the apical preparation. Cement consistency retrofilling materials, such as SuperEBA, are mixed to a putty consistency and carried to the apical preparation in small truncated cones 1 to 2 mm in size on a #12 spoon excavator (Figure 16.32). The cross-sectional diameter of this instrument is 1 mm and therefore does not block the visual access to the apical preparation. The tip of the cone reaches the base of the preparation as the sides of the cone contact the walls. Between each aliquot of material, a small plugger (JEDMED Instrument Company, St. Louis, MO) that will fit inside the apical preparation is used to condense the SuperEBA (Figure 16.33). Additional aliquots of material are added and condensed until there is a slight excess mound of material on the beveled

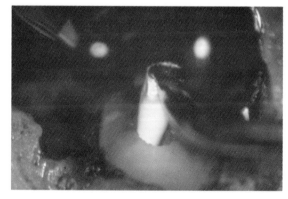

Figure 16.32 Placing SuperEBA™ into the apical preparation with a number 12 spoon excavator at 16×.

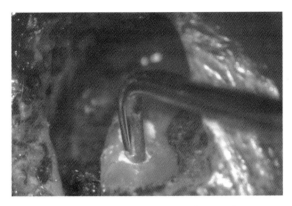

Figure 16.33 Plugging SuperEBA™ into the apical preparation with a small plugger at 16×.

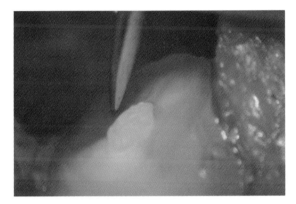

Figure 16.34 Checking for marginal integrity with a CX-1 explorer at 20×.

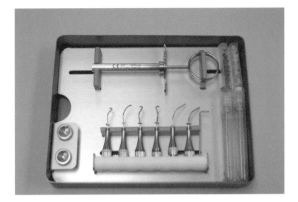

Figure 16.35 Microapical Placement System.

surface of the root. Final compaction is accomplished with a ball burnisher. When the cement has set, a finishing bur or smooth diamond is used to finish the retrofilling. After the SuperEBA has been finished, a CX-1 explorer is used under high magnification to check for marginal integrity and adaptation. Final examination of the retrofilling is performed after the surface has been dried with a Stropko Irrigator, because it is more accurate to check the margins of the preparation when the beveled surface of the root is dry (Figure 16.34).

Materials such as ProRoot MTA are best delivered to the apical preparation with a carrier-based system. The problems with carriers in the past were that the diameters were too large to fit into the apical preparation, bends were inadequate, and they plugged easily. The Micro Apical Placement (MAP)

System (Roydent, Johnson City, TN) (Figure 16.35) addresses these problems. This system consists of several delivery tips with cross-sectional diameters ranging from 0.9 mm for small preparations to 1.5 mm for use in immature roots. The plungers are made of a PEEK (polyetheretherketone) material, which has a coating similar to Teflon™ and therefore retrofilling materials will not stick to the surface. The PEEK plunger can easily navigate a triple bended carrier. When in use the carriers should not be packed too tightly, and gentle pressure should be used to express the material. The carriers should be disassembled and cleaned immediately after use.

When placing ProRoot MTA, select a carrier that will fit into the apical preparation (Figure 16.36). This will avoid spilling material into the bony crypt. This is mostly a cosmetic issue, because ProRoot

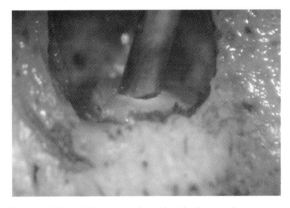

Figure 16.36 MAP carrier placed inside the apical preparation at 16×.

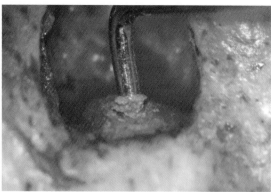

Figure 16.37   ProRoot™ MTA being pulled out of the apical preparation at 16×.

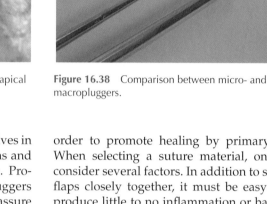

Figure 16.38   Comparison between micro- and macropluggers.

MTA is a tricalcium compound. Once it dissolves in tissue fluids, it combines with phosphate ions and produces CaPO4, which is osteoconductive. Pro-Root MTA is then condensed with small pluggers that will fit into the apical preparation to assure thorough compaction and less chance of leakage. As ProRoot MTA is cohesive to itself and only slightly adhesive to the walls of the preparation, care must be exerted to avoid pulling the material out of the preparation (Figure 16.37). Gentle teasing and wiping of the material along the walls of the preparation will assure its complete placement.

The ProRoot MTA retrofilling is finished by wiping the beveled surface with a moist cotton pellet. Visual inspection at mid-range magnification is used to check for any remaining cotton fibrils and marginal integrity.

Emphasis has been placed on using small pluggers. However, when apical surgery involves immature roots using small diameter pluggers to condense, retrofilling materials can be inefficient and a waste of time. JEDMED recently introduced three new pluggers. These pluggers incorporate 60° and 90° angles and cross-sectional diameters of 1.5, 2.0, and a 1 mm ball that address these needs (Figure 16.38). The combination of using a large 1.5 mm diameter MAP carrier and a large diameter plugger provides for efficient retrofilling and condensing of apical preparations made in immature roots.

The final stage of apical microsurgery is flap closure. Suturing is a critical part of this procedure. Care must be taken to reapproximate the flap in order to promote healing by primary intention. When selecting a suture material, one needs to consider several factors. In addition to securing the flaps closely together, it must be easy to handle, produce little to no inflammation or bacterial contamination, and not dissolve before initial healing is complete. Traditionally, silk has been the suture of choice for many clinicians because of its excellent handling properties. However, it is a multifilament material, which produces considerable wicking and increased bacterial contamination. Parirokh *et al.* (48), showed significantly more bacterial contamination and physical debris with silk sutures compared to polyvinylidene fluoride (PVDF), a monofilament suture, at 3, 5, and 7 days postplacement. However, PVDF is difficult to handle and needs to be pulled several times to erase the stiff memory. In addition, patients often complain that the tag ends of the suture are stiff and irritating to the oral mucosa. Tevdek (Teleflex Medical, NC USA) is a polytetrafluorethylene (PTFE) coated multifilament suture, which acts like a monofilament. This material produces less inflammation and contamination than silk and has the added benefit of handling like silk. Because Tevdek is such a soft material that it is suggested that the clinician place an additional throw when tying the surgical knot.

While selection of suture material is important, it is also necessary to consider needle design. Manufacturers have suggested various needle configurations to help the clinician reapproximate the flap and cause as little trauma as possible. Among the choices are reverse-cutting needles and tubular side-cutting needles. Reverse-cutting needles are more traumatic than tubular side-cutting needles. Because they are sturdier than tubular side-cutting needles, they can withstand occasional contact with interproximal bone if resistance is met while redirecting the needle. On the other hand, tubular side-cutting needles may bend if contact is made with bone. Tevdek suture material offers the choice of a double-needled 3/8 in circle. The KT-1 needle has a length of 12.1 mm making it ideal for reapproximating the vertical incision and attached gingival flap suturing. The KT-2 needle has a length of 17.8 mm making it ideal for interproximal suturing.

Once the sutures are placed, the flap should be compressed with a saline soaked gauze and firm finger pressure for a minimum of 3 min. If this is not performed properly, there is a possibility that bleeding may occur under the flap, a hematoma may form, and an impaired healing may occur.

The key to suture removal is in the healing of the epithelium. Harrison and Jurosky (49) reported that a thin epithelial seal was established in the horizontal wound at 24 h and a multilayered epithelial seal was established in the vertical incisional wound between 24 and 48 h. While some clinicians might infer from this study that sutures could be removed at 48 hours, one must understand that it does not take into account personal habits of patients and their willingness to comply with postoperative directions. Therefore, most clinicians would agree that sutures could be left in place up to 7 days without causing significant soft tissue irritation. The SOM can be used to facilitate suture removal at low-range magnification. Microsurgical scissors and tweezers should be used to cut and remove the sutures. Care should be exercised during removal so as not to damage the suture sight.

Does apical microsurgery really make a difference?

The SOM was originally introduced as a surgical tool. Almost immediately after its introduction, many clinicians realized its benefit in conventional treatment and nonsurgical retreatment. Consequently, many instruments and devices were developed for use in disassembly, postremoval, and removal of separated instruments.

Gorni and Gagliani (50) reported the outcome of 452 nonsurgical retreatment cases 2 years after treatment. The range of magnification used during the treatment of the cases was 3.5× to 5.5×. They reported a success rate of 47% when the root canal morphology had been altered and a success rate of 86.8% when the root canal morphology was respected. The overall success rate reported was 69%. The difficult question to answer when considering a nonsurgical versus a surgical approach is whether the clinician can readdress the original biology of the case. This question may be impossible to answer without actually reentering the case and possibly rendering the tooth nonrestorable after disassembly. Considering this possible outcome, apical microsurgery may have been a better and more conservative approach.

As mentioned previously, Frank et al. reported that success rate in apical surgeries sealed with amalgam, which had been considered successful, dropped to 57.7% after 10 years (51). Friedman et al. (52) reported successful treatment results as 44.1% in 136 premolar and molar roots that were observed over a period of 6 months to 8 years. Kvist and Reit (53) in a randomized study compared results of surgically and nonsurgically treated cases. They could find no systematic difference in the outcome of treatment, which ranged in success from 56% to 60%. These studies all used conventional surgical protocol without the benefit of an SOM and microsurgical armamentarium.

Setzer et al. (54), in a meta-analysis of the literature, compared endodontic microsurgical techniques with and without the use of higher magnification. Weighted pooled success rates calculated from extracted raw data showed an 88% positive outcome for traditional root-end surgery and a 94% positive outcome for apical microsurgery. The difference in probability was statistically significant for molars.

Rubinstein and Kim (55, 56) reported the short-term and long-term success rates for apical surgery using the SOM and SuperEBA as retrofilling material as 96.8% and 91.5%, respectively. The rate of healing independent of lesion size was 7.2 months. Unlike most early conventional surgical studies (57–62), which reported the pooled results of multiple clinicians, and consisted mostly of anterior teeth, 60% of the cases reported by Rubinstein and Kim consisted of premolar and molar teeth.

Several studies (63–67) have demonstrated a favorable outcome of apical surgery performed with ultrasonic technology similar to that used by Rubinstein and Kim (55, 56). However, none of these studies used the SOM. Furthermore, the follow-up periods in these studies were considerably shorter and it must be emphasized that because of variations in treatment and evaluation methods, direct comparisons to the cited studies cannot be made.

More recently, Song *et al.*, (68) reported on the long-term outcome of apical microsurgery cases classified as successful when more followed from a previous short-term study. The success rates from the 5-year short-term study were 91.5%. The healed population was then followed for a period from 6 to 10 years. The long-term success for these cases after 6 years was 93.3%. von Arx *et al.*, (69) demonstrated similar results in a 5-year longitudinal assessment of the prognosis of apical microsurgery as 8% poorer than assessed at 1 year.

Assuming that the surgery has been done properly, it is important to understand the reasons for the regression of healing. Some of the reasons for regression have been reported as fracture, periodontal disease, lateral canals, and leaky restorations (55, 68). These are not endodontic in origin and may skew statistics.

Setzer *et al.* (70) showed in a meta-analysis of traditional root-end surgery and endodontic apical microsurgery that the success rate of traditional surgery was 59% and that of apical microsurgery was 94%. The difference was statistically significant and the relative risk ratio showed that the probability for success for apical microsurgery was 1.58 times the probability of success for traditional surgery.

References

1. Nair, P.N. (2004) Pathogenesis of apical periodontitis and the causes of endodontic failures. *Critical Reviews in Oral Biology and Medicine: An Official Publication of the American Association of Oral Biologists*, **15** (6), 348–381.
2. Siqueira, J.F. Jr. (2001) Aetiology of root canal treatment failure: why well-treated teeth can fail. *International Endodontic Journal*, **34** (1), 1–10.
3. Sunde, P.T., Olsen, I., Lind, P.O. & Tronstad, L. (2000) Extraradicular infection: a methodological study. *Endodontics & Dental Traumatology*, **16** (2), 84–90.
4. Tronstad, L., Kreshtool, D. & Barnett, F. (1990) Microbiological monitoring and results of treatment of extraradicular endodontic infection. *Endodontics & Dental Traumatology*, **6** (3), 129–136.
5. Ricucci, D. & Siqueira, J.F. Jr. (2008) Apical actinomycosis as a continuum of intraradicular and extraradicular infection: case report and critical review on its involvement with treatment failure. *Journal of Endodontics*, **34** (9), 1124–1129.
6. Ricucci, D. & Siqueira, J.F. Jr. (2010) Fate of the tissue in lateral canals and apical ramifications in response to pathologic conditions and treatment procedures. *Journal of Endodontics*, **36** (1), 1–15.
7. Kronfeld, R. (1974) *Histopathology of teeth and their surrounding structures*, 2nd edn. Lee & Febiger, Philadelphia.
8. Stewart, G.G. (1947) A study of bacteria found in root canals of anterior teeth and the probable mode of ingress. *Journal of Endodontia*, **2** (3), 8–11.
9. Hedman, W.J. (1951) An investigation into residual periapical infection after pulp canal therapy. *Oral Surgery, Oral Medicine, and Oral Pathology*, **4** (9), 1173–1179.
10. Tronstad, L., Barnett, F., Riso, K. & Slots, J. (1987) Extraradicular endodontic infections. *Endodontics & Dental Traumatology*, **3** (2), 86–90.
11. Vigil, G.V., Wayman, B.E., Dazey, S.E., Fowler, C.B. & Bradley, D.V. Jr. (1997) Identification and antibiotic sensitivity of bacteria isolated from periapical lesions. *Journal of Endodontics*, **23** (2), 110–114.
12. Siqueira, J.F. Jr., Rocas, I.N., Baumgartner, J.C. & Xia, T. (2005) Searching for Archaea in infections of endodontic origin. *Journal of Endodontics*, **31** (10), 719–722.
13. Noiri, Y., Ehara, A., Kawahara, T., Takemura, N. & Ebisu, S. (2002) Participation of bacterial biofilms in refractory and chronic periapical periodontitis. *Journal of Endodontics*, **28** (10), 679–683.
14. Leonardo, M.R., Rossi, M.A., Silva, L.A., Ito, I.Y. & Bonifacio, K.C. (2002) EM evaluation of bacterial biofilm and microorganisms on the apical external root surface of human teeth. *Journal of Endodontics*, **28** (12), 815–818.
15. Stashenko, P. (1990) Role of immune cytokines in the pathogenesis of periapical lesions. *Endodontics & Dental Traumatology*, **6** (3), 89–96.
16. Stashenko, P., Teles, R. & D'Souza, R. (1998) Periapical inflammatory responses and their modulation. *Critical Reviews in Oral Biology and Medicine : An Official Publication of the American Association of Oral Biologists*, **9** (4), 498–521.

17. Nair, P.N. (1997) Apical periodontitis: a dynamic encounter between root canal infection and host response. *Periodontology 2000*, **13**, 121–148.

18. Ricucci, D. & Siqueira, J.F. Jr. (2010) Biofilms and apical periodontitis: study of prevalence and association with clinical and histopathologic findings. *Journal of Endodontics*, **36** (**8**), 1277–1288.

19. Hirshberg, A., Tsesis, I., Metzger, Z. & Kaplan, I. (2003) Periapical actinomycosis: a clinicopathologic study. *Oral Surgery, Oral Medicine, Oral Pathology, Oral Radiology, and Endodontics*, **95** (**5**), 614–620.

20. Sabeti, M., Valles, Y., Nowzari, H., Simon, J.H., Kermani-Arab, V. & Slots, J. (2003) Cytomegalovirus and Epstein-Barr virus DNA transcription in endodontic symptomatic lesions. *Oral Microbiology and Immunology*, **18** (**2**), 104–108.

21. Slots, J., Sabeti, M. & Simon, J.H. (2003) Herpesviruses in periapical pathosis: an etiopathogenic relationship? *Oral Surgery, Oral Medicine, Oral Pathology, Oral Radiology, and Endodontics*, **96** (**3**), 327–331.

22. Sabeti, M., Simon, J.H. & Slots, J. (2003) Cytomegalovirus and Epstein-Barr virus are associated with symptomatic periapical pathosis. *Oral Microbiology and Immunology*, **18** (**5**), 327–328.

23. Takahashi, K. (1998) Microbiological, pathological, inflammatory, immunological and molecular biological aspects of periradicular disease. *International Endodontic Journal*, **31** (**5**), 311–325.

24. Nair, P.N. (2006) On the causes of persistent apical periodontitis: a review. *International Endodontic Journal*, **39** (**4**), 249–281.

25. Thoma, K.H. & Goldman, H.M. (1946) Odontogenic tumors: a classification based on observations of the epithelial, mesenchymal, and mixed varieties. *The American Journal of Pathology*, **22** (**3**), 433–471.

26. Hess, W.Z.E. (1925) *The anatomy of root canals of the permanent dentition*. William Wood and Company, New York.

27. Kim, S., Pecora, G. & Rubinstein, R. (2001) *Color Atlas of Microsurgery in Endodontics*. WB Saunders, Philadelphia.

28. Weller, R.N., Niemczyk, S.P. & Kim, S. (1995) Incidence and position of the canal isthmus. Part 1. Mesiobuccal root of the maxillary first molar. *Journal of Endodontics*, **21** (**7**), 380–383.

29. West, J.D. (1975) The Relationship between the three-dimensional endodontic seal and endodontic failures. Thesis, Boston University Goldman School of Graduate Dentistry.

30. Veksler, A.E., Kayrouz, G.A. & Newman, M.G. (1991) Reduction of salivary bacteria by pre-procedural rinses with chlorhexidine 0.12%. *Journal of Periodontology*, **62** (**11**), 649–651.

31. Lin, L.M., Gaengler, P. & Langeland, K. (1996) Periradicular curettage. *International Endodontic Journal*, **29** (**4**), 220–227.

32. Kakehashi, S., Stanley, H.R. & Fitzgerald, R.J. (1965) The effects of surgical exposures of dental pulps in germ-free and conventional laboratory rats. *Oral Surgery, Oral Medicine, and Oral Pathology*, **20**, 340–349.

33. Layton, C.A., Marshall, J.G., Morgan, L.A. & Baumgartner, J.C. (1996) Evaluation of cracks associated with ultrasonic root-end preparation. *Journal of Endodontics*, **22** (**4**), 157–160.

34. Beling, K.L., Marshall, J.G., Morgan, L.A. & Baumgartner, J.C. (1997) Evaluation for cracks associated with ultrasonic root-end preparation of gutta-percha filled canals. *Journal of Endodontics*, **23** (**5**), 323–326.

35. Min, M.M., Brown, C.E. Jr., Legan, J.J. & Kafrawy, A.H. (1997) In vitro evaluation of effects of ultrasonic root-end preparation on resected root surfaces. *Journal of Endodontics*, **23** (**10**), 624–628.

36. Morgan, L.A. & Marshall, J.G. (1999) A scanning electron microscopic study of in vivo ultrasonic root-end preparations. *Journal of Endodontics*, **25** (**8**), 567–570.

37. Rainwater, A., Jeansonne, B.G. & Sarkar, N. (2000) Effects of ultrasonic root-end preparation on microcrack formation and leakage. *Journal of Endodontics*, **26** (**2**), 72–75.

38. Carr, G.C. (1992) Microscopes in endodontics. *Journal of the California Dental Association*, **11**, 55–61.

39. Brent, P.D., Morgan, L.A., Marshall, J.G. & Baumgartner, J.C. (1999) Evaluation of diamond-coated ultrasonic instruments for root-end preparation. *Journal of Endodontics*, **25** (**10**), 672–675.

40. Gilheany, P.A., Figdor, D. & Tyas, M.J. (1994) Apical dentin permeability and microleakage associated with root end resection and retrograde filling. *Journal of Endodontics*, **20** (**1**), 22–26.

41. Siqueira, J.F. Jr. (2005) Reaction of periradicular tissues to root canal treatment: benefits and drawbacks. *Endodontic Topics*, **10**, 123–147.

42. Nair, P.N., Henry, S., Cano, V. & Vera, J. (2005) Microbial status of apical root canal system of human mandibular first molars with primary apical periodontitis after "one-visit" endodontic treatment. *Oral Surgery, Oral Medicine, Oral Pathology, Oral Radiology, and Endodontics*, **99** (**2**), 231–252.

43. Teixeira, F.B., Sano, C.L., Gomes, B.P., Zaia, A.A., Ferraz, C.C. & Souza-Filho, F.J. (2003) A preliminary in vitro study of the incidence and position of the root canal isthmus in maxillary and mandibular first molars. *International Endodontic Journal*, **36** (**4**), 276–280.

44. Mannocci, F., Peru, M., Sherriff, M., Cook, R. & Pitt Ford, T.R. (2005) The isthmuses of the mesial root of mandibular molars: a micro-computed tomographic study. *International Endodontic Journal*, **38** (8), 558–563.

45. Degerness, R. & Bowles, W. (2008) Anatomic determination of the mesiobuccal root resection level in maxillary molars. *Journal of Endodontics*, **34** (10), 1182–1186.

46. Gutarts, R., Nusstein, J., Reader, A. & Beck, M. (2005) In vivo debridement efficacy of ultrasonic irrigation following hand-rotary instrumentation in human mandibular molars. *Journal of Endodontics*, **31** (3), 166–170.

47. Song, M., Shin, S.J. & Kim, E. (2011) Outcomes of endodontic micro-resurgery: a prospective clinical study. *Journal of Endodontics*, **37** (3), 316–320.

48. Parirokh, M., Asgary, S., Eghbal, M.J., Stowe, S. & Kakoei, S. (2004) A scanning electron microscope study of plaque accumulation on silk and PVDF suture materials in oral mucosa. *International Endodontic Journal*, **37** (11), 776–781.

49. Harrison, J.W. & Jurosky, K.A. (1991) Wound healing in the tissues of the periodontium following periradicular surgery. I. The incisional wound. *Journal of Endodontics*, **17** (9), 425–435.

50. Gorni, F.G. & Gagliani, M.M. (2004) The outcome of endodontic retreatment: a 2-yr follow-up. *Journal of Endodontics*, **30** (1), 1–4.

51. Frank, A.L., Glick, D.H., Patterson, S.S. & Weine, F.S. (1992) Long-term evaluation of surgically placed amalgam fillings. *Journal of Endodontics*, **18** (8), 391–398.

52. Friedman, S., Lustmann, J. & Shaharabany, V. (1991) Treatment results of apical surgery in premolar and molar teeth. *Journal of Endodontics*, **17** (1), 30–33.

53. Kvist, T. & Reit, C. (1999) Results of endodontic retreatment: a randomized clinical study comparing surgical and nonsurgical procedures. *Journal of Endodontics*, **25** (12), 814–817.

54. Setzer, F.C., Kohli, M.R., Shah, S.B., Karabucak, B. & Kim, S. (2012) Outcome of endodontic surgery: a meta-analysis of the literature--Part 2: comparison of endodontic microsurgical techniques with and without the use of higher magnification. *Journal of Endodontics*, **38** (1), 1–10.

55. Rubinstein, R.A. & Kim, S. (2002) Long-term follow-up of cases considered healed one year after apical microsurgery. *Journal of Endodontics*, **28** (5), 378–383.

56. Rubinstein, R.A. & Kim, S. (1999) Short-term observation of the results of endodontic surgery with the use of a surgical operation microscope and Super-EBA as root-end filling material. *Journal of Endodontics*, **25**, 43–48.

57. Dorn, S.O. & Gartner, A.H. (1990) Retrograde filling materials: a retrospective success-failure study of amalgam, EBA, and IRM. *Journal of Endodontics*, **16** (8), 391–393.

58. Finne, K., Nord, P.G., Persson, G. & Lennartsson, B. (1977) Retrograde root filling with amalgam and Cavit. *Oral Surgery, Oral Medicine, and Oral Pathology*, **43** (4), 621–626.

59. Grung, B., Molven, O. & Halse, A. (1990) Periapical surgery in a Norwegian county hospital: follow-up findings of 477 teeth. *Journal of Endodontics*, **16** (9), 411–417.

60. Hirsch, J.M., Ahlstrom, U., Henrikson, P.A., Heyden, G. & Peterson, L.E. (1979) Periapical surgery. *International Journal of Oral Surgery*, **8** (3), 173–185.

61. Mattila, K. & Altonen, M. (1968) A clinical and roentgenological study of apicoectomized teeth. *Odontologisk Tidskrift*, **76** (6), 389–408.

62. Rud, J., Andreasen, J.O. & Jensen, J.E. (1972) A follow-up study of 1,000 cases treated by endodontic surgery. *International Journal of Oral Surgery*, **1** (4), 215–228.

63. Sumi, Y., Hattori, H., Hayashi, K. & Ueda, M. (1996) Ultrasonic root-end preparation: clinical and radiographic evaluation of results. *Journal of Oral and Maxillofacial Surgery*, **54** (5), 590–593.

64. Sumi, Y., Hattori, H., Hayashi, K. & Ueda, M. (1997) Titanium-inlay--a new root-end filling material. *Journal of Endodontics*, **23** (2), 121–123.

65. Testori, T., Capelli, M., Milani, S. & Weinstein, R.L. (1999) Success and failure in periradicular surgery: a longitudinal retrospective analysis. *Oral Surgery, Oral Medicine, Oral Pathology, Oral Radiology, and Endodontics*, **87** (4), 493–498.

66. von Arx, T. & Kurt, B. (1999) Root-end cavity preparation after apicoectomy using a new type of sonic and diamond-surfaced retrotip: a 1-year follow-up study. *Journal of Oral and Maxillofacial Surgery*, **57** (6), 656–661.

67. Zuolo, M.L., Ferreira, M.O. & Gutmann, J.L. (2000) Prognosis in periradicular surgery: a clinical prospective study. *International Endodontic Journal*, **33** (2), 91–98.

68. Song, M., Chung, W., Lee, S.J. & Kim, E. (2012) Long-term outcome of the cases classified as successes based on short-term follow-up in endodontic microsurgery. *Journal of Endodontics*, **38** (9), 1192–1196.

69. von Arx, T., Jensen, S.S., Hanni, S. & Friedman, S. (2012) Five-year longitudinal assessment of the prognosis of apical microsurgery. *Journal of Endodontics*, **38** (5), 570–579.

70. Setzer, F.C., Shah, S.B., Kohli, M.R., Karabucak, B. & Kim, S. (2010) Outcome of endodontic surgery: a meta-analysis of the literature--part 1: comparison of traditional root-end surgery and endodontic microsurgery. *Journal of Endodontics*, **36** (11), 1757–1765.

Index

Disinfection of Root Canal Systems: The Treatment of Apical Periodontitis, First Edition. Edited by Nestor Cohenca.
© 2014 John Wiley & Sons, Inc. Published 2014 by John Wiley & Sons, Inc.